Portland Comm

FIFTH EDITION

Barrow & McGee's

Practical Measurement and Assessment

FIFTH EDITION

Barrow & McGee's

Practical Measurement and Assessment

Kathleen Tritschler, Ed.D.

Associate Professor of Sport Studies
Guilford College
Greensboro, North Carolina

LIPPINCOTT WILLIAMS & WILKINS
A **Wolters Kluwer** Company

Philadelphia · Baltimore · New York · London
Buenos Aires · Hong Kong · Sydney · Tokyo

Editor: Peter Darcy
Managing Editor: Linda S. Napora
Marketing Manager: Chris Kushner
Production Editor: Bill Cady

351 West Camden Street
Baltimore, Maryland 21201-2436 USA

530 Walnut Street
Philadelphia, Pennsylvania 19106-3621 USA

Printed in the United States of America

First Edition, 1964	Lea & Febiger	Third Edition, 1979	Lea & Febiger
Second Edition, 1971	Lea & Febiger	Fourth Edition, 1989	Lea & Febiger

Library of Congress Cataloging-in-Publication Data

Tritschler, Kathleen A.
  Barrow & McGee's practical measurement and assessment   /   Kathleen Tritschler.—5th ed.
    p. cm.
  Rev. ed. of: Practical measurement in physical education and sport   /   Harold M. Barrow, Rosemary McGee, Kathleen A. Tritschler. 4th ed. 1989.
    Includes index.
    ISBN 0-683-08393-7
    1. Physical fitness—Testing. I. Title: Practical measurement and assessment. II. McGee, Rosemary, 1926–   III. Barrow, Harold M. (Harold Marion), 1909–   Practical measurement in physical education and sport. IV. Title.

GV436 .B3 2000
613.7—dc21   99-058429

The publishers have made every effort to trace the copyright holders for borrowed material. If they have inadvertently overlooked any, they will be pleased to make the necessary arrangements at the first opportunity.

To purchase additional copies of this book, call our customer service department at **(800) 638-3030** or fax orders to **(301) 824-7390.** International customers should call **(301) 714-2324.**

Lippincott Williams & Wilkins customer service representatives are available from 8:30 am to 6:00 pm, EST, Monday through Friday, for telephone access. *Or visit Lippincott Williams & Wilkins on the Internet:* **http://www.lww.com.**

00 01 02 03 04
1 2 3 4 5 6 7 8 9 10

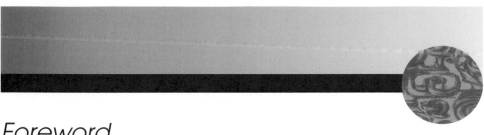

Foreword

One of the supreme satisfactions of a professional career is seeing your work perpetuated, enlarged, and greatly enhanced. Our original measurement and evaluation text was published in 1964. This is the fifth edition.

The study of measurement and evaluation started as a subdiscipline of physical education designed primarily for the teacher-student in school settings. Over the years its growth has paralleled the development of the exercise science field as we know it today. Each edition of our text, including this one, has reflected the ever-enlarging scope of the discipline. We began our work with the aim that all textbook content be practical and complete. Dr. Tritschler has continued that commitment and in addition has included materials pertinent to the many subdisciplines now included under the exercise science umbrella. Also noteworthy is Dr. Tritschler's exceptional ability to present information in an interesting and down-to-earth manner while keeping the content challenging and thought provoking.

We knew we were fortunate to have Dr. Tritschler join our authorship team for the fourth edition. Now, as she assumes sole responsibility for this edition, we feel even more rewarded. We are delighted, both with Kathy and with her work on this fifth edition.

June 1999
Harold M. Barrow, Winston-Salem, NC
Rosemary McGee, Greensboro, NC

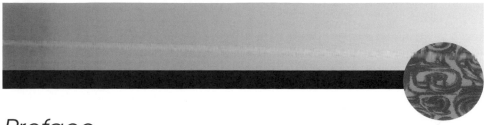

Preface

Up-to-date knowledge and skills in measurement are expected of all professionals in fitness and sport careers. Thus, course work in measurement is a hallmark of our undergraduate and graduate programs. Yet to stay abreast of the many changes in the dynamic field of measurement is no easy task.

Barrow & McGee's Practical Measurement and Assessment is written for the beginning student of measurement and for the busy in-service professional. Like earlier editions of this textbook, the fifth edition is characterized by its practical approach and content. Explanations of how to select, administer, and interpret a wide variety of measurement and assessment tools for evaluation of physical fitness, motor skills, knowledge, and affects are straightforward. And this text features complete, ready-to-use test descriptions and scoring information, so the busy practitioner does not have to make time to go to a library to get the information necessary to actually administer and interpret tests.

Harold Barrow, of Wake Forest University, and Rosemary McGee, of the University of North Carolina at Greensboro (UNCG), together wrote the first edition of this text in 1964. Kathleen Tritschler studied under Rosemary McGee during Tritschler's doctoral work at UNCG and was invited to join Drs. Barrow and McGee as an author of the fourth edition. Now professors emeriti of their universities, Drs. Barrow and McGee entrusted the writing of the fifth edition to Dr. Tritschler.

Content Features

Section 1, Assessment Fundamentals, contains three chapters that introduce the use of measurement and assessment (Chapter 1) and present fundamental information for selection and administration of measurement and assessment tools (Chapter 3). Chapter 2 offers an historical perspective on the use of measurement and assessment. While this content interests most readers, some instructors may choose to skip this chapter if time is limited.

Section 2, Data Analysis and Evaluation, is designed to teach the reader to make sense of test scores and other quantitative information. Chapter 4 explains options for nonstatistical data analysis, such as frequency distribution tables, polygons, and histograms. Chapters 5 and 6 describe when and how to use common descriptive and inferential statistics. Chapter 7 describes how to use measurement and assessment data for grading. Instructors who do not have preservice physical education students in their classes may skip Chapter 7.

Section 3, Assessment of Physical Fitness and Motor Skills, consists of four chapters. Chapter 8 is a focused presentation of practical methods of body composition assessment for adults of various ages and children. Also addressed in Chapter 8 are several screening tools for body composition, such as body mass index. Chapter 9 offers detailed descriptions of maximal and submaximal procedures for the practical assessment of cardiorespiratory fitness. Chapter 10 presents practical assessments of musculoskeletal fitness, that is, for assessment of muscular strength, muscular endurance, and flexibility. Also described in Chapter 10 are several practical tools for the assessment of selected aspects of motor fitness, that is, agility, balance, coordination, muscular power, and speed. Chapter 11 provides a comprehensive review of tools for the assessment of sport skills. Included in this chapter are 25 sport skill tests or observation tools.

Section 4, Special Assessment Concerns, comprises nine chapters that focus on topics of interest to many fitness and sport practitioners, such as nutrition assessment, body image assessment, sport facility risk reviews, and dance assessment. Each chapter is by a renowned authority on the topic. These chapters add depth and breadth to the beginner's study of measurement and assessment.

Four appendices conclude the text. Appendix A presents detailed information on the administration and interpretation of several of the most popular physical fitness tests for children, young adults, and older adults. Appendix B provides contact information for a variety of sources of measurement and assessment resources. Appendix C lists URLs (universal resource locators) for Web sites and ListServes of interest to sport and fitness practitioners. Appendix D reproduces the Compendium of Physical Activities, a listing of more than 500 activities with their standardized MET intensity levels.

Pedagogical Features

Scattered through the text are "*What Do YOU Think?*" boxes that present topics to challenge the reader to consider the ethical dimensions and controversies related to the use of measurement. Examples of these topics are why Americans haven't embraced the metric system, whether Michael Jordan is an all-around athlete, and the ethics of using health and fitness scores collected in a corporate wellness program to deny a worker's compensation claim.

The personal computer has become an invaluable tool for the test administrator. Instead of isolating **computer applications** in a single chapter, *Barrow & McGee's Practical Measurement and Assessment* has embedded pertinent information on computer applications throughout the text. Applications are discussed in a natural way, that is, within the context of related material.

Each chapter begins with a list of **keywords** that are defined for the reader later in the chapter and that appear in the **Glossary. Self-test questions** (with answers provided) allow the reader to check comprehension of key concepts in each chapter. At the end of each chapter are **Doing Projects for Further Learning.** These are ideas for hands-on learning opportunities.

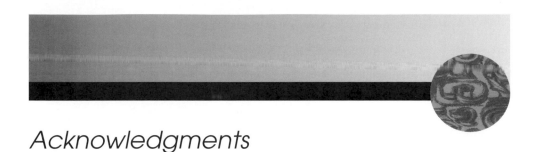

Acknowledgments

First and foremost is my indebtedness to Harold Barrow and Rosemary McGee for their generous trust in my ability to carry on their work. I hope that they will always be proud of their legacy.

Many thanks to numerous academic colleagues who supported my work and assisted in this project, most especially Mitch Craib and Liz Hart. Heartfelt appreciation also goes to "CD" (Carolyn Dunn), Barb Ainsworth, Jerry Hawkins, Todd Seidler, Mary Lou Veal, Sue Combs, and Rayma Beal—valued colleagues whose expertise is evident in the wonderful special concerns chapters they contributed to this text. And to my students at Guilford College: I cannot thank you enough for all that you have taught me.

This text was produced over several years, and during that time I received assistance and advice from many individuals associated with the publisher (Lea & Febiger, Williams & Wilkins, and now Lippincott Williams & Wilkins). Very special thanks to Linda Napora, a consummate professional, who found just the right balance between nudging and nagging. Thanks also to Eric Johnson, Donna Balado, and Vicki Vaughn for never losing faith in this project.

Last but not least, thanks to my family and friends who encouraged me and tolerated my excuses during the many, many months of the textbook creation. So, tennis anyone?

Kathy Tritschler
Greensboro, NC

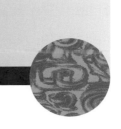

Contributors

Barbara E. Ainsworth, Ph.D., MPH
Associate Professor
Department of Epidemiology & Biostatistics
Department of Exercise Science
School of Public Health
University of South Carolina
Columbia, South Carolina

Rayma K. Beal, Ed.D.
Associate Professor of Dance
University of Kentucky
Lexington, Kentucky

Sue Combs, Ph.D.
Associate Professor
Department of Health, Physical Education, and Recreation
University of North Carolina at Wilmington
Wilmington, North Carolina

Carolyn Dunn, Ph.D.
Associate Professor
Department of Family and Consumer Sciences
North Carolina Cooperative Extension Service
North Carolina State University
Raleigh, North Carolina

Elizabeth A. Hart, Ph.D.
HealthMagic
Denver, Colorado

Jerald D. Hawkins, Ed.D., ATC, FACSM
Professor, and Director of Sports Medicine Education
Department of Physical Education and Exercise Studies
Lander University
Greenwood, South Carolina

Rosemary McGee, Ph.D.
Professor Emeritus of Exercise and Sport Science
University of North Carolina at Greensboro
Greensboro, North Carolina

Todd L. Seidler, Ph.D.
Associate Professor
Department of Sports Administration
University of New Mexico
Albuquerque, New Mexico

Mary Lou Veal, Ed.D.
Associate Professor
Department of Exercise and Sport Science
University of North Carolina at Greensboro
Greensboro, North Carolina

Contents

SECTION **THREE**

Assessment of Physical Fitness and Motor Skills   201

SECTION **FOUR**

Special Assessment Concerns   407

18 *Assessment for Physical Education Teachers*   *591*

Mary Lou Veal

19 *Assessment of Special-Needs Populations*   *615*

Sue Combs

20 *Assessment in Dance Education*   *653*

Rayma K. Beal

Appendices

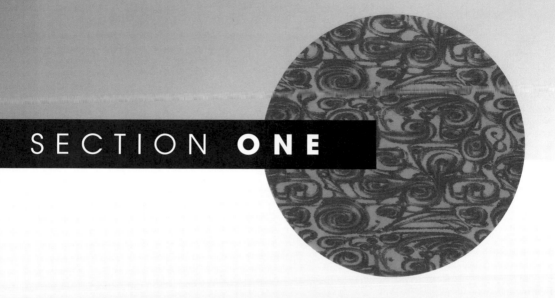

Assessment Fundamentals

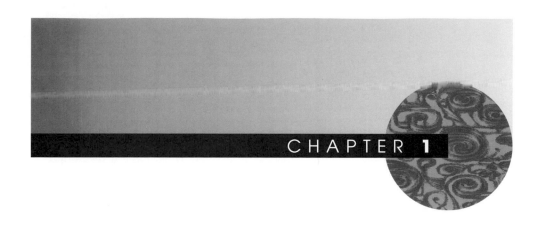

Introduction to Modern Assessment

Course work in assessment has long been a hallmark of graduate programs in exercise and sport studies (ESS). Today, however, knowledge and skills in assessment are also deemed essential to the professional preparation of undergraduates aspiring to careers as physical education teachers, athletic coaches, sports medicine specialists, and sport managers. *Your* future employers will expect *you* to have a good grounding in assessment. They will assume that you are familiar with and can administer a wide variety of assessment instruments. Furthermore, they will count on you to be able to evaluate the results of assessment data. The purpose of this textbook is to aid you in developing the requisite knowledge and skills for competence in 21st-century assessment.

This chapter provides an overview of the study of assessment. The overview is organized into three main sections. The first section introduces terminology, that is, the language of assessment. The second section clarifies the processes of assessment by answering the newspaper reporter's standard questions—who, what, why, when, and how—regarding the role of assessment in modern exercise and sport programs. The final section examines ethical and legal principles that guide practitioners in their use of assessment.

As you read this chapter, watch for the following keywords:

Assessment	Formative assessment	Prognostic assessment
Battery	Inventory	Rating scale
Checklist	Laboratory test	Self-referenced
Criterion-referenced	Measurement	Summative assessment
Diagnostic assessment	Norm-referenced	Test
Evaluation	Proficiency assessment	Test consumer
Field assessment		

The Language of Assessment

Learning the language of assessment is not as difficult as learning a foreign language, but it is challenging. To get a taste for this language, read the following paragraph, paying special attention to the boldface and italic words. These words are terms that you need to understand. You may want to return to this paragraph after you have read a little further in this chapter.

The *Y's Way to Fitness* (1) adult physical fitness battery includes a series of tests to assess the four major aspects of health-related physical fitness. Included in the battery is a skinfold *field test* to assess body composition. The test protocol specifies that skinfold thickness is to be *measured* at each of four anatomical sites using Harpenden calipers. Body fat percentage is read from a chart by comparing the sum of the four skinfold thicknesses with gender- and age-appropriate values. The subject's body composition is *assessed* as the percentage of fat weight that contributes to his or her total body weight. Body composition is *evaluated* according to theoretical and epidemiological guidelines. The YMCA guidelines recommend use of 16% and 23%, respectively, as *criterion-referenced standards* for body composition for healthy men and women.

Test and Related Terms

What does the word **test** conjure up in your mind? For many students and former students it elicits a grumble in the stomach and an image of pages filled with questions (sometimes obscure ones!) to which one is expected to respond. While a test *can* be a written evaluation of knowledge, in the language of assessment, *test* is interpreted in a much broader sense. For example, think about how this term is used in the context of blood test, pregnancy test, eye test, and drivers license test.

In exercise and sport venues, testing goes well beyond use of traditional paper-and-pencil formats. Sport testing evaluates physical fitness, sport skills, exercise stress, and athletic injury. *Test administrators* observe examinees' physical responses, time the objects they project, palpate their body parts, and analyze their body fluids. Many of these tests require special tools, such as the skinfold caliper, goniometer, and force platform; others use common tools such as cones, yardsticks, and stopwatches. Such testing can occur in laboratories or in gymnasia and on athletic fields. Test subjects may be single individuals or groups, such as an entire athletic team. Regardless of the specific test protocol, the purpose of all testing is to gain information about some characteristic of the test subject.

> A test is an instrument or procedure that elicits an observable response to provide information about a specific attribute of a person or persons.

Examination is synonymous with test. *Examinees* are persons who take or are given tests or examinations. Those who give tests or examinations are called *test administrators*, *examination administrators*, or simply *examiners*. A test administrator is not needed for a *self-administered test*. This text employs the term **test consumer** to denote a person who uses test results to make informed decisions. The author of a test is called the *test developer*.

A test consumer is someone who uses test results to make informed decisions.

Police officers know all about assault and battery! ESS specialists use the term **battery** to refer to a collection of related tests administered together to assess a multidimensional attribute of an examinee. For example, in the sample paragraph that began this discussion, *health-related physical fitness* (HRPF) was used. HRPF is commonly considered to have four component parts: cardiovascular endurance, body composition, muscular strength and endurance, and flexibility. An HRPF battery therefore consists of at least four tests. All four tests are administered to examinees; then a composite score for HRPF is determined. Ideally, all the tests in a battery are standardized on the same population so that results on the component tests can be compared.

A battery is a collection of related tests administered within a specified time frame to obtain information about a multidimensional attribute.

Other forms of tests include *rating scales*, *checklists*, and *inventories*. Questions such as "on a 10-point scale, how do you rate the gymnast's routine?" and "on a 7-point scale, how severe is your pain?" represent the essence of **rating scales**. Because rating scales require a significant degree of human judgment, they are usually considered to be more subjective than other types of tests. Well-designed rating scales are structured to reduce subjectivity by providing detailed descriptions of observable behaviors that define points along the scale. Good scale point definition increases the likelihood of agreement among raters. Rating scales are commonly used for evaluation of the process or technique of performance. Figure 1-1 shows a well-designed rating scale.

A rating scale is a type of test that provides a subjective estimate of an attribute based on observation and/or self-appraisal; it provides for degrees of the attribute being examined.

Checklists are usually rating scales that are dichotomous, that is, in which each element in the checklist is rated as present or absent. Checklists are commonly used as aids to observation. Figure 1-2 is a checklist.

A checklist is a dichotomous rating scale used to aid observation.

Although *test* is a term that can be applied very broadly, it is most often associated with protocols for which the examinee's responses can be evaluated in terms of correctness. Instruments or procedures that assess affective qualities such as interests, attitudes, beliefs, and personal values can be included within the general definition of *test* but are usually assessed by means of an **inventory**. Figure 1-3 is an inventory.

An inventory is an assessment instrument used to obtain information about an affective attribute of an examinee; examinee responses typically are *not* judged as correct or incorrect.

CODE FOR PHYSICAL ACTIVITY

*Select the one value that best represents your
general ACTIVITY LEVEL for the PREVIOUS MONTH.*

DO NOT PARTICIPATE REGULARLY IN PROGRAMMED
RECREATION SPORT OR HEAVY PHYSICAL ACTIVITY.

0 = Avoid walking or exertion, e.g., always use elevator, drive
whenever possible instead of walking.
1 = Walk for pleasure, routinely use stairs, occasionally exercise
sufficiently to cause heavy breathing or perspiration.

PARTICIPATE REGULARLY IN RECREATION OR WORK
REQUIRING MODEST PHYSICAL ACTIVITY, SUCH AS GOLF, HORSEBACK
RIDING, CALISTHENICS, GYMNASTICS,
TABLE TENNIS, BOWLING, WEIGHT LIFTING, YARD WORK.

2 = 10 to 60 minutes per week.
3 = Over 1 hour per week.

PARTICIPATE REGULARLY IN HEAVY PHYSICAL EXERCISE SUCH
AS RUNNING OR JOGGING, SWIMMING, CYCLING, ROWING,
SKIPPING ROPE, RUNNING IN PLACE, OR ENGAGING
IN VIGOROUS AEROBIC ACTIVITY-TYPE EXERCISE
SUCH AS TENNIS, BASKETBALL, OR HANDBALL.

4 = Run less than 1 mile per week or spend less than 30 minutes
per week in comparable physical activity.
5 = Run 1 to 5 miles per week or spend 30 to 60 minutes per
week in comparable physical activity.
6 = Run 5 to 10 miles per week or spend 1 to 3 hours per week in
comparable physical activity.
7 = Run over 10 miles per week or spend over 3 hours per week
in comparable physical activity.

FIGURE 1-1

A well-constructed rating scale, developed for use at NASA/Johnson Space Center, Houston, TX. (Reprinted with permission from Ross, R.M., and Jackson, A.S.: Exercise Concepts, Calculations, & Computer Applications. Carmel, IN, Benchmark Press, 1990, p. 109.)

Techniques of Beginning Fencing Skills Checklist—Parry 4

Directions: Observe the fencer perform the skill several times, then check (✓) each of the actions below that is consistently present in performance of the skill.

_____ Parry occurs as tip of opponent's foil passes fencer's bell guard
_____ Parry occurs with lower one-third of foil blade
_____ Foil tip remains high (just above opponent's head)
_____ Foil tip remains in line with midline of opponent's torso
_____ Bell guard moves in a horizontal plane
_____ Parry is just sufficient (parry carries tip of opponent's foil just beyond fencer's torso)
_____ Change in hand position from fingers up to thumb up

FIGURE 1-2

A checklist. (Reprinted with permission from Tritschler, K.A.: Techniques of a beginning fencing skills checklist. Unpublished paper. University of North Carolina at Greensboro, 1981.)

Measurement and Assessment

Measurement is the process of administering a test. Measurement assumes precision of the data obtained. Generally we speak of administering a test to measure some tangible attribute of interest, such as time or distance, or a physiological attribute, such as body weight, limb girth, heart rate, or blood pressure. Quantitative data, characteristically expressed in numerical form as *scores*, are the usual outcome of measurement.

> Measurement is the process of systematically assigning numerical values to an attribute of interest.

In recent years the term **assessment** has gained favor as an umbrella term for the process of obtaining data by administration of a test, rating scale, checklist, or inventory. There is, however, a subtle but very important distinction in use of the terms *measurement* and *assessment*. We use *assessment* to acknowledge our understanding that the attribute we are studying is too elusive to measure objectively. For example, while we can confidently *measure* skinfold thicknesses, we use these measures to *assess* body composition (Fig. 1-4). *Assessment* communicates awareness of the subjectivity involved in attempts to quantify or qualitatively describe an attribute. ESS addresses many attributes that defy objective measurement, such as body image, sportsmanship, aggression, adherence to exercise, pain, level of orthopaedic dysfunction, team cohesion, basketball skill, teaching excellence, and coaching effectiveness.

Feelings About Physical Activity

Directions: Circle the appropriate letter (SD, strongly disagree; D, disagree; U, uncertain; A, agree, SA, strongly agree) to indicate how well the statement describes *your feelings most of the time.* There are no right or wrong answers. Physical activity is interpreted to include all individual and dual sports, all team sports, and all individual exercises.

1.	I look forward to physical activity.	SD	D	U	A	SA
2.	I wish there were a more enjoyable way to stay fit than vigorous physical activity.	SD	D	U	A	SA
3.	Physical activity is drudgery.	SD	D	U	A	SA
4.	I do not enjoy physical activity.	SD	D	U	A	SA
5.	Physical activity is vitally important to me.	SD	D	U	A	SA
6.	Life is so much richer as a result of physical activity.	SD	D	U	A	SA
7.	Physical activity is pleasant.	SD	D	U	A	SA
8.	I dislike the thought of doing regular physical activity.	SD	D	U	A	SA
9.	I would arrange or change my schedule to participate in physical activity.	SD	D	U	A	SA
10.	I have to force myself to participate in physical activity.	SD	D	U	A	SA
11.	To miss a day of physical activity is sheer relief.	SD	D	U	A	SA
12.	Physical activity is the high point in my day.	SD	D	U	A	SA

Scoring: Items 1, 5, 6, 7, 9, and 12 are scored 1 to 5; items 2, 3, 4, 8, 10, and 11 are scored 5 to 1; 36 is the middle score. The following scale gives some interpretative information:

54–60	Very favorable feelings about physical activity
42–53	Favorable feelings
30–41	Neutral feelings
18–29	Unfavorable feelings
12–17	Very unfavorable feelings about physical activity

FIGURE 1-3

An inventory. (Reprinted with permission from Nielsen, A.B., and Corbin, C.B.: Physical activity commitment. Conference Abstracts, North American Society for the Psychology of Sport and Physical Activity Conference, Scottsdale, AZ, June 1986, p. 93.)

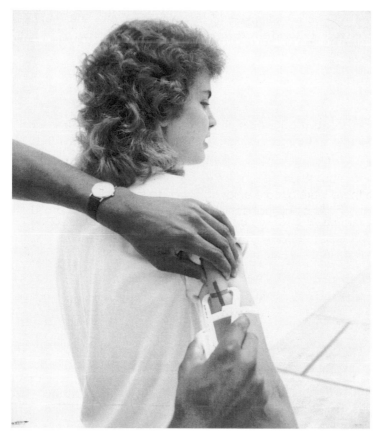

FIGURE 1-4

Skinfolds measured to assess body composition. (Photo by Dr. Karen Uhlendorf, University of Vermont, Burlington, VT.)

> Assessment is the process of subjectively quantifying or qualitatively describing an attribute of interest; it can also refer collectively to both measurement and assessment.

The title of this textbook employs the term *assessment* in addition to the more narrow term *measurement*. In this text, assessment instruments (or the abbreviated assessments) refers collectively to tests, rating scales, checklists, and inventories used in measurement and assessment. Subsequent chapters examine many types of assessment instruments. Some yield precise, objective data; others yield subjective data.

Evaluation

Evaluation is the process of interpreting the results of measurement and/or assessment. Both quantitative and qualitative data are evaluated by comparing them with guidelines or standards to make judgments about some aspect of a person and/or to make appropriate decisions about a course of action. The process of evaluation uses one of three reference systems. The three systems of evaluation are known as **norm-referenced**, **criterion-referenced**, and **self-referenced**.

> Evaluation is the process of making judgments based on quantitative and/or qualitative measurement or assessment data.

Norm-referenced evaluation allows for identification of individual differences among examinees. This means that a person's score on a norm-referenced test can be compared with the scores of similar persons who have taken the same test. These comparative scores are known as *norms*. The standardized achievement tests that you took in elementary and secondary school were probably norm-referenced tests. Perhaps you remember being told that you scored, for example, at the 92nd percentile, meaning that you scored as well as or better than 92% of your peers who took the same test. Many physical fitness and sport skill tests provide for norm-referenced evaluations.

> Norm-referenced evaluation entails interpretation of an examinee's score by comparing it with the scores of similar examinees.

In recent years there has been increased interest in the development of tests that are **criterion-referenced**. These assessments evaluate a person's performance by comparing his or her score with a *standard* of performance. The criterion is a defined satisfactory level of performance. For example, several health-related physical fitness batteries have established being able to reach one's toes as the criterion standard for a sit-and-reach test. On criterion-referenced tests, examinees whose scores meet or exceed the standard are judged to be *masters*, while examinees whose scores fall below the standard are judged *nonmasters.* Theoretically there are no limits to the number of persons who may achieve mastery on a criterion-referenced test. In fact, for some tests the desired outcome is a 100% mastery rate; such a test is the American Red Cross cardiopulmonary resuscitation test. Other common criterion-referenced tests include referee certification tests and other professional certification tests. Criterion-referenced approaches to assessment of the physical fitness of children have also been developed in recent years.

> Criterion-referenced evaluation entails interpretation of an examinee's score by comparing it with a predetermined standard defined by a behavior.

It is also sometimes useful to consider **self-referenced** evaluations. Sometimes appropriate interpretation of a test entails comparing a person's test score with a score that he or she obtained earlier or under different conditions. Such comparisons allow judgments regarding improvement or deterioration of an attribute for a single individual. Athletic injury tests are a good example of self-referencing. Athletic trainers and physical therapists palpate a joint or move a joint through a motion to ascertain the existence and/or extent of an injury and/or progress in rehabilitation. The only appropriate interpretation is comparison of the score with the score from a previous administration of the test to the same person and/or a score on the contralateral limb of the injured person (Fig. 1-5). Similarly, medical doctors administer

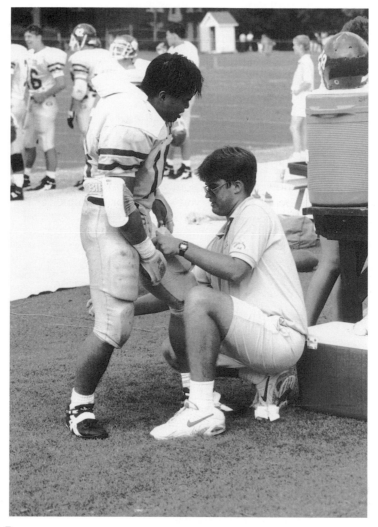

FIGURE 1-5

Athletic trainers use bilateral comparisons to evaluate some types of injuries. (Photo by John Bell, Touch a Life Photography, Greensboro, NC.)

to their middle-aged clients chest radiographs, electrocardiograms (ECGs), and mammograms to provide baseline data that can be used later for comparison.

> Self-referenced evaluation entails interpretation of an examinee's score by comparing it with his or her score from another administration of the same assessment instrument.

Laboratory Tests and Field Assessments

Many performance instruments are so sophisticated and/or costly that they seldom are administered except in university laboratories, medical clinics, and hospitals. Examples include graded exercise tests of cardiac function, hydrostatic body composition (underwater weighing) tests, and bone density tests. Also, **laboratory tests** are usually administered to only one examinee at a time. These features make most laboratory tests impractical for use in real-world exercise and sport settings.

> Laboratory tests are tests that require specialized equipment and specialized training of examiners and/or evaluators; laboratory tests may also be time consuming because only one examinee is tested at a time.

Alternatives to laboratory tests are **field assessments**, including some tests, rating scales, checklists, and inventories. Compared with laboratory assessments, field assessment instruments generally employ inexpensive equipment and require less training of the administrator and/or evaluator. Additionally, field assessments are often time efficient, because many allow for *mass testing*; that is, they can be administered simultaneously to several examinees. Valid field assessments must, of course, yield correct information about the attribute under investigation, but the data from field assessments are assumed to be less precise than laboratory test data. This lack of precision, however, is acceptable if appropriate judgments and decisions can be made despite the lesser precision. Because of their administrative feasibility, practitioners often prefer field assessments to laboratory assessments.

> Field assessments are assessments that require no prohibitively expensive equipment or extremely specialized training of the administrator or evaluator.

This textbook features field assessments that are employed by a wide variety of exercise and sport practitioners. You can learn more about laboratory tests by taking additional courses in exercise physiology, kinesiology, and advanced exercise psychology.

Formal and Informal Assessments

Assessments can be *formal*, characterized by careful preparation, precise timing and scoring, and standardization. Formal assessments are typically constructed with great care and are subjected to testing to ensure that all items are unambiguous and that the scores have consistent meaning. Many formal tests are standardized on national populations. Examples of such tests are the Scholastic Achievement Test (SAT) and the Graduate Record Examination (GRE). Formal assessments should be used when findings are to be used to make decisions that may significantly affect an examinee's life.

Assessments can also be *informal*. Actually, it is probably best to think of a continuum with extremes of highly formal and highly informal assessments. Informal assessments are often designed locally and are seldom tested during development. For example, at the end of a practice a basketball coach may ask team members to raise their hands if they understand their responsibilities in the three new plays that were taught that day. Or a physical educator may ask students to help evaluate a teaching unit in softball by writing three adjectives on an index card. Informal assessments are especially useful in providing feedback about learning and instruction.

Who, What, Why, When, and How of Assessment in ESS

This section of text answers the questions who, what, why, when, and how in respect to assessment practices in ESS.

Who Uses Assessment?

Assessment is a universal practice, something that all persons engage in either formally or informally. Professionals in ESS are no exception. Literally every one of us uses assessment in our jobs, but for a variety of purposes and in a variety of settings. To illustrate how widespread measurement and assessment are, offered next are testimonials from actual ESS professionals. Each statement was given in response to the question, "What is one way in which you use testing or measurement in your job?"

66 We have three physical education teachers who share the responsibilities for about 60 students each class period. We begin every teaching unit the same way—with a series of tests that all the students take. Based on their test scores, we then divide the students into three instructional groups. When the next unit begins, we do new tests, and the groupings and the teachers change."

—High School Physical Education Teacher

66 Most of my students love taking physical fitness tests each fall and each spring. I keep their records from year to year and make them available to the students. They really enjoy seeing how they are getting stronger and faster."

—Elementary School Physical Education Teacher

66 The YMCA national office has developed a physical fitness test battery that we administer to our members to help them set realistic exercise goals."

—Director of YMCA Branch

66 We are currently working on an instrument that will be used to more fairly evaluate the effectiveness of our coaching staff. Our goal is to eliminate some of the subjectivity and overreliance on win-loss records."

—College Athletic Director

66 My staff uses a 40-yard dash, a mile run, the vertical jump, bench press, and squats to help us make initial cuts for the team. The tests also serve as a great motivator for the returning players, so they come back in playing shape."

—High School Football Coach

66 In my research, I use graded exercise tests to assess how different persons respond to the stresses of different kinds of exercise."

—Exercise Physiologist

66 We do some sort of testing nearly every day. We test to evaluate injuries, and then we test to check on how well rehab is going. We also administer a battery of range-of-motion and strength tests to all athletes during their preseason. We

use the test results to identify the athletes who have a high risk of injury because of limited flexibility or muscle imbalances."

—Professional Team Athletic Trainer

66 Measurement is fundamental to clinical practice. We need this information to make sound decisions about interventions."

—Sports Physical Therapist

66 In occupational therapy, we use what we call work-hardening tests during the process of rehabilitation. The tests tell us how well the client is responding to the program of planned exercise and how successful task adaptations are."

—Occupational Therapist

66 People at our school use testing to develop IEPs—individualized education plans. The tests help us decide what to work on with each child. They also help us to show progress concerning the guidelines of the IEP."

—Adapted Physical Educator

66 I've developed a gymnastics potential test that we give free of charge to any child who is interested in learning gymnastics. We have many parents bring preschoolers to us. They all hope that they have a potential Olympic star! Occasionally I tell a parent to let the child mature and learn to follow directions before they start lessons, but usually they sign up for lessons after they take the test. I think the test is really a great way to market our program."

—Owner of a Private Gymnastics Academy

66 I use soccer skills tests for dribbling and kicking practice. I think the tests add a gamelike and fun element to our practices."

—Youth Soccer Coach

66 My training partner and I have learned to do skinfold tests so we can check our body fat percents. We help each other monitor body fat in the weeks before a contest so we know that we're losing body fat, not muscle."

—Professional Body Builder

66 Every few days before getting out of bed, I check my resting heart rate and body temperature. If either of these is abnormally high, it may mean I'm overtraining. My coach will have me cut back some on my workouts."

—Collegiate Swimmer in Training for the 2000 Olympics

66 I was required to take a bear of a test to get my National Strength and Conditioning certification. It was tough! That muscle physiology stuff made my brain swell! One rep max tests are the blood and guts of our program. The guys max out every few weeks. I adjust their workouts accordingly."

—Collegiate Football Strength Coach

66 During the aerobic conditioning part of my class, we do 10-second counts to see if everyone is working in the target heart rate zone."

—Aerobic Dance Instructor, Private Health Club

TABLE 1-1	Examples of Phenomena Assessed by ESS Researchers and Practitioners	
PSYCHOMOTOR ASSESSMENTS (MOVEMENT)	**COGNITIVE ASSESSMENTS (KNOWLEDGE)**	**AFFECTIVE ASSESSMENTS (INTERESTS, ATTITUDES, VALUES)**
Sport skill	Knowledge of sport rules and strategies	Attitudes toward physical activity
Fundamental motor skill	Knowledge of fitness development	Exercise adherence
Physical fitness	Knowledge of principles of injury rehabilitation	Body image
Physical activity level	Nutrition knowledge	Sport aggression
Dance ability	Knowledge of biomechanical principles	Team cohesion
Severity of athletic injury	Knowledge of sport techniques	Pain of injury

What Is Assessed?

ESS has existed as an academic discipline for more than a century. During this time researchers and practitioners have developed assessment tools and procedures for nearly every phenomenon that interests us. Assessment is critical to this research because it is the means by which the discipline's body of knowledge grows and is refined. We have figured out ways to assess phenomena that we want to learn more about and to understand better—with the ultimate purpose of improving our professional practices as physical educators, coaches, athletic trainers, sports therapists, sport managers, and so on. Table 1-1 gives several examples of attributes for which assessment tools have been developed.

Why Assess?

There are many reasons to assess. Most intentional human behavior that entails choice consists of a four-step process of (*a*) establishing a criterion, (*b*) making an assessment, (*c*) evaluating assessment data, and (*d*) choosing among possible courses of action. Very often the assessment aspect of the decision making process is informal. For instance, in all sports, assessments occur whenever a player or coach

What Do YOU Think?

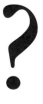

Robert Thorndike, a famous theoretician and pioneer in the field of measurement, is known for his claim that everything that exists can be measured. His reasoning went like this: *If something exists, then it exists in some quantity. If it exists in some quantity, then it can be measured.* Do you agree with Thorndike? Can we really measure everything that exists? Can humans measure quantities of love, courage, integrity, sense of humor, sex appeal, and so on? What do YOU think?

must make a choice, such as when a golfer selects a 5-iron rather than a 6-iron, when a basketball player shoots rather than passes, when a football coach decides to go for fourth-down yardage instead of punting. ESS practitioners face a myriad of choices each day. Although many choices are based on informal assessments, formal assessments are essential to consistent, quality decisions. Formal assessments increase accuracy and reduce bias in decision making. So perhaps a general answer to "why assess?" is "to formalize the evaluation process to make better decisions."

In addition to the general answer a number of more specific answers are worth discussing. These answers are based upon the ways in which assessment data are used by ESS professionals to aid in certain types of decision making.

Selection. Coaches often use performance tests to add objectivity to tryouts. Performance test scores help to identify the athletes who are most likely to contribute to the team. Similarly, performance tests are used in tryouts for cheerleaders, dance teams, jump rope teams, and other such performance-oriented groups.

Classification. Classification results in the grouping of individuals to enhance opportunities for activity or instruction. Grouping of similar individuals is based on the assumption that a homogeneous grouping better meets the needs of the participants than would a heterogeneous grouping. Heterogeneous groupings are also sometimes created to form teams of near-equal abilities or to enhance interpersonal relationships. Classification is accomplished by administering and evaluating the results of appropriate assessments.

Motivation. The value of using assessment results to motivate should not be underestimated. Human beings often can be motivated to perform at higher levels because of our inherent desire to make a good showing and/or in response to a spirit of competition. The keys to effective use of motivation are self-improvement and self-realization. Assessment can therefore be used to motivate clients to perform well and/or to adhere to an exercise prescription, a special diet, and so on.

Learning. Motor learning researchers have determined that performance feedback is essential for learning. Through the use of targets, ropes, and cones, sport skill tests often provide greater performance feedback than is available in the natural sport environment. Therefore, sport skill tests can be used to create an effective and interesting practice for learners. The same is true for fitness tests. Many fitness tests require a maximum effort on the part of the examinee. As such, the tests themselves can be used for fitness development. Paper-and-pencil tests and inventories can be used by the physical education instructor to stimulate class discussions about issues such as personal health, sportsmanship, and attitudes toward competition. Furthermore, learning will sometimes occur concomitantly with the taking and scoring of a test.

Guidance. Guidance concerns are so interwoven through the realm of assessment that it is difficult to delineate them. Assessment data can be accumulated over time to provide a complete picture of the changing status of a person. Diagnostic, prognostic, and proficiency assessments are particularly valuable to instructional counseling in physical education and sport.

On the basis of **diagnostic assessment**, fitness instructors, physical education teachers, and coaches can recommend exercises, learning activities, or skill drills that are needed to remediate an identified weakness.

Diagnostic assessments are assessments designed to identify weaknesses.

Prognostic assessments are concerned with the examinee's capacity to develop a skill and ultimate development of a skill and/or fitness. Prognostic tests can be especially valuable to coaches if they accurately predict persons who will develop into highly skilled athletes. These assessments may, however, run counter to democratic sensibilities in Western societies, so relatively little attention has been paid to this area of assessment and few good prognostic tests have been developed.

Prognostic assessments are assessments designed to predict the potential for development of a human attribute.

Proficiency assessments are used to determine placement at an appropriate level and/or to justify exemption from a particular program. For example, a score on a swimming proficiency test may determine placement of a student in an intermediate swimming class or excuse the person from a required beginning swimming class.

Proficiency assessments are assessments designed to determine placement in or exemption from a required program.

Grading. In schools, assessment scores are used more often for grading than for any other single purpose. In one sense this appears to be a sound practice because it ensures at least some objectivity in the assignment of grades. On the other hand, grading is just one of the many ways in which assessment can contribute to education. Grades should never be based exclusively on test scores, nor should test scores be relegated to this narrow purpose. Grading is discussed further in Chapter 7.

Vocational Suitability. Employers increasingly use preemployment tests to determine an applicant's suitability for a particular job (2). In many municipalities around the country, military, fire, and police personnel are required to take physical performance tests (3). And over the past decade performance testing has become commonplace in the private business sector. A 1990 survey by the Center for Workplace Trends found that more than 60% of the 577 companies surveyed were using or planned to begin use of skills testing as a condition for employment (4). Some companies also use knowledge tests and/or health assessments that include drug, alcohol, and physical fitness testing. ESS professionals are often recruited to assist in the development of valid and reliable vocational suitability tests that have physical dimensions.

Program Evaluation. Assessment data can be used to evaluate many aspects of ongoing programs in schools and other settings (Fig. 1-6). Status and progress in relation to program goals can be assessed to determine a program's strengths and weaknesses. Assessment data can also allow for comparisons between a particular program and standards established by program certifying agencies. Similarly, several programs can be compared by using formal assessment approaches.

Personnel Evaluation. Teachers, coaches, and others often can be evaluated more fairly by use of formal assessment tools than otherwise. They must, however,

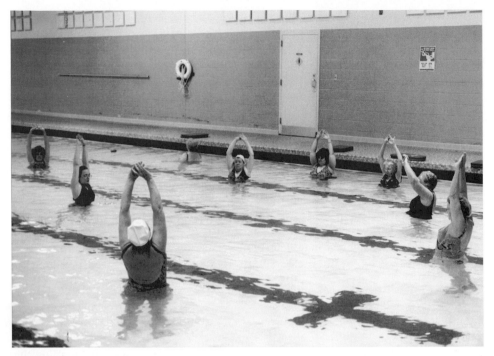

FIGURE 1-6

The water exercise program at a YWCA can be evaluated to determine its strengths and weaknesses. (Photo by Dr. Karen Uhlendorf, University of Vermont, Burlington, VT.)

be evaluated only on variables over which they have a significant degree of control. For example, a physical education teacher could be evaluated by assessing student learning in relation to stated program goals.

Public Relations.   Assessment results can be used to develop interest in and support for physical activity and other types of programs. For example, youth physical fitness test results can provide the ammunition needed to justify quality daily physical education in a school curriculum. A sports medicine clinic in Greensboro, North Carolina, offers comprehensive fitness assessments free of charge to local residents. The owner of the clinic readily admits that improved public relations is the reason for this program.

Research.   ESS researchers use assessment results in many and varied ways. The variables under investigation are often operationally defined in terms of scores generated by a particular assessment tool. Thus, test results provide data that are analyzed to answer the problem under investigation. For example, the Eating Attitude Test, a 40-item inventory, can be administered to subjects to assess disturbed eating attitudes (5). Assessment results are also sometimes used by researchers to assign subjects to control and treatment groups. Researchers realize that the quality of their investigations hinges on the quality of the data they collect. They therefore are concerned that assessment tools are good and that they are administered accurately.

When to Assess?

Anytime! Assessments can be conducted on a one-time basis, or daily, monthly, annually, or over even longer units of time. However, assessments should be done only when they contribute positively to instructional, recreational, athletic, or personal growth goals. They should never detract from more important goals. *As a general guideline, it is recommended that formal assessments take up no more than 10% of the allotted instructional time for a program.*

An important distinction exists between summative and formative assessments. These terms have to do with the timing of the testing. **Summative assessments** occur at the conclusion of a program or unit of study. This is the common testing practice when assessment results are to be used for grading or for program evaluation.

> Summative assessments are assessments conducted at the end (summation) of an identified program.

Both assessment and learning specialists, however, strongly encourage more use of **formative assessments**. Many students appreciate being tested and told about their performance while they still have opportunities to work on problem areas. Formative assessments are given to obtain data to be used for classification, motivation, and diagnosis. Testing for practice to support learning is another type of formative assessment.

> Formative assessments are assessments that occur while skills, knowledge, and/or attitudes are still being formed, not at the end of a program.

How Is Assessment Done?

Data derive from a variety of assessment methods. Some of these methods yield data that are numerical, that is, quantitative; these data can be tabulated and statistically summarized. Other methods yield data in the form of written words or phrases, that is, qualitative data. No single technique is best for all situations. Following are brief descriptions of several types of assessment methods used by ESS professionals.

Physical Performance Tests. Physical performance tests require examinees to perform a gross motor response under strictly specified conditions. The assessment focuses on the *product* of the examinee's performance or motor behavior. Sport skill and physical fitness tests are common types of physical performance tests, but also in this category are tests such as graded exercise tests (GXTs). During a GXT the examinee walks or runs on a treadmill or cycles on an ergometer while his or her heart rate, blood pressure, and/or other physiological parameters are measured.

Bodily Function and Status Indicator Tests. Evaluations of an examinee's health status rely on assessments of attributes of bodily fluids or tissues. Blood tests of all kinds, such as blood cholesterol tests, are examples of this category of test.

Other examples are blood pressure tests, muscle biopsy tests, and drug tests performed on urine specimens.

Rating Scales and Checklists.   When using rating scales and checklists, the examiner observes a physical performance or behavior and rates the *process* used by the examinee. For example, the form of a tennis serve is rated on a numerical scale, or the pattern used by a child in an overarm throw is rated according to level of maturity, or the gait of a stroke victim is rated in comparison with normal walking.

Paper-and-Pencil Knowledge Tests.   Paper-and-pencil tests require a written response by the examinee. Objective items typically require the examinee to indicate the true or best selection from among two or more choices. Subjective items require the examinee to provide a word, phrase, or essay in response to a question. Paper-and-pencil tests are used to assess the examinee's achieved knowledge or aptitude for cognitive learning.

Self-Report Scales and Inventories.   Self-report scales and inventories are used to assess attitudes, beliefs, feelings, and values held by the examinee (respondent). Although desirable responses are generally identified, responses cannot be evaluated strictly in terms of correctness. Scores from self-report scales and inventories are typically compared with norms and/or self-referenced scores.

Questionnaires and Interviews.   Written questionnaires and oral interviews are similar to self-report scales and inventories, but they differ in that they are often broader in scope of coverage than scales and inventories. Additionally, they are seldom subjected to formal testing to determine whether the questions actually yield consistent and honest answers that can be interpreted without bias. Homemade questionnaires and interviews are often used in informal assessments. Questionnaires and interviews have been used extensively in ESS research, especially in studying administrative concerns.

Anecdotal Records.   An anecdotal record is a written account of an incident in the life of a student, athlete, or client. Carefully recorded, detailed anecdotal records may reveal patterns of conduct and behavior trends, providing insight into problems and adjustments of program participants. Anecdotal records are based on observation and are maintained by the program leader. The key to effective use of anecdotes for assessment is to be selective but consistent in the recording of significant incidents. For example, a coliseum manager might choose to keep anecdotal records of all incidents of spectator violence in which someone is ejected from the stands. Records may include details such as gender, age, and race of the person ejected, whether alcohol consumption was believed to be a factor, and time and exact nature of the incident.

Portfolios.   Another valuable assessment technique is the portfolio. Portfolios can be created to assess the work of students or other clients. The portfolio is a collection of work samples. In physical education, the student portfolio may include written assignments, papers, and photographs or videos of performances. An applicant for a position as a sports information director may be asked to provide a portfolio of sample press releases.

Guidelines for Ethical Assessment Practices

Like everything else that humans do, assessment can be done well or poorly. When it is done well, it both informs the examiner and benefits the examinee. The following are caveats that the test administrator and the test consumer should consider to ensure ethical treatment of examinees. Since ethics is "about getting human life right" (6), ethical treatment of students, clients, and research subjects is clearly an important goal for all ESS professionals.

Cause No Physical Harm

The Hippocratic oath taken by medical doctors can also be applied to ESS assessment practices. As ESS practitioners and researchers, we explicitly understand that we must *never* do anything—or fail to do something—that directly or indirectly causes harm to those in our charge. This is true whether we are using assessment while teaching a class, working one on one with a client, or conducting research. This also is true whether our students, clients, or research subjects are 2, 22, 42, or 82 years of age.

Harm can be either physical or psychological; both types must be avoided. The test administrator must realize that physical harm can result from asking an examinee to overextend himself or herself while taking a physical performance test. The American College of Sports Medicine (ACSM) has provided safety guidelines for exercise testing (7). These guidelines are presented in detail and discussed in Chapter 9. We should all understand and closely follow these guidelines when administering fitness tests. The ACSM guidelines recommend maximal exertion tests of fitness only for apparently healthy young adults. When in doubt about an examinee's health status, you should obtain medical clearance before proceeding with your testing. Although the ACSM guidelines were developed specifically for exercise testing, the spirit of the guidelines can and should be followed for all types of physical performance testing. When in doubt about an examinee's physical safety, proceed with caution. No test result can be worth the risk of personal injury to an examinee.

Cause No Psychological Harm

Psychological harm resulting from an assessment is a bit more nebulous. It can occur through the deliberate actions of the test administrator, but more often it is inadvertent. A casual, offhand comment by a test administrator can be taken by an examinee as a harsh criticism (Fig. 1-7). Two major concerns are violations of privacy and violations of confidentiality in disclosure of test scores. Test administrators must be sensitive to the feelings of examinees. No one likes to be poked or probed, and certainly no one wants to be embarrassed, especially in front of his or her peers. In many cases, a preassessment explanation of test procedures and testing purposes reduces examinees' anxiety. Beyond that, simple common sense can help. In some cases you should arrange the test environment so the examinee will have privacy while measurements are being taken. You should also be aware of how the assessment process may affect examinees of different genders, races, ages, and abilities. Scores should be recorded quietly, then discussed in a professionally con-

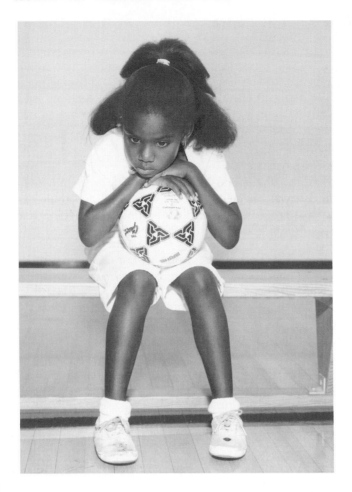

FIGURE 1-7

A test administrator's comments can inadvertently hurt an examinee's feelings. (Photo by Marvin Arrington, Heritage Photography, Greensboro, NC.)

ducted, one-on-one meeting with the examinee. This discussion should probably occur sometime after the original assessment period. Never rush through assessments; allow examinees time to ask questions and express their feelings. Professional attitudes and behaviors are a must during all aspects of assessment and evaluation.

Use Assessments Only for the Purposes for Which They Were Designed

The Code of Fair Testing Practices in Education was developed by the Joint Committee on Testing Practices by representatives of The American Educational Research Association, the American Psychological Association, and the National Council on Measurement in Education (8). The code emphasizes the importance of using tests only for the purposes for which they were designed and for which they have been validated. The test consumer should always keep the intended examinees in mind and should carefully match assessment tools with appropriate objectives for the population of examinees. Although the code was written for educational settings, its recommendations can be generalized to all assessment conditions. Test scores and other assessment data must never be used in simplistic or capricious ways. Remember that assessment ideally benefits the examinee; it should not be used to punish the examinee or to deny him or her opportunities.

Maintain Confidentiality of Assessment Data

The Family Educational Rights and Privacy Act of 1974, commonly known as the Buckley Amendment, was enacted to protect children and their parents from the misuse of educational records. The Buckley Amendment gives parents the right to inspect assessment data that are part of educational records. This law also limits access to those who have legitimate educational needs for the information in educational records. In this case, the law of the land and ethical principles are in sync with each other. Unfortunately, no such legal standard protects examinees in nonschool settings.

Assessment Is Not an End in Itself

The test consumer should always have a valid objective in mind when undertaking assessment. Refer to the purposes of assessment earlier in this chapter. Testing should never be done merely for the sake of testing. Assessment is a means to some other end. Assessment data that are collected and evaluated and then filed away in a drawer or a computer are relics of wasted time and opportunities. Remember that assessment is a valuable tool for making sounder, better-informed decisions. Base changes in what you do as a program leader on assessment data. Use assessment data to help achieve sound program goals.

What Do YOU Think?

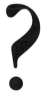

Assume that you are the director of a voluntary in-house wellness program for a large corporation. As part of your program services, you perform comprehensive health and fitness assessments of employees. Your program records include medical histories, lifestyle inventories, resting ECGs, blood pressures, body composition measures, aerobic capacity measures, and so on. The director of human resources approaches you one day and asks for copies of your records for a particular employee to investigate a "suspicious" workers compensation claim that the employee filed. Should you comply with the request? Why or why not? What are the implications of providing the information or refusing? (What if your company wanted access to everyone's records so it could raise the health insurance premiums paid by the high–health risk employees? Does this change your answer?)

P.S. If this issue intrigues you, see "Open Secrets," by Ellen E. Schultz, *The Wall Street Journal,* May 18, 1994 (9).

No Test Is Perfect

No assessment tool is completely accurate in every setting for every individual. Assessment scores must be interpreted with full awareness of the fallibility of the tool. In a later chapter you will learn about the standard error of measurement. This is a statistical value that indicates the assumed accuracy of a particular assessment tool. But even a tool that has a very small standard error cannot offer a definitive measurement for any single individual. Measurement error can never be eliminated; some error of some unknown magnitude always exists. Test administrators and test consumers sometimes forget these important facts. Conscientious test consumers choose the most valid and reliable available assessment tools that are administratively feasible, but they remember that even the best tests come with some errors. Validity, reliability, and administrative feasibility are discussed in Chapter 3.

Do Not Confuse Test Scores and Personal Worth

It is important that you as a test administrator and evaluator never subconsciously ascribe low personal worth to an examinee who scores poorly on a particular assessment. A young woman who has a very high body fat percentage is simply overfat; she is not necessarily a glutton or undeserving of love and respect. A man who has low muscular strength scores cannot be assumed to be unmasculine or lazy. A low test score tells us nothing about a person's worth as a human being. Similarly, a high test score tells us nothing about a person's worth as a human being. All assessment data must be interpreted within the context of the whole individual. Do not allow yourself to make inferential leaps from assessment data to unfounded generalizations.

Chapter Summary

The study of assessment requires familiarity with a number of special terms. A test is used to measure or assess a specified attribute of the examinee. Quantitative or qualitative assessment data are interpreted to evaluate the attribute. All professionals in ESS employ assessment in their work; thus, assessment skills and knowledge are deemed essential to professional preparation in ESS. ESS professionals use many widely varied methods and tools of assessment. This text emphasizes field assessments that are practical rather than assessments that require expensive equipment and/or highly specialized training. The chapter concludes with several caveats that if adhered to, will help all professionals use assessment to serve their students, athletes, or clients without causing physical or psychological harm.

It is hoped that you now feel oriented to the study of assessment and have begun to develop fluency in the language of assessment. Concepts presented in this chapter will help you develop insight into the discussions in the rest of the book. I hope your journey through our text is a rewarding one.

SELF-TEST QUESTIONS

1. Which of the following could best be assessed using a battery of tests?
   A. Knowledge of nutrition
   B. Sportsmanship

    C. Physical fitness

    D. Softball batting skill

2. Which of the following types of tests should be used when you want to find out how an examinee compares with his or her peers on a particular attribute?

    A. A criterion-referenced test

    B. A norm-referenced test

    C. A diagnostic test

    D. A prognostic test

3. A field assessment is likely to have all of the following characteristics *except*

    A. Good administrative feasibility

    B. Simple administrator training requirements

    C. Precision in scoring

    D. Inexpensive equipment

4. When a test is used to group examinees by their ability levels, the purpose of the test is best described as

    A. Classification

    B. Diagnosis

    C. Motivation

    D. Selection

5. When a test is given to predict performance, the purpose of the test is best described as

    A. Diagnosis

    B. Prognosis

    C. Program cvaluation

    D. Public relations

6. Which of the following purposes of testing uses summative evaluation?

    A. Diagnosis

    B. Grading

    C. Motivation

    D. Vocational suitability

7. Which of the following attributes is better evaluated from a criterion-referenced than a norm-referenced perspective?

    A. Agility

    B. Blood pressure

    C. Height

    D. Intelligence

8. Which of the following attributes is best assessed by use of an inventory?

    A. Cardiorespiratory endurance

    B. Knowledge of the benefits of good cardiorespiratory endurance

    C. Knowledge of how to improve cardiorespiratory endurance

    D. Beliefs about the value of good cardiorespiratory endurance

ANSWERS

1. C	2. B	3. C	4. A
5. B	6. B	7. B	8. D

DOING PROJECTS FOR FURTHER LEARNING

1. Develop your own informal word association test that includes terms like *examination*, *spelling test*, *SAT*, *physical fitness test*, *score*, and *grade*. Administer your test to a few friends. (In a word association test, the examinee is to respond to each term with the first word or thought that comes to mind.) Reflect on your examinees' responses, then summarize what you have learned about memories and feelings about educational assessment practices.

2. Schedule an appointment and interview a person who is employed in a career that you may wish to pursue yourself. Prepare for your interview by developing a set of questions that will help you learn more about the use of assessment in this career area. Summarize what you have learned in a short paper, then share your learning with a classmate who interviewed someone in a different career.

3. Examine the ethical dimensions of testing college athletes for drug use. Begin by reading the guest editorial "Drug Testing of College Athletes" in *Sports Medicine* (10) and an article by Stanley Eitzen, "The Paradox of Sport: The Contradictory Lessons Learned" in *World & I* (11). Then discuss the ideas presented by these authors with a college athlete, coach, or athletic director.

REFERENCES

1. Golding, L.A., Myers, C.R., and Sinning, W.E. (eds.): Y's Way to Physical Fitness. 3rd Ed. Champaign, IL, Human Kinetics for the YMCA of the USA, 1989.
2. Tritschler, K.A.: Ethical and legal considerations in HPERD assessment practices. Unpublished paper. AAHPERD National Convention, Portland, OR, 1995.
3. Morris, A.F.: Status of research in testing public safety officers for physical performance. AAHPERD Research Consortium: Research Tracks, February 1998.
4. Randall, I.: The great debate. Black Enterprise, February 1992, p. 141.
5. Haase, A.M., and Prapavessis, H.: Social physique anxiety and eating attitudes: moderating effects of body mass and gender. Psychology, Health & Medicine, 3:201, 1998.
6. Kretchmar, R.S.: Philosophy of ethics. Quest, 45(1):3, 1993.
7. American College of Sports Medicine: ACSM's Guidelines for Exercise Testing and Prescription. 5th ed. Baltimore, Williams & Wilkins, 1995.
8. Joint Committee on Testing Practices: Code of Fair Testing Practices in Education. Washington, American Psychological Association, 1988.
9. Schultz, E.E.: Open secrets. Wall Street Journal, May 18, 1994.
10. Albrecht, R.R., Anderson, W.A., and McKeag, D.B.: Drug testing of college athletes: the issues. Sports Medicine, 14:349, 1992.
11. Eitzen, S.D.: The paradox of sport: the contradictory lessons learned. World & I, 11:306, 1996.

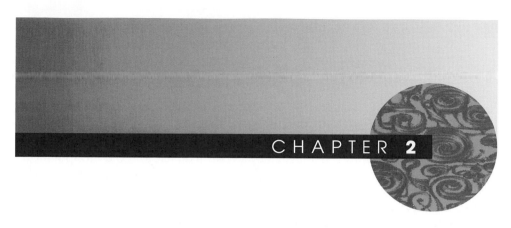

CHAPTER **2**

Historical Perspectives

Many people are surprised to learn that the ancient Greeks did not measure and record performance scores for victors in their major festivals such as the Olympic Games. What a contrast this is to the profusion of sport statistics that are kept in most modern societies! Similarly, medical practitioners in ancient cultures practiced their craft without measuring temperatures, heart rates, blood pressures, cholesterol levels or other such indicators of body function, as is common medical practice today. History reveals that as humans became more civilized, they also became more scientific and consequently sought exact ways to measure phenomena that interested them. In the United States the history of measurement and assessment practices in exercise and sport studies (ESS) has paralleled the growth of research and development of the field as an academic discipline. This chapter presents some of the highlights in the history of formal assessment practices in ESS.

As you read this chapter, watch for the following keywords:

Anthropometry	Dynamometer	Motor capacity
Athletic ability	Grade exercise test (GXT)	Motor educability
"Authentic" assessment	Motor ability	

The Beginnings of Assessment: Anthropometry

The oldest form of assessment, known as **anthropometry**, dates to the ancient cultures of India, Egypt, and Greece. The early practice of anthropometry entailed measurement of human body parts and examination of relationships among the body parts. In ancient India and later in Egypt, study was undertaken to find a single body part or component of the body that could be used as a common measure for all body parts. Egyptians, for example, believed that the length of one's middle finger could be used as a common measure. According to their investigations, the knee ideally should be five finger lengths from the ground, and one's arm reach should be eight finger lengths. (Check it out on yourself or a friend. Are you proportioned according to the Egyptian physical ideal?)

Anthropometry is the science of measuring the human body.

The ancient Greeks practiced anthropometry both in their study of medicine and in their art. Hippocrates, the father of modern medicine, developed a method of anthropometry by dividing subjects into two body types. His dichotomy included two body types, the phthisic, dominated by a vertical dimension, and the apoplectic, dominated by a horizontal dimension. Hippocrates believed that symmetry and proportionality in both the vertical and horizontal dimensions were related to good health, while asymmetry and improper proportions were believed to be both a reflection of poor health and a potential cause of ill health.

Greek artists were similarly concerned with anthropometry. Sculptors studied body symmetry and proportions for aesthetic reasons, and they often looked to the athlete as the physical ideal. The Greek athlete alone rivaled the gods as subjects for sculpture. It was Greek custom to carve marble statues of Olympic victors in their honor. Ancient Greek sculptures were and still are recognized for their artistic elegance. Over the centuries anthropometry has been studied by many artists and sculptors, including da Vinci, Michelangelo, and later, Joshua Reynolds.

Historical Highlights of Measurement and Assessment Practices in ESS

Formal measurement and assessment in ESS began only about a century and a half ago in the United States. It is noteworthy, however, that interest and research in several areas of assessment have waxed and waned over the years. Some early areas of assessment today are no longer practiced. Other types of assessment are only a few years old. So we will begin an examination of the history of assessment in ESS by tracing the patterns of predominant interests from about 1860 to the present (Table 2-1).

Anthropometry

Interest in anthropometry also initiated the measurement and assessment movement in American physical education. In 1861 Edward Hitchcock, a medical doctor, was hired at Amherst College as the director of student health. Hitchcock instituted a program of yearly measurements of the all-male student body. His detailed records included height, weight, reach, girth, *vital capacity*, and selected strength measures. The expressed purpose of Hitchcock's measurements was to define the ideal physical proportions of the adult man.

Further contributions to anthropometry were made by another medical doctor, Dudley Allen Sargent. Sargent was hired at Harvard University in 1878 to oversee the health of Harvard students. During his tenure there, Sargent defined more than 40 anthropometric measures and used them to prescribe a program of exercise for each student. Sargent's system was subsequently adopted for use in several other colleges and in public schools and Young Men's Christian Associations (YMCAs) across the nation. Sargent actively promoted physical assessment by publishing the first administrative manual and by writing numerous articles for professional journals.

TABLE 2-1	Predominant Focus of Assessment Practices in Exercise and Sport Studies in the United States, 1860 to Present

PREDOMINANT FOCUS	APPROXIMATE YEARS OF EMPHASIS
Anthropometry	1860–1890
Muscular strength	1880–1910
Cardiovascular function	1900–1925
General athletic and motor ability	1900–1930
Social qualities	1920–1970
Sport skills	1920–present
Program evaluation	1930–present
Cognitive knowledge	1940–present
Physical fitness	1940–present
Systematic observation in physical education	1970–present
Sport and exercise affects	1980–present
"Authentic" educational assessment	1990–present
Physical activity	1990–present

Anthropometry is still practiced today in ESS, although there are comparatively few physical educators or exercise scientists who identify themselves as specialists in this area. Most current anthropometric research is conducted by athletic trainers, strength and conditioning specialists, exercise physiologists, and the like. Current investigations often focus on corporeal characteristics of elite athletes and dancers, including measures of body composition, along with the traditional measures of height, weight, limb lengths, and girths (1, 2) (Fig. 2-1). The reader interested in learning more about the modern techniques of anthropometry should read and study the *Anthropometric Standardization Reference Manual*, the modern bible of anthropometry (3).

Muscular Strength

In the last couple of decades of the 19th century, interest in anthropometry waned as interest in strength testing grew. Although Hitchcock included some strength testing in his program at Amherst, the acknowledged pioneer in strength testing was Sargent. Along with an anthropologist, William T. Brigham, Sargent experimented with the newly invented **dynamometer**. They designed a battery composed of measures of the strength of the legs, back, arms, and hand grip.

A dynamometer is a spring-loaded device for measuring muscular force; force in pounds or kilograms is read off an index or recording scale.

The strength test battery designed by Sargent and Brigham also included a test of lung vital capacity, made possible by the recent invention of the spirometer. (Vital capacity is the total volume of air that can be expelled from the lungs after a full in-

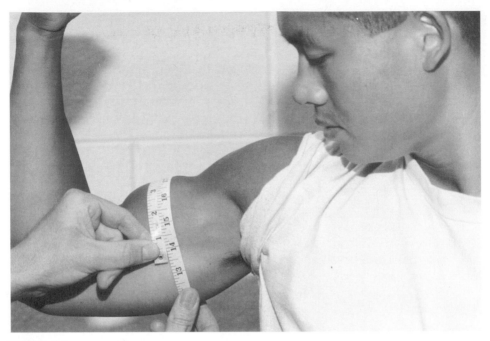

FIGURE 2-1

Upper arm girth, a common anthropometric measure. (Photo by Marvin Arrington, Heritage Photography, Greensboro, NC.)

spiration.) Today it seems odd that a lung function measure was considered to be an aspect of strength, but lung vital capacity remained at least vestigially a part of strength testing for several decades.

Strength testing has never gone out of vogue, although it is unlikely that it will ever receive the attention that it did from 1880 to 1910. In the 1920s interest in the measurement of strength was revived to some extent, and several new test batteries were developed. The best-known of these was one by Frederick Rand Rogers (4). His scheme of testing differed from that of others in his manner of test construction. Rogers's strength test was designed in a scientific manner and was demonstrated as having a high correlation with general athletic ability. Rogers's development of a strength index and a physical fitness index made his test one of the classics in this field.

Today strength measurement occurs in a variety of venues, including exercise physiology laboratories, gymnasia and weight training rooms, athletic training rooms, and physical and occupational therapists' offices. The National Strength and Conditioning Association publishes two journals, *Strength and Conditioning* and the *Journal of Strength and Conditioning Research*, to facilitate communication about strength and conditioning among both practitioners and researchers. It is deemed important to measure strength in its own right but also because it is an important aspect of both health-related physical fitness and motor physical fitness (Fig 2-2). Today's laboratory tests of strength employ various types of instruments, including dynamometers, cable tensiometers, and isokinetic machinery such as the

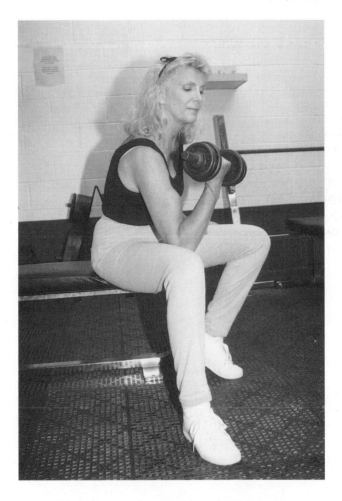

FIGURE 2-2

Strength measurement, an important aspect of both health-related physical fitness and athletic ability. (Photo by Marvin Arrington, Heritage Photography, Greensboro, NC.)

Cybex, Orthotron, and Kin-Com. Most modern field tests of strength require the performer to lift maximal loads of free weights or weighted plates on Universal or Nautilus exercise machines.

Cardiovascular Function

At the turn of the 20th century, assessment interests again began to shift. New interests concerned the efficiency of heart and blood vessel function. Just as strength assessment was inspired by the invention of the dynamometer, cardiovascular assessment was spurred on by the invention of the ergograph. While physiologists studied the effects of fatigue and the relationship between muscular work and the circulatory system, physical educators searched for methods to assess cardiovascular efficiency. In 1905 C. W. Crampton published the Blood Ptosis Test (5). Crampton's seminal test was based upon changes in heart rate and blood pressure as an examinee stood up from a supine position. E. C. Schneider designed a similar but more sophisticated test that was used during World War I to assess the fitness of military aviators (6). This test assessed the rate of cardiovascular recovery after a measured exercise bout. In 1931 W. W. Tuttle developed a block stepping protocol to standardize exercise bouts for his Pulse-Ratio Test (7). Tuttle's work influenced Brouha and his coworkers in their 1943 development of the well-known Harvard Step Test (8).

The Balke Treadmill Test, developed in 1952, was the first successful maximal effort **graded exercise test** (GXT) (9). Balke's work signaled the way for a dramatic increase in the sophistication of laboratory assessments of cardiovascular function related to exercise stress. Many maximal and submaximal GXTs were subsequently developed for standard workloads performed on either a treadmill or a bicycle ergometer. These tests are used widely today in both research and medical examinations. Despite their strong validity and reliability, GXTs are used less often among ESS practitioners because most of these tests require fairly expensive equipment and significant administrator training (Fig 2-3).

> A graded exercise test (GXT) is a laboratory test of cardiovascular functioning; cardiovascular and respiratory responses of the GXT examinee are monitored during progressive increases in workload.

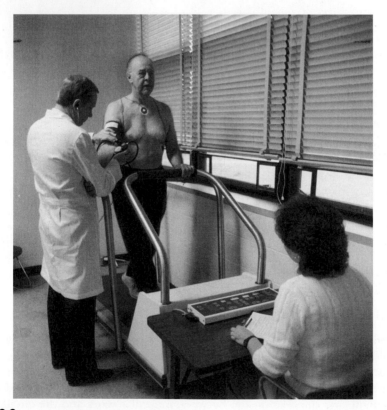

FIGURE 2-3

A treadmill used to standardize workloads for a graded exercise test. (Photo by Dr. Karen Uhlendorf, University of Vermont, Burlington, VT.)

The need for a valid and reliable field assessment of cardiovascular function was met by Kenneth Cooper. In 1968 Cooper's popular book, *Aerobics*, was published (10). In *Aerobics*, Cooper promoted use of a practical field test that he and his colleagues had developed for the United States Air Force. Cooper's assessment instrument specified a 12-minute walk and/or run on a measured track, during which examinees tried to cover as much distance as possible. Scores on the 12 Minute Walk/Run Test were shown to be positively correlated with test results from laboratory GXT testing.

In recent years numerous other field assessments of cardiovascular function have been developed for persons of all ages. Cooper himself developed several other versions of his original 12 Minute Walk/Run Test, including a 1.5 Mile Run Test, a 3 Mile Walk Test, a 12 Minute Swim Test, and a 12 Minute Cycle Test (11). Rockport, makers of quality walking shoes, commissioned development of the Rockport Fitness Walking Test (12). The Rockport Fitness Walking Test is based on a one-mile timed walk. This test is promoted by American College of Sports Medicine as a field test of aerobic fitness appropriate for adults aged 20 to 60 and older (13). An especially unusual assessment was developed at Ball State University for use in its water aerobic classes. This test requires examinees to run or walk 500 yards as quickly as possible—against the resistance of chest-high water in a swimming pool (14).

Athletic and Motor Ability

Interest in **athletic ability** testing was largely a result of the "new physical education" movement inspired by the philosophies of T. D. Wood, Luther Gulick, and Clark Hetherington, early leaders in American physical education. As sports and games became more central to the school physical education curriculum, a concomitant interest evolved in athletic ability assessment.

> Athletic ability refers to one's acquired level of learning in skills common to athletic performance.

Interest in athletic ability assessment, however, soon spread well beyond the schools. Even before the turn of the 20th century, the YMCA and the Turners developed batteries of athletic achievement. In 1913 the Athletic Badge Tests, with standards for both boys and girls, were developed by the American Playground Association. Test items in all of these early athletic achievement assessments were based on traditional track and field events, along with items such as the rope climb and vault. Colleges also adopted programs to assess athletic ability, sometimes replacing their programs of traditional strength assessment. Many people were realizing that strength per se was not necessarily as important as the way strength could be used for effective performance.

The 1920s were particularly significant for the field of assessment. During this era new statistical techniques were employed to construct tests that were more scientifically sound. Test accuracy (i.e., validity) and consistency (i.e., reliability) were improved, and better ways of developing scoring tables were devised. C. H. McCloy pioneered scientific test construction at the University of Iowa. His contributions included athletic achievement scales for boys in track and field, gymnastics, games, and swimming.

Over the next several decades, considerable research interest was focused on the notions of **motor capacity**, **motor ability**, and **motor educability**. These defined human attributes were considered to be separate but related.

> Motor capacity is a person's innate potential for motor performance.

> Motor ability is the level to which a person has developed his or her innate capacity.

> Motor educability is the ease with which one learns new motor skills.

Major contributors to motor ability assessment were McCloy and David K. Brace. In 1927 Brace developed a motor ability test that consisted of 20 novel stunts (15). Brace's test items included a variety of stunts such as jumping through the loop formed by grasping the toes of one foot with the opposite hand. (Try it!) In 1937 McCloy revised Brace's stunt test, and the new test became known as the Iowa-Brace Test (16). Another stunt test, it was purported to measure motor educability. Figure 2-4 has a list of sample test items from the Iowa-Brace Test.

McCloy also borrowed some of Brace's ideas about how to assess motor capacity and ability, and he put them to use in his General Motor Capacity Test (17). This test was presumably a test of innate performance; it yielded a motor quotient that was interpreted as the motor equivalent of the intelligence quotient. Research on this construct continued into the 1950s. In 1953 Harold Barrow developed a motor ability test for college men and junior and senior high school boys that was widely used (18). Barrow's test was structured around motor abilities that are needed for success in many athletic endeavors, such as agility and power. (Yes, this is the same Barrow whose name graces the title of this textbook. Barrow, a professor emeritus from Wake Forest University, and Rosemary McGee, a professor emeritus from the University of North Carolina at Greensboro, published the first edition of this textbook in 1964.)

During the 1960s, research and test development in motor capacity, motor ability, and motor educability came to a screeching halt. New motor learning theories and research cast a dark shadow on the idea of general motor capacities or abilities. Research evidence supported a hypothesis of high task specificity of motor skills (19, 20). Today, despite the conceptual appeal of these ideas and commonly held be-

What Do YOU Think?

Is Michael Jordan, the legendary basketball player, an "all-around athlete"? If Jordan had put in the practice time, could he have been as great in baseball and golf as he was in basketball? What do you think about the notion of an all-around athlete? Do you know anyone who you think qualifies as one? How did she or he become one? Does the attribute of general motor ability exist or not? Or do you suppose the problem is that we just don't know how to assess general motor ability in an accurate and reliable way?

Iowa-Brace Test

Scoring: Two points are given for successful completion of each stunt on the first trial, and one point is given for success in the second trial. Zero points are given if the test item is not passed in the first two trials. *No practicing is allowed.*

Item 1. One Foot—Touch Head. Stand on left foot. Bend forward and place both hands on the floor. Raise the right leg and stretch it back. Touch the head to the floor and regain the standing position without losing the balance. It is a failure:
1. Not to touch head to the floor.
2. Losing the balance and having to touch the right foot down or step about.

Item 2. Side-Leaning Rest. Sit down on the floor, legs straight out and feet together. Put the right hand on the floor behind you. Turn to the right and take a side-leaning rest position, resting on the right hand and the right foot. Raise the left arm and keep this position for five counts. It is a failure:
1. Not to take the proper position.
2. Not to hold the position for five counts.

Item 6. Double Heel Click. Jump into the air and clap the feet together twice and land with the feet apart (any distance). It is a failure:
1. Not to clap the feet together twice.
2. To land with the feet touching each other.

Item 7. Cross-Leg Squat. Fold the arms across the chest. Cross the feet and sit down cross-legged. Get up without unfolding the arms or having to move the feet about to regain the balance. It is a failure:
1. To unfold the arms.
2. To lose the balance.
3. To be unable to get up.

Item 16. Kneel, Jump to Feet. Kneel on both knees. Extend the toes of both feet out flat behind. Swing the arms and jump to the feet without rocking back on the toes or losing the balance. It is a failure:
1. To have the toes curled under and rock back on them.
2. Not to execute the jump and to stand still on both feet.

Item 21. Jump Foot. Hold the toes of either foot in the opposite hand. Jump up and jump the free foot over the foot that is held, without letting go. It is a failure:
1. To let go of the foot that is held.
2. Not to jump through the loop made by holding the foot.

FIGURE 2-4

Selected items from the Iowa-Brace Test of Motor Educability. (Reprinted with permission from McCloy, C.H.: An analytical study of the stunt type test as a measure of motor educability. Research Quarterly, 28:46, 1937.)

liefs about the existence of all-around athletes, general motor assessments are seldom administered.

Social Qualities

During the 1920s attention was first directed toward some of the intangibles that had been attributed to quality physical education programs. Since character, personality, and other social values were stated objectives of the new sports and games programs, it seemed logical that their status and improvement should be assessed. McCloy again made a major contribution by developing one of the first character inventories for physical education (21). Another early contributor to this area was B. E. Blanchard, who devised a behavior rating scale for the measurement of character and personality for use in physical education programs (22).

Prosocial behaviors of participants in physical education, sports, and recreation programs were studied through the late 1970s and 1980s (23). Behaviors such as winning without gloating, abiding by the rules of the game, and sharing equipment are identified as prosocial. Unfortunately, research has failed to provide convincing support for the claims that physical education and athletic programs encourage development of socially positive attitudes and behaviors. Sage (24) has concluded that the effect of sport on character development depends on the social context in which sport takes place. One of the continuing lines of research in social qualities that continues today focuses on the assessment of moral reasoning and moral development among student athletes (25, 26). Unfortunately, in most of this research student athletes score lower than their nonathletic peers.

Sport Skills

Sport skills testing dates to the Athletic Badge Tests developed in 1913, but interest in this assessment area boomed during the 1920s. One of the earliest skills tests of this era was an assessment of basketball playing ability developed by David K. Brace. Skills tests to assess achievement in specific sports were devised by statistically determining a few simple test items that could effectively represent the total activity of that sport. During the 1920s, 1930s, and 1940s, batteries were developed for nearly every sport, with norms for high school and college students of both genders. These early tests were designed to reflect the rules and performance techniques of their day, so many are inappropriate for use today. Since most sports have undergone major rule and technique changes, older tests have lost some of their original claims of validity. Furthermore, norms of decades ago may no longer match the skills of modern sports participants (Fig. 2-5).

Today's sport skills tests are being developed according to more stringent test construction standards. The American Alliance for Health, Physical Education, Recreation and Dance (AAHPERD) has provided leadership in the development of sport skills batteries for school and college populations (27–29). Experts from across the nation are brought together by AAHPERD to develop quality tests; norms are developed from data from national samples. The AAHPERD tests are also characterized by conscientious presentation of evidence of validity and reliability. University graduate programs are another source of new sport skills tests. A number of excellent tests have been developed to fulfill requirements for masters and doctoral degrees in ESS or related programs. And faculty of physical education and ESS around the world

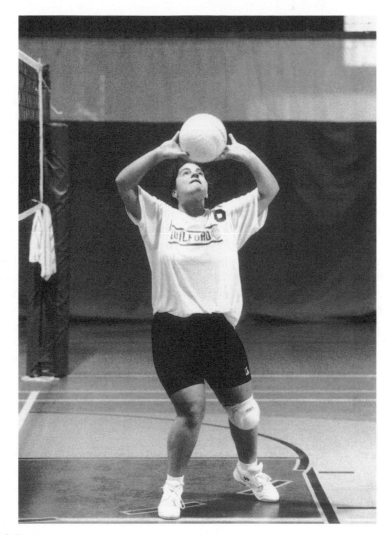

FIGURE 2-5

Volleyball setting assessed by a sport skill test. (Photo by John Bell, Touch a Life Photography, Greensboro, NC.)

continue independent development of new sport skills tests for a variety of athletic populations (30). Undoubtedly, sport skill test research and development will continue indefinitely.

Program Evaluation

As school programs in physical education grew in popularity, there was a corresponding need to determine valid ways to evaluate them to justify tax expenditures. In the 1930s the subjective elements of program evaluation began to be quantified. W. R. LaPorte (31) devised for the California schools the first school program evaluation instrument to receive wide recognition. Subsequently assessment instruments have been developed for nearly all school, public, and private physical activity and sport programs, including intramurals, athletics, and youth sport. Instruments have also been developed to assess the quality of services of athletic support programs such as athletic training. Program evaluation instruments typically take the form of checklists that are used to evaluate administrative aspects of a program against standards recommended by professional organizations or defined by a consensus of the professional literature. Administrative concerns addressed in program evaluations include finances, personnel, facilities, services, and marketing.

Cognitive Knowledge

Knowledge testing has historically been a part of school physical education programs. Most knowledge assessments employ locally developed teacher-made tests. The first formal knowledge test reported in the professional literature was a test of basketball knowledge, developed by J. C. Bliss in 1929 (32). Scientifically constructed and standardized tests are, however, still relatively rare in physical education. Noteworthy exceptions are the Cooperative Physical Education Tests, developed for the American Association of Health, Physical Education, and Recreation (AAHPER) by the Educational Testing Service, the same organization that developed the Scholastic Aptitude Test and the newer Scholastic Achievement Test (33). It was hoped that the Cooperative Physical Education Tests would be used across the country in school programs; unfortunately, they never gained much popularity. Much of their content is now outdated, and published norms are no longer appropriate. New in 1999, however, is the National Youth Physical Fitness Knowledge test of basic health-related fitness knowledge for high school students. It is available on FitSmart software in either CD-ROM format or disks with two 50-item parallel versions (34).

An examination of recently published ESS literature reveals some knowledge tests in selected areas, such as nutrition. However, most of these tests were developed for use in research studies in which cognitive learning was a dependent variable. As a result, few of these tests have published norms. Nonetheless, the tests may be useful to someone interested in assessing a specific area of cognitive learning on a local level.

Criterion-referenced assessments of knowledge are now popular for all types of professional certifications. For example, to become a certified athletic trainer the examinee must demonstrate knowledge (and skills) on comprehensive written and practical sections of the National Athletic Trainers Association certification examination. The American College of Sports Medicine has developed examinations for the professional designations that they offer, such as exercise test technologist. The American Coaching Effectiveness Program assesses cognitive knowledge for aspiring youth sport coaches. Similarly, the American Red Cross and other such organizations have designed tests for certifications in cardiopulmonary resuscitation, first aid, and aquatic safety.

Physical Fitness

World War II inspired national concern for "fitness for war," and a rush to develop fitness tests ensued. All branches of the armed forces devised fitness tests, geared to the needs of the war era. These tests could be mass administered and easily scored and interpreted. During this same period a number of fitness tests were also developed for school and college populations. Among the latter were Bookwalter's Indiana University Motor Fitness Index and Cureton's 14-Item Motor Fitness Test developed at the University of Illinois (35, 36).

After World War II President Dwight Eisenhower advocated for the improved physical fitness of American schoolchildren. His advocacy was largely in response to the shocking results of the international testing of children using the Kraus-Weber Tests of Minimal Fitness (37). Results suggested that most American children were less than minimally fit, significantly less fit than European children. The Kraus-Weber Tests of Minimal Fitness are shown in Figure 2-6. (How do *you* score on these tests? Are you "minimally fit"?)

In 1958 AAHPER published its first Youth Fitness Test and promoted its use in schools nationwide (38). This test has been revised several times in the past 4 decades. However, during this time there has been a paradigm shift in the definition of physical fitness used for development of these tests. Until the 1980 publication of the Health Related Physical Fitness Test, this national organization used a composite definition of physical fitness that included assessments of physical characteristics related to effective athletic performance. Since 1980 all physical fitness test batteries sponsored by AAHPERD have included only components related to health fitness and functional capacity. Additionally, in 1988, AAHPERD switched to a criterion-referenced approach to physical fitness assessment (39).

During the 1980s and early 1990s, many public and private organizations devised and promoted their own children's physical fitness batteries. These tests varied in the definition of physical fitness employed by the test developers and by specific items used to assess each component. Many children's fitness leaders were baffled by the array of available fitness batteries and were unsure which assessment they should use. In December 1993 AAHPERD simplified this decision by their endorsement of the Prudential FITNESSGRAM, a computerized assessment system designed by the Dallas-based Cooper Institute for Aerobics Research (40). The FITNESSGRAM was designed to assess the principal components of health-related physical fitness, that is, aerobic fitness, body composition, muscle strength, muscle endurance, and flexibility. This assessment was supplemented by AAHPERD's Physical Best educational materials. In 1999 the American Fitness Alliance released a new version of the FITNESSGRAM with updated standards for some tests and a new aerobic test alternative (41). (The FITNESSGRAM and other youth fitness tests are described in Appendix A.) Fitness assessments for special populations of schoolchildren have also been developed. Most notable is the new Brockport Physical Fitness Test (BPFT) for physically and mentally disabled youth (42). (The BPFT is described in Appendix A; other fitness tests for disabled populations are described in Chapter 19.)

Interest in the assessment of the physical fitness and the functional capacity of college students and other adults has continued. Again, AAHPERD made important contributions, most notably with its 1985 publication of a health-related physical fitness battery for college students and its 1990 *Functional Fitness Assessment for Adults Over 60 Years* (43, 44). A comprehensive health-related physical fitness test battery for healthy adults aged 18 to 65 and older was published by the YMCA (45). A similar test battery has been published by the American College of Sports Medicine (ACSM) (13). The *ACSM Fitness Test* is a compilation of four individual tests for adults that were developed by other organizations.

Kraus-Weber Tests of Minimum Muscular Fitness

Directions: Administer six tests in the order given. Tests are typically graded on a pass-fail basis; however, partial movements on each test can be scored from 0 to 10 as described below.

Test 1. Abdominal plus psoas. Examinee lies in supine position with hands behind neck; examiner holds feet down. Scoring: 0 if examinee cannot raise shoulders from surface, 10 if examinee performs full sit-up.

Test 2. Abdominal minus psoas. Examinee in same position as test 1 except knees are bent; examiner holds feet down. Scoring same as test 1.

Test 3. Psoas and lower abdomen. Examinee in supine lying position with hands behind neck. Examinee raises feet 10 inches with knees straight, while examiner counts to 10 seconds. Scoring: 0 to 10, depending on number of seconds position is held.

Test 4. Upper back. Examinee in prone position with pillow under hips and lower abdomen and hands behind neck; examiner holds feet down. Raise chest, head, and shoulders while examiner counts to 10 seconds. Scoring: 0 to 10, depending on number of seconds position is held.

Test 5. Lower back. Examinee in same position as test 4, except feet are raised with knees straight. Scoring: 0 to 10, depending on number of seconds position is held.

Test 6. Length of back and hamstring muscles. In stocking or bare feet, examinee stands erect, with hands at sides and feet together. Bend slowly and touch floor with fingertips; hold for 3 seconds. Bouncing is not permitted. Examiner holds knees to detect any bend of knees. Scoring: 0 if distance reached is 10 or more inches from floor, 10 if examinee reaches floor and holds for 3 seconds.

FIGURE 2-6

Kraus-Weber Tests of Minimum Muscular Fitness. (Reprinted with permission from Kraus, H., and Hirschland, R. P.: Minimum muscular fitness tests. Research Quarterly, 25:178, 1954.)

Systematic Observation in Physical Education

Systematic observation instruments have added another dimension to program evaluation in physical education. Researchers have identified several behaviors of physical education teachers that are consistently associated with effective teaching and student learning. These behaviors include use of specific performance feedback; liberal praising of students; enthusiastic teaching; active supervision; and organization of classes to achieve high levels of activity and success (46). During the past 2 decades physical education pedagogy specialists have developed a number of assessment instruments with the purpose of identifying and increasing positive behaviors by teachers (47). The most informative of these are known as systematic observation instruments. They are a hybrid of checklists and rating scales. These assessment instruments identify and quantify specific behaviors of the physical education teacher during instructional periods.

Systematic observation instruments have also been developed to assess the behaviors of students during their physical education classes. Most of these instruments are designed to assess the amount of available class time that is actually spent by children in active, productive, successful learning experiences, that is, time spent on task.

Sport and Exercise Affects

In recent years, affective assessments have focused less on social qualities and more on the interests, motivations, self concepts, and body images of participants in physical activity programs. As researchers in sport and exercise psychology identified new psychological constructs they desired to study, they typically had to develop new assessment instruments because existing instruments were not sufficient for their purposes. In the 1980s and 1990s literally hundreds of psychological instruments were developed by sport and exercise researchers (48). By and large these are scientifically constructed instruments that employ paper-and-pencil formats.

Researchers from other disciplines also contributed new instruments useful to ESS professionals. A number of self-report pain inventories have been developed and are being used in athletic training, occupational therapy, and physical therapy. The most popular of these is the McGill Pain Questionnaire, in which the examinee responds to a scries of questions that will elicit an accurate description of his or her pain (49). Part 2 of the McGill Pain Questionnaire is shown in Figure 2-7. Exercise physiologists, test technologists, and fitness leaders use Borg's Perceived Exertion Scale to assess their clients' perceptions of the intensity of their physical exertion during exercise (50). Many tools to assess and study body image have been developed; these are reviewed in Chapter 12. Sport management specialists have been active in the development of instruments to assess leadership qualities of administrators and coaches (51). Chapter 16 examines methods for the assessment of risk in exercise and sport settings.

"Authentic" Educational Assessment

The 1990s are being energized by educational reform. Educators are realizing the shortcomings and artificiality of many of our traditional modes of student assessment. In physical education, end-of-unit sport skills tests and multiple-choice knowledge tests are giving way to assessment modes that are more "authentic" (52, 53). **Authentic assessments** (*a*) are consistent with curricular emphases, (*b*) are logical extensions of the work done in the physical education classroom, (*c*) provide information that teachers can use to make further instructional choices to benefit the learners, and (*d*) provide the learners information that they can use to aid their own learning. Examples of assessments that meet these criteria are structured observations during game play, logs of fitness activities, projects, and exhibitions. Also popular are portfolios of written work and videotaped samples of student work. A key mode of authentic knowledge assessment is the performance task, that is, a realistic task that is complex and requires divergent thinking on the part of the student. The

Part 2. What Does Your Pain Feel Like?

Some of the words below describe your **present** sensations. Circle **ONLY** those words that best describe it. Leave out any category that is not suitable. Use only a single word in each appropriate category—the one that applies best.

1	2	3	4
Flickering	Jumping	Pricking	Sharp
Quivering	Flashing	Boring	Cutting
Pulsing	Shooting	Drilling	Lacerating
Throbbing		Stabbing	
Beating		Lancinating	
Pounding			

5	6	7	8
Pinching	Tugging	Hot	Tingling
Pressing	Pulling	Burning	Itchy
Gnawing	Wrenching	Scalding	Smarting
Cramping		Searing	Stinging
Crushing			

9	10	11	12
Dull	Tender	Tiring	Sickening
Sore	Taut	Exhausting	Suffocating
Hurting	Rasping		
Aching	Splitting		
Heavy			

13	14	15	16
Fearful	Punishing	Wretched	Annoying
Frightful	Grueling	Blinding	Troublesome
Terrifying	Cruel		Miserable
	Vicious		Intense
	Killing		Unbearable

17	18	19	20
Spreading	Tight	Cool	Nagging
Radiating	Numb	Cold	Nauseating
Penetrating	Drawing	Freezing	Agonizing
Piercing	Squeezing		Dreadful
	Tearing		Torturing

FIGURE 2-7

Part 2 of the McGill Pain Questionnaire. Categories 1 to 10 address sensory components of pain; categories 11 to 15 cover affective components of pain; category 16 addresses pain intensity; and categories 17 to 20 indicate combinations of two or more types of pain. (Reprinted with permission from Melzack, R.: The McGill pain questionnaire: major properties and scoring methods. Pain, 1:277, 1975.)

performance task is scored by means of standardized rubrics that define varying levels of students' insight into the task content.

Authentic assessments are assessments characterized by their lack of artificiality.

Authentic assessments have not yet developed beyond the domain of school physical education. It is exciting to think, however, about how this new way of envisioning assessment may contribute to assessment practices in many exercise and sport settings. Imagine how useful a coaching portfolio could be in the annual coach performance review!

Physical Activity

Recently, considerable research attention has been focused on the relationship between health and various modes and intensities of physical activity. As a result of this line of research, active lifestyles are promoted for persons of all ages, and ESS practitioners are encouraged to monitor their client's levels of physical activity (54). Many direct and indirect methods are being used to measure or assess physical activity in research investigations in the field (55). Direct methods (measurement) include use of mechanical and electronic motion detectors, observations, and physical activity record books and logs. Indirect methods (assessment) employ survey questionnaires and interview techniques (56, 57).

Chapter Summary

Formal assessment practices began in ancient cultures with the study of anthropometry, that is, measurements of the human body. In the United States the predominant assessment interests of ESS researchers and practitioners have varied from 1860 to the present. During the last few decades of the 19th century, anthropometry and strength assessment commanded great interest. Today considerable interest continues in the assessment of sport skills, program evaluation, cognitive knowledge, and physical fitness. Developments in assessment during the past 2 decades include systematic observation in physical education, sport and exercise affects, and physical activity, along with "authentic" educational assessment.

The historical perspectives you have gained in this chapter may help you appreciate the content of this textbook. In subsequent chapters you will learn much more about topics introduced in this section.

SELF-TEST QUESTIONS

1. Which of the following is *not* a modern "anthropometric" measure?
   A. Arm span
   B. Body fat
   C. Thigh girth
   D. Lung capacity
2. Who pioneered development of strength measurements using devices such as dynamometers and spirometers?
   A. David Brace

    B. Edward Hitchcock
    C. C. H. McCloy
    D. Dudley Allen Sargent

3. The Blood Ptosis Test, developed by C. W. Crampton in 1905, assessed cardiovascular function by measuring pulse and blood pressure as the examinee
    A. Stepped up and down repeatedly from a block.
    B. Recovered from 1 minute of stationary running.
    C. Moved from a supine to a standing position.
    D. Hung by his or her ankles in an inverted position.

4. The "new physical education" movement of the early 20th century inspired which new area of assessment?
    A. Athletic ability
    B. Physical fitness
    C. Program evaluation
    D. Social qualities

5. Which area of testing has gone out of vogue because of criticisms of its validity?
    A. Anthropometric testing
    B. Motor capacity testing
    C. Muscular strength testing
    D. Sport skill testing

6. Which is *not* true of the 1954 Kraus-Weber Test?
    A. European children performed better than American children.
    B. Test items provided a comprehensive assessment of physical fitness.
    C. One of the test items was a standing toe touch.
    D. The test was criterion-referenced.

7. Who developed the first successful maximal effort GXT?
    A. Balke
    B. Brouha
    C. Cooper
    D. Rockport

8. Which of the following assessment methods is probably *least* authentic?
    A. Game play rating scales
    B. Portfolios of completed work
    C. Sport skill tests
    D. Self-evaluations

ANSWERS

1. D	2. D	3. C	4. A
5. B	6. B	7. A	8. C

DOING PROJECTS FOR FURTHER LEARNING

1. Use the references at the end of this chapter to locate the original source for an assessment tool published in the first half of the 20th century. (Alternatively, locate the

test description in an old measurement textbook.) Review the test carefully, and if possible, administer it to yourself or a willing partner. Report to the class about what you learned.

2. Considering what you know about current interests and trends in exercise and sport, brainstorm with a partner about the future. What do you predict for the 21st century? Will any new types of tests or areas of assessment be developed? Will some of the existing tests lose their present popularity?

REFERENCES

1. Greene, J.J., Best, T.M., Leverson, G., and McGuine, T.A.: Anthropometric and performance measures for high school basketball players. Journal of Athletic Training, 33:229, 1998.
2. Snow, T. K., Millard-Stafford, M., and Rosskopf, L.B.: Body composition profile of NFL football players. Journal of Strength and Conditioning Research, 12:146, 1998.
3. Lohman, T.G., Roche, A.F., and Martorell, R. (eds.): Anthropometric Standardization Reference Manual. Abridged edition. Champaign, IL, Human Kinetics, 1991.
4. Rogers, F.R.: Physical capacity tests in the administration of physical education. New York, Teachers College, Columbia University, Contribution to Education, No. 173, 1925.
5. Crampton, C.W.: A test of condition. Medical News, 88:529, September, 1905.
6. Schneider, E.C.: A cardiovascular rating as a measure of physical fatigue and efficiency. Journal of the American Medical Association, 74:1507, 1920.
7. Tuttle, W.W.: The use of the pulse-ratio test for rating physical efficiency. Research Quarterly, 2:5, May 1931.
8. Brouha, L. The step test: A simple method of measuring physical fitness for muscular work in young men. Research Quarterly, 14:31, March 1943.
9. Balke, B.: Correlation of static and physical endurance. I. A test of physical performance based on the cardiovascular and respiratory response to gradually increased work. Air University, USAF School of Aviation Medicine, Project No. 21-32-004, Report No. 1, April 1952.
10. Cooper, K.H.: Aerobics. New York, Bantam, 1968.
11. Cooper, K.H.: The Aerobics Program for Total Well-Being. New York, Bantam, 1982.
12. Rockport Walking Institute: Rockport Fitness Walking Test. Marlboro, MA, Rockport Walking Institute, 1986.
13. American College of Sports Medicine: ACSM Fitness Book. 1st and 2nd Ed. Champaign, IL, Human Kinetics, 1992 and 1998.
14. Robbins, G., Powers, D., and Burgess, S.: A Wellness Way of Life. Dubuque, IA, William C. Brown, 1991.
15. Brace, D.K.: Measuring Motor Ability. New York, A.S. Barnes, 1927.
16. McCloy, C.H.: An analytical study of the stunt type test as a measure of motor educability. Research Quarterly, 28:46, 1937.
17. McCloy, C.H.: The measurement of general motor capacity and general motor ability. Research Quarterly, 5:46, 1934.
18. Barrow, H.M.: Motor Ability Tests for College Men. Minneapolis, Burgess, 1957.
19. Henry, F.M.: Specificity versus generality in learning motor skills. Proceedings of the College Physical Education Association, 61:127, 1958.
20. Henry, F.M.: Increased response for complicated movements and a memory drum theory of motor reaction. Research Quarterly, 31:448, 1960.
21. McCloy, C.H.: Character building through physical education. Research Quarterly, 2:41, October 1931.
22. Blanchard, B.E.: A behavior frequency rating scale for measurement of character and personality in physical education. Research Quarterly, 7:56, May 1936.

23. Horrocks, R.N.: Horrocks prosocial play behavior inventory. In Barrow, McGee, & Tritschler's Practical Measurement in Physical Education. 4th Ed. Baltimore, Williams and Wilkins, 1989.

24. Sage, G.: Character development: Does sport affect character development in athletes? Journal of Physical Education, Recreation and Dance, 69(1):15, 1998.

25. Baldizan, L., and Frey, J.H.: Athletes and moral development: Regulatory and ethical issues. College Student Affairs Journal, 15(1):33, 1995.

26. Stoll, S., et al.: Moral reasoning of division III and division I athletes: Is there a difference? ERIC Document ED382618. Paper presented at the Annual Meeting of the American Alliance of Health, Physical Education, Recreation and Dance, Portland, OR, March 30, 1995.

27. Hopkins, D.R., Shick, J., and Plack, J.J.: Basketball Skills Test Manual. Reston, VA, American Alliance of Health, Physical Education, Recreation, and Dance, 1984.

28. Hensley, L. (ed.): Tennis Skills Test Manual. Reston, VA, American Alliance of Health, Physical Education, Recreation, and Dance, 1989.

29. Rikli, R.E. (ed.): Softball Skills Test Manual. Reston, VA, American Alliance of Health, Physical Education, Recreation, and Dance, 1991.

30. Vergauwen, L., Spaepen, A.J., Lefevre, J., and Hespel, P.: Evaluation of stroke performance in tennis. Medicine & Science in Sports & Exercise, 30:1281, 1998.

31. LaPorte, W.R.: The Physical Education Curriculum. Los Angeles, College Book Store, 1955.

32. Bliss, J.C.: Basketball. Philadelphia, Lea & Febiger, 1929.

33. Cooperative Tests and Services: American Association of Health, Physical Education, and Recreation Cooperative Physical Education Tests. Princeton, NJ, Educational Testing Service, 1970.

34. FitSmart: High School Edition. Champaign, IL, Human Kinetics, 1999.

35. Bookwalter, K.W.: Test manual for Indiana University motor fitness indices for high school and college age men. Research Quarterly, 14:356, 1943.

36. Cureton, T.K.: Physical Fitness Appraisal and Guidance. St. Louis, Mosby, 1947.

37. Kraus, H., and Hirschland, R.P.: Minimum muscular fitness tests. Research Quarterly, 25:178, 1954.

38. American Association of Health, Physical Education, and Recreation: Youth Fitness Test Manual. Washington, American Alliance of Health, Physical Education, Recreation, and Dance, 1958.

39. American Alliance for Health, Physical Education, Recreation and Dance: Physical Best: The American Alliance Physical Fitness Education & Assessment Program. Reston, VA, American Alliance of Health, Physical Education, Recreation, and Dance, 1988.

40. Cooper Institute for Aerobics Research: The Prudential FITNESSGRAM Test Administration Manual. 1st and 2nd eds. Dallas, CIAR, 1992 and 1994.

41. Cooper Institute for Aerobics Research: The FITNESSGRAM Test Administration Manual. Champaign, IL, Human Kinetics for the American Fitness Alliance, 1999.

42. Winnick, J.P., and Short, F.X.: The Brockport Physical Fitness Test Manual. Champaign, IL, Human Kinetics for the American Fitness Alliance, 1999.

43. American Alliance for Health, Physical Education, Recreation and Dance: Health Related Physical Fitness Test: Norms for College Students. Reston, VA, AAHPERD, 1985.

44. American Alliance for Health, Physical Education, Recreation and Dance: Functional Fitness Assessment for Adults Over 60 Years. 1st and 2nd Ed. Reston, VA: AAHPERD, 1990 and 1996.

45. Golding, L.A., Myers, C.R., and Sinning, W.E. (eds.): Y's Way to Physical Fitness. Champaign, IL, Human Kinetics for YMCA of USA, 1989.

46. Faucette, N.: Evaluating and improving teachers' instructional skills. In J. Rink (ed.). Critical Crossroads: Middle and Secondary School Physical Education. Reston, VA, National Association for Sport and Physical Education, 1993.

47. Darst, P.W., Zakrajsek, D., and Mancini, H.H.: Analyzing Physical Education and Sport Instruction. Champaign, IL, Human Kinetics, 1989.

48. Ostrow, A.C. (ed.): Directory of Psychological Tests in the Sport and Exercise Sciences. Morgantown, WV, Fitness Information Technology, 1990.

49. Melzack, R.: The McGill Pain Questionnaire: Major properties and scoring methods. Pain, 1:277, 1975.

50. Borg, G.A.V.: Perceived exertion: a note on "history" and methods. Medicine and Science in Sports, 5:90, 1973.

51. Abraham, A., and Collins, D.: Examining and extending research in coach development. Quest, 50(1):59, 1998.

52. Veal, M.L.: The role of assessment in secondary physical education: a pedagogical view. Journal of Physical Education, Recreation, and Dance, 63(7):88, 1992.

53. Schiemer, S.: Authentic Assessment Strategies for Elementary Physical Education. 2nd ed. Champaign, IL, Human Kinetics, 1999.

54. Hensley, L.D., Ainsworth, B.E., and Ansorge, C.J.: Assessment of physical activity: professional accountability in promoting active lifestyles. Journal of Physical Education, Recreation, and Dance, 64(1):56, 1993.

55. Ainsworth, B.E., Montoye, H.L., and Leon, A.S.: Methods of assessing physical activity during leisure and at work. In C. Bouchard, R.J. Shephard, & T. Stephens (eds.). Physical Activity, Fitness, and Health: International Proceedings and Consensus Statement. Champaign, IL, Human Kinetics, 1994.

56. Kriska, A.M., and Caspersen, C.J. (eds.): A collection of physical activity questionnaires for health-related research. Medicine and Science in Sports and Exercise, 29:S1, 1997.

57. Ainsworth, B.E.: Measurement of physical activity questionnaires. Research Tracks from the AAHPERD Research Consortium, October 1998.

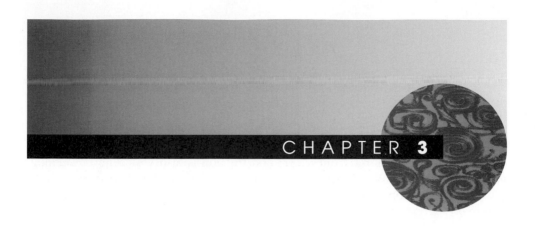

CHAPTER **3**

Selection and Administration of Assessment Instruments

This chapter addresses two how-to concerns. First, it instructs you on how to find and select a quality assessment instrument to achieve your goals. Second, it discusses administrative guidelines to help you learn to conduct assessments in an efficient and effective manner.

Both of these concerns are essential to your development as a skilled and knowledgeable assessment professional. The concerns of selection and administration are interrelated; both must be done well to obtain quality assessment data from which good decisions can be made. The best test in the world cannot give you good information if it is administered poorly. And conversely, accurate and efficient administration of a poor assessment instrument will not give you quality data. Exercise and sport studies (ESS) professionals must know how to find and select good assessment instruments—and must know how to administer them efficiently and effectively.

As you read this chapter, watch for the following keywords:

CD-ROM	ListServe	Reliability
Electronic reference database	Mass testing	Search engine
	NewsGroup	URL
Freedom from assessment bias	Objectivity	Validity
	Psychometry	World Wide Web
Internet		

Where and How to Find Assessment Instruments

The process of finding tests is relatively easy. There are many readily available sources and reference guides to help you locate all different types of tests, rating scales, checklists, and inventories.

Sources of Assessment Instruments

New instruments to assess attributes of interest to ESS professionals are being developed literally every day. This is not, however, a quick or easy task. Quality test construction requires considerable knowledge of measurement theory. Persons who have not had at least one course in assessment should probably refrain from developing their own assessment tools, especially if the decisions to be based on the assessment data are important ones. Test construction is also very time consuming. For these reasons, most ESS practitioners who plan to do formal assessment turn to instruments developed and validated (i.e., determined to be sound) by others. Where do we find these instruments?

ESS Assessment Textbooks.   Before you read any further, you should take several minutes to explore the wide variety of tests, rating scales, checklists, and inventories described in later chapters of this textbook. Perhaps the most obvious source of assessment instruments for ESS professionals is the assessment textbook. Besides the one that you are now reading, there are many other such texts (1–6). These texts usually present abbreviated descriptions of existing assessment instruments but give references to find or purchase the complete instrument. Many texts' authors also provide helpful, informative critiques of the instruments.

Other Assessment Books.   Some ESS assessment instruments are published in book form, complete with the instrument and directions for administration, scoring, and interpretation. Examples include the Sport Competitive Anxiety Scale by Martens and the Perceived Exertion scales developed by Borg (7, 8). Also available in book form are the American Alliance of Health, Physical Education, Recreation, and Dance (AAHPERD) series of sport skill tests for elementary- and high-school age youth (9–11). In contrast to these single-test publications, there are also books that review collections of assessments in areas such as health fitness, sport skills, and physical activity and energy expenditure (12–14). While most of these books focus on assessment of adolescents and adults, some are designed for other populations, such as children (15). These books can usually be found in university libraries and may also be purchased for personal use directly from the publisher. The two biggest publishers of ESS assessment instruments are the AAHPERD and Human Kinetics Publishers.

Journals, Dissertations, and Theses.   The instruments described in ESS assessment texts often can be located in their original form in professional journals, dissertations, and theses. A reference guide, *Completed Research in Physical Education*, is helpful in locating specific tests, rating scales, checklists, and inventories that originally were produced as dissertations or theses. Many periodical guides may be used to locate tests published in professional journals. An especially valuable journal reference source for the ESS professional is *The Physical Education Index*. The *Index* catalogs journal articles from most of our physical education, sports medicine, sport management, health education, dance education, and recreation journals.

The Buros Guides.   A comprehensive approach for locating commercially published assessment instruments are *The Mental Measurement Yearbooks,* published by the Buros Institute of Mental Measurements. Volumes of these yearbooks are housed in the reference section of most university libraries. They are an invaluable source of test information for persons in all areas of education, psychology, and some other disciplines. Each volume contains information on new and substantially revised tests, rating scales, checklists, and inventories published since the previous volume of the yearbook. A typical entry includes title, author, publisher, price, a brief description of the instrument, a description of the persons for whom the instrument was developed, administration time requirements, and reliability and validity data (concepts to be discussed later in this chapter). The entry may also include references for further information and one or more critical evaluations by a knowledgeable reviewer. Buros reviews address concerns about the development, administration, interpretation, and scoring of the instrument. Figure 3-1 shows two examples of entries from a recent yearbook (16).

A

[128]

Functional Fitness Assessment for Adults Over 60 Years.

Purpose: Designed to "assess the functional fitness of adults over 60 years of age."
Population: Adults over age 60.
Publication Date: 1990.
Scores, 7: Body Composition (Body Weight, Standing Height Measurement), Flexibility, Agility/Dynamic Balance, Coordination, Strength, Endurance.
Administration: Group.
Price Data, 1993: $7.50 per manual (24 pages).
Time: Administration time not reported.
Authors: Wayne H. Osness, Marlene Adrian, Bruce Clark, Werner Hoeger, Diane Rabb, and Robert Wiswell.
Publisher: American Alliance for Health, Physical Education, Recreation and Dance.

Review of the Functional Fitness Assessment for Adults Over 60 Years by MATTHEW E. LAMBERT, Research Psychologist, Neurology Research and Education Center, St. Mary Hospital, Lubbock, TX:

.
.
.

Review of the Functional Fitness Assessment for Adults Over 60 Years by CECIL R. REYNOLDS, Professor of Educational Psychology & Professor of Neuroscience, Texas A&M University, College Station, TX:

.
.
.

B

[348]

TestWell: Wellness Inventory—College Version.

Purpose: "Designed to address lifestyle choices facing today's college students."
Population: College students.
Publication Date: 1993.
Scores, 11: Physical Fitness, Nutrition, Social Awareness, Self-Care and Safety, Emotional and Sexuality, Intellectual Wellness, Environmental Wellness, Emotional Management, Occupational Wellness, Spirituality and Values, Total.
Administration: Group.
Manual: No manual.
Price Data, 1993: $89.95 per interactive version, single user license; $299.95 per interactive version, multiuser license; $249.95 per group/batch version; $.50 per group/batch entry questionnaire booklet; $750 per reproduction rights (for educational institutions only); $395 per scanner support capability.
Time: (20) minutes.
Comments: Requires IBM or compatible computer hardware.
Author: National Wellness Institute, Inc.
Publisher: National Wellness Institute, Inc.

Review of the TestWell: Wellness Inventory—College Version by DAVID L. BOLTON, Assistant Professor, West Chester University, West Chester, PA:

.
.
.

Review of the TestWell: Wellness Inventory—College Version by RICHARD E. HARDING, Senior Vice President, The Gallup Organization, Lincoln, NE:

.
.
.

FIGURE 3-1

Sample entries from *The Thirteenth Mental Measurement Yearbook.* **A.** Entry 128. Functional Fitness Assessment for Adults Over 60 Years. **B.** Entry 348. TestWell: Wellness Inventory—College Version. (Reprinted with permission from Impara, J.C., and Plake, B.S. (Eds.): The Thirteenth Mental Measurements Yearbook. Lincoln, NE, The Buros Institute of Mental Measurements, 1998, pp. 442, 1097.)

Supplementing *The Mental Measurement Yearbooks* is Buros' *Tests in Print*. This reference aid is a bibliography of all tests that have appeared in preceding volumes of the yearbooks. *Tests in Print* can also be found in the reference section of most university libraries.

Specialized ESS Reference Texts.   As the numbers of assessment instruments have proliferated, specialized reference texts have appeared on the market. Two references of particular interest to the ESS professional are *Kirby's Guide to Fitness and Motor Performance Tests* and *A Reference Manual for Human Performance Measurement in the Field of Physical Education and Sports Sciences* (17, 18). Practitioners and researchers will also find the *Directory of Psychological Tests in the Sport and Exercise Sciences* of interest (19). *Kirby's Guide* provides descriptions and reviews of 193 fitness and motor performance tests; the guide is organized by fitness parameters such as agility, balance, coordination, and cardiorespiratory endurance. Brodie's *Reference Manual* reviews and supplies research results from 30 tests. Ostrow's *Directory* presents summaries of nearly 200 sport- or exercise-specific psychological tests, organized by psychological constructs such as achievement orientation, body image, leadership, and motivation to exercise. Only self-report paper-and-pencil psychological tests are included in this reference. Test summaries include information about the construction and validation of the test, review references, and information about obtaining copies of instruments. Figure 3-2 is a sample entry.

Professional Colleagues.   One's professional colleagues are always a great source for all sorts of information and advice. Ask personal acquaintances for their recommendations about assessment instruments. Also attend sessions at professional conferences and conventions where newly developed assessment instruments are presented and discussed by professionals working in the areas of your interests. At AAHPERD conventions, most assessment sessions are sponsored by the Measurement and Evaluation Council of AAALF (American Association for Active Lifestyles and Fitness).

 ## Computer-Assisted Searches

There are several ways computers can assist us in searches for quality assessment instruments and related information. These include the use of electronic reference databases, reference databases on CD-ROM, the World Wide Web, ListServes, and NewsGroups.

Use of Electronic Reference Databases

Computerized searches for assessment instruments are often highly productive and sometimes even fun. If you're like most other people, you prefer computerized searches to the alternative of hand searches of hard print sources. The reference librarian at your local university library or a person from your computer services can help you if you are a novice computer user. They can assist you or teach you to search online information retrieval systems such as the Lockheed DIALOG system, OCLC First Search, or EBSCOhost. By using these online retrieval systems, you can gain access to journal articles and other written reference materials from a wide variety of **electronic reference databases**.

REHABILITATION ADHERENCE QUESTIONNAIRE [RAQ]
A. Craig Fisher and Mary A. Domm

Source: Fisher, A. C., Domm, M. A., & Wuest, D. A. (1988). Adherence to sports-injury rehabilitation programs. The Physician and Sportsmedicine, 16(6), 47-54.

Purpose: To identify the personal and situational factors related to rehabilitation adherence among athletes.

Description: The RAQ contains six scales: perceived exertion, pain tolerance, apathy, support from significant others, scheduling of rehabilitation, and environmental conditions. For example, subjects are asked to respond to the item "I worked out until I felt pain and then stopped" (pain tolerance). Subjects respond to the 40-item questionnaire using a 4-point Likert scale, with the anchors strongly agree to strongly disagree.

Construction: Items were derived from an analysis of the content of the adherence literature.

Reliability: Not reported.

Validity: Discriminant validity was supported in that the RAQ differentiated between college athlete adherents ($\underline{n}$=21) and nonadherents ($\underline{n}$=20), with the adherents perceiving they worked harder at rehabilitation, were more self-motivated, and made a greater effort to fit rehabilitation into their schedules.

Norms: Not reported. Psychometric data were cited for 41 college athletes ($\underline{n}$=21 males; $\underline{n}$=20 females) who had been injured in sports.

Availability: Contact A. Craig Fisher, Department of Exercise and Sport Sciences, Ithaca College, Ithaca, NY 14850. (Phone # 607-274-3112)

FIGURE 3-2

Sample entry from *Directory of Psychological Tests in the Sport and Exercise Sciences.* (Reprinted with permission from Ostrow, A.C. (ed.): Directory of Psychological Tests in the Sport and Exercise Sciences. Morgantown, WV, Fitness Information Technology, 1990, pp. 206–207.)

An electronic reference database is an extremely large file of reference information that is accessible via a networked computer.

Most electronic reference databases are searched by means of keywords, titles, author names, or combinations of these. Searches can be limited to selected years, types of material, language, and so on. Some especially useful electronic databases for ESS practitioners and researchers include the following:

ERIC—Citation and abstract information from more than 750 education journals, books, theses, curricula, conference reports, standards and guidelines,

and related documents from the Educational Resource Information Center;
includes educational symposium report literature back to 1967.

MasterFILE Premier—Abstracts and indexing for more than 3100 periodicals,
searchable full text for more than 1500 active periodicals; subjects include
general reference, business, health, multicultural, and more.

MEDLINE—Abstracted articles from medical journals published internationally,
covering all areas of medicine.

Health Source Plus—Abstracts and indexing for nearly 500 consumer health,
nutrition, and professional periodicals; more than 200 periodicals and more
than 1000 health pamphlets are covered in full text; includes patient-oriented
drug information and 17 health books published by the People's Medical Society.

CINAHL—Cumulative Index to Nursing & Allied Health Literature covers
nursing, allied health, biomedical, and consumer health journals back to
1982.

Fact Search—Facts and statistics on social, economic, political, environmental,
and health issues.

SocSciAbs—Abstracts of international English-language periodicals in sociology,
anthropology, geography, economics, political science, and law.

PsychInfo—Comprehensive international index of psychology journals, dissertations, book chapters, books, technical reports, and other documents from
1887 to the present plus relevant materials from related disciplines such as
medicine, psychiatry, education, social work, law, criminology, social science, and organizational behavior.

GPO—U.S. government publications with records on subjects of interest to the
U.S. government.

ABI/Inform Global—Database of abstracts and full text articles on national and
international business, management, advertising, economics, human resources, finance, taxation, marketing, and computers; also information on
more than 60,000 companies.

Reference Databases on CD-ROM

Your university library may also subscribe to a **CD-ROM** information service that
condenses large volumes of reference information onto small sets of CD-ROMs.
SPORT is one of the most useful CD-ROM sources for ESS professionals; it is
searched by topic much as one searches a hard print source. *The Physical Education Index* is also now available in CD-ROM. (Gosh! It's *so* much easier than using
the hard print version! Encourage your reference librarian to purchase it.)

> A CD-ROM is a laser disk that stores large volumes of information accessed by
> computer. CD-ROM is short for compact disk read-only memory.

Searching the World Wide Web

Information about assessment instruments is also available through searches of the
World Wide Web on the **Internet**. Using browser software (e.g., Netscape Naviga-
tor or Microsoft Internet Explorer), the user can navigate the Web and read files
stored on millions of computers worldwide. Each of these computer files has an address, called a universal resource locator (**URL**). Appendix C lists URLs that may be

of particular interest to ESS professionals, including URLs for professional organizations, public nonprofit organizations, and government agencies. Appendix B contains additional URLs for private companies that sell measurement and assessment tools. Once you have a URL for a Web site that you wish to visit, you simply type the address in the Go To line, and then press Enter. The browser in your computer will link your computer to the computer that houses the files of interest. (Almost like magic!)

> The Internet is a vast network of computers linking individual and organizational computers in most parts of the world.

> The World Wide Web, one of the newest and most exciting Internet applications, allows the user to access information from computers anywhere in the world.

> A URL, or universal resource locator, is an address for a particular computer file that can be accessed via the World Wide Web.

To find additional URLs for Web sites that you may like to visit, you can use one or more of the **search engines** on your browser. Common search engines are Alta Vista, Excite, HotBot, InfoSeek, Lycos, Magellan, Snap, and Webcrawler. Additionally, you may choose to use Yahoo!, a directory of Web sites organized into a voluminous set of categories and subcategories. Yahoo! is often a good first place to start an Internet search. The Yahoo! directory and the search engines make it possible for you to conduct a global search on a topic of interest in a matter of minutes. To use the directory and the search engines, you simply enter a keyword or keywords as you would when using a periodical index.

> A search engine is a device that scans Web sites to find matches with the keyword or keywords entered for a search. The Web site rated as the best match is listed first on the results list.

ListServes and NewsGroups

Two other sources that can help in a search for assessment instruments are **ListServes** and **NewsGroups**. Both ListServes and NewsGroups allow you to communicate with others who share your interest in a particular topic, such as running, weight training, baseball, youth sports, or dieting. ListServes use electronic mail, so you must have a current e-mail account to participate in a ListServe and must subscribe (i.e., sign up) by sending a message to the organization or person who manages the ListServe. Appendix C provides information on several ListServes.

NewsGroups are a separate Internet application, one of the oldest areas of the Internet. There are several thousand NewsGroups, created to allow Internet users to exchange news and views about a variety of topics. When you do a keyword search with the Alta Vista search engine, the results include both traditional Web sites and NewsGroups. Some NewsGroup entries are written by experts and some are merely opinions of the "man (or woman) on the street." It is suggested that you listen in on a NewsGroup before you post a message, and then only post on topic.

ListServes are electronic mailing lists that allow subscribers (i.e., those who sign up through an e-mail account) to communicate with each other about a common topic of interest.

NewsGroups, another Internet application, also allow Internet users to exchange news and views about a common topic of interest.

Both ListServes and NewsGroups can be excellent sources of information. Both allow you to ask specific questions and receive a variety of responses, some from folks who *may* be knowledgeable about the topic. Internet sources, however, are *not* refereed. This means that you must be very selective about the information you use from any Internet source.

To learn more about Internet applications, you should consider taking courses, getting one-on-one assistance, and/or reading self-help computer books. Despite the insult of their titles, the "Dummy" series of books on the Internet and on e-mail are excellent references for the beginner (20, 21).

Evaluation of Assessment Instruments

Before buying a new car, most people go car shopping. They learn about the qualities of various cars, then evaluate the qualities based on how they intend to use the car. An expensive car that has superior road handling, sleek lines, plush interior, and a great sound system is right for some persons, but others need a less expensive car with good gasoline mileage and a roomy interior for the family or the camping equipment. So it is with assessment instruments. Each instrument must be evaluated in terms of its intended use. Some tests must be very accurate and precise because they will be used to make critical decisions, such as whether a particular patient is a good candidate for a risky surgery. Other tests must be quick and easy to administer and can be less accurate because they will be used for less important decisions, such as grouping for instruction in a physical education class.

Two broad categories of qualities must be taken into consideration when evaluating a test, rating scale, checklist, or inventory for possible use. These are *administrative feasibility* and *psychometric qualities*.

Administrative Feasibility

The test consumer should examine an assessment instrument carefully before selecting it for use. The best way to do this is to take the test yourself if possible. The test consumer also should pay close attention to (*a*) what the test developer has specified regarding the population for whom the test was developed, (*b*) the stated purpose of the test, and (*c*) recommended administration procedures.

Assessment Population.   For whom was the instrument developed? Many assessment instruments are developed for high-school and college age students; far fewer instruments are designed for young children, adults, the elderly, and disabled populations (Fig. 3-3). Some tests have been developed for both genders; others are designed only for a single gender. A test originally developed for one population is often inappropriate for use with a different population.

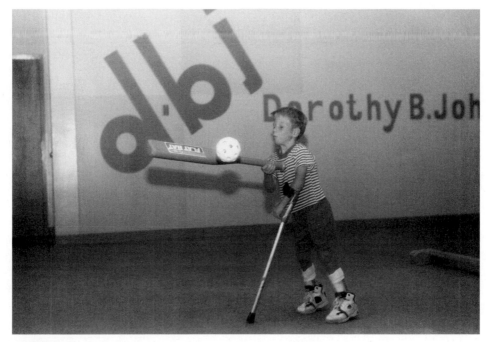

FIGURE 3-3

Relatively few motor tests have been developed for disabled populations. (Photo courtesy of Dr. Sue Combs, University of North Carolina at Wilmington.)

Purpose of Assessment. What is the stated purpose of the assessment instrument? What exactly is it supposed to assess? The answers to these questions are critical to the instrument selection process. For example, is a "physical fitness" test designed to measure health-related physical fitness or athletic performance? Is the test designed to diagnose specific areas of weakness or simply to classify? Is a basketball knowledge test intended to assess strategic knowledge or just knowledge of rules? An instrument cannot assess something it is not intended to assess. Using an assessment instrument inappropriately is like trying to use a hammer to saw a board. It simply will not do the job.

Administration Group Size. How is the assessment instrument to be administered? May the test, rating scale, checklist, or inventory be given to a group of examinees (mass testing), or must it be administered individually to each examinee? How many administrators are needed for efficient and effective administration for a particular number of examinees?

Administrator Training. What, if any, special training is needed to administer the instrument and/or interpret results? For example, because of medical risks, maximal-effort graded exercise tests should be administered only by trained individuals. Interpretations of electrocardiographic (ECG) printouts and projective psychological tests such as inkblot tests should be done only by trained individuals.

Administration Time. How much time is needed to conduct the assessment? When is the assessment to be done? Is a particular test to be given before or after initial instruction? Is the test, rating scale, checklist, or inventory to be given on one day, two days, or longer?

Administration Environment. What are the recommended testing conditions or environment? Is the assessment to be conducted in a classroom, a gymnasium, or an outside field? Is privacy required? Is noise likely to affect results? Is high temperature or humidity likely to affect results? Are special floor or wall markings or special pieces of equipment required?

Administrative Costs. What, if any, is the fee for use of the assessment instrument? What is the cost of equipment that must be purchased? How expensive are the awards given for top performers? Are there any other fees associated with the assessment?

Administrative feasibility is evaluated by comparing the match between characteristics of the assessment instrument and your intended use of it. The closer the match, the better the administrative feasibility. While some of the areas of mismatch can be lived with, others prohibit the use of a particular instrument. There are, however, no clear-cut rules by which to evaluate the administrative feasibility of an assessment instrument. Ultimately, you, the test consumer, must decide what is or is not feasible in your particular situation.

Psychometric Qualities

Psychometry is the academic specialization in testing and assessment. Validity, reliability, objectivity, and freedom from assessment bias are psychometric qualities. These fancy-sounding terms are qualities that are considered in the process of evaluating an assessment instrument. It is the responsibility of the assessment author to communicate information about validity, reliability, objectivity, and assessment bias to potential consumers. Just as the car manufacturer evaluates a car for gasoline mileage, braking ability, impact resistance, and other such qualities, the test's author evaluates an assessment instrument for validity, reliability, objectivity, and freedom from assessment bias. Both the car buyer and the test consumer use this information in deciding the value to them of a particular product.

> Psychometry is the academic specialization in testing and assessment; validity, reliability, objectivity, and freedom from assessment bias are psychometric qualities.

A good assessment instrument always has a significant degree of all four of the psychometric qualities (Fig. 3-4). While validity is the most important of the psychometric qualities, it is impossible for an assessment instrument to have a high degree of validity unless it also has significant degrees of reliability, objectivity, and freedom from assessment bias. So ultimately all four psychometric qualities are important.

Validity, reliability, objectivity, and freedom from assessment bias are important for all types of assessment instruments. There is a difference, however, in how validity and reliability are defined and evaluated for norm-referenced (N-R) and criterion-referenced (C-R) assessment instruments. (In Chapter 1 you learned that N-R tests compare the performances of individuals, while C-R tests compare performances with a standard that represents the level of mastery.)

Psychometric Qualities		
Validity	⇔	*veracity, integrity, soundness*
Reliability	⇔	*dependability, consistency*
Objectivity	⇔	*scoring accuracy, scoring consistency*
Freedom from assessment bias	⇔	*impartiality, fairness, equity*

FIGURE 3-4

Psychometric qualities of good assessment instruments.

Validity of Norm-Referenced Assessments

Validity is the single most important consideration in evaluating assessment instruments. Validity is the degree to which an assessment instrument really does what it is designed to do. In other words, how accurately does an assessment instrument assess the attribute it claims to assess? More technically, the concept of **validity** refers to the "appropriateness, meaningfulness, and usefulness of the specific inferences made from test scores" (22). In other words, can a particular assessment instrument be used to make good decisions?

> Validity refers to the veracity of an assessment instrument. A valid instrument accurately assesses the attribute it claims to assess and allows meaningful inferences to be made from the assessment results.

It is important to realize that no assessment instrument is ever completely valid or valid in all circumstances. Validity always refers to the *degree* to which accumulated evidence supports specific inferences made from scores. Validity, therefore, can be evaluated only in terms of a particular purpose and for a particular population. Validation entails gathering different types of evidence to support different types of inferences made from the assessment scores. The three categories of evidence used to demonstrate validity of norm-referenced assessment instruments are *content validity*, *criterion validity*, and *construct validity*.

Content Validity. Content validity evidence demonstrates the "degree to which the sample of items, tasks, or questions on a test are representative of some defined universe or domain of content" (22). Perhaps this is best explained by nonexamples. What would you think about a final examination that included questions about topics not taught in the course? (What a nightmare, huh?) What would you think of a "comprehensive" physical examination that did not include an assessment of your cardiorespiratory system? Chances are that you would not think either of these tests was very good—because they lack content validity.

Evidence of content validity can take many forms. Consider the following two examples:

EXAMPLE 1

Content validity was established for a basketball skill test battery by a committee of measurement experts who identified the four essential skills of basketball as shooting, passing, dribbling, and defensive movement. This was deduced from a survey of professional, college, high school, and elementary school basketball coaches. The coaches were asked to identify essential basketball skills and to suggest performance tests to measure those skills. (See the AAHPERD Basketball Test for Boys and Girls in Chapter 11.)

EXAMPLE 2

For a written test of intermediate tennis knowledge, the test author demonstrated content validity by providing a guide that identified the items that test knowledge of rules, history, skill and technique, strategy, and equipment, and facilities. (See Intermediate Tennis Test by Reynolds in Chapter 17.)

Criterion Validity.   Criterion validity evidence demonstrates "that test scores are systematically related to one or more outcome criteria" (22). The outcome criteria may be future behaviors (predictive) or behaviors in the present (concurrent).

Predictive validity evidence demonstrates the degree of accuracy with which an assessment predicts how examinees will perform in a future situation. For example, the Scholastic Achievement Test (SAT) is taken during one's junior or senior year in high school; the scores are used to predict success in college. The test developers collected evidence to demonstrate predictive validity by following into their first year of college hundreds of students who had taken their examination. The students' SAT scores were correlated with their freshman grade point averages. (Correlation is explained in Chapter 5. If you are not familiar with this term, you may want to turn to the appropriate section of Chapter 5 now. A correlation determines the direction and strength of linear relationships between two quantifiable variables.) Predictive validity was claimed by the developers of the SAT because in their validation studies students who scored high on the SAT also tended to receive high grades in college. Conversely, students with low SAT scores tended to receive low grades. (How did the SAT do in predicting your freshman grade point average?)

Concurrent validity evidence demonstrates the degree to which assessment scores are related to some other valid criterion. When validating ESS assessment instruments, criteria assumed to be valid include such things as laboratory measurements, expert ratings by knowledgeable persons, and competition scores. Criteria can also be scores from an existing test that has already been shown to be valid.

Many new tests are developed because existing assessment methods are unsatisfactory in some way. The new test is validated by correlating scores from the new test with scores from the original test or some other concurrent valid criteria. Concurrent validity is claimed if the correlation demonstrates a strong relationship between the scores. The value of the correlation coefficient represents the strength of the linear relationship between the assessment instrument scores and the scores representing the criterion. The higher the correlation coefficient, that is, the closer it is to the maximal value of ± 1.00, the stronger the validity evidence is believed to be. *Usually a coefficient of .70 is interpreted as adequately demonstrating concurrent validity, while a correlation of .60 is considered acceptable for predictive validity.* These values are only guidelines, however, because acceptability of a validity coefficient really depends on many factors including the appropriateness of the criterion and the purpose and intended use of the assessment. Consider the following examples of concurrent validity evidence:

EXAMPLE 1

The author of a field hockey ball control skill test demonstrated concurrent validity by correlating test scores with expert rankings of players based upon subjective evaluations of their stickwork skills. The value of this correlation was .63 (23). (See the Chapman Ball Control Test in Chapter 11.)

EXAMPLE 2

The validity of skinfold measurements to estimate percentage of body fat was demonstrated by correlating skinfold measurement sums with body fatness assessed in the laboratory by underwater weighing techniques. The concurrent validity coefficients ranged between .70 and .90 for male and female subjects in grades K through college (24). (See the *FITNESSGRAM* in Appendix A.)

Construct Validity. The evidence to demonstrate construct validity can be either logical or statistical. This validation process, however, relies on indirect evidence because the attribute of interest cannot be measured in a direct way. If an assessment score has real meaning, a person who is believed to possess a lot of the attribute should theoretically receive a high score on the test, while a person with little of the attribute should receive a low score. Validity is claimed when the assessment scores tend to agree with the expectations.

The following examples illustrate evidence collected to demonstrate construct validity:

EXAMPLE 1

One would expect golfers with low handicaps to score better than high-handicap golfers on a valid test of golf skill. (Right?) Construct validity was claimed by the author of a golf skill test battery when the mean score (the arithmetic average) for golfers with handicaps between 0 and 12 was significantly better than the mean score for golfers with handicaps between 13 and 18. Golfers with handicaps of 19 and greater performed worse than the other two groups of golfers on the golf skill test battery (25).

EXAMPLE 2

Children's scores on an inventory designed to assess attitudes toward physical activity were found to be positively related to active involvement in physical activity. In other words, children who expressed positive attitudes on the inventory tended to be physically active, while children who had negative attitudes tended to be less active. Construct validity was claimed on the basis of this evidence (26).

Validity of Criterion-Referenced Tests

Validity is also the most important psychometric concern for evaluating criterion-referenced (C-R) assessments. The definition of validity is, however, slightly different when applied to C-R instruments, and there are different types of validity evidence. C-R validity can be demonstrated through the use of either logical or statistical evidence. The logical approach is termed *domain-referenced validity*; the statistical approach is called *decision validity*.

Domain-Referenced Validity.   Every C-R assessment has a performance measure referenced to a criterion behavior that distinguishes masters from nonmasters. Domain validation of C-R tests, rating scales, checklists, and inventories entails demonstrating that the items sampled by the assessment instrument adequately represent the criterion behavior. "Domain" is used to represent the criterion behavior.

Consider the task of validating an officiating rules examination for volleyball officials. The first step in the validation process is to identify in detail the complete domain of volleyball rules. The next step is to classify the rules into categories such as ball handling, serving, rules about positions and interchange, and substitution rules. Next, a procedure is developed to sample systematically from the domain in such a way that the entire domain is well represented by the sample of items.

Domain-referenced validity may sound very similar to content validity. It should, for there are many similarities. The differences lie in the precise definition of the domain that represents the criterion behavior and the systematic sampling from the domain.

Decision Validity.   Decision validity evidence demonstrates that the assessment instrument can accurately classify individuals as masters or nonmasters. One method by which this is done is through identification of contrasting groups, that is, groups of individuals who are assumed to be either masters (e.g., professionals) or nonmasters (e.g., amateurs) on the attribute of interest. These persons are given the assessment instrument and classified as masters or nonmasters based on whether their scores are above or below a specified cutoff score. Validity is established if the test accurately classifies most of the assumed masters as masters and assumed nonmasters as nonmasters.

Decision validity can be numerically estimated by a *contingency coefficient*, symbolized by C, that represents the proportion of the total test group who are accurately classified by the test (6). A value that approaches 1.00 indicates nearly perfect classification, while a coefficient of .50 indicates that the test classification was no better than chance. *Krippendorff (27) suggested that values of .80 or higher are desirable.* The C value is easily calculated from a contingency table by summing the number of accurate master-master classifications plus the number of nonmaster-nonmaster classifications, then dividing by the total group size to find a proportion.

The following shows how the contrasting groups method was used to establish decision validity in the development of a C-R skill test for archery. In this example the contrasting groups were students who had received at least eight classes of archery instruction and those who had received fewer than eight classes.

EXAMPLE 1

The authors tested instructed students and uninstructed students on their newly developed Criterion-Referenced Test for Archery. After determining the cutoff score that maximized correct classifications, the authors reported that 42 of the 47 instructed group students were accurately classified as masters and 26 of the 31 uninstructed students were accurately classified as nonmasters (28). This yielded a C value of .87. Figure 3-5 shows calculation of the C value. (See the McKenzie-Shifflett Archery Test in Chapter 11.)

A Few More Words About Validity.   Remember that validity is the single most important psychometric quality of an assessment instrument. Each of the validity procedures presented here is merely a different way to demonstrate that an assessment instrument works as it should. Figure 3-6 summarizes the major types of validity evidence.

In the next section we turn to a discussion of reliability, the second most important psychometric quality. It is not sufficient for a test to assess accurately; it must do so consistently, that is, nearly every time it is used. Reliability and validity are, however, related. *A valid assessment is always reliable, but a reliable assessment is not necessarily valid.* (Can you reason why this is so?)

Reliability of Norm-Referenced Tests

Are you a reliable person? Reliability as a measurement concept means approximately the same as it does in everyday English. A reliable person is dependable and consistent; a reliable test, rating scale, checklist, or inventory is also dependable and consistent. **Reliability** denotes the consistency with which an assessment instrument assesses whatever it assesses. This is why a test can be reliable without being valid. The test may actually assess something other than what it claims to assess, but as long as it does so consistently, it is considered reliable. (I have a bathroom scale that is reliable. It consistently measures people as 3 lb less than their true body weight. Assessing body weight by use of this instrument is reliable but not valid.) A reliable assessment instrument gives us confidence that an examinee's score would be approximately the same if the test, rating scale, checklist, or inventory were read-

| | Criterion Groups | |
	Instructed (n = 47)	Uninstructed (n = 31)
Masters	42	5
Nonmasters	5	26

$$C = \frac{(42 + 26) = 68}{(47 + 31)\quad 78} = .87$$

FIGURE 3-5

Calculation of the contingency coefficient (C) to demonstrate decision validity.

Validity for Norm-Referenced Assessment Instruments

Content validity—degree to which the items or tasks sampled from an N-R assessment instrument are representative of a defined universe or "domain" of content

Criterion validity—degree to which an N-R assessment instrument assesses the true or "criterion" behavior of examinees

    Predictive—validity based upon correlation between N-R assessment scores and a predicted future behavior

    Concurrent—validity based upon correlation between N-R assessment scores and a criterion variable that is assessed at about the same time

Construct validity—degree to which an N-R assessment instrument accurately assesses an attribute that cannot be measured directly

Validity of Criterion-Referenced Assessment Instruments

Domain-referenced validity—degree to which items or tasks sampled by a C-R assessment instrument adequately represent the domain of items or tasks

Decision validity—degree to which a C-R assessment instrument accurately classifies examinees as masters or nonmasters

FIGURE 3-6

Major types of validity evidence.

ministered. It also gives us confidence that there is consistency in the magnitude of score differences between any two examinees.

> Reliability refers to the dependability of an assessment instrument. A reliable instrument assesses an attribute consistently such that scores consistently reflect differences between examinees.

A reliable assessment instrument is not affected to any large degree by random errors that might improve an examinee's score on one day but hurt it on another day. Examples of such random errors are boredom and fatigue, inconsistent administration, distracting noises, uncomfortable temperatures, lack of warm-up, and cheating. High reliability can be achieved only if sources of error are reduced or eliminated.

As is true of validity, reliability can be demonstrated by any of several types of evidence (Fig. 3-7).

Reliability of Norm-Referenced Assessment Instruments

Test-retest reliability—degree to which an N-R assessment instrument yields consistent scores over time

Internal consistency reliability—degree to which examinee scores are consistent across parts or trials of an N-R instrument

    Split half reliability—consistency of examinees' scores on two halves of an N-R assessment instrument

Parallel forms reliability—degree of consistency in scores on two forms of an N-R assessment instrument

Reliability of Criterion-Referenced Assessment Instruments

Repeated mastery reliability—degree to which a C-R assessment instrument consistently classifies examinees as masters and nonmasters

---

FIGURE 3-7

Major types of reliability evidence.

A reliability coefficient, a numerical value, is calculated from the evidence. The theoretical range of reliability coefficients varies from a low of .00 to a high of 1.00. No assessment instrument is perfectly reliable. There are always measurement or assessment errors that cannot be eliminated even under the best administrative conditions. Reliability is, however, usually easier to achieve than validity, so reliability coefficients are usually expected to be higher than corresponding validity coefficients.

Since reliability can be determined in several ways, reliability coefficient is a generic term. Each reliability coefficient estimates a different type of consistency. For N-R assessment instruments we will discuss test-retest, internal consistency, split half, and parallel forms reliability. This will be followed by a discussion of the reliability of C-R instruments.

Test-Retest Reliability.   Test-retest reliability coefficients estimate stability, or consistency, over time. In this process of test evaluation, the same individuals are administered an assessment instrument twice within a relatively short period. The relationship between the two sets of scores is determined by one of two statistical methods. One method is to use a statistical procedure called analysis of variance (ANOVA) to calculate an *intraclass correlation coefficient*. This reliability estimate is symbolized by $R_{xx'}$. (If you are not familiar with ANOVA, you may want to turn now to the description of this statistical technique in Chapter 6. It is not, however, necessary that you fully understand this term as yet. ANOVA compares differences between two or more arithmetic averages; in the case of test-retest reliability, it compares the average test score with the average retest score.) The second method for evaluating test-retest reliability is to correlate the two sets of scores by the Pearson product-moment correlation (i.e., the same correlation statistic that is used for estimating predictive and concurrent validity). The resulting correlation coefficient is reported as the test-retest reliability coefficient, symbolized by $r_{xx'}$.

You may be wondering why there are two methods of estimating reliability and whether one method is better than the other. The intraclass correlation coefficient calculated by ANOVA is preferred for estimating reliability. The product-moment correlation is actually designed to establish the relationship between two *different* variables, such as SAT scores and freshman year grade point averages. It is not appropriate for use in univariate situations, such as we have when correlating repeated measures (test and retest) on the same variable. You will, however, find the $r_{xx'}$ reliability coefficient reported in older tests, for it was used exclusively until the late 1970s.

Test-retest reliability is the most commonly reported type of reliability for ESS assessment instruments because it is well suited for assessments that require motor responses. One of the important decisions that must be made when attempting to demonstrate test-retest reliability is the length of time between the administrations of the assessment. If too little time passes, scores are likely to be affected by fatigue. If too much time passes, scores may vary because of learning or physical changes. So ideally, both the size of the test-retest coefficient and the length of the test-retest interval should be reported and considered in evaluating reliability.

An example of how test-retest reliability was estimated for an actual test follows:

EXAMPLE 1

In development of a basketball test battery, male and female subjects between age 10 and college age were tested and a few days later were retested on the four basketball tests that constitute the battery. Test-retest reliability was reported for each of the tests by means of the intraclass correlation coefficient. For the Control Dribble Test, $R_{xx'}$ ranged from .93 to .97 for females and from .88 to .95 for males (29). (See AAHPERD Basketball Test for Boys and Girls in Chapter 11.)

Internal Consistency Reliability.   Reliability of a test, rating scale, checklist, or inventory can be estimated from a single administration of an assessment instrument. This measure of reliability refers to the consistency of examinee performance across parts of a test or from trial to trial within a test.

A common type of single-administration reliability is termed *split half reliability*. The total test is divided into two comparable halves with an equal number of questions or trials per half. Each examinee's score is determined for each half, and then the two half-scores are correlated. Split half reliability is established to the extent that there is consistency between performances on the two halves of the test.

The split half reliability coefficient must be interpreted with care, however, because long tests are usually more reliable than short tests. The correlation coefficient for the two halves of a test underestimates the reliability of the full test. The split half reliability coefficient must therefore be adjusted by the *Spearman-Brown prophecy formula* so the reliability of the complete test is reflected. This formula is:

$$\text{r of total test} = \frac{2 \, (\text{r of halves})}{1 + (\text{r of halves})} \qquad \text{Formula 3-1}$$

For example, suppose a 10-trial pitching accuracy test is divided into two halves, with the odd-numbered trials making up half and the even-numbered trials, the other half. If the split half reliability coefficient is calculated to be .60, the Spearman-Brown formula estimates the reliability of the 10-trial test to be .75. (Check this by plugging .60 into the formula.)

Internal consistency reliability can also be estimated by calculating an intraclass correlation coefficient. Again, it is actually preferred over reliability estimates that use the Pearson product-moment correlation. Not only is the ANOVA a more appropriate procedure for this univariate situation but it is not necessary to reduce the trials to two sets to calculate the intraclass correlation coefficient. This is a distinct advantage when evaluating the reliability of motor tests that have many trials. Reducing the trials to two groups sometimes masks systematic increases or decreases across trials. The ANOVA approach is sensitive to differences across the trials and thus gives a lower but more honest estimate of internal consistency reliability.

Computer-Assisted Calculations of Internal Consistency Reliability

Since the advent of computers to handle the long, involved arithmetic, internal consistency reliability can be determined easily by other approaches. These approaches employ one of the Kuder-Richardson formulas, KR-20 or KR-21, or Cronbach's formula for coefficient alpha. These approaches for demonstrating the internal consistency of an assessment instrument are similar to that of the split half method. Essentially they provide a reliability coefficient that represents the average of all possible split halves. For example, for a 10-trial test, the internal consistency reliability is the average of all the split half reliabilities that can be calculated for every possible combination of five-trial sets. See why a computer is needed for these calculations? (More complete discussions of using computers for statistical analyses will follow in Chapters 5 and 6.)

Parallel Forms Reliability. Parallel forms of an assessment instrument are designed to be identical in every way except the actual items. Parallel forms have the same number of items, the same levels of difficulty, and the same directions for administration, scoring, and interpretation. Parallel forms reliability, also known as equivalent forms and/or alternate forms reliability, implies consistency from one form to another. Parallel forms are used almost exclusively with written assessment instruments. Parallel forms are especially useful for research studies in which one form is used for pretesting and the other form is used for posttesting following a treatment of some kind. Whenever parallel forms are available, it is important to know that an examinee's score will be minimally affected by the form of the test that is taken. The *coefficient of equivalence*, $r_{ab'}$, is calculated by correlating the scores of examinees who have taken both forms of the test during the validation process. $R_{ab'}$, the corresponding intraclass correlation coefficient, is calculated by ANOVA.

Interpreting Reliability Coefficients. Although it is rare to accept a reliability coefficient lower than .70, the different types of reliability estimates cannot be interpreted identically. Remember that they represent different types of consistency, some of which may be relatively simple or hard to achieve for different types of assessment instruments and for different groups of individuals. For example, muscular strength tests often report reliabilities of .95 or higher, while motor accuracy tests such as pitching or putting tests usually report reliabilities less than .85. Additionally, motor skill tests for beginners are often higher in reliability than tests designed for intermediates. And as already mentioned, long tests tend to be more reliable than short tests. *As a general guideline, reliability coefficients should be .80 or higher.*

    Standard Error of Measurement. It is sometimes desirable to know the precision of a single examinee's performance. This is done by calculating the *standard error of measurement*, symbolized SE_m, from the following formula:

$$SE_m = s\sqrt{1-r} \hspace{4cm} \text{Formula 3-2}$$

where s is the standard deviation and r is a reliability coefficient. (The standard deviation is discussed in Chapter 5. Turn to that chapter now if you are not familiar with this term. It represents average variability of individuals' scores from the group average score.)

    For example, suppose the standard deviation for a set of vertical jump scores is 2 inches and the test-retest reliability coefficient is .91. In this case, the standard error of measurement is estimated to be 0.6 inch.

$$SE_m = 2\sqrt{1-.91} = .6'' \hspace{3cm} \text{Formula 3-3}$$

    What does this mean? The standard error of measurement, a reflection of the measurement error in each test score, tells how precise any particular examinee's score is. Assume a volleyball player jumped 15 inches. According to measurement theory, if he were to retake this vertical jump test 100 times, his score would fall between 14.4 and 15.6 inches on 68 of the 100 jumps. In other words, the obtained score ± 1 SE_m creates a 68% confidence interval for any examinee's test score. Similarly, the obtained score ± 2 SE_m creates a 95% confidence interval, and the obtained score ± 3 SE_m creates a 99% confidence interval. In other words, the *smaller* the standard error of measurement, the more reliance we have on the precision of the obtained scores. Small measurement errors usually produce high reliability coefficients; large measurement errors produce imprecise scores and low reliability coefficients.

Reliability for Criterion-Referenced Tests

Criterion-referenced reliability is defined as consistency of classification. *Repeated mastery reliability* is evaluated by the consistency with which examinees are classified as masters or nonmasters by a C-R test. This is determined by administering a mastery test to the same examinees on two different occasions. The test results are then entered on a contingency table as depicted in Figure 3-8. In this example, 80 examinees took a mastery test twice; 34 were judged to be masters on both test administrations, 30 were judged to be nonmasters on both occasions, 9 were judged to be masters on day 1 but nonmasters on day 2, and 7 were judged to be nonmasters on day 1 but masters on day 2.

    The reliability is estimated by calculation of the *proportion of agreement*, symbolized by P. The calculation of P is identical to that of C (i.e., the contingency coefficient used to estimate decision validity). The number of consistent classifications is divided by the total number of examinees. In this example, P is .80. Interpretation is

Day 2

	Masters	Nonmasters
Masters (Day 1)	34	9
Nonmasters (Day 1)	7	30

$$P = \frac{(34 + 30)}{(34 + 30 + 7 + 9)} = \frac{64}{80} = .80$$

FIGURE 3.8

Calculation of the proportion of agreement (P) to demonstrate repeated mastery reliability.

the same as for C. The interpretable range of P are values between .50 and 1.00, because values less than .50 indicate classification poorer than that of chance.

Objectivity

Objectivity is also a consistency measure, but it implies consistency in the scoring of an assessment instrument, not consistency of examinee performance. An estimate of the consistency in scoring is especially important when scoring requires subjectivity, such as in scoring essays, gymnastic or dance performances, or using a rating scale of most any kind.

> Objectivity refers to the accuracy of the scoring system of an assessment instrument. An objective assessment instrument can be used consistently by different scorers to obtain similar results.

Interscorer objectivity refers to the consistency of scoring for independent raters; *intrascorer objectivity* refers to the consistency of scoring for a single rater. Objectivity estimates are obtained through use of correlation and are interpreted like reliability coefficients. *Correlation coefficients for objectivity should generally be .80 or higher.*

Freedom From Assessment Bias

Assessment bias is related to validity but deserves special note because of its potential to damage our society. Assessment bias is a concern whenever an assessment instrument is administered to examinees who have experiential backgrounds that are noticeably different from those of the population for whom the test was developed and on whom the test was standardized (30). Experiential backgrounds can differ by ethnic heritage, nationality, socioeconomic status, gender, age, and physical or mental abilities. Unfairness can result when the use of scores requires large inferential leaps, such as when scores on standardized tests are used as the sole criterion for admission to desirable educational programs, for awarding of scholarships, or for job opportunities.

> Freedom from assessment bias refers to the impartiality of an assessment instrument. An instrument that is free of assessment bias is appropriate for examinees from all groups for whom the instrument is intended.

Assessment bias can be identified both at the level of a single item and for a complete test. One of the indicators of *item bias* is that a particular item is disproportionately hard or easy for the special group. Indicators of *test bias* can be differences in mean scores, group differences in reliability, and group differences in prediction of a criterion variable. Freedom from assessment bias is a worthy goal in the development and validation of assessment instruments that are intended to be used for testing of a broad spectrum of individuals. *Good assessment instruments accurately reflect real differences among members of different groups, but they do not unfairly or artificially discriminate against them.*

In exercise and sport settings, one of the major concerns is gender difference. Especially when selecting a physical performance or bodily function or status test that was designed for use with both genders, the consumer should try to determine whether the test is truly gender appropriate. Is the test equally fair to males and females in how it is designed, scored, and interpreted? Test developers sometimes account for gender differences by providing separate norm tables for the interpretation of the scores for males and females. Test developers may also specify differences in test administration to account for real gender differences in strength, oxygen uptake capacity, and other physiological differences. For example, females may use shorter distances or lighter weights in physical performance tests that have a significant strength or power element. The test consumer should carefully examine how gender differences are treated in ESS assessment instruments.

Selecting From the Alternatives

After identifying as many instruments as you can that could serve your purpose, it is time to conduct a comparative evaluation. In most cases, the following step-by-step evaluation process will help you to select the best instrument from among the alternatives.

What Do YOU Think?

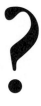

Researcher Phyllis Rosser concluded that the November 1987 version of the SAT was biased against female examinees (31). Her conclusion was based on research findings that 21 of the 145 items on the test favored men but only 2 of the items favored women. For example, Rosser found that women were more likely to answer correctly the analogy, "Love is to requite as attack is to retaliate," and men were more likely to answer correctly the analogy, "Dividends is to stock as royalties is to writer." Rosser called on the Educational Testing Service, developers of the SAT, to remove questions that favor one gender or to balance them with items that favor the other gender. Rosser pointed out that although men consistently outscore women on the SAT, women earn higher grades both in high school and college. Rosser claimed that when SAT scores are used for awarding scholarships or for admitting applicants to special academic programs, women are cheated! The ETS countered Rosser's charges, claiming that the differences in male and female scores reflect legitimate educational differences between the genders. What do YOU think?

Step 1. Eliminate from consideration all of the instruments that are administratively unfeasible for one reason or another. Does the instrument require too much time? Does it require unavailable equipment?

Step 2. Carefully consider validity. Are the inferences to be made from the test scores appropriate? Is one instrument better than the rest for testing the population you are interested in? If content validity is a major concern, do the items in one of these tests best match the content that you wish to test? Or simply, does one instrument have a higher validity coefficient than any of the others?

Step 3. The next factor to consider is reliability. All else being equal, one would naturally select the most reliable measurement instrument. Seldom, however, is the decision this simple. The most reliable test may be considerably longer than a test that has an only slightly lower reliability coefficient. Remember also that reliability coefficients that have been determined by different methods (e.g., test-retest or split halves) are not directly comparable.

Step 4. Return to the factor of administrative feasibility to reconsider any other information about an instrument. Rethink the requirements for administration, scoring, and interpretation. Also consider objectivity and assessment bias.

At this point, you probably have selected an instrument. But what if you haven't? If you have narrowed the choices to a couple of possibilities, you might proceed by trying out the two assessment instruments on a small sample of persons drawn from or similar to the intended population.

If you cannot locate any acceptable instruments, the solution is to develop your own instrument. But remember that quality test construction requires special knowledge and a considerable time investment. Perhaps at this point you should try to locate an expert who can assist you in the development of an assessment instrument. Don't be too shy to ask for help in the design of your instrument or in conducting a validation study. Anyone who understands assessment will appreciate your situation and is likely to come to your aid.

Administration of Assessments

Now that you've selected an instrument, how can you administer it to get the most out of it? Administering an assessment instrument can be deceptively easy. On the surface it appears that all one has to do is follow the directions. But unfortunately, strict adherence to written directions is only half the battle. This is because each testing situation has numerous variables, not all of which can be anticipated or adequately addressed in the printed directions. Similarly, there is no one set of administrative guidelines that can be applied to all assessment instruments and all testing situations. Nonetheless, the following are general suggestions for effective and efficient collection of assessment data. The guidelines are organized by three time periods, the preparation period, the data collection period, and the posttest period.

Preparing for Administration

Before one can administer an assessment instrument, a number of tasks must be performed. This is true whether one is administering a physical performance test, a function and status test, or a paper-and-pencil test, rating scale, checklist, or inventory.

Become Very Familiar With the Assessment Instrument.   The test administrator is like a referee. It is essential that the test administrator be in command of the testing situation and know every single rule for administration. Valuable time can be wasted if the test administrator has to put everything on hold while he or she refers to printed directions to clarify a question. On the other hand, if a question comes up and time is not taken to clarify the question, data may be erroneously collected and/or recorded. The test administrator must be a walking rule book. There are often many details to know and remember. How many trials are to be given? In what order are test items to be taken? Are practice trials allowed? Is warm-up recommended or allowed? Are scores measured to the nearest inch, half-inch, or centimeter? How is a ball that lands on a target line scored? Is the final score the average of the trials or the best of all trials? Under what conditions should the testing be terminated?

How can you become a good referee of administrative protocols? In the process of instrument selection you undoubtedly read the test directions or watched a video that described and demonstrated assessment methods (32). You probably also spent some time visualizing yourself actually administering the assessment instrument to the population that you serve. These processes are important first steps toward developing administrative proficiency, but they are seldom sufficient. There is no substitute for physical practice to learn all of the ins and outs of an assessment tool. The practitioner learning to administer an instrument should either (*a*) practice administering the instrument to sample subjects and/or (*b*) self-administer the instrument. It may also be helpful to arrange to assist someone who is already proficient in use of a particular assessment instrument. This is especially good when learning to administer one of the more complex ESS instruments, such as a graded exercise test, skinfold measurements, a 24-hour dietary recall, or selected orthopaedic injury tests.

Plan the Physical Layout for the Testing Site.   The test administrator must be an efficiency expert. Wasted time in a class or program is lost forever. So before data collection begins, every aspect of the testing situation must be examined and planned with efficiency in mind. This begins with plans for the physical layout.

Make detailed plans, complete with a diagram. Keep in mind the logical order of data collection and the flow of traffic. Also keep safety in mind as you plan the layout, especially if the testing involves flying objects or quickly moving persons. Whenever possible, make use of existing lines or structures to facilitate the testing and scoring. For example, the end line for the basketball court can be used for a starting line. A field, gym floor, or laboratory can be laid out and marked for rapid scoring in events such as throws, jumps, and kicks for distance. Modify distances and markings only when you are sure that the changes will not invalidate the scores or the intended use of the scores (Fig. 3-9).

Make Plans for Organizing Examinees for Testing.   Even if one-on-one testing is to be done, decisions must be made about time, place, order of examinees, order of test items, and so on. When testing large groups of examinees, however, the decisions are more complicated.

There are three main ways to organize groups for testing. The most efficient use of time is made when examinees are tested *en masse*. **Mass testing** is possible,

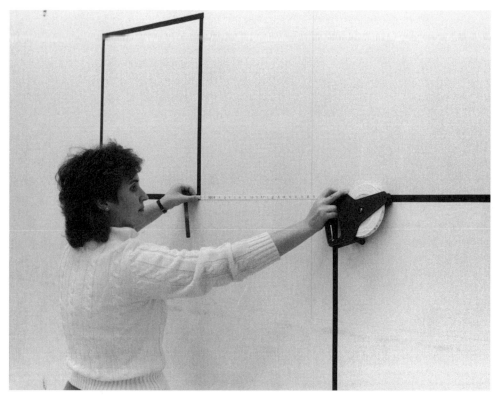

FIGURE 3-9

Targets must be measured accurately and marked clearly. (Photo by Dr. Karen Uhlendorf, University of Vermont, Burlington, VT.)

however, only when equipment and administrative personnel are sufficient to meet the test's demands. For example, distance run tests can often be administered simultaneously to a large group of examinees. A variation of this method pairs examinees; while one partner is tested, the other partner serves as scorer and recorder (Fig. 3-10). Another organizational scheme is to divide the large group into smaller groups, or squads. *Squad testing* works well when several stations are to be used for data collection for a battery of tests. The entire squad moves as a unit to the next station. This method of organization should *not* be used, however, if the order of tests in the battery would handicap certain squads. When groups are large and the order of events is not important or when some stations require more time than others, the best method of organization and rotation is on a station-to-station basis. In *station-to-station testing* examinees rotate from one station to another as individuals. For some situations a combination of these three basic methods can be used. No single plan of organization fits all situations, so the test administrator must apply a large dose of common sense.

> Mass testing is the practice of simultaneously administering an assessment instrument to a group of examinees.

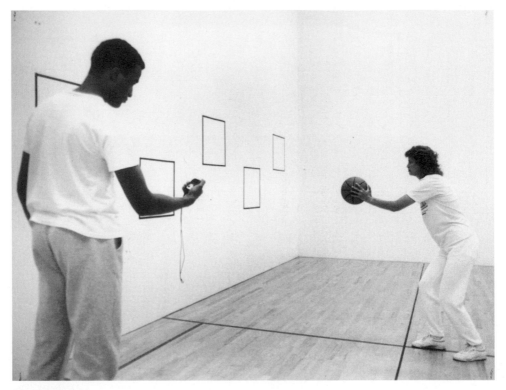

FIGURE 3-10

Partners take turns timing and scoring each other on a basketball passing test. (Photo by Dr. Karen Uhlendorf, University of Vermont, Burlington, VT.)

Plan for Assistants.   Related to decisions about how to organize examinees for data collection are plans for assistants. How many assistants are needed to administer the assessment efficiently and effectively? What skills or knowledge do they need? When testing groups, the examinees themselves sometimes can be asked to retrieve balls, score, record performances, and so on. If assistants must be trained, their training must also be planned. When will it be done? What exactly will they be taught to do?

Plan for Scoring and Record Keeping.   Some assessment instruments come with suggested score sheets, but in most circumstances test administrators must design their own. What information should be recorded? Where will it be recorded? Besides the assessment data, what additional information will be needed to evaluate the assessment data? It is a real headache to have to track down examinees to get a piece of information, such as their age, that could easily have been recorded at the time of testing. Whenever possible, all information about an examinee should be recorded together in such a way as to facilitate data analysis and evaluation. Space should be left on the score sheet for calculations related to statistical analyses. When mass testing is done, it often makes sense to use a class list or enrollment form to collect scores. In other cases, individual score sheets or scorecards are

Data Sheet

7

FUNCTIONAL FITNESS ASSESSMENT FOR ADULTS OVER 60 YEARS
INDIVIDUAL DATA COLLECTION FORM

Name _____ Testing Date _____

Sex: F M Age: ____yrs. Location: _____ D/M/Y

Test Administrator: _____

Administer the 5 item test battery in the suggested sequence. (Endurance Walk and Agility/Dynamic Balance tests should not be given consecutively.)

Test Item	Test Trials/Score		
	Trial 1	Trial 2	Final Recorded Score
1. Ponderal Index (to nearest .1 of Unit)			
Weight [ ] [ ] [ ] [ ] lb.			
Height [ ] [ ] [ ] in.			
Ponderal Index [ ] [ ] [ ] Units			
2. Flexibility (score to .5 inch) Practice given, not recorded.	[ ] [ ] [ ]	[ ] [ ] [ ]	[ ] [ ] [ ]
3. Agility/Dynamic Balance - Score seconds & tenths of seconds.	[ ] [ ] [ ]	[ ] [ ] [ ]	[ ] [ ] [ ]
4. Coordination - Score seconds & tenths of seconds. Practice given, not recorded	[ ] [ ] [ ]	[ ] [ ] [ ] [ ] [ ] [ ]	[ ] [ ]
5. Strength - Score # of repetitions in 30 sec. 4# Women. 8# Men (single lift practice)			[ ] [ ]
6. Endurance Walk - Time in minutes and seconds		[ ] [ ] [ ] [ ]	

Note: Convert to seconds and tenths of seconds to use profile and norms.

FIGURE 3-11

Sample individual scoresheet. (Reprinted with permission from Osness, W.H., et al.: Functional Fitness Assessment for Adults Over 60 Years: A Field Based Assessment. 2nd ed. Reston, VA, AAHPERD, 1996, p. 37.)

best. If using squad organization, scores for all squad members can be recorded on the same score sheet. Figure 3-11 is an example of an individual score sheet.

Plan to Use Computers to Facilitate Data Collection and Record Keeping.   A discussion of efficiency and effectiveness is incomplete without mention of computers. There are no ifs, ands, or buts about it. The modern ESS professional *must* be computer literate. Computers are important tools of our trade. They are used in many of our professional tasks—and in most cases help us to do those tasks faster, easier, and even better.

In your role as a test consumer, computers will facilitate several key functions. This chapter mentions how computers can be used to locate information about assessment instruments. Future chapters explain how computers are used in data analysis, in evaluation and grading, and in reporting assessment results. For now, just recognize that computers can be part of your administrative plans for efficient and effective data collection and record keeping.

In North Carolina, applicants for a driver's license now take a rules-of-the-road test at a computer terminal instead of a desk. State officials replaced the traditional paper-and-pencil test with a computerized test because they recognized that there are several distinct advantages to computerized testing. ESS professionals can make good use of computers both for knowledge testing and for collecting self-report data from examinees about health and exercise habits, attitudes, values, and so on.

Advantages to computerized assessments include the following: (*a*) Cheating is minimized because multiple parallel versions of the test are created simply by programming the computer to shuffle test items and present them in a random fashion. (*b*) Test results are virtually immediate because a computer can evaluate responses as quickly as they are made. (*c*) Human scoring errors are eliminated. (*d*) Test items can be changed and updated easily by loading a new program into the computer. (*e*) Individual examinees' responses can be analyzed so appropriate instruction can follow to remediate the problems. For some types of content, there are advantages inherent in the graphic and sound capabilities of computers. Illustrations are more realistic when they are presented with movement, color, and sound. Objects can also be made to appear three-dimensional and can be rotated on the monitor screen to show different perspectives.

Computerized assessment is also perceived by many examinees as being user friendly, meaning that they are easy to use. Computerized assessment allows great flexibility in scheduling because computer terminals can be set up for use throughout the day in locations that are convenient for examinees. Anonymity and confidentiality are possible when using computers to collect data that are sensitive or potentially embarrassing. Anonymous data collection can be important when evaluating programs and behaviors or attitudes of a group, because program participants or group members can respond to questions with complete honesty. Even when it is necessary to associate responses with particular examinees, computers can create a feeling of confidentiality. Examinees can enter their social security number instead of their name, then tell a computer things that they might hesitate to share in writing or when face to face with an interviewer.

Computers can also be interfaced with other pieces of measurement equipment to facilitate assessment of muscular strength, body composition, oxygen consumption, postural balance, and movement mechanics. Although today we are most likely to see computerized interfaces in a research laboratory or a medical clinic, we will undoubtedly see increased practitioner use as equipment prices drop. Already it is not unusual to see bioelectrical impedance analysis (BIA) for assessing body composition in health clubs. BIA uses a computer to predict an examinee's body fat percentage by analyzing resistance to a low-level electrical current that is passed between electrodes anchored to the examinee's wrist and ankle.

As an aid to record keeping, computers really shine. This is the sort of function they do far better than humans. Most database systems allow great flexibility in entry of data. They also make it possible to sort and order entries by any variable that is part of the database. For example, a corporate wellness director might create a database that includes fitness test scores, medical histories, exercise records, and demographic information. The computer can then sort the records by gender, age, regularity of exercise, cardiovascular risk, or any other fitness parameter. And this can be done in a matter of seconds to minutes, depending on the power of the computer and the number of records in the database.

Collect and Inspect All Equipment. Write out a list of *everything* that will be needed for the assessment, making sure that numbers of items are sufficient for the number of examinees and for the number of testing stations to be used. How many skinfold calipers are needed? How many tape measures? How many marking pens? How many privacy screens? How many score sheets, pencils, clipboards? How many computer terminals?

After making the equipment list, physically collect the items and check that every piece of equipment is in proper working order. Replace old batteries with fresh ones. Sharpen pencils. Calibrate equipment so measurements will be accurate.

Make Plans for Makeups. Count on the fact that some examinees will not be able to attend the scheduled testing period. If you already have a makeup session planned, you can inform examinees of the new date when they call to tell you that they will be absent. This saves time in the long run.

Plan and Rehearse Your Explanation and Demonstration. Don't leave your explanation to chance. It is strongly recommended that you plan what you will say and/or do to explain the purposes for testing and the assessment protocol. Write out what you plan to say to the examinees as if it were a script. Plan and practice the physical demonstration that will accompany verbal directions for performance tests. The demonstration should be practiced under actual test conditions. Be clear and concise about the response that is desired. Give tips for good performance. Also explain what you want examinees to do while they are waiting to be tested. *But keep all of this explaining and demonstrating as brief as possible.*

Data Collection Period

If you have planned well, the actual data collection period should go well. Follow the plans you have developed for effective and efficient administration. If an unexpected occurrence occurs, don't panic. Use common sense and make the appropriate in-flight adjustments. Also consider the following suggestions for the data collection period.

Brief Examinees on the Reasons for the Assessment. Explain why you are administering the assessment instrument and how the results will be used. Allow ample opportunities for questions. Clarify how the assessment will benefit the examinees, and inform examinees of their rights. In a research study, examinees must sign an informed consent form. In other settings, you may also choose to ask for signed consent. Be especially careful when administering assessments to children; parental consent is definitely needed.

Behave in Ways Consistent With the Intended Use of the Results.   Examples will explain what is meant by this statement. If a sport skill test is being used for skill practice, be a teacher and do all the things that a good teacher does. Give encouragement, correct performances, and modify the test for the high- and low-performance students. On the other hand, if a test is being given as part of a research study or for assigning grades, you must be precise about timing, scoring, distance markings, and so on. Treat all examinees alike. In a research or grading situation it is inappropriate to offer encouragement selectively to some examinees but not to others.

Spot-Check for Accuracy in Administration and Scoring.   During the data collection period, spot-check the work of all assistants. Check for accuracy in methods and scoring at all stations. Also watch for dangerous situations. Position yourself in such a way that you can visually survey the test site with a quick glance.

Post–Data Collection Period

Several tasks also have to be accomplished after data collection. In most cases the sooner these tasks are done, the better.

Dismantle the Test Area.   Put equipment away, store supplies, and return desks and tables to their original locations. And by all means, don't forget to peel tape off floors, rugs, and walls. When possible, get assistance from the last group of examinees.

Check Recorded Scores.   As soon after completing the data collection as possible, check all data for readability and completeness. Also spot-check for accuracy. You can sometimes catch errors in recording while performances are still fresh in your mind or that of the examinee.

Tabulate Results and Perform Statistical Analyses.   Using appropriate nonstatistical and/or statistical procedures, summarize quantitative assessment data. Qualitative data are usually summarized by performing a content analysis. In either case, do the analyses as soon as possible.

Report Results to Examinees.   Results in written and/or oral form should be reported to examinees and other concerned parties, such as parents and administrators. In addition to assessment results, discuss recommendations and decisions that can be made on the basis of this information. *Remember that assessment is not conducted for its own sake; it is conducted for the purpose of making decisions that will serve clients and/or improve professional practice.*

File All Pertinent Information.   Create a paper or computer filing system for all assessment data. Clearly label records with dates, locations, and so on. Also retain copies of assessment procedures used in data collection. This is especially important if assessment instruments were modified. Even a couple of months after testing, you are unlikely to remember all the details of how the data were collected.

Chapter Summary

A wide variety of reference sources can be used to locate assessment instruments. The selection of a quality assessment instrument is based on both administrative feasibility and the psychometric qualities of the instrument. The most important psychometric quality is validity, that is, the degree to which an instrument assesses what it is claimed to assess. Reliability, the consistency of assessment, is also important. Objectivity is the psychometric concern that has to do with scoring consistency. A good assessment instrument is valid, reliable, objective, and free of assessment bias. Freedom from assessment bias means that the instrument is free of unfair or artificial scoring discrimination against members of a particular gender, ethnic background, or other distinguishing feature. There are many different types of evidence that can demonstrate each of these psychometric characteristics for norm-referenced and for criterion-referenced assessment instruments.

Once a good instrument is selected, it must be administered well, or the resulting data will not be of good quality. A test administrator should carefully plan for the administrative process, then carry out the plan. In-flight adjustments are made when needed.

SELF-TEST QUESTIONS

1. An assessment tool that seems illogical in its design is probably lacking in
   A. Concurrent validity
   B. Construct validity
   C. Content validity
   D. Predictive validity

2. When a test is considered to be a good substitute for a criterion test, the test has a high degree of
   A. Concurrent validity
   B. Construct validity
   C. Content validity
   D. Predictive validity

3. A gymnastics coach develops a new test of abdominal muscular endurance that he thinks is better than a traditional curl-up test. He administers his new test to a group of college gymnasts, then administers a curl-up test to the same gymnasts a few days later. He correlates the scores. What psychometric quality is he trying to demonstrate?
   A. Concurrent validity
   B. Construct validity
   C. Predictive validity
   D. Test-retest reliability

4. When a test is administered on 2 days and the test scores are correlated, the reliability coefficient is called
   A. An equivalent (parallel) forms coefficient
   B. A proportion of agreement coefficient
   C. A split half coefficient
   D. A test-retest coefficient

5. The Spearman-Brown prophecy formula is used in conjunction with which method of calculating reliability coefficients?
   A. Parallel forms
   B. Proportion of agreement
   C. Split half
   D. Test-retest

6. If a split half reliability coefficient is .80, what is the reliability coefficient for the full-length test? _____

7. What is the 68% confidence interval for an examinee who scores 70 on a test with a standard error of measurement of 5? _____

8. Which of the following reflects *interscorer* objectivity?
   A. One judge scores 20 skaters on each of two different days; she compares her scores for each of the skaters on the two different days.
   B. Two judges each score 20 skaters on one day; the judges compare their scores for each of the 20 skaters.
   C. Two judges each score 20 skaters on each of two different days; each judge compares his or her own scores for the two days for each of the 20 skaters.
   D. One judge scores 20 skaters from a videotape on each of two different days; he or she compares his or her scores for each of the 20 skaters.

9. Which of the following assessment instruments has acceptable levels of both concurrent validity and test-retest reliability?
   A. Test A: concurrent validity .56; test-retest reliability .86
   B. Test B: concurrent validity .60; test-retest reliability .92
   C. Test C: concurrent validity .66; test-retest reliability .99
   D. Test D: concurrent validity .72; test-retest reliability .82

10. The validity of a criterion-referenced test is best defined as
    A. The accuracy of classifications
    B. The consistency of classifications
    C. The mastery of classifications
    D. The objectivity of classifications

Consider the following contingency tables:

TABLE A

| | | DAY 2 | |
		MASTERS	NONMASTERS
DAY 1	MASTERS	50	20
	NONMASTERS	10	20

TABLE B

| | | DAY 2 | |
		MASTERS	NONMASTERS
DAY 1	**MASTERS**	50	10
	NONMASTERS	10	30

11. Which contingency table reflects a more reliable test?
    A. Table A
    B. Table B
    C. Both are equally valid.
    D. More information is needed.

12. Which method of organizing examinees is usually most time efficient?
    A. Partner testing
    B. Mass testing
    C. Squad testing
    D. Station-to-station testing

ANSWERS

1. C	2. A	3. A	4. D	5. C	6. .89
7. 65–75	8. B	9. D	10. A	11. B	12. B

DOING PROJECTS FOR FURTHER LEARNING

1. In the reference section of your college or university library, locate a recent volume of Buros' *Mental Measurements Yearbook* or *Tests in Print*. Use the Index at the back of the book to locate a published test in an area of your personal or professional interests (e.g., nutrition, leadership, stress, eating disorders, motor development). Read about the test.

2. In the reference section of your college or university library, locate the *Physical Education Index*, then
    A. Scan the list of periodicals in the index service. (This list is found near the front of each year's index.) Write the names of a couple of periodicals that relate to your personal or professional interests.
    B. Select at least two subject heading terms that are of interest to you (e.g., eating disorder, coaching, psychology, aerobics, injury), then search the listings under those terms for the last 5 years or so, looking for articles that describe or discuss an assessment instrument.

C. Using the listings found in B, locate one or more articles in the holdings of your library. If the periodical is not available at your library, use the interlibrary loan system to obtain the article or articles.

D. Read what is said in the article about validity and reliability. What evidence is given to convince you that the assessment instrument is sound and dependable?

3. Find an ESS professional who is willing to let you observe or help with testing. Pay special attention to the administration of the assessment instrument or instruments. Is the administration efficient and effective? How are data collected and recorded? Are computers used? What suggestions do you have for improving the testing?

REFERENCES

1. Baumgartner, T.A., and Jackson, A.S.: Measurement for Evaluation in Physical Education and Exercise Science. 6th ed. Brown & Benchmark, Madison, WI, 2000.
2. Dunham, P.: Evaluation for Physical Education. Englewood, CA, Morton, 1994.
3. Hastad, D.N., and Lacy, A.C.: Measurement and Evaluation in Physical Education and Exercise Science. 3rd ed. Needham Heights, MA, Allyn & Bacon, 1998.
4. Miller, D.K.: Measurement by the Physical Educator: Why and How. 3rd Ed. Madison, WI, Brown & Benchmark, 1997.
5. Morrow, J.R., Jackson, A.W., Disch, J.G., and Mood, D.P.: Measurement and Evaluation in Human Performance. Champaign, IL, Human Kinetics, 1995.
6. Safrit, M.J., and Wood, T.M.: Introduction to Measurement in Physical Education and Exercise Science. 3rd ed. St. Louis, Mosby–Year Book, 1995.
7. Martens, R., Vealey, R.S., and Burton, D.: Competitive Anxiety in Sport. 2nd ed. Champaign, IL, Human Kinetics, 1990.
8. Borg, G.: Borg's Perceived Exertion and Pain Scales. Champaign, IL, Human Kinetics, 1998.
9. Hopkins, D.R., Shick, J., and Plack, J.J.: Basketball for Boys and Girls: Skills Test Manual. Reston, VA, American Alliance of Health, Physical Education, Recreation, and Dance, 1984.
10. Hensley, L. (ed.): Tennis for Boys and Girls: Skills Test Manual. Reston, VA, American Alliance of Health, Physical Education, Recreation, and Dance, 1989.
11. Rikli, R.E. (ed.): Softball for Boys and Girls: Skills Test Manual. Reston, VA, American Alliance of Health, Physical Education, Recreation, and Dance, 1991.
12. Heyward, V.H.: Advanced Fitness Assessment & Exercise Prescription. 3rd ed. Champaign, IL, Human Kinetics, 1997.
13. Strand, B.N., and Wilson, R.: Assessing Sport Skills. Champaign, IL, Human Kinetics, 1993.
14. Montoye, H.J., Kemper, H.C.G., Saris, W.H.M., and Washburn, R.A.: Measuring Physical Activity and Energy Expenditure. Champaign, IL, Human Kinetics, 1996.
15. Docherty, D.: Measurement in Pediatric Exercise Science. Champaign, IL, Human Kinetics, 1996.
16. Impara, J.C., and Plake, B.S. (eds.): The Thirteenth Mental Measurements Yearbook. Lincoln, NE, The Buros Institute of Mental Measurements, 1998.
17. Kirby, R.F.(ed.): Kirby's Guide to Fitness and Motor Performance Tests. Cape Girardeau, MO, BenOak, 1991.
18. Brodie, D.A.: A Reference Manual for Human Performance Measurement in the Field of Physical Education and Sports Sciences. Lewiston, NY, Edwin Mellen Press, 1995.
19. Ostrow, A.C. (ed.): Directory of Psychological Tests in the Sport and Exercise Sciences. 2nd ed. Morgantown, WV, Fitness Information Technology, 1996.
20. Levine, J.R.: The Internet for Dummies. Indianapolis, IDG Books Worldwide, 1999.

21. Levine, J.R.: Internet E-Mail for Dummies. Indianapolis, IDG Books Worldwide, 1998.

22. American Educational Research Association, American Psychological Association, and National Council on Measurement in Education: Standards for Educational and Psychological Testing. Washington, American Psychological Association, 1985, pp. 9–11.

23. Chapman, N.L.: Chapman ball control test—field hockey. Research Quarterly for Exercise and Sport, 53:239, 1982.

24. Morrow, J.R., Falls, H.B., and Kohl, H.W. (eds.): The Prudential *FITNESSGRAM* Technical Reference Manual. Dallas, Cooper Institute for Aerobics Research, 1994.

25. Rowlands, D.J.: A Golf Skills Test Battery. Doctoral dissertation, University of Utah, 1974.

26. Schutz, R.W., et al.: Inventories and norms for children's attitudes toward physical activity. Research Quarterly for Exercise and Sport, 56:256, 1985.

27. Krippendorff, K.: Content Analysis: An Introduction to Its Methodology. Thousand Oaks, CA, Sage, 1980.

28. Shifflett, B., and Schuman, B.J.: A criterion-referenced test for archery. Research Quarterly for Exercise and Sport, 53:330, 1982.

29. Hopkins, D.R., Shick, J., and Plack, J.J.: Basketball Skills Test Manual for Boys and Girls. Reston, VA, American Alliance of Health, Physical Education, Recreation, and Dance, 1984.

30. Thorndike, R.L.: Applied Psychometrics. New York, Houghton Mifflin, 1982.

31. Rosser, P.: The SAT Gender Gap: Identifying the Causes. Washington, Center for Women Policy Studies, April 1989.

32. Lohman, T.: How to Do Skinfolds (video). Champaign, IL, Human Kinetics, 1995.

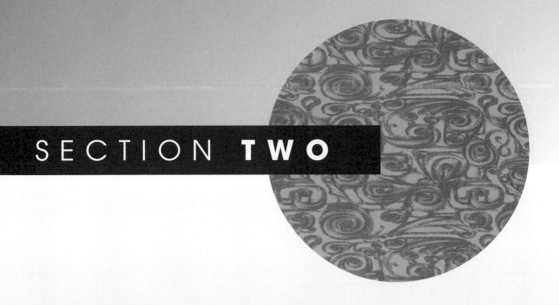

SECTION **TWO**

Data Analysis and Evaluation

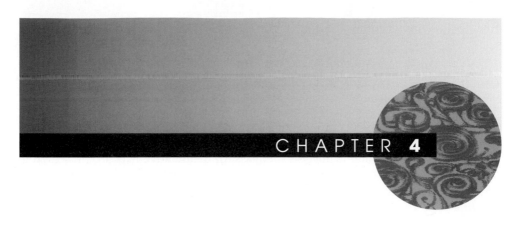

CHAPTER **4**

Nonstatistical Data Analysis

After assessment data are collected, they must be analyzed to reveal their meaning. Analyses vary according to the nature of the assessment data, so the first step in data analysis is to examine the collected data to determine their characteristics. The second step is to apply one or more nonstatistical data analysis techniques. These topics are addressed in this chapter.

As you read this chapter, watch for the following keywords:

Content analysis	Frequency table	Microcomputer
Continuous data	Grouped frequency	Power (of a computer)
Discrete data	distribution	Quantitative data
Frequency distribution	Histogram	Qualitative data
Frequency polygon	Mainframe computer	

Characteristics of Assessment Data

Because of the wide variety of available assessment instruments, assessment data themselves vary greatly. Discussed next are several of the ways in which data vary. Before analyzing data, you should determine which of the following characteristics apply to your data.

Are Data Qualitative or Quantitative?

The usual result of measurement is **quantitative data,** that is, data in the form of numbers. **Qualitative data** take the form of words or illustrations that describe data according to kind or quality. Qualitative data typically result from administration of open-ended questionnaires, anecdotal records, video records, and some rating scales.

> Quantitative data are numerical information. They describe an attribute according to amount or number.

> Qualitative data are words or illustrations used to describe an attribute according to kind or quality.

Both quantitative and qualitative data must be analyzed to discern meanings and patterns in the data, however the methods of analysis for these two types of data differ. Quantitative data are analyzed by a combination of nonstatistical and statistical methods; the more common analysis methods for quantitative data are presented in this and the next two chapters. Qualitative data are analyzed by a process called **content analysis.** An excellent reference for learning to conduct a content analysis is *Content Analysis* by Krippendorff (1).

> Content analysis is a research technique for making replicable and valid inferences from qualitative data.

What Are the Units of Measurement?

When working with quantitative data, it is extremely important to pay attention to the measurement units of the scores used to represent the attribute. For example, do data represent the time to walk a mile measured in minutes and seconds, the distance of a standing long jump in feet and inches, pulse rate after 1 minute of recovery from a step test protocol, or perhaps a judge's rating of a dive from the 3-meter platform? It is also important to know the range of possible score values, especially noting the highest and lowest possible scores. Similarly, for performance data it is

What Do YOU Think?

For the past several decades the U.S. Commerce Department has struggled with Americans to persuade them to accept the metric system. The main selling point is that the base 10 system is easier than the English system. To no avail; Americans have resisted metrication. We just don't seem to like metric speed limit signs, and we won't buy Celsius thermometers.

Gene Zirkel, past president of the Dozenal Society of America and a math professor at Nassau Community College in Washington, D.C., offered an explanation for the failure of metrication in the United States (2). According to Zirkel, it has failed because the metric system is a second-best system, because human beings count by tens only because of the "unfortunate biological accident" of having 10 fingers. When humans measure things, they tend to use units of 12. As evidence, Zirkel pointed out that there are 12 inches to a foot, 12 items per dozen, 12 dozen per gross, 12×2 hours per day, 12×5 minutes per hour, 12×5 seconds per minute, 12×30 degrees in a circle, and 12 tones in a musical scale. A colleague of Zirkel challenges the metric fan to try to divide 10 eggs into thirds and quarters; of the common fractions, only halves work. It gets pretty messy! But dividing 12 eggs, one gets whole numbers for all of the common fractions. Hmm. Is the Dozenal (dozen-all?) Society of America on to something? What do YOU think?

important to clarify whether a high score or a low score represents better performance. A score of 72 is a better golf score than a score of 82, but 82 is a better archery score than a 72.

Before data can be analyzed, some quantitative data have to be converted to other units of measurement to facilitate mathematical manipulation of values. For example, a set of scores for the standing long jump recorded in feet and inches may have to be converted to inches or centimeters for subsequent analyses. Knowledge of measurement conversions is therefore a necessity. Table 4-1 provides some of the common measurement conversions used by the ESS professional. You should become facile in calculating conversions. Some hand calculators, such as Texas Instruments 36X, have built-in metric-to-English and English-to-metric conversions.

Are Data Continuous or Discrete?

Quantitative data can reflect measurement of either a continuous or a discrete variable. **Continuous data** have a potentially infinite number of possible score values because the precision of measurement is limited only by the precision of the measurement instrument. Between any two recorded score values are countless other values that could be expressed as fractions of these numbers. For example, using a hand-held stopwatch, one would probably measure a downhill ski run to the nearest tenth of a second; with an electronic timer the same score would be recorded in thousandths of a second. **Discrete data** are limited to specific score values that are seldom expressed as a fraction. Golf scores, numbers of successful free throws, and heartbeats per minute are all examples of variables that yield discrete data.

> Continuous data can take on any value within a range.

> Discrete data take on only distinct values, usually representing whole events.

When summarizing continuous data, it is appropriate and logical to use fractions or decimals to report average values. Using fractions or decimals to summarize discrete data is often artificial and sometimes even nonsensical, especially when the numbers are carried out to several decimal places to imply a level of precision that doesn't exist. (The average number of students in the classes I teach is 18.6237!)

What Is the Scale of Measurement?

Numbers are not all created equal. Some are more "sophisticated" than others; they can be used to represent exact values. Other less sophisticated numbers merely classify or identify persons or objects. Numbers are categorized according to their *scale of measurement*. There are four measurement scales, *ratio*, *interval*, *ordinal*, and *nominal*. Each scale has its own characteristics, as shown in Table 4-2. *It is important for the test consumer to know the scale of measurement of the data, because certain statistical operations are valid only for data measured on certain scales.* (Read that sentence again. It communicates a very important concept.)

Ratio. The ratio scale is the most sophisticated of the measurement scales. Data measured on a ratio scale have the following characteristics: (*a*) a constant in-

TABLE 4-1	Common Measurement Conversions

UNITED STATES CUSTOMARY SYSTEM	METRIC SYSTEM AND SCIENTIFIC UNITS
Units of Weight	
1 lb = 16 oz	0.4536 kg
2.2046 lb	1 kg = 1000 g
1 oz	28.3495 g
35.274 oz	1 kg
Units of Length	
1 mi = 1760 yd	1.6093 km
0.6214 mi	1 km = 1000 m
1 yd = 3 ft = 36 in	0.9144 m
1.09 yd = 39.37 in	1 m = 100 cm
1 ft	0.3048 m
1 in	2.54 cm
0.3937 in	1 cm = 10 mm
Units of Volume	
1 gal = 4 qt	3.785 L
1 qt = 32 fl oz	0.9461 L
1.0567 qt	1 L = 1000 mL = 1000 cc
1 fl oz	29.573 mL
Temperature Scales	
32°F	0°C
212°F	100°C
°F	(°C × 1.8) + 32
(°F − 32) ÷ 1.8	°C
Units of Force	
1 lb	4.448 N
0.2248 lb	1 N
Units of Work or Energy	
1 ft-lb	0.13825 kgm
7.23 ft-lb	1 kgm
1 ft-lb	1.35582 J
1 C	4186 J
0.2389 C	1 J

lb, pound; oz, ounce; kg, kilogram; g, gram; yd, yard; km, kilometer; in, inch; m, meter; cm, centimeter; ft, foot; mm, millimeter; gal, gallon; qt, quart; L, liter; fl oz, fluid ounce; mL, milliliter; cc, cubic centimeter; F, Fahrenheit; C, Celsius (centigrade); N, newton; ft-lb, foot-pound; kgm, kilogram-meter; C, Calorie (kilocalorie); J, joule. All abbreviations of measurement have the same singular as plural form.

TABLE 4-2	Characteristics of the Scales of Measurement			
CHARACTERISTIC	RATIO SCALE	INTERVAL SCALE	ORDINAL SCALE	NOMINAL SCALE
Has a true and meaningful zero	√			
Has constant score intervals	√	√		
Can be ordered logically by size	√	√	√	
Can be used to classify or identify	√	√	√	√

terval of measurement between each possible score value and (*b*) a *true zero* point at which 0 means no amount of the attribute being measured. Also, ratio score values can be logically ordered in terms of amount of the attribute. Because of these characteristics, ratio scale data permit comparisons of score values. For example, one may correctly conclude that a grip strength score of 80 lb represents twice as much strength as a grip strength score of 40 lb. One may also conclude that an increase from 80 to 90 lb is the same amount of increased muscular strength as an increase from 40 to 50 lb.

Distances, times, weights, and points scored are examples of ratio scale data commonly collected in exercise and sport settings. Many measures of physiological functions, such as heart rate, blood pressure, blood cholesterol, and force of muscular contraction, are also ratio data.

Interval. Like ratio data, data measured on an interval scale have a constant interval of measurement between score values, and the score values can be logically ordered. Interval data do not, however, have a true zero point. If a 0 is recorded for an interval scale score, it does not mean that absolutely no amount of the attribute exists. The Fahrenheit scale for temperature is an interval scale. The degree units have a constant interval at all points along the scale and temperatures can be logically ordered in terms of amount of heat. However, 0°F is not a true zero because some heat exists at 0°F. The Kelvin scale for temperature is a ratio scale; absolute zero (no thermal energy) occurs at 0°K.

In ESS, many affective inventories and psychological scales use interval scales of measurement. A person who scores a 0 on a sportsmanship inventory generally is not completely devoid of sportsmanship. Because zero cannot be used as a meaningful reference point, it is incorrect to conclude that someone who receives 80 points on a sportsmanship inventory has double the amount of sportsmanship as someone who scores 40. Similarly, 80°F is not twice as warm as 40°F.

Ordinal. Score values for data measured on an ordinal scale can be logically ordered, but the scores do not have a constant interval between possible score values. Nor do they have a true zero. Ordinal scores allow judgments that one examinee has performed better or worse than another or that a score is greater or less than another. Finishes in a cross-country race, team standings in a league, and rank order preferences for favorite types of physical activity (e.g., cross-country skiing, 1; running, 2; race walking, 3) are all measured on ordinal scales. A ranking of 1 is (usually) better, stronger, more than a ranking of 2, but it is unclear how much better, stronger, or more. Because the intervals between the ranked values are not constant, ordinal data should never be summed and arithmetically averaged. (This is a common error committed even by some experienced researchers.)

Nominal. The nominal scale of measurement uses numbers to classify persons or objects into two or more categories; they can also be used for identification. The nominal scale is the least sophisticated of the scales of measurement. Nominal scale data cannot be ordered in terms of size, nor can the values be summed and arithmetically averaged. For example, a researcher who uses a 1 to code gender for female athletes and a 2 for male athletes would be incorrect to conclude that the average gender of subjects is 1.7. A nominal scale 1 merely represents a different category from a nominal scale 2. It is appropriate to report frequencies for each category.

Numbers used for identification, such as social security numbers, license plate numbers, and numbers on team jerseys are also nominal. They cannot be interpreted or ordered logically in any numerical sense. Figure 4-1 shows two football players. It is incorrect to conclude that the player wearing number 50 is 10 times as good as his teammate wearing number 5. We can't conclude anything meaningful about the two men on the basis of their numbers. We know only that player 50 is different from player 5.

SELF-TEST QUESTIONS: PART A

1. Data from administration of the McGill Pain Questionnaire (see Fig. 2-5) are
   A. Quantitative
   B. Qualitative

2. Data from body weight measurement are
   A. Quantitative
   B. Qualitative

3. What does a 150-lb athlete weigh in kilograms? _____ kg

4. Approximately how many miles does one run in a 5-km race?

   _____ miles

5. Which one of the following variables yield discrete data?
   A. A vertical jump
   B. Height
   C. RBI (runs batted in)
   D. Temperature

6. What measurement scale is used to measure blood pressure?
   A. Ratio
   B. Interval
   C. Ordinal
   D. Nominal

7. Intelligence (IQ score) is measured on what scale?
   A. Ratio
   B. Interval
   C. Ordinal
   D. Nominal

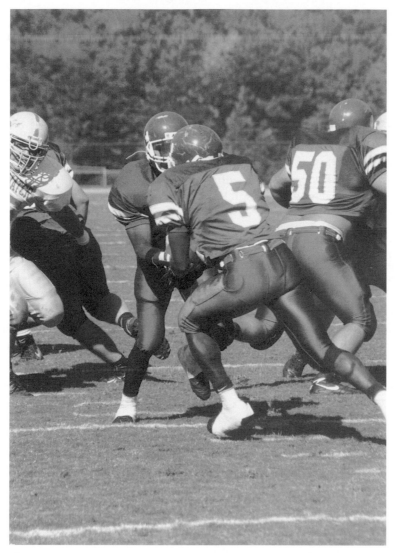

FIGURE 4-1

Uniform numbers: nominal scale numbers. (Photo by John Bell, Touch a Life Photography, Greensboro, NC.)

8. Score values for the Code for Physical Activity (see Fig. 1-1) are measured on what scale?
   A. Ratio
   B. Interval
   C. Ordinal
   D. Nominal

ANSWERS

1. B	2. A	3. 68 kg	4. 3.1 mi
5. C	6. A	7. B	8. C

Nonstatistical Data Analysis

The number of scores to be analyzed usually determines which of several nonstatistical and/or statistical techniques is used. In general, the larger the data set, the more helpful it is to precede statistical analyses with use of one or more of the techniques presented here.

Frequency Distributions

Developing a frequency distribution is a simple and straightforward method of quantitative data analysis. The **frequency distribution** is a tabular method of organizing scores to help you see patterns in the data. Frequency distributions can be developed for discrete and continuous data and for data that are at least ordinal. Frequency distributions cannot be developed in any meaningful way for nominal data.

> A frequency distribution is a tabulation of scores from high to low or low to high, showing the number of occurrences of each score value.

Listed in Table 4-3 are vertical jump scores for a group of junior high school girls attending a summer volleyball camp. The scores are rounded to the nearest inch of fingertip reach at the height of the jump. As they are listed, the scores are hard to interpret. The camp director is unable to tell the girls much about the average performance of the group or about the performance of individual girls.

Simple Frequency Distributions. Contrast the random lists of scores in Table 4-3 with the frequency distribution presented in Table 4-4. In Table 4-4, the *score* column lists all obtained score values in descending order, with the best score always listed first. The *f* column indicates the frequency of occurrence of each particular score value (consistent with the result of the hand tally). The column labeled *cum f* lists the cumulative frequency, starting at the bottom of the frequency table and accumulating frequencies up to the total number of scores at the highest obtained score value. The % and *cum* % columns give the same information as the *f* and *cum f* columns, but the information is expressed in terms of percentage of the total number of scores.

From this table it is easy to see that scores ranged from a high of 95 inches to a low of 83 inches, a difference of 12 inches. It is also easy to see that most scores fell

TABLE 4-3	Vertical Jump Scores in Inches for 50 Junior High School Girls								
88	86	88	90	90	91	87	89	91	89
87	87	85	85	88	91	95	89	87	87
86	87	85	89	91	86	88	87	83	90
90	86	86	88	89	89	86	94	88	92
92	90	89	90	89	91	90	88	89	88

	TABLE 4-4	Simple Frequency Table for Vertical Jump Scores in Inches for 50 Junior High School Girls				

SCORE	TALLY	f	cum f	%	cum %
95	/	1	50	2	100
94	/	1	49	2	98
92	//	2	48	4	96
91	/////	5	46	10	92
90	///// //	7	41	14	82
89	///// ////	9	34	18	68
88	///// ///	8	25	16	50
87	///// //	7	17	14	34
86	////// /	6	10	12	20
85	///	3	4	6	8
83	/	1	1	2	2

between 86 and 91 inches, with the single most common score being 89 inches. From the *cum %* column one can easily determine that half (50%) of the girls jumped a height of no more than 88 inches, the height of the standard volleyball net for girls and women. What decisions do you think the camp director can now make regarding net height for setting and spiking practices?

Grouped Frequency Distributions.   A variation of the simple frequency distribution is the **grouped frequency distribution**. This analysis serves the same purposes as the simple frequency distribution but differs in definition of the score values, that is, the *score* column values. Instead of identifying the frequencies for individual score values, frequencies are recorded for specified *score intervals*. This becomes necessary when there are many score values with low incidences of recurrence. For such a data set, the simple frequency table would be excessively cumbersome and difficult to interpret.

> A grouped frequency distribution is a tabulation of score intervals from high to low or low to high, showing the number of occurrences within each score interval.

A grouped frequency distribution is constructed by forming 10 to 20 score intervals that include all obtained score values. *Fifteen score intervals with an odd-numbered interval size is usually considered ideal.* A grouped frequency distribution can be constructed by following these steps:

Step 1.   The score intervals are determined by dividing the difference between the largest and smallest scores by 15 and rounding the result to the nearest whole number. This number defines the score interval that should probably be used.

Step 2.   The next step is to define the top interval to contain the best score. If the interval size is odd, the midpoint of this top interval should be a multiple of the

TABLE 4-5		Number of Bent-leg Curl-ups in 1 Minute by High School Boys							
47	60	72	37	26	48	74	51	52	39
30	76	60	57	57	49	50	44	38	64
67	55	50	58	81	66	57	61	69	29
16	64	47	5	36	61	51	53	38	55
56	34	44	52	50	48	59	45	46	41

interval size. If the interval size is even, the smallest score of this top interval should be a multiple of the interval size.

Step 3.   Tally scores that fall into each of the defined score intervals.

Step 4.   Complete columns *f*, *cum f*, %, and *cum %*.

Using these guidelines, try to construct a grouped frequency table for the scores in Table 4-5. After you finish, compare your grouped frequency table to the one in Table 4-6.

Do we agree on the grouped frequency table? Did you also decide to use an interval size of 5? Do you see that the top interval of 78 to 82 includes the best score of 81? Do you also see that the top interval is defined so that the midpoint of the interval (that is, 80) is a multiple of 5, the interval size? Good for you! If you used a dif-

TABLE 4-6	Grouped Frequency Table for Number of Bent-leg Curl-ups in 1 Minute by High School Boys				
SCORE INTERVAL	**TALLY**	**f**	**cum f**	**%**	**cum %**
78–82	/	1	50	2	100
73–77	//	2	49	4	98
68–72	//	2	47	4	94
63–67	////	4	45	8	90
58–62	///// /	6	41	12	82
53–57	///// //	7	35	14	70
48–52	///// ////	9	28	18	56
43–47	///// /	6	19	12	38
38–42	////	4	13	8	26
33–37	///	3	9	6	18
28–32	//	2	6	4	12
23–27	/	1	4	2	8
18–22	/	1	3	2	6
13–17	/	1	2	2	4
8–12		0	1	0	2
3–7	/	1	1	2	2

ferent interval size, it doesn't necessarily mean that your grouped frequency table is wrong. The interval size of 5 does, however, fit the guidelines and produce a highly interpretable frequency distribution.

Frequency Tables. Since nominal scale values cannot be ordered in any meaningful way, no frequency distribution can be developed. *Nominal data may, however, be summarized by a frequency table.* The **frequency table** is developed by tallying frequencies for each category, then listing the category names and respective frequencies and/or percentages in a logical order. For example, one might choose to list categories from high to low in order of their frequencies. Alternatively one might list categories in alphabetical order, chronological order, or some other scheme. Table 4-7 is an example of a frequency table from a survey question about social betting (3).

> A frequency table is a tabulation of nominal scale data, showing the number of occurrences within each category.

Frequency Polygons and Histograms

It has been said that a picture is worth a thousand words, so a graphic representation is sometimes used to communicate the scores of a group of examinees. Types of graphs include frequency polygons, histograms, pie graphs, ogive graphs, picture graphs, and so on. The most popular types of graphs for summarizing assessment data are the **frequency polygon** and the **histogram.**

Frequency Polygons. Frequency polygons are line graphs of a frequency distribution in which score values or score intervals are charted on the horizontal axis

TABLE 4-7	A Frequency Table	
SPORTS BET ON IN THE PAST 12 MONTHS		
Sport	Number of Bettors	Percent of Bettors[a]
Professional football	441	72
Baseball	331	51
College football	172	28
Thoroughbred horse racing	141	23
Professional boxing	98	16
Professional basketball	61	10
Harness horse racing	61	10
College basketball	49	8
Ice hockey	25	4

[a]Percent of 613 respondents who admitted betting in past 12 months. Percentages total greater than 100% because respondents could check more than one sport. Modified with permission from Sports Illustrated: Sports Poll '86. New York: Lieberman Research, 1986, p. 93.

and the associated frequencies are given on the vertical axis. Individual scores are plotted at the intersection of the appropriate points on the two axes. If score intervals greater than 1 are used to form the frequency polygon, the points used to plot the score should be midpoints of the intervals given on the horizontal axis.

> A frequency polygon is a line graph of a frequency distribution in which score values or score intervals are charted on the horizontal axis and the associated frequencies are given on the vertical axis.

Histograms.   Histograms are bar graphs of a frequency distribution that either chart scores or score intervals on the horizontal axis and frequencies on the vertical axis, or vice versa. The width of each bar usually represents the width of the score interval.

> A histogram is a bar graph of a frequency distribution that charts either scores or score intervals on one axis and frequencies on the other axis.

Figures 4-2 and 4-3 depict the curl-up scores given in Table 4-5. Figure 4-1 displays this information as a frequency polygon, and Figure 4-2 is a histogram. Both graphs use the test score intervals that were calculated for the construction of the grouped frequency table in Table 4-6. Also, the score intervals are ordered from low to high as one reads from left to right across the horizontal axis. Whether to use a frequency distribution, a frequency polygon, or a histogram to display assessment data is largely a matter of personal preference.

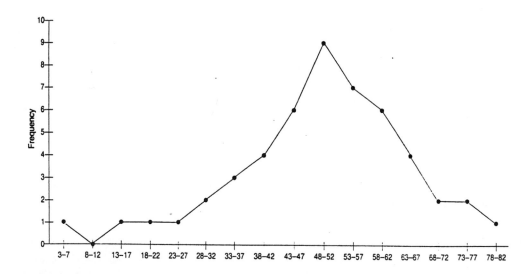

Test Score Intervals (number of curl-ups in 1 minute)

FIGURE 4-2

Frequency polygon of frequency distribution in Table 4-6.

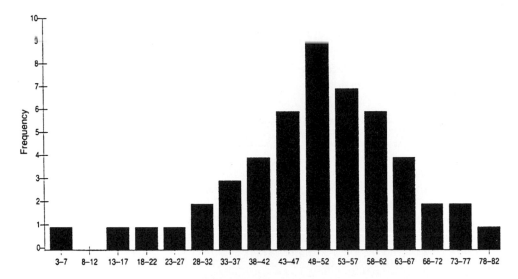

Test Score Intervals (number of curl-ups in 1 minute)

FIGURE 4-3

Histogram of frequency distribution in Table 4-6.

1. A frequency distribution can be developed for all *except* which of the following types of data:
   A. Continuous
   B. Nominal
   C. Quantitative
   D. Ratio

2. Which column in a frequency distribution should be consulted to find the total *percentage* of examinees who received scores of *at least* a particular value?
   A. The *f* column
   B. The *cum f* column
   C. The % column
   D. The *cum* % column

3. What is the ideal interval size for a grouped frequency distribution for which scores range from 88 to 40?
   A. 2
   B. 3
   C. 4
   D. 5

4. If the best score received by an examinee is 77 and the interval size is 3, how should the top score interval be defined?
   A. 75–77
   B. 76–78

C. 77–79

D. Cannot be determined from this information alone.

Questions 5 to 8 refer to the following frequency distribution. Complete the missing data, then answer the questions.

FREE THROWS (20 ATTEMPTS)	f	cum f	%	cum %
16	1			
13	2			
10	3			
8	2			
7	6			
5	2			
4	3			
2	1			

5. *How many* examinees were tested on the free throw test?

   _____

6. *How many* examinees scored *at least* 50% of the free throws that they attempted? _____

7. What *percentage* of examinees scored *exactly* 10 free throws?

   _____%

8. What *percentage* of the examinees scored *at least* 10 free throws?

   _____%

ANSWERS

1. B   2. D   3. B   4. C
5. 20   6. 17   7. 15%   8. 85%

Use of Computers for Nonstatistical Data Analysis

In the last chapter we posited that the computer is a valuable tool for the test consumer. With large data sets, constructing the nonstatistical data analysis techniques presented in this chapter by hand can be time consuming and tedious. Unlike most humans, computers are great at repetitive, tedious work. Luckily, many computer programs can construct frequency distributions, frequency polygons, histograms, and a number of other types of graphs. These programs are available for **mainframe computers** and **microcomputers** (Macintosh and IBM compatibles) (Fig. 4-4). When using programs for frequency analyses, typically all the user has to do is to enter the raw data (i.e., the score values) either from the keyboard or by accessing a file where the data have been stored, and then request a particular analysis or graph.

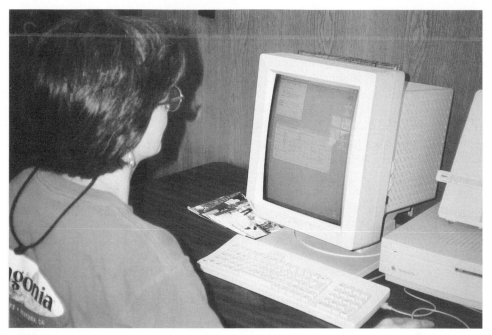

FIGURE 4-4

An ESS professional now spends a part of each workday at the computer. (Photo by Dr. Kathy Tritschler, Greensboro, NC.)

A mainframe computer is a multiuser system composed of large pieces of hardware that have huge memory capacities; the system is accessed through a terminal consisting of a keyboard and a monitor.

A microcomputer is a stand-alone computer to serve a single user; it consists of hardware including a central processing unit, a keyboard, a monitor, and sometimes a printer and other peripheral devices.

Available for use on mainframe computers at many universities, colleges, agencies, and corporations are large, extremely powerful statistical packages such as SPSS (Statistical Package for the Social Sciences) and SAS (Statistical Analysis System). These packages are said to be **powerful** because they can have huge memory capacities that make it possible to conduct complicated analyses on extremely large data sets in seconds or minutes.

Power of a computer refers to its memory capacity and processing speed.

Both SPSS and SAS have programs for nonstatistical data analysis and graphing and a host of other programs for different functions. The SPSS program for nonstatistical analyses is called FREQUENCIES; the SAS program is FREQ (4, 5). Another popular statistics package for the mainframe computer is MINITAB (6). This is a particularly good package for novices in statistics and/or computer usage. MINITAB is easy to use because it is interactive (i.e., it shows results on the terminal screen as one works), uses commands that are like spoken English, and accepts variations in command language. For example, to create a histogram from data entered into column 1, one may type "histogram C1," "histogram from data in C1," or "draw histogram from C1."

Many software programs conduct nonstatistical data analyses on a microcomputer. SPSS, SAS, and Minitab all have developed microcomputer versions of their statistical packages. The SPSS and Minitab packages are available in both IBM and Macintosh versions; the SAS microcomputer package runs only on IBM-compatible machines. These packages handle less data and are slower than their mainframe counterparts. Nonetheless, they provide the average test consumer and even the average researcher with plenty of computer power. The major drawbacks are that they are fairly expensive and that some novices will find them somewhat intimidating and not especially user friendly.

Good options do exist, however, for the novice user who does not want to invest a lot of money. Certainly one option is to recruit the assistance of someone who knows one or more computer languages and can write a program to do the functions that you need. Far easier is to take advantage of one or more of the professionally developed software programs available for a minimal fee from Softshare, a software clearinghouse for programs developed by professors and others in physical education and exercise and sport studies. The fee to cover the cost of copying and mailing disks is less than $10 per disk. All software from Softshare is in the public domain; some programs are freeware and some are "shareware." Shareware programs may be freely copied and distributed, but an adoption fee is paid to the author of the program by anyone who, after trying out the program, finds it useful enough to continue to use it. The adoption fee is often only about $20. In exchange for this fee, you receive technical support and notices of improvements to the program. So for less than $30 you can have your own data analysis program. You can purchase a Softshare catalog that lists software for IBM, MacIntosh, and Apple computers from the AAHPERD Bookstore. The toll free phone number is 800-321-0789.

The Softshare catalog lists more than two dozen statistical packages, most of which can construct frequency distributions and histograms. One of the easiest programs to use is Statistics on Software (S.O.S.) (7). The authors of the program designed it "specifically for the person with a limited understanding of the subject material or computers." S.O.S. calculates the most common statistics on small data sets (fewer than 100 cases). Figure 4-5 is a grouped frequency distribution created by S.O.S. for the data in Table 4-6. Compare this computer-generated distribution with the hand-calculated distribution. There are some differences. Most notable is that the computer version lists the score intervals from low to high rather than high (best score) to low. (Perhaps in the next version of the program, the authors will correct this.) You may also notice that all numbers other than frequencies are reported to two decimal places. All in all, however, the distributions are essentially the same. The generation of the grouped frequency table using S.O.S. took only a couple of minutes from start to finish. The most time-consuming part was entering the 50 score values. In this program the user is asked to define the interval size and the values of the first interval. The user also can title the distribution. Since it is so easy to generate frequency distributions by computer, if the user is unsure about the best interval size, a trial and error approach can be used until a distribution that fits the guidelines for grouped frequency distributions is created.

Figure 4-6 is the S.O.S. version of a histogram based on these same data, that is, the curl-up data for high school boys. This graph was assembled from the grouped

```
¤               F R E Q U E N C Y     D I S T R I B U T I O N                ¤
¤     MEASUREMENT CLASSES           F          RF%      CF            CF%    ¤
¤        3.00 up to     7.00        1        2.04%       1          2.04%   ¤
¤        8.00 up to    12.00        0        0.00%       1          2.04%   ¤
¤       13.00 up to    17.00        1        2.04%       2          4.08%   ¤
¤       18.00 up to    22.00        0        0.00%       2          4.08%   ¤
¤       23.00 up to    27.00        1        2.04%       3          6.12%   ¤
¤       28.00 up to    32.00        2        4.08%       5         10.20%   ¤
¤       33.00 up to    37.00        3        6.12%       8         16.33%   ¤
¤       38.00 up to    42.00        4        8.16%      12         24.49%   ¤
¤       43.00 up to    47.00        6       12.24%      18         36.73%   ¤
¤       48.00 up to    52.00       10       20.41%      28         57.14%   ¤
¤       53.00 up to    57.00        7       14.29%      35         71.43%   ¤
¤       58.00 up to    62.00        6       12.24%      41         83.67%   ¤
¤       63.00 up to    67.00        4        8.16%      45         91.84%   ¤
¤       68.00 up to    72.00        2        4.08%      47         95.92%   ¤
¤       73.00 up to    77.00        2        4.08%      49        100.00%   ¤
¤                                                                           ¤
¤     GROUPED FREQUENCY DISTRIBUTION FOR CURL-UPS IN 1 MIN. BY H.S. BOYS    ¤
```

FIGURE 4-5

Frequency distribution created by S.O.S. microcomputer program. (Reprinted with permission from Timko, J., and Downie, J.: Statistics on Software, Version 2.0. Orange, CA, Statistics for Management, 1992.)

frequency distribution by the pressing of *one* key! The numbers along the horizontal axis of the histogram represent score intervals, or measurement classes, ordered from left to right, with 1 representing the first interval in the distribution. There are no values printed along the vertical axis, but one can nonetheless get a fairly clear sense of the patterns in the data. And after all, that is the purpose of the nonstatistical data analysis techniques.

```
¤               F R E Q U E N C Y     H I S T O G R A M                     ¤
¤                                                                           ¤
¤             Y                                                             ¤
¤          10¤                            ÜÜÜ                               ¤
¤            ¤                            ÜÜÜ                               ¤
¤            ¤                            ÜÜÜ                               ¤
¤            ¤                         ÜÜÜÜÜÜ                               ¤
¤            ¤                      ÜÜÜÜÜÜÜÜÜÜÜÜ                            ¤
¤            ¤                      ÜÜÜÜÜÜÜÜÜÜÜÜ                            ¤
¤     f      ¤                   ÉÉÉÜÜÜÜÜÜÜÜÜÜÜÜÜÉÉÉ                        ¤
¤            ¤                ÉÉÉÜÜÜÜÜÜÜÜÜÜÜÜÜÜÜÜÜÜ                         ¤
¤            ¤                ÜÜÜÜÜÜÜÜÜÜÜÜÜÜÜÜÜÜÜÜ                         ¤
¤            ¤             ÜÜÜÜÜÜÜÜÜÜÜÜÜÜÜÜÜÜÜÜÜÜÜÜÜÜ                      ¤
¤            ¤  ÜÜÜ    ÜÜÜ  ÜÜÜÜÜÜÜÜÜÜÜÜÜÜÜÜÜÜÜÜÜÜÜÜÜÜ                    ¤
¤            ¤  ÜÜÜ    ÜÜÜ  ÜÜÜÜÜÜÜÜÜÜÜÜÜÜÜÜÜÜÜÜÜÜÜÜÜÜ                    ¤
¤           0                                                   X         ¤
¤               1   2   3   4   5   6   7   8   9  10 11 12 13 14 15        ¤
¤                                                                           ¤
¤     GROUPED FREQUENCY DISTRIBUTION FOR CURL-UPS IN 1 MIN. BY H.S. BOYS    ¤
```

FIGURE 4-6

Histogram created by S.O.S. microcomputer program. (Reprinted with permission from Timko, J., and Downie, J.: Statistics on Software, Version 2.0. Orange, CA, Statistics for Management, 1992.)

Chapter Summary

Both quantitative and qualitative assessment data must be analyzed to give them meaning. A frequency distribution can be developed for quantitative data that are measured on a ratio, interval, or ordinal scale. The frequency distribution is a tabular method of organizing data so that patterns of meaning can be discerned. Simple frequency distributions use a score interval of 1 unit; grouped frequency distributions used score intervals of 2 or greater. A grouped frequency distribution is usually constructed so that it has 10 to 20 score intervals that include all obtained score values. Frequency polygons and histograms are common ways to graph the information from a frequency distribution. Computer programs can assist in the generation of these nonstatistical data analysis techniques. A variety of programs are available for both mainframe computers and microcomputers.

DOING PROJECTS FOR FURTHER LEARNING

1. The following data are 30 yard dash times for boys trying out for a Pop Warner football team. The data are recorded in seconds.

8.1	7.7	6.8	9.2	8.1
7.0	8.7	8.2	7.2	8.0
8.2	6.8	8.3	9.0	9.4
6.9	8.6	6.7	8.1	8.3

   A. Develop a grouped frequency distribution for these data. (How about a couple of hints? Since a low score represents better performance than a high score, construct the distribution with the lowest scores at the top. Try a score interval of 0.2 seconds.)

   B. Construct either a frequency polygon or a histogram for these data. Use graph paper or a computer program.

2. Call the AAHPERD Bookstore at 800-321-0789 and request a copy of the SOFTSHARE catalog. When it arrives, read through the descriptions of programs under Statistics. If you feel inspired, order a statistics program that will run on your microcomputer. (Happy computing!)

REFERENCES

1. Krippendorff, K.: Content Analysis: An Introduction to Its Methodology. Thousand Oaks, CA, Sage Publications, 1980.
2. Gugliotta, G.: People dislike the metric system, so why make them use it? (Greensboro, NC) News & Record, June 30, 1995.
3. Sports Illustrated: Sports Illustrated Poll '86. New York, Lieberman Research, 1986.
4. SPSS. Staff: SPSS Base 7.5 for Windows: User's Guide. Paramus, NJ, Prentice Hall, 1996.
5. SAS Institute: SAS/ETS User's Guide, Version 6. Cary, NC, SAS Institute, 1998.
6. Minitab Staff: Stat 101: Software for Statistics Instruction. Reading, MA, Addison Wesley Longman, 1993.
7. Timko, J., and Downie, J.: Statistics on Software, Version 2.0. Orange, CA, Statistics for Management, 1992.

CHAPTER **5**

Descriptive Statistics

Every measurement and assessment textbook on the market has one of these—a chapter on statistics. Now tell the truth: are you holding your breath, anticipating something akin to having your teeth drilled without novocaine? Well, believe it or not, this will not be too unpleasant even for those of you with mathematics anxiety. The statistics needed to analyze quantitative assessment data require little more numerical literacy than knowledge of addition, subtraction, multiplication, and division. Occasionally you will have to determine square roots, but please feel free to use a calculator to obtain those values. In fact, please use your calculator or a computer any time you wish, because we think that it is unproductive for you to get bogged down in statistical formulas and calculations. ESS practitioners should focus instead on (*a*) learning to select appropriate descriptive statistics for a given situation, (*b*) learning to interpret statistical values, and (*c*) understanding the decisions that can be made on the basis of available evidence.

As you read this chapter, watch for the following keywords:

Descriptive statistics	Parameter	Scattergram
Inferential statistics	Population	Semi-interquartile range
Median	Range	Skewness
Mode	Real limits	Standard deviation
Normal distribution	Sample	Statistic

How to Read a Statistical Formula

Statisticians use a shorthand system of communicating. Called *summation notation*, it uses symbols with constant meanings. If you know just a few basic symbols, you can be ready to calculate many statistics from written formulas. Basic symbols used in summation notation are summarized in Table 5-1.

Symbols are used to represent a mathematical function (e.g., Σ means to add) or to represent a characteristic of a population or a sample. A **population** is a group of persons or objects that have at least one quality in common that is used to determine membership to the population. The only way to know the exact characteristics of a population is to measure all of its members. Characteristics of populations are **para-**

TABLE 5-1	Common Symbols used in Statistical Formulas

SYMBOL	MEANING
N	Number of cases in a population
n	Number of cases in a sample
X	A particular variable
Y	A different variable
X_i	An individual X score
X_3	Third X score
X_n	Last X score
Σ	Sum (add)
ΣX	Sum the X scores
$\sqrt{}$	Calculate the square root
$\sqrt{X}$	Square root of X
XY or (X)(Y)	Cross-product of X and Y (multiply X by Y)
X/Y or $\dfrac{X}{Y}$	Divide X by Y
μ	Population mean
$\overline{X}$ or M	Sample mean (arithmetic average) of X
χ	Deviation score of X ($X_i - \overline{X}$)
σ	Population standard deviation
s	Sample standard deviation

meters. When it is impossible or impractical to measure all members of a population, a **sample** is drawn from the population and measured. Characteristics of a sample are **statistics.** If the sample is drawn according to specific guidelines that ensure adequate representation, the sample statistic provides a good estimate of the population parameter. In summation notation, Greek letters are usually used to denote population parameters and Roman letters are used to represent sample statistics. Statistics is also used in a less formal sense to refer inclusively to characteristics of both populations and samples.

A population is a complete group of persons or objects that have in common at least one defining characteristic.

A sample is a portion of a population.

A parameter is a characteristic of an entire population.

A statistic is a characteristic of a sample that may be used to estimate the value of a population parameter.

Statistical formulas are written to convey to the user how to calculate a particular parameter or statistic. The symbol to the left of the equal sign names the parameter or statistic that will be calculated by following the procedure on the right of the equal sign. Mathematical operations named in the formula must be executed in a particular order according to precedence rules. The general precedence rules for formulaic calculations are:

1. Before doing any calculations, identify all symbols used in the formula.
2. Begin calculations at the extreme right-hand side of the formula, then work from right to left through the calculations. (This is the reverse of what we do when we read words.)
3. When there are parentheses in the formula, do all operations indicated inside the parentheses before doing other calculations.
4. When there are exponents, do what they direct before continuing. (An exponent is written as a superscript, e.g., the 2 in X^2 tells one to square the value of X, that is, multiply X by itself.)
5. Addition and subtraction are performed before multiplication and division.
6. When formulas are written with directions above and below a horizontal line, perform all operations above the line and all operations below the line before dividing.
7. If there is an inclusive symbol, such as a square root radical, that contains other symbols, perform the operation only on the included symbols.

SELF-TEST QUESTIONS: PART A

Consider the X scores of 6, 8, 5, 2, 1, and 3 for the following questions:

1. What is the value of $(\Sigma X)^2$? (This formula tells you to sum all of the X scores and then to square the sum.) _____

2. What is the value of ΣX^2? (This formula tells you to square each of the X scores, then add the six squared values.) _____

3. What is the value of $\sqrt{\dfrac{\sum X^2 - 11}{2}}$? _____

4. What is the value of $\dfrac{\sqrt{\sum X^2 + 5}}{2}$? _____

ANSWERS

1. 625   2. 139   3. 8   4. 6

Branches of Statistics

Statistical data analysis entails the calculation of values or indices that summarize various characteristics of assessment data. Two broad categories of statistics are used in analyses to achieve different purposes. **Descriptive statistics** are used to summarize and describe characteristics of a data set. Descriptive statistics are an integral part of every quantitative assessment analysis. **Inferential statistics** are used only when assessment personnel are interested in making inferences from a sample to a population, that is, applying inferences derived from the group of persons who were measured to similar persons who were not measured.

Sound confusing? Perhaps an example will help. A coach who takes a set of pre-season fitness measurements on the team members probably is interested only in summarizing and describing the measurements of the group. The coach is not immediately concerned with any athletes other than those who are playing on the team. As such, the coach should calculate appropriate descriptive statistics. Another coach has been using a new training technique for some players. This coach wants to know whether the observed and measured improvements are due to chance or are real improvements likely to occur with other players subjected to the new technique. This coach should calculate one or more inferential statistics to answer the question. Do you see that the second coach is interested in drawing inferences from the group of players who were measured and applying those inferences to similar players who were not measured?

> Descriptive statistics are statistics used to describe or summarize characteristics of a set of data.

> Inferential statistics are statistics used to make inferences about populations based on characteristics of the sample data.

The calculation and interpretation of descriptive statistics are fairly straightforward, and the limitations for their appropriate use are easily grasped. Common descriptive statistics are discussed in this chapter. Selected inferential statistics are discussed in Chapter 6.

All descriptive statistics describe characteristics of a set of assessment data. *Measures of central tendency* are used to describe the average or typical score in a set of scores. *Measures of variability* describe the extent of similarity or difference among the scores in a set. *Measures of relative position* describe how a particular examinee's score compares with the scores of other examinees. The fourth category is *measures of association*. These statistics describe the relationship between two sets of assessment data. Table 5-2 summarizes the major categories of descriptive statistics.

TABLE 5-2	Major Categories of Descriptive Statistics	
CATEGORY	**FUNCTION**	**STATISTICS**
Central tendency	Describe the average or "typical" score in a data set	Mean, median, mode
Variability	Describe the extent of similarity or difference among scores in a data set	Standard deviation, interquartile range, range
Relative position	Describe an individual score in comparison to other scores in a data set	Percentile rank, z-score, T-score
Association	Describe a relationship between two sets of data	Pearson product moment, Spearman rank order

Measures of Central Tendency

Since about fourth grade you have been computing and using the arithmetic *mean* to report the average or typical score. In sport settings you have calculated batting averages, free-throw averages, volleyball kill averages, and the like to represent typical performances of sport skills during athletic competitions (Fig. 5-1). In school you have tracked your grade point average. Although the mean is the most frequently used measure of central tendency, it is not the only statistic that can be used to represent a typical score. The median and the mode are two other commonly used measures of central tendency.

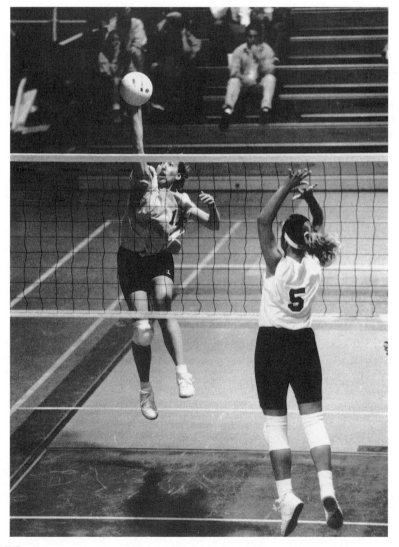

FIGURE 5-1

The mean is calculated to report volleyball kill averages. (Photo by John Bell, Touch a Life Photography, Greensboro, NC.)

Mode

The mode, symbolized by *Mo*, is defined as the most commonly occurring value. No formula is required to determine this value. One simply inspects a frequency distribution, frequency polygon, histogram, or even the raw scores themselves and notes which score appears most often. The mode for the data set of 8, 6, 6, 6, 5, 3, 3 is 6. The mode for the data tabulated in the frequency distribution in Table 4-4 is 89 inches. (Of the 50 junior high school girls at the volleyball camp, 9 scored 89 inches on a vertical jump test.)

The **mode** gives a quick but rough sense of the typical score. It is, however, a relatively unstable measure of central tendency because it can be affected to a large extent by the value of one or two scores. In other words, changing one or two scores may change the value of the mode. Another problem with using the mode to describe the central tendency of data is that the data can be *bimodal*, that is, they can have two (or more) modes. Therefore, the mode has limited value and is only occasionally used for describing the central tendency of ratio, interval, and ordinal scale data. The mode is, however, the only appropriate measure of central tendency for nominal scale data. For example, the mode is used to describe the typical pattern of voting for all-star players in a tournament, the typical ethnic background of participants in a wellness program, and the typical response to a survey question about one's favorite spectator sport.

> The mode is the most frequently occurring value in a data set.

Median

Just as a median on a highway divides a road into two halves, the statistical median divides a data set into two equal halves. The median, symbolized by *Mdn*, is a single value that is greater than half of the scores and smaller than the other half of the scores. The median of a set of scores is found by ordering all the data values from best to worst, then finding the middle point of this distribution, that is, the value of the 50th percentile. *The scores must be ordered before one can find a middle value.*

Although researchers often need to know the exact value of the median, physical education teachers, coaches, exercise specialists, and other practitioners usually find the approximate median by following these simple guidelines:

1. If the number of scores in the data set is odd, the approximate median is the value of the single score in the middle position of the distribution. For example, the median of 15, 12, 9, 9, 7, 5, 4 is 9, the value of the fourth of seven scores.
2. If the number of scores in a data set is even, the approximate median is the arithmetic average of the two middle scores of the distribution. The median of 15, 12, 9, 9, 7, 5, 4, 2 is 8, the arithmetic average of 9 and 7.

The **median** is more stable than the mode because data are ordered. What it gains in stability, however, it loses in precision because the median considers only the position and not the exact value of each score. The median is the ideal measure of central tendency for ordinal data. It is also the most appropriate measure of central tendency for interval and ratio data sets that have one or more extreme scores or that are skewed (discussed in the section after next). The median may *not* be used to report the central tendency of nominal data because nominal data cannot be ordered by numerical value. (Had you already figured that out?)

> The median is the value that divides an ordered data set into two equal halves so that half of the scores are greater than the median and the other half of the scores are less than the median.

Mean

The mean is the arithmetic average of the scores in a distribution. It is calculated by summing the values of all the scores, then dividing by the number of scores that were summed. This is expressed by the formula

$$\mu = \overline{X} = \frac{\sum X}{N}$$

Formula 5-1

Since the mean takes into account every score value, it is considered a more stable and precise index than either the median or the mode. The mean is the appropriate measure of central tendency for most interval and ratio data sets. *It should never, however, be used for describing the central tendency of ordinal or nominal data.*

Central Tendency for Extreme Score and Skewed Data

If there are extremely high or extremely low scores in a distribution, the mean is artificially inflated or deflated. The mean is somewhat "dishonest" because the typical score appears to be higher or lower than it is. In these cases, the median is the preferred measure of central tendency over the mean.

How about an example to illustrate this point? Imagine a high school basketball team that advertises that the average height of its starting lineup is 6 feet even. They got this figure by calculating the mean of the five players' heights. Suppose they have four starters who are 5 feet 9 inches and one starter who measures in at 7 feet even. In this case, the height of the 7-footer artificially inflates the mean. The mean is "dishonest" as a measure of central tendency because it does not do a good job of representing the typical height of the starting team, one player actually being taller than 6 feet. The median value of 5 feet 9 inches gives a more honest representation of the typical height of the starting lineup. Be sure to inspect interval and ratio data for extreme scores before reporting a mean as the measure of central tendency.

Similarly, the median is a better measure of central tendency for skewed data. **Skewness** is associated with asymmetrical distributions in which the majority of scores cluster either at the high end or low end of the scale of scores. Normally we expect most scores in a data set to cluster approximately in the middle of the obtained score values. Skewness affects the mean more than the median or mode (1) (Fig. 5-2).

> Skewness is the tendency of a distribution to depart from symmetry of balance around the mean. If more than half of the scores fall below the mean, the distribution is positively skewed. If more than half of the scores fall above the mean, the distribution is negatively skewed (2).

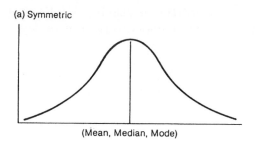

(a) Symmetric

(Mean, Median, Mode)

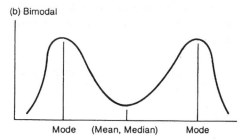

(b) Bimodal

Mode   (Mean, Median)   Mode

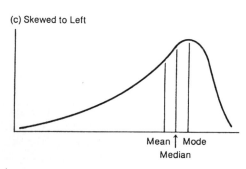

(c) Skewed to Left

Mean ↑ Mode
Median

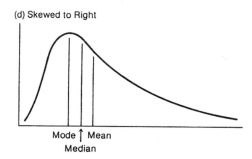

(d) Skewed to Right

Mode ↑ Mean
Median

FIGURE 5-2

Comparisons of the mode, median, and mean in four distributions. (Reprinted with permission from Hinkle, D.E., Wiersma, W., and Jurs, S.G.: Basic Behavioral Statistics. New York, Houghton Mifflin, 1982, p. 56.)

Table 5-3 summarizes recommendations for use of the mean, median, and mode with ratio, interval, ordinal, and nominal data.

SELF-TEST QUESTIONS: PART B

The following scores are bench press scores in pounds for healthy, active men over age 65.

420
140
130
120
100
100
100
90

1. What is the scale of measurement of these data? _____

2. Are there any extreme scores in this data set? _____

3. What is the mode of these data? _____

4. What is the median? _____

5. What is the mean? _____

6. What is the appropriate, most honest measure of central tendency for these data?

_____

TABLE 5-3	Relationship Among Central Tendency Statistics and Measurement Scales		
	NOMINAL SCALE DATA	**ORDINAL SCALE DATA**	**INTERVAL AND RATIO SCALE DATA**
Mode	BEST	OK	OK
Median	WRONG	BEST	OK; BEST if extreme scores or skewed data
Mean	WRONG	WRONG	BEST if no extreme scores and if data are normal or not skewed

ANSWERS

1. Ratio scale
2. Yes; 420 lb
3. Mo = 100 lb
4. Mdn = 110 lb
5. $\overline{X}$ = 150 lb
6. Median

P.S. The gentleman who pressed 420 lb was a competitive weight lifter most of his life.

Measures of Variability

Measures of central tendency describe the typical score for a group, but alone they do not sufficiently describe a set of scores. *To describe a set of scores, at least one* measure of central tendency *and one* measure of variability *are needed.*

Consider the following example comparing the heights of the starters on two basketball teams:

Team A	5' 4"	5' 5"	6' 0"	6' 7"	6' 8"
Team B	5' 10"	5' 11"	6' 0"	6' 1"	6' 2"

The mean height of both teams' players is 6 feet, and the median height for both is 6 feet, yet the teams are markedly different in terms of their players' heights. Team A is blessed with two very tall players, a 6-footer, and two very short players. Team B players all hover close to the 6-foot mark. Measures of variability describe the characteristic of spread in the scores; they describe how similar or different the scores within a data set are. The three most commonly used measures of variability are the *range,* the *semi-interquartile range,* and the *standard deviation.*

Range

The **range** is simply the numerical difference between the highest and the lowest scores. (In some assessment texts the range is defined as the highest score minus the lowest score plus 1. This variation in the definition takes into account the real limits of the score values. For practical purposes you may use either definition of the range.) If the range is small, like that for team B, one knows that the scores are grouped close together and that the scores are relatively homogeneous. If the range is large, it indicates more heterogeneity in the scores.

For ratio, interval, and ordinal data, the range can give a very quick, rough estimate of the spread of the scores. However, it is unstable because it takes into account only two score values, those at the extremes. Frequent or large gaps in the distribution of scores can easily distort this measure of variability.

> Range is the value of the spread of scores in a distribution; it is the numerical difference between the highest and lowest scores.

Semi-Interquartile Range

The **semi-interquartile range,** symbolized by Q, is used to determine the spread of the middle 50% of the scores taken from the median. The formula for calculating the semi-interquartile range is:

$$Q = \frac{Q_3 - Q_1}{2}$$ Formula 5-2

The values Q_3 and Q_1 refer, respectively, to the 75th percentile ($P_{.75}$) and the 25th percentile ($P_{.25}$).

In most cases exercise and sport practitioners may approximate the values of the 75th and 25th percentiles in a manner similar to finding the median, or the 50th percentile. One simply finds the points that define the upper and lower fourths of the distribution. The value of Q_3 and Q_1 is either the value of the score that represents that point or the average of the two scores on either side of the defined point. Subtract Q_1 from Q_3 and divide by 2 to get this measure of variability. Table 5-4 shows a sample calculation of Q.

A small Q value indicates a small spread in scores, whereas a large Q indicates a large spread in scores. To interpret the semi-interquartile range, this value can be added to and subtracted from the median. For example, if Q is equal to 20 and Mdn is 100, approximately 50% of scores fall between 80 and 120. The median plus Q approximates the value of Q_3 but does not equal it unless the distribution is symmetrical around the median. The same is true of the median minus the Q value and Q_1. Thus, Q can help to interpret the skewness in a set of ordered scores.

The semi-interquartile range is a more stable measure of variability than the range because it does not take into account the extreme scores in the upper and lower quarters of the distribution. It is used appropriately when the median is reported as the measure of central tendency.

> The semi-interquartile range is a measure of the variability of the middle 50% of the scores in a distribution.

Standard Deviation

The standard deviation is the appropriate measure of variability whenever the mean is selected to report central tendency. It is the most stable of all variability measures because its calculation takes into account the value of every score in the distribution.

The **standard deviation,** symbolized by *s* or *SD* (for a sample) or σ (for a population), is a theoretical measure of the spread of the middle 68% of the scores taken from the mean. However, it is commonly defined as the average deviation of the

TABLE 5-4	Sample Calculation of the Semi-Interquartile Range

$$X$$
100
90
80
80_____ $Q_3 = 80$
80
70
70
70____ Mdn = 70
70
70
60
60_____ $Q_1 = 55$
50
30
30
10

$$Q = \frac{Q_3 - Q_1}{2} = \frac{80 - 55}{2} = 12.5$$

scores about the mean. If you read that statement carefully, you may guess what is necessary to calculate this value. First calculate the *deviation scores* by subtracting the mean from each score. To find an average deviation, add the deviations and then divide by the number of scores. Close, but not quite right, because the sum of the deviation scores would always equal zero. Instead, square each deviation score before summing them, then divide by the number of score values, and finally take the square root (or "unsquare") the obtained value.

> Standard deviation is a theoretical measure of the spread of the middle 68% of the scores taken from the mean.

The formula is:

$$\sigma = s = \sqrt{\frac{\sum (X - \overline{X})^2}{N}}$$
Formula 5-3

Since Formula 5-3 can be cumbersome with anything but whole numbers, you are likely to find this alternative formula easier for most calculations of standard deviation:

$$\sigma = s = \sqrt{\frac{\sum X^2}{N} - \overline{X}^2}$$
Formula 5-4

Sample calculations in Table 5-5 show use of both standard deviation formulas. As demonstrated, these formulas are computationally equivalent.

Regardless of the formula used to calculate the value of the standard deviation, the interpretation is the same. A small standard deviation indicates that scores are close together, while a large standard deviation indicates that the scores are widely spread.

Relationship of Mean and Standard Deviation

If you know both the mean and standard deviation of a set of scores, you can get a good idea how the frequency polygon built from this distribution will look. This is true especially if the distribution is a **normal distribution** or bell-shaped. (You may be familiar with such a distribution in relation to grading. Teachers who grade on the curve give most students C's, and only a small percentage of students receive A's and F's; a slightly larger percentage of students get B's and D's.) If a set of scores is normally distributed, there is a curious relationship between the mean and standard deviation. Virtually all the scores, that is, more than 99% of them, fall within three standard deviations above and below the mean. Furthermore, about 95% of scores fall within two standard deviations above and below the mean, and about 68% of the scores fall within one standard deviation on either side of the mean.

> A normal distribution produces a bell-shaped frequency polygon with known characteristics.

As an example, suppose that you have analyzed a set of scores and found the mean to be 63 and the standard deviation to be 8. In this case, the mean plus 3 stan-

TABLE 5-5	Sample Calculation of Standard Deviation Using Formulas 5-3 and 5-4

X	$(X - \bar{X})$	$(X - \bar{X})^2$	
2	−1	1	
1	−2	4	$s = \sqrt{\dfrac{\Sigma(X-\bar{X})^2}{N}}$
4	1	1	
3	0	0	$= \sqrt{\dfrac{10}{5}}$
5	2	4	
$\Sigma =$ 15		$\Sigma =$ 10	
$\bar{X} =$ 3			$= 1.4$

X	X^2	
2	4	
1	1	$s = \sqrt{\dfrac{\Sigma X^2}{N} - \bar{X}^2}$
4	16	
3	9	
5	25	$= \sqrt{\dfrac{55}{5} - 9}$
$\Sigma =$ 15	$\Sigma =$ 55	
$\bar{X} =$ 3		
$\bar{X}^2 =$ 9		$= 1.4$

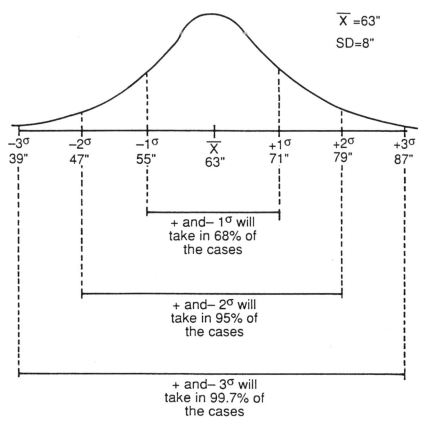

$\overline{X}$ =63"

SD=8"

+ and– 1^σ will take in 68% of the cases

+ and– 2^σ will take in 95% of the cases

+ and– 3^σ will take in 99.7% of the cases

FIGURE 5-3

Percentage of area under the normal curve associated with 1, 2, and 3 standard deviation units.

dard deviations $(63 + 8 + 8 + 8)$ equals 87. The mean minus 3 standard deviations $(63 - 8 - 8 - 8)$ equals 39. To the extent that the scores are normally distributed, we can expect virtually all of the scores to fall between 39 and 87. Approximately 95% of the scores will fall between 47 and 79, and 68% of the scores, between 55 and 71 (Figure 5-3).

Each distribution has its own mean and standard deviation that are calculated according to the particular scores in that distribution. It is also important to realize that not all distributions are normal, especially those of samples or small populations. However, many of the variables of interest in exercise and sport settings have normally distributed underlying populations even though the sample distributions are not normal. Understanding the theoretical relationship between the mean and the standard deviation for normal distributions can help one interpret the standard deviation of any distribution.

SELF-TEST QUESTIONS: PART C

Let's look again at the bench press scores for the older gentlemen. Their bench press scores in pounds are:

420
140
130
120
100
100
100
90

1. What is the range of these data? _____

2. What is the semi-interquartile range? _____

3. What is the standard deviation? _____

4. Since the median was reported to describe the central tendency of the data, which of the three measures of variability should be reported?

_____

ANSWERS

1. 330 lb
2. 17.5 lb
3. 103.3 lb
4. Semi-interquartile range

Measures of Relative Position

Measures of relative position are statistics that describe how a single score compares with the rest of the scores in a distribution. A major advantage of such measures is that they standardize the interpretation of scores by converting raw scores to a common scale. This allows us to compare how an individual performed on two or more different types of assessments. (In other words, it creates a way for us to compare apples and oranges.) For example, imagine that Angela has participated in a track and field unit and has obtained the following scores: Shot put, 38 feet; 50 yard dash, 8.2 seconds; and running long jump, 14 feet. How do Angela's scores compare with those of her classmates? Which was Angela's best event? The raw scores themselves are not sufficient to answer either of these questions. The questions are answered easily, however, once we convert the raw scores to measures of relative position. Two common measures of relative position are *percentile ranks* and *standard scores*.

Percentile Ranks

A percentile rank, symbolized by *PR*, tells the percentage of scores in the distribution that are equal to or poorer than a given score. If you are told that a score of 32 has a percentile rank of 85, this means that 85% of the scores in the distribution are 32 or poorer. If a score of 68 has a *PR* of 95, then 95% of the scores are equal to or poorer than 68. In other words, a person who scored 68 performed as well as or better than 95% of the examinees. Conversely, only 5% of the examinees performed better than the person who scored 68. Got it? It should be clear to you that percentile ranks for each of Angela's track and field scores will help show how she performed on each event in comparison with her classmates.

So how do we find *PR* values? Percentile ranks are easily determined from a set of ordered scores or from a frequency distribution of size interval one. From a simple frequency table we can read the *PR* for any score directly from the *cum* % column. If the data are not in a frequency distribution, one can simply order the raw scores and divide the order score by the total number of examinees. For example, assume Angela's 14-foot long jump was the 33rd longest jump in a class of 40 students. The *PR* for a score of 14 feet is about 82.5%, calculated by dividing 33 by 40.

Percentile ranks can also be calculated for any score from data presented in a grouped frequency distribution. This calculation is a bit tricky. The formula:

$$\text{PR for X} = \frac{\cfrac{\text{cum f in}}{\text{interval below}} + \cfrac{X - \text{LRL}}{\text{interval size}}(\text{f of interval})}{N}(100) \qquad \text{Formula 5-5}$$

In this formula X is the score of interest, that is, the score for which we are trying to find the *PR*. The phrase *cum f in interval below* refers to the cumulative frequency in the interval immediately below the interval within which the score of interest falls. *LRL* is the lower real limit of the interval within which the score of interest falls. And *f of interval* is the frequency of the interval within which the score of interest falls.

Time out! What is a **real limit?** In a grouped frequency distribution each score interval is defined in terms of the actual scores obtained on the test. There should be no confusion regarding the interval within which a particular score falls. However, if you think about the defined score intervals as if they were plotted along a number line, you will realize that there are small spaces between each of the defined score intervals. Real limits for each score interval are created by halving these small spaces between the defined score intervals and adding the extra numerical value to each of the adjacent score intervals.

> Real limits are the upper and lower values of score intervals in a frequency distribution, defined so that no numerical area is unaccounted for between the score intervals.

Using the grouped frequency distribution in Table 4-6, calculate the *PR* for a score of 60. The score of 60 falls in the score interval of 58 to 62, which has a frequency of 6. The interval immediately below is defined as 53 to 57; the cumulative frequency of this interval is 35. The lower real limit of the interval of 58 to 62 is 57.5, that is, half of the space between the score limits of 57 and 58. Now you can calculate:

$$\text{PR of 60} = \frac{35 + \cfrac{60 - 57.5}{5}(6)}{50}(100)$$

$$= \frac{35 + \cfrac{2.5}{5}(6)}{50}(100)$$

$$= 76\%$$

According to this calculation, a score of 60 has a *PR* of 76%. A person who scored 60 has performed equal to or better than 76% of the other examinees. In other words, only 24% of the examinees performed superiorly.

Percentile ranks are appropriate especially for ordinal data because the only requirement is that the scores can be logically ordered by numerical value. It is also perfectly appropriate to use them for interval and ratio data. One caution is in order, however. Be careful with these calculations if a low score represents a better performance than a high score. Make the necessary adjustments to your thinking and to your calculations.

A Word About National and Local Norms. Percentile ranks are frequently used to interpret the performance of individual students on published tests such as the AAHPERD Basketball Skill Test for Boys and Girls (3). But calculations of these percentile ranks are based upon the performances of hundreds of youth across the nation; thus they are usually called national norms. For most sport skill and fitness tests separate norms are presented according to age and gender. Before any table of published norms is used by a test consumer, it must be determined that the norms will provide an appropriate comparison. Specifically, it must be determined that the sample on which the norms are based is similar to local performers who will be taking the test. Norms based on a dissimilar group and norms that are over a decade old or older are suspect and should not be used.

The exercise and sport professional may choose to develop local norms. The procedure for developing local norms requires a minimum of 100 scores. After a frequency distribution is constructed, the cumulative frequency values are rounded to whole numbers.

Standard Scores

Norms may also be reported as standard scores. There are many types of *standard scores*. All standard scores transform raw scores into derived scores that describe how far, in standard deviation units, the raw score is from some reference point such as the mean. These measures of relative position are appropriate only for use with interval and ratio data. Two of the more common standard scores are the *z-score* and the *T-score*. (Notice that z is lowercase and T is uppercase.)

z-Score.   A raw score is transformed to a z-score by subtracting the mean from the raw score, then dividing by the standard deviation. The formula:

$$z = \frac{X = \overline{X}}{s} \hspace{4cm} \text{Formula 5-6}$$

where X is the value of the individual raw score, $\overline{X}$ is the group mean, and s is the group standard deviation. A raw score exactly equal to the group mean is transformed to a z-score of 0. A raw score that is exactly one standard deviation above the mean is equivalent to a z-score of +1.00. A raw score that is exactly two standard deviations below the mean equals a z-score of −2.00. Remember the relation between the mean and standard deviation for normal distributions? Since z-scores are expressed in standard deviation units, virtually all raw scores yield z-scores between −3.00 and +3.00.

Let's go back to Angela and her track and field performances in the shot put, the 50 yard dash, and the running long jump. We want to know (*a*) how she did in each event in comparison with her classmates, and (*b*) which event was Angela's best. Suppose, based on the class mean and standard deviation for each event, we calculate Angela's z-scores for these events as +2.46, −0.12, and +1.08. Since the performances are now expressed in standard units of measurement, we can see that Angela's best event was the shot put. We can also conclude that Angela was one of the very top performers on the shot put, that she performed a little below the class mean in the dash, and that she performed equal to or better than about 84% of her classmates on the running long jump. (Do you see where the 84% comes from? The area of the normal curve to the left of the mean includes 50% of the distribution of scores, and the area between the mean and +1 standard deviation includes another 34%.)

Table 5-6 is used to calculate the exact percentage of cases associated with any particular z-score. For positive z-scores, remember to add 50% to the tabled value. For negative z-scores, the percentage of cases is calculated by subtracting the tabled percentage for any given z-score from 50%. Assuming that a set of scores is normally distributed, what percentage of examinees would score equal to or lower than a z-score of +1.08? The answer is 85.99%. (This comes from adding 50% to the tabled value of 35.99%.) What percent of cases are represented by a z-score of −0.12? The answer is 45.22%. (Hint: The tabled value of 04.78% was subtracted from 50%.)

T score. A T score is a z score expressed in a form that does not require negative values or decimals. A z-score is transformed into a T-score by multiplying the z-score by 10 and adding 50:

$$T = 10\,(\,z\,) + 50 \qquad\qquad \text{Formula 5-7}$$

Let's try a couple. A z-score of +1.00 is equivalent to a T-score of 60, because 10 (+1.00) + 50 = 60. A z-score of −1.50 becomes a T-score of 35 because 10 (−1.50) + 50 = 35. A z-score of 0.00, the mean score, is equivalent to 50. When raw scores are transformed to T-scores, the new distribution has a mean of 50 and a standard deviation of 10. Virtually all raw scores yield T-scores between 20 and 80. Figure 5-4 depicts the relationships among raw score standard deviations, z-scores, and T-scores.

SELF-TEST QUESTIONS: PART D

1. For the data given in the simple frequency distribution in Table 4-4, what is the *PR* for a girl whose vertical jump was 86 inches? _____

2. For the data given in the grouped frequency distribution in Table 4-6, what is the exact *PR* for a boy who performed 36 curl-ups in one minute? (Use Formula 5-5.) _____

3. If a group mean is 25 and the standard deviation is 2, what is the z-score for a raw score of 30? _____

4. If a z-score is −1.52, what is the equivalent T-score? _____

5. A z-score of +0.50 is equal to or greater than what percentage of cases in a normal distribution? _____

TABLE 5-6	Percentage Parts of the Total Area Under the Normal Probability Curve, Corresponding to Distances on the Baseline Between the Mean and Successive Points From the Mean in Units of Standard Deviation[a]

UNITS	.00	.01	.02	.03	.04	.05	.06	.07.	08	.09
0.0	00.00	00.40	00.80	01.20	01.60	01.99	02.39	02.79	03.19	03.59
0.1	03.98	04.38	04.78	05.17	05.57	05.96	06.36	06.75	07.14	07.53
0.2	07.93	08.32	08.71	09.10	09.48	09.87	10.26	10.64	11.03	11.41
0.3	11.79	12.17	12.55	12.93	13.31	13.68	14.06	14.43	14.80	15.17
0.4	15.54	15.91	16.28	16.64	17.00	17.36	17.72	18.08	18.44	18.79
0.5	19.15	19.50	19.85	20.19	20.54	20.88	21.23	21.57	21.90	22.24
0.6	22.57	22.91	23.24	23.57	23.89	24.22	24.54	24.86	25.17	25.49
0.7	25.80	26.11	26.42	26.73	27.04	27.34	27.64	27.94	28.23	28.52
0.8	28.81	29.10	29.39	29.67	29.95	30.23	30.51	30.78	31.06	31.33
0.9	31.59	31.86	32.12	32.38	32.64	32.90	33.15	33.40	33.65	33.89
1.0	34.13	34.38	34.61	34.85	35.08	35.31	35.54	35.77	35.99	36.21
1.1	36.43	36.65	36.86	37.08	37.29	37.49	37.70	37.90	38.10	38.30
1.2	38.49	38.69	38.88	39.07	39.25	39.44	39.62	39.80	39.97	40.15
1.3	40.32	40.49	40.66	40.82	40.99	41.15	41.31	41.47	41.62	41.77
1.4	41.92	42.07	42.22	42.36	42.51	42.65	42.79	42.92	43.06	43.19
1.5	43.32	43.45	43.57	43.70	43.83	43.94	44.06	44.18	44.29	44.41
1.6	44.52	44.63	44.74	44.84	44.95	45.05	45.15	45.25	45.35	45.45
1.7	45.54	45.64	45.73	45.82	45.91	45.99	46.08	46.16	46.25	46.33
1.8	46.41	46.49	46.56	46.64	46.71	46.78	46.86	46.93	46.99	47.06
1.9	47.13	47.19	47.26	47.32	47.38	47.44	47.50	47.56	47.61	47.67
2.0	47.72	47.78	47.83	47.88	47.93	47.98	48.03	48.08	48.12	48.17
2.1	48.21	48.26	48.30	48.34	48.38	48.42	48.46	48.50	48.54	48.57
2.2	48.61	48.64	48.68	48.71	48.75	48.78	48.81	48.84	48.87	48.90
2.3	48.93	48.96	48.98	49.01	49.04	49.06	49.09	49.11	49.13	49.16
2.4	49.18	49.20	49.22	49.25	49.27	49.29	49.31	49.32	49.34	49.36
2.5	49.38	49.40	49.41	49.43	49.45	49.46	49.48	49.49	49.51	49.52
2.6	49.53	49.55	49.56	49.57	49.59	49.60	49.61	49.62	49.63	49.64
2.7	49.65	49.66	49.67	49.68	49.69	49.70	49.71	49.72	49.73	49.74
2.8	49.74	49.75	49.76	49.77	49.77	49.78	49.79	49.79	49.80	49.81
2.9	49.81	49.82	49.82	49.83	49.84	49.84	49.85	49.85	49.86	49.86
3.0	49.865									
3.1	49,903									
3.2	49.93129									
3.3	49.95166									
3.4	49.96631									
3.5	49.97674									
3.6	49.98409									
3.7	49.98922									
3.8	49.99277									
3.9	49.99519									

[a]Reprinted with permission from Pearson, E. S., and Hartley, H. O. (eds.): Biometrika Tables for Statisticians. Cambridge, England, Cambridge University Press, 1956.

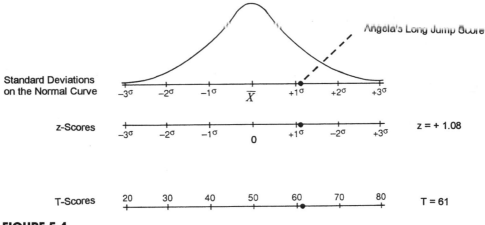

FIGURE 5-4

Comparison of z-score and T-score scales.

ANSWERS

1. 20%   2. 16.2%   3. +2.5   3. 35   5. 69.15%

Measures of Association

The final category of descriptive statistics to be discussed is *measures of association*. These statistics describe whether and to what degree a relationship exists between two sets of measurement scores. The degree of relationship is expressed as a correlation coefficient. A correlation coefficient close to +1.00 or −1.00 is obtained if the two sets of scores are highly related. A coefficient close to .00 will be obtained when the scores are not related in any systematic way (Fig. 5-5).

Different measures of association are appropriate for use with different scales of measurement and to describe different patterns of quantitative relationships. Described here are the *Spearman rank order correlation* and the *Pearson product moment correlation*. Both measures of association describe the strength and the direction of linear relationships between two quantifiable variables. The Spearman correlation was developed for use when one or both of the variables to be correlated are expressed in ranks, representing ordinal data. The Pearson correlation is for use only with interval and ratio level data.

Two cautions must be issued prior to discussing the calculation of these measures of association. First, the data that you are working with must be paired. That is, you must have a score for each person, object, and so on for each of the two variables. The relationship that will be described is that of the assessment on variable X for examinee 1 with that of variable Y for examinee 1, variable X for examinee 2 with variable Y for examinee 2, and so on. If your data are not in this form, there is no logical way to pair the data. The second caution is that the data should be bivariate. In other words, X and Y should be measures of two different attributes, not two measures of the same variable.

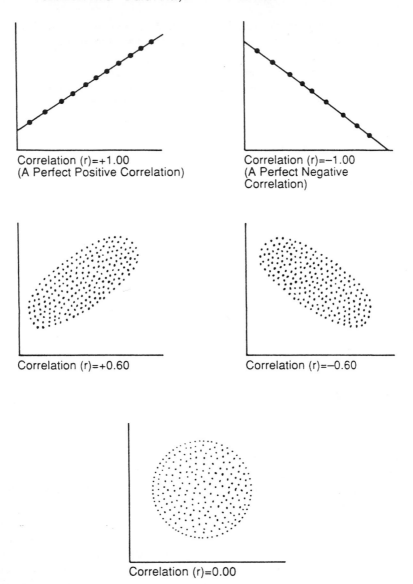

FIGURE 5-5

Scattergrams associated with correlation coefficients of various magnitudes and directions. (Reprinted with permission from Hinkle, D.E., Wiersma, W., and Jurs, S.G.: Basic Behavioral Statistics. New York, Houghton Mifflin, 1982, p. 107.)

Spearman Rank Order Correlation

The first step in calculating the Spearman correlation is to report both variables in terms of ranks. If one variable is expressed in ranks and the other variable is reported as an interval or ratio variable, the interval or ratio variable must be transformed to ranks before calculating the Spearman correlation. When ranking scores, the best score is assigned a rank of 1. If more than one person receives a given score, the tied ranks are averaged. For example, if two performers share the third highest score, each is assigned a rank score of 3.5, the average of ranks 3 and 4. If three performers share the third highest score, they are each assigned the rank of 4, the average of ranks 3, 4, and 5.

The next step is to determine the numerical difference between the rank on variable X and the rank on variable Y for each examinee. For example, if one examinee has a rank of 6 on variable X and a rank of 2 on variable Y, the difference between the ranks (DR) is 4. Each DR value is squared, and the squared values are summed across all examinees.

The final step is to plug the appropriate values in to the formula to calculate the Spearman correlation coefficient, called *rho*:

$$rho = 1 - \frac{6\sum(DR)^2}{N(N^2-1)}$$

Formula 5-8

In this formula, DR is the difference between the ranks, N refers to the number of examinees or pairs of data, and 6 is a constant.

Table 5-7 is a sample calculation of the Spearman rank order correlation. In this example the variable X represents team standing in a small college football league.

TABLE 5-7	Sample Calculation of Spearman Rank Order Correlation			
TEAM	**LEAGUE STANDING X**	**AVERAGE ATTENDANCE Y**	**Y IN RANKS**	**DR**	**(DR)²**
A	1	850	2	−1	1
B	2	1000	1	1	1
C	3	600	3.5	−.5	.25
D	4	600	3.5	.5	.25
E	5	500	5	0	1
F	6	200	8	−2	4
G	7	250	7	0	0
H	8	400	6	2	4
					Σ = 11.5

$$rho = 1 - \frac{6\,\Sigma(DR)^2}{N(N^2-1)}$$

$$= 1 - \frac{6\,(11.5)}{8\,(64-1)}$$

$$= 1 - \frac{69}{504}$$

$$= 1 - .12$$

$$= +.88$$

The variable Y is average game attendance, rounded to the nearest 50. Note that X is already in rank form, but Y scores must be converted to ranks.

The Spearman rank order correlation coefficient of *rho* varies between −1.00 and +1.00. A plus sign indicates a positive relation between the two variables. In other words, high ranks on one variable tend to be associated with high ranks on the other variable, and low ranks are associated with low ranks. A minus sign preceding the value of *rho* indicates a negative or inverse relationship, meaning that high ranks on one variable are associated with low ranks on the other variable and vice versa. The numerical value of *rho* tells the strength of the relation between the two variables. Table 5-8 will give you a general idea of how to interpret the magnitude of *rho*. These are, however, rough estimates that vary with the nature of the actual variables that are measured.

Pearson Product Moment Correlation

The Pearson product moment correlation, symbolized by r, is the most appropriate measure of association when the scores to be correlated are both interval or ratio scale scores. The data must also be paired and should be bivariate. The Pearson correlation gives a more precise estimate of relationship than the Spearman because the actual values of every score are taken into account in the calculation of the Pearson r. The Spearman procedures should be used only on interval and ratio data when a quick, rough estimate of the measure of association is desired.

The purpose of the Pearson correlation is identical to that of the Spearman. The only real difference is that interval or ratio scores are used rather than ranks. The Pearson r correlation coefficient will range from −1.00 to +1.00. It is interpreted identically to that of the Spearman *rho*.

The major problem with the Pearson correlation procedure is that the formula is long, hence highly susceptible to errors. A hand calculator is a must if working with large data sets, and use of a computer is better. The Pearson r is calculated thus:

$$r = \frac{N \sum (XY) - (X)(Y)}{\sqrt{\left[N \sum X^2 - \left(\sum X \right)^2 \right]\left[N \sum Y^2 - \left(\sum Y \right)^2 \right]}}$$ Formula 5-9

TABLE 5-8	Guidelines for Interpretation of the Magnitude of Spearman *rho* and Pearson *r* Correlation Coefficients
CORRELATION COEFFICIENT	**STRENGTH OF RELATIONSHIP**
±.90 or greater	Very strong
±.70 to .89	Strong
±.50 to .69	Moderate
±.30 to .49	Weak
less than ±.30	Little if any correlation

In this formula X represents the scores on one variable and Y represents the paired scores on the second variable; XY is the cross product of the paired X and Y scores; and N is the number of examinees or paired data sets. Table 5-9 is a sample calculation of the Pearson r correlation coefficient. In this example X scores are the number of golf putts sunk in 10 trials at 5 feet. The Y scores are the number of putts sunk in the same number of tries from twice the distance. The resulting r value indicates the strength and direction of the relationship between putting performances at these two distances. (Before you look at Table 5-9, what is your guess? Will the r value be positive or negative? How strong is the relationship?)

SELF-TEST QUESTIONS: PART E

1. The Spearman rank order correlation is most appropriate for which of the following category of data?
   A. Ratio
   B. Interval
   C. Ordinal
   D. Nominal

TABLE 5-9	Sample Calculation of Pearson Product Moment Correlation			
GOLFER	PUTTS AT 5 FEET X	PUTTS AT 10 FEET Y	X^2	Y^2	XY
A	9	7	81	49	63
B	7	7	49	49	49
C	7	4	49	16	28
D	6	5	36	25	30
E	5	2	25	4	10
	$\Sigma = 34$	$\Sigma = 25$	$\Sigma = 240$	$\Sigma = 143$	$\Sigma = 180$

$$r = \frac{N\Sigma(XY)-(\Sigma X)(\Sigma Y)}{\sqrt{[N\Sigma(X^2)-(\Sigma X)^2][N\Sigma(Y^2)-(\Sigma Y)^2]}}$$

$$= \frac{5(180)-(34)(25)}{\sqrt{[5(240)-(34)^2][5(143)-(25)^2]}}$$

$$= \frac{900-850}{\sqrt{[1200-1156][715-625]}}$$

$$= \frac{50}{\sqrt{3960}}$$

$$= +.79$$

2. Which of the following represents a weak linear relationship between two variables?
    A. $r = +.59$
    B. $r = -.99$
    C. $r = +.29$
    D. None of the above

3. For an inverse (or negative) relationship, a high score on Variable X is likely to be related to
    A. A high score on variable Y
    B. A moderate score on variable Y
    C. A low score on variable Y
    D. No score on variable Y

ANSWERS

1. C
2. C
3. C

 # Use of Computers

The computing options for descriptive statistics are very similar to those for nonstatistical data analyses discussed in the last chapter. Most mainframe and microcomputer packages include an assortment of nonstatistical and statistical programs. Very few statistics programs are written to do just one type of analysis.

On the mainframe computer, options are again the SPSS, SAS, and MINITAB packages (4–6). For calculation of descriptive statistics, refer to the CONDESCRIPTIVE program in SPSS. Refer to the MEANS and SUMMARY programs in SAS. But unless you are an experienced computer user, you will probably find the MINITAB approach to descriptive statistic analyses far more compelling.

When using MINITAB, one must begin by entering data or accessing data in a previously created file. Then a simple command, DESCRIBE DATA IN C1, gives values for most measures of central tendency and measures of variability. If you have more than a single variable to analyze, then the command is modified to DESCRIBE DATA IN C1, C2. Standard scores are obtained by typing the command Z-SCORES FOR DATA IN C1. MINITAB will calculate a Pearson product moment correlation with the command CORRELATE C1 WITH C2. If data in columns 1 and 2 are in ranks, the same command gives a Spearman rank order correlation coefficient. MINITAB will also create a **scattergram** (like those in Figure 5-5) from the command PLOT C1 WITH C2.

> A scattergram is a type of graph that visually depicts the relationship between two quantifiable variables whose values are paired. Individual data points are plotted at the intersection of the appropriate values for the variables charted on the horizontal and vertical axes.

There are many statistical programs written for microcomputers. As mentioned in Chapter 4, microcomputer versions of SPSS, SAS, and MINITAB are available for purchase. Another excellent package that is surprisingly powerful and affordable is MYS-

```
DESCRIPTIVE   STATISTICS
VERTICAL JUMP SCORES (IN INCHES)

n        =    50

MEAN     =    88.52000            s       =    2.34077

MEDIAN   =    88.50000            s²      =    5.47918

MODE     =    89                  σ       =    2.31724
f(o)     =    9
                                  σ²      =    5.36960
SKEWNESS =    0.02563
                                  X(Low)  =    83.00000
VARIATION =   2.64434%
                                  X(High) =    95.00000
S.E. of X̄ =   0.33103
                                  Range   =    13.00000


          ᵃᵃᵃ---ᵃᵃᵃ  S O S  ᵃᵃᵃ---ᵃᵃᵃ  S O S  ᵃᵃᵃ---ᵃᵃᵃ  S O S  ᵃᵃᵃ---ᵃᵃᵃ
```

FIGURE 5-6

Descriptive statistics calculated by S.O.S. microcomputer program. (Reprinted with permission from Timko, J., and Downie, J.: Statistics on Software, Version 2.0. Orange, CA, Statistics for Management, 1992.)

TAT (7). This package makes use of spreadsheet technology for data management. Versions are available for IBM-PC and Macintosh computers.

Last but not least, do not overlook the many very affordable and user-friendly statistical programs from SOFTSHARE. In Chapter 4 we demonstrated the ease of frequency distribution and histogram construction using Statistics on Software (S.O.S.) (8). Calculation of descriptive statistics using S.O.S. is similarly easy and straightforward. Figure 5-6 is a sample printout of central tendency and variability statistics calculated by S.O.S. for the 50 vertical jump scores given in Table 4-3. The mean is 88.52 inches, the median is 88.5 inches, and the mode is 89, with 9 the frequency of observations. The population standard deviation is 2.32 inches; this was calculated by Formula 5-3 or 5-4. Since these are descriptive statistics and we are not concerned with sampling, this is the standard deviation we want. The high score was 95 inches; the low score was 83 inches. S.O.S. reports the range as 13 inches, the high score minus the low score plus 1.

S.O.S. also has options to calculate z-scores. The printout gives the value of the z-score and designates the area under the normal curve associated with this z-score. This is the information determined from Table 5-6. A sample printout of the z-score calculation for the score 83 inches is given in Figure 5-7. S.O.S. also calculates Pearson and Spearman correlations for up to 48 pairs of data.

Chapter Summary

This chapter describes several techniques for analysis of quantitative measurement and assessment data. It shows how to develop frequency distributions and graphs to summarize a data set. It also discusses statistical techniques to describe the central tendency and variability of a data set. It has additional techniques to describe how an individual examinee performs in relation to a group and to describe the linear re-

```
                      N O R M A L   D I S T R I B U T I O N




                      MEAN:        88.5200

                      STANDARD DEVIATION:        2.3172

                      X VALUE      83.0000

   THE Z-SCORE IS -2.38219
   THE AREA INSIDE THE MEAN AND THE Z-SCORE IS 0.491398
   THE AREA OUTSIDE THE Z-SCORE IS 0.008602
   THE AREA ABOVE THE Z-SCORE IS 0.991398


            S O S            S O S            S O S
```

FIGURE 5-7

Calculation of z-scores by S.O.S. microcomputer program. (Reprinted with permission from Timko, J., and Downie, J.: Statistics on Software, Version 2.0. Orange, CA, Statistics for Management, 1992.)

lation between two paired data sets. These techniques can be performed by hand or by use of appropriate computer programs.

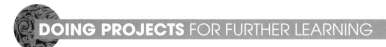

DOING PROJECTS FOR FURTHER LEARNING

Test your new knowledge of data analysis by working the problems in Table 5-10. You may, of course, do these problems by hand or by computer. Perhaps best of all would be to do the problems both ways so you can compare the answers and the

TABLE 5-10	Practice in Data Analysis	
	VERTICAL JUMP (INCHES)	**STANDING LONG JUMP (INCHES)**
Student	X	Y
A	9	65
B	10	72
C	7	62
D	6	55
E	4	44
F	7	62
G	7	56
H	9	70
I	4	54

procedures. Don't be distressed if there are small numerical differences between the hand calculations and the computer results; some computer programs use slightly different formulas for some of the statistical procedures. You will find our answers to the problems at the end of this chapter. Good luck!

REFERENCES

1. Hinkle, D.E., Wiersma, W., and Jurs, S.G.: Basic Behavioral Statistics. New York, Houghton Mifflin, 1982.
2. Jaeger, R.M.: Statistics: A Spectator Sport. Thousand Oaks, CA, Sage, 1983.
3. Hopkins, D.R., Shick, J., and Plack, J.J.: Basketball Skills Test Manual for Boys and Girls. Reston, VA, American Alliance of Health, Physical Education, Recreation, and Dance, 1984.
4. Statistical Package for the Social Sciences Staff: SPSS Base 7.5 for Windows: User's Guide. Paramus, NJ, Prentice Hall, 1996.
5. Statistical Analysis System Institute: SAS/ETS User's Guide, Version 6. Cary, NC, SAS Institute, 1998.
6. Minitab Staff: Stat 101: Software for Statistics Instruction. Reading, MA, Addison Wesley Longman, 1993.
7. Aczel, A.D.: Complete Business Statistics MYSTAT Software with QC Tools. Burr Ridge, IL, McGraw-Hill Higher Education, 1994.
8. Timko, J., and Downie, J.: Statistics on Software, Version 2.0. Orange, CA, Statistics for Management, 1992.

QUESTIONS

1A. Calculate the mean, median, and mode for the vertical jump for the nine elementary school students.

1B. Which measure of central tendency is preferred for these data? Explain.

2A. Calculate the range, semi-interquartile range, and standard deviation for the vertical jump scores.

2B. Which of the variability measures is preferred? Explain.

3A. Calculate the percentile rank, z-score, and T-score for Student D on the vertical jump.

3B. Describe how Student D performed on the vertical jump in comparison to the other children.

4A. Construct a scattergram showing the relationship between the vertical jump and the standing long jump scores.

4B. From the pattern of data points on the scattergram, verbally describe the relationship between the two jumps.

5A. Calculate the Pearson's product moment correlation between the vertical jump scores and the scores on the standing long jump.

5B. Interpret the Pearson's r value.

6A. Convert both sets of scores to ranks, then calculate Spearman's rank order correlation.

6B. Which of the two correlation measures is preferred for these data? Explain.

ANSWERS

1A. $\overline{X} = 7$, Mdn = 7, and Mo = 7

1B. Since these are ratio level data and the data have no extreme scores and are normally distributed (as evidenced by the common mean, median, and mode), the
mean is preferred.

2A. Range = 6.0, Q = 1.5, and s = 2.0

2B. Since the mean is the preferred measure of central tendency, the standard deviation is the preferred measure of variability.

3A. *PR* of 33, z-score = −.50, and T-score = 45

3B. The *PR* tells us that Student D performed equal to or better than 33% of the
other children; the z and T values tell that his vertical jump was one-half standard deviation below the class mean.

4A. Scattergram of vertical jump and standing long jump scores:

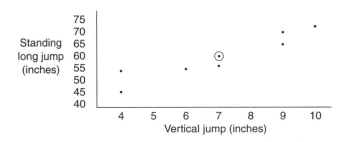

4B. In general, students who received high scores on the vertical jump also tended
to receive high scores on the standing long jump; students who scored lower
on the vertical jump also scored lower on the standing long jump. The scattergram suggests a strong positive correlation.

5A. r = +.92 (ΣX = 63, ΣY = 540, $\Sigma X2$ = 477, $\Sigma Y2$ = 33010, and ΣXY = 3917)

5B. The r value suggests that there is a very strong positive correlation between vertical jump and standing long jump scores.

6A. *rho* = +.98

6B. The Pearson product moment is preferred because the data are ratio. There is
loss of precision in reducing the actual values to ranks, so the r value is actually
more precise than the *rho* value.

CHAPTER **6**

Inferential Statistics

In Chapter 5 you learned that inferential statistics are used when the test consumer wants to generalize from a sample to a population. Okay, but *why* would you want to? There are two primary reasons: because results that are true only for samples usually have limited value and because it is often impractical to take measurements on all members of a population. There are many situations in which exercise and sport studies (ESS) practitioners and researchers measure members of a sample and then make inferences about the population from which the sample was drawn. Making formal inferences from carefully collected sample data is at the heart of professional decision making and research. This chapter shows how to calculate and interpret inferential statistics that are commonly used by ESS practitioners and researchers.

As you read this chapter, watch for the following keywords:

ANOVA	Null hypothesis	Standard error
Between-group variance	Paired samples t-test	Statistical significance
Chi square	Post hoc multiple	t-Test
Confidence interval	comparison	Test of significance
Critical value	Prediction	Type I error
Degrees of freedom	Random sampling	Type II error
Independent samples	Sampling error	Within-group variance
t-test		

Essential Concepts for Understanding Inferential Statistics

Several concepts underlie the use of all inferential statistics. It is necessary to understand these concepts to appreciate the power and the limitations of statistical inference.

Concept 1: Samples Must Be Representative

By definition, a sample consists of *any* portion of a population. However, some samples are essentially worthless for making good inferences. To make a trustworthy inference from a sample to a population, the sample must be *representative* of the

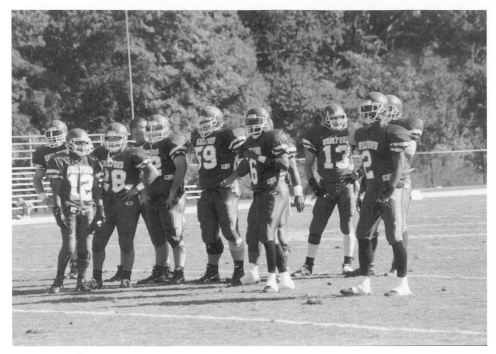

FIGURE 6-1

A good sample is representative of the population from which it was drawn. (Photo by John Bell, Touch a Life Photography, Greensboro, NC.)

population (Fig. 6-1). Whether a sample is representative is a function of both (*a*) the size of the sample relative to the size of the population and (*b*) the method used to select the sample.

Sample Size

For a population of a given size, how big must a representative sample be? Assume that we are interested in the population of NCAA Division III football players. Surely a one-man sample wouldn't be representative. Would it? Nor would a two-man sample be representative. How about 11? 12? 25? 50? 100? How big is big enough? The complete answer to this question is quite complicated and is beyond the scope of this textbook. For our purposes, though, let's just say that appropriate sample size depends upon several factors, including the type of question being asked (that is, the research method), the degree of accuracy desired, and the amount of variability of the attribute being assessed. Results from a very small sample are seldom generalizable to a large population.

Research specialists have developed rough guidelines that the novice can use as a starting point for consideration of sample size. Table 6-1 presents these guidelines (1).

Selection Method

Several valid methods can be used to select samples. They differ, however, in the level of assurance of representativeness that they offer. For many situations the best method is **random sampling.** Random sampling procedures are similar to those

TABLE 6-1	Rough Guidelines for Determination of Sample Size
TYPE OF RESEARCH	**SAMPLE SIZE GUIDELINE**
Descriptive, e.g., estimate population parameter such as the arithmetic average	Sample should be ≥ 10% of the population; 20% is better if population is small (e.g., <150)
Correlational, e.g., estimate correlation between two numerical variables in population	30-member sample usually minimum
Experimental, e.g., theorized causal variable manipulated by researcher to see how it affects another variable	At least 15 sample members for each comparison group; 30 sample members per group if experimental controls are loose
Quasi-experimental, e.g., causal variable that cannot be manipulated by researcher observed for its effect on another variable	At least 30 sample members for each comparison group

used to select bingo numbers. In its simplest form random sampling entails drawing names from a container that has one name card for each member of a population. The primary requirement of random sampling is that each member of the population has an equal chance of being selected for the sample. Random sampling cannot *guarantee* that the resulting sample will be representative, but it increases the likelihood that it will be. *Differences between a randomly drawn sample and the population are usually small and unsystematic.* Random sampling is a theoretical requirement for use of inferential statistics. In practice, however, inferential statistics are commonly used with other sampling methods.

Random sampling is the process of selecting a sample in such a way that each member of the population has an equal chance of being selected.

To be avoided are hand-picked samples, groups of volunteers, and samples consisting only of easily accessible persons. Samples formed by these methods are seldom representative. Less problematic but also not ideal are samples that consist of intact groups such as classes and teams. Again, however, in practice intact groups are sometimes used in educational and sport research.

Concept 2: Sampling Errors Are Normally Distributed

Before this concept can be addressed, it is necessary to explain sampling error. Assume you know the arithmetic average of a particular attribute in a population. (This is for illustrative purposes only, because in real situations this information would not be available.) How likely is it that the mean of a random sample of adequate size drawn from this population would be *identical* to the population average? The answer is pretty unlikely. It would not be surprising if the sample mean and the population average were close, but it would be very unusual if they were *exactly* the same. How about using another sample? How about another? What if 100 or more samples were drawn and the

What Do YOU Think?

Assume that the director of the student health center at a large Midwestern university wants to know more about the sexual practices of its students. He wants this information so he can design effective informational programs to prevent the spread of AIDS and other sexually transmitted diseases. He places the following ad in the student newspaper:

> 66   VOLUNTEERS WANTED FOR SEX SURVEY TO BE CONDUCTED BY THE UNIVERSITY HEALTH CENTER. $5 FEE TO THE FIRST 50 STUDENTS WHO VOLUNTEER TO BE INTERVIEWED. CALL THE HEALTH CENTER TODAY AT 888-8888!"

What types of students do you think will respond to this solicitation? What students are *not* likely to volunteer for this study? Do you think that the 50 volunteers will be representative of the university student population as a whole? Will the director of the student health center be able to draw valid conclusions about the sexual practices of the university students? Explain.

---

mean for each of these samples found? No doubt the sample means would vary considerably. Perhaps one or two or maybe none of the sample means would *exactly* match the population average. Many would be a little larger or a little smaller than the population average, and a few would be considerably larger or considerably smaller. These chance variations among sample means are called **sampling errors.** Sampling errors are not mistakes and are not the fault of the researcher or anyone else; they are expected variations that occur with every sample.

> Sampling error is the expected variation in statistical values that occurs when a sample is selected from a population.

Sampling errors are normally distributed. In other words, a plot of the deviations from the actual population average takes on the shape of a normal curve. That is, 68% of the sample means are within one standard deviation of the true population average, 95% fall within two standard deviations, and 99% fall within three standard deviations. Furthermore, the arithmetic average of all of the sample means provides a good estimate of the population average, and the standard deviation of the sample means provides a good estimate of the standard deviation of the population. Neat, huh? But remember that in actual practice, we draw only one sample, not 100. Nonetheless, it is important to understand this concept whenever you make an inference on the basis of an observed characteristic of a sample.

Concept 3: The Standard Error Can Be Estimated and Used to Create Confidence Intervals

The standard deviation of the distribution of sample estimates of a population parameter is called the **standard error**. When estimating a population average, the standard error of the mean ($SE_{\overline{x}}$) informs us how likely sample means of various magnitudes are. Based on the normal curve, we can expect approximately 68% of all sample means to be within ±1 $SE_{\overline{X}}$ of the true population average, 95% of sample means to be within ±2 $SE_{\overline{X}}$ of the population average, and 99% of sample means to be within ±3 $SE_{\overline{X}}$ of the population average. Thus, a small standard error increases confidence when estimating a population parameter; a large standard error decreases confidence in the estimation.

> The standard error is the standard deviation of the distribution of sample estimates of a population parameter.

The standard error of the mean can be estimated by dividing the sample's standard deviation by the square root of the sample size minus one:

$$SE_{\overline{X}} = \frac{s}{\sqrt{n-1}}$$

Formula 6-1

This estimate of the standard error of the mean along with the sample mean allows calculation of the probable limits within which the true population average can be expected to fall. These limits create a **confidence interval.** The 68% confidence interval is created by subtracting and adding one standard error estimate to either side of the sample mean. This means that the researcher is 68% confident that the true population parameter falls somewhere within this confidence interval. The 95% confidence interval is created by subtracting and adding two standard error estimates to either side of the sample mean. The 99% confidence interval is created by subtracting and adding three standard error estimates to either side of the sample mean (Table 6-2).

> A confidence interval, bounded by a lower and an upper limit, provides the estimated bounds for the true population parameter.

Need an example? Assume you want to know the average shoulder girdle strength of NCAA Division III women tennis players. You could draw a random sample of players from the population, then administer a maximum bench press test to each woman (Fig. 6-2). You could then calculate a mean and standard deviation for the sample. Assume you find the mean bench press to be 100 lb and the standard deviation to be 21 lb. Plugging these values into Formula 6-1, the standard error of the mean is found to be 3 lb. So if the population average falls between 97 and 103 pounds, you have a 68% chance of being correct. If the population average falls be-

TABLE 6-2	Confidence Intervals for Estimation of a Population Average
CONFIDENCE INTERVAL (%)	**FORMULA**
68	$\overline{X} \pm 1SE_{\overline{X}}$
95	$\overline{X} \pm 2SE_{\overline{X}}$
99	$\overline{X} \pm 3SE_{\overline{X}}$

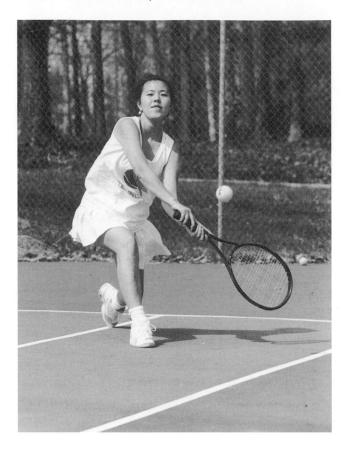

FIGURE 6-2

What is the average shoulder girdle strength of NCAA Division III female tennis players? How confident can you be that your estimate is correct? (Photo by John Bell, Touch a Life Photography, Greensboro, NC.)

tween 94 and 106, you are 95% likely to be correct. And of course, you are almost sure, or 99% confident, that the population average falls somewhere between 91 and 109 pounds. These confidence intervals are created by adding and subtracting one, two, or three standard error estimates to the sample mean. What are the 68%, 95%, and 99% confidence limits for this example if the sample standard deviation is 28 lb? Do you see that a smaller standard error of the mean allows greater confidence when you are estimating a population average from a sample mean?

If you are insightful about numbers and formulas, you probably figured out that sample size inversely affects the magnitude of the standard error of the mean. (See the denominator of Formula 6-1.) As sample size increases, the standard error of the mean decreases. This makes sense because a large sample is usually more representative than a small one. The standard deviation also affects the standard error of the mean. (See the numerator of Formula 6-1.) If the population standard deviation is large, the sample deviation is also likely to be large. Hence confidence limits will be large and estimates of the population average will lack precision. Unlike sample size, however, this factor is not controllable by the practitioner or researcher.

Standard errors can also be computed for other statistics. For example, standard errors can be calculated for estimates of proportions, correlations, and even for the difference between means. The difference between two means is used in the t-test, a common statistical procedure described later in this chapter. It is fairly common to compare two groups to see whether it is likely that they are different. For example, researchers commonly give a treatment (e.g., a new diet, a new training program, or a new drug) to one group; another group, the control group, does not receive the treatment. At the end of the treatment period the researchers measure both groups and record the sample means to discover whether the treatment made a real difference. If a difference between the two groups is observed, how likely is it that such a difference might occur by chance if there is no difference between these groups? Differences in the two sample means are normally distributed around the average difference in the population. Most of the differences are close to the true difference, and a few are way off.

Concept 4: The Null Hypothesis Is Tested

For two sample means to be different, the observed difference must be caused by the independent variable (i.e., the treatment or causal variable). If the difference is a result of sampling errors, we say that the difference is not true. The **null hypothesis,** symbolized by H_O, is a statement that the observed difference was due to chance and therefore does not reflect a true difference in the population averages. In other words, the observed difference in the sample means was probably caused by sampling errors. Although the research hypothesis might claim that a real difference exists, in statistics one always tests the null hypothesis, not the research hypothesis. The sample evidence either supports or fails to support—that is, the researcher accepts or rejects—the null hypothesis. Support of the null hypothesis means that observed differences in the samples are probably due to chance variations. Failure to support the null hypothesis means the evidence *suggests* that observed sample differences are *probably* due to true differences in the population.

Note the use of the words *suggests* and *probably*. We can never really know *for sure* because we have not measured all members of the population or populations. Remember, this entire chapter is about making inferences—that is, likely guesses.

> The null hypothesis (H_O) is the initial statement about the value of the population parameter; it states that there is no difference (or relationship) between variables. Any observed difference (or relationship) is a chance difference (or relationship) caused by sampling errors.

Null hypotheses are evaluated by **tests of significance.** Tests of significance determine whether to accept or reject the null hypothesis. With differences between two sample means, if the observed difference is too large to be attributable to chance, reject the null hypothesis. If the observed difference in the sample means is small enough to be due to chance variations, accept the null hypothesis and conclude that the population averages are likely not to differ.

> A test of significance is a statistical test used to determine whether or not a sample statistic is likely to represent a particular population parameter.

Concept 5: Tests of Significance Are Conducted at Preselected Probability Levels

Tests of significance are conducted at preselected *probability levels*, symbolized by p or α. In most ESS research and evaluation studies, we use a probability level of .05. A p of .05 means that if you reject the null hypothesis on the basis of the observed sample differences, you expect to find a difference of this magnitude by chance only 5 in 100 times. Or conversely, 95 in 100 times differences in sample means of the observed magnitude reflect a true difference in the population averages.

When a null hypothesis is accepted or rejected on the basis of sample evidence, there are several possible outcomes. The decision to accept or reject may be correct or incorrect. Table 6-3 summarizes the four possible outcomes. Rejection of a true null hypothesis is a **type I error.** Acceptance of a false null hypothesis is a **type II error.**

> A type I error occurs if a true null hypothesis is rejected on the basis of the sample evidence.

> A type II error occurs if a false null hypothesis is accepted on the basis of the sample evidence.

It would be great if we could eliminate both type I and type II errors. Unfortunately, this is not possible. The likelihood of making a type I error can be reduced by selecting a more stringent probability level, that is, p = .01 instead of p = .05. However, this causes a concomitant increase in the likelihood of making a type II error. It's a trade-off. For many ESS studies, a probability level of .05 provides a reasonable balance between type I and type II errors.

The p value should be preselected, that is, it should be selected before conducting a test of significance. It is theoretically wrong to conduct a test of significance and wait to see how significant the findings are. The practitioner or researcher should preselect a p value by weighing the relative seriousness of committing a type I versus a type II error. A stringent p value, that is, p = .01 or .001, may be selected for medical research, since committing a type I error may result in a decision with the potential to cause serious injury or death. A less stringent p value, that is, p = .10,

TABLE 6-3	Four Possible Outcomes of Decisions to Reject or Accept the Null Hypothesis (H_o)

RESEARCHER'S DECISION ON THE NULL HYPOTHESIS	ACTUAL STATUS OF THE NULL HYPOTHESIS	OUTCOME OF RESEARCHER'S DECISION
Rejects H_o	H_o is **true**	Type I **error**
Rejects H_o	H_o is **false**	**Correct** decision
Accepts H_o	H_o is **true**	**Correct** decision
Accepts H_o	H_o is **false**	Type II **error**

might be selected for an exploratory study. Use of a less stringent *p* value makes any difference or relationship more likely to be identified.

Concept 6: Most Tests of Significance Are Two-Tailed

Most tests of significance are two-tailed. This means that rejection of the null hypothesis occurs regardless of the direction of the deviations. For example, when two sample means are compared, the null hypothesis is rejected if the mean of sample A is sufficiently larger than the mean of sample B, and vice versa. A one-tailed test of significance is used when the researcher is sure that differences can occur only in one direction. When this is the case, for a particular probability level a smaller magnitude of difference will result in rejection of the null hypothesis (Fig. 6-3).

Concept 7: Sample Size Affects Degrees of Freedom

After a probability level and a two-tailed or one-tailed test of significance are selected, the test of significance is conducted. The result of the test of significance is a calculated value. In and of itself this calculated value is relatively meaningless. To make a decision about the null hypothesis, it is necessary to compare the calculated value with a **critical value.** This critical value is determined by consulting one of several statistical distribution tables.

> The critical value is the value of the test statistic at and beyond which the null hypothesis is rejected.

When using a distribution table, the practitioner or researcher must find the critical value associated with the preselected probability level and the appropriate **degrees of freedom,** symbolized by *df*. In general, the degrees of freedom are a function of sample size and the number of groups. Each test of significance has its own formula for determining the degrees of freedom, but in general the larger the number of subjects, the greater the degrees of freedom.

> The degrees of freedom (*df*) are the number of observations minus the number of restrictions placed on them.

*If the calculated value is less than the critical value, the null hypothesis is accepted. If the calculated value equals or exceeds the critical value, the null hypothesis is rejected—and **statistical significance** is claimed*. (Read those two sentences again.)

> Statistical significance is the conclusion that results are unlikely to be due to chance; the observed difference or relationship is probably real.

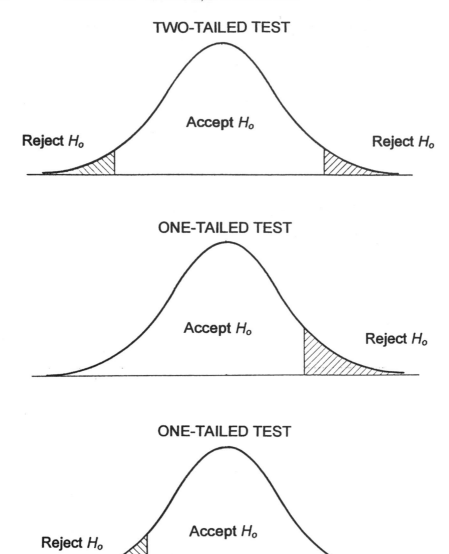

FIGURE 6-3

Areas of rejection of the null hypothesis (H_o) for one-tailed and two-tailed tests of significance.

Concept 8: Statistical Significance Is Not the Same as Practical Significance

The final concept that you must learn is that statistical significance does not guarantee practical significance. The test consumer or researcher must apply judgment to statistical results to determine whether the findings have any real meaning. For example, assume you conclude that a new training program is statistically better than the program now in use. Should you adopt this new training program? Maybe;

maybe not. If the new program is extremely costly and/or if the expected gains are relatively small, then despite statistical significance, you may decide to stick with the current program.

1. Which of the following *can* constitute a sample of a 120-person population?
   A. 1 person
   B. 30 persons
   C. 100 persons
   D. All of the above

2. How large a sample is generally recommended for a correlational study?
   A. At least 15 persons
   B. At least 30 persons
   C. 100 persons
   D. None of the above

3. Which of the following terms indicates the differences between observed scores in a sample and true scores in a population?
   A. Measurement errors
   B. Errors due to bias
   C. Sampling errors
   D. Standard errors

4. As sample size increases, what theoretically happens to the standard error?
   A. It increases
   B. It decreases
   C. It stays the same
   D. It varies in an unpredictable fashion

5. What is the estimate of $SE_{\bar{X}}$ if $n = 82$ and $s = 18$? _____

6. What is the 95% confidence interval for this example if the sample mean is 70?
   _____ to _____

7. How often is the conclusion for a test of significance likely to be correct if the researcher selects a p value of .05? _____ of 100 times

8. If a researcher accepts a false null hypothesis, what type of error is committed?
   A. Type I
   B. Type II

ANSWERS

1. D	2. B	3. C	4. B
5. 2.0	6. 66 to 74	7. 95	8. B

Selected Tests of Significance

It's time to try actual calculations for several tests of significance. The following pages show you how to calculate several common inferential statistics. An example is given for each test of significance. The example is for demonstration purposes, so unusually small sample sizes and score values are used. Even if you don't consider yourself a number whiz, please try to do the computations. The purpose of working a few examples by hand is to help you understand the conceptual bases for these tests.

t-Test

The most common purpose of a t-test is to determine whether two sample means are significantly different at a preselected probability level. The strategy of a t-test is to compare the observed difference in the sample means with the difference expected by chance. This is done by calculating the ratio between these two values. The numerator of a t-test formula is the observed difference in the two sample means; the denominator is the standard error of the difference between the means. The calculated t value is compared with the critical value. If the calculated t equals or exceeds the critical t, the null hypothesis is rejected, and the conclusion is that the difference is significant. The assumption is that the observed difference was due to a real difference in the populations, not to mere sampling variations. If the calculated t is less than the critical t, the null hypothesis is accepted or retained; the conclusion is that the difference is nonsignificant. The assumption is that the observed difference was due to chance variations caused by sampling. Make sense?

> The t-test is a statistical test used to determine whether two sample means are significantly different at a preselected probability level.

There are two versions of the t-test, the *independent samples t-test* and the *paired samples t-test*. The two tests are conceptually similar but computationally different. They are used for different types of samples.

The **independent samples t-test** is used when the two groups to be compared have been randomly formed or when the members of the two groups are not related to each other in any systematic way. For example, two completely separate groups of women volleyball players might be randomly selected from the population of NCAA Division I volleyball players. One group is given a special weight training program to increase vertical jumping; the other group is given the traditional weight training program. It is assumed that initially the vertical jumping ability of the two groups is essentially the same. Therefore, if they are essentially the same at the end of the study, the null hypothesis is probably true. If the two groups are sufficiently different at the end of the study, the null hypothesis is probably false. An independent samples t-test would similarly be used to compare scores on an attribute for two different groups such as men and women, whites and nonwhites, old and young adults, and beginners and nonbeginners.

The **paired samples t-test** is used for comparing the means of two samples that were formed by some type of matching. For example, if 20 persons are ranked on some characteristic, two approximately equal groups could be formed by assigning persons with the ranks of 1, 4, 5, 8, 9, 12, 13, 16, 17, and 20 to one group, and assigning persons with ranks of 2, 3, 6, 7, 10, 11, 14, 15, 18, and 19 to the other group. Another example of paired samples is two samples of the same people at different times. This can occur when a group is pretested and later posttested.

The independent samples t-test is a statistical test used to compare the means of two samples that were randomly formed.

The paired samples t-test is a statistical test used to compare the means of two samples formed by some type of matching.

Calculation of the Independent Samples t-Test

Suppose we have the following test scores for variable X for two groups that *were formed by random sampling*. Note that the samples for this example are not the same size; the independent samples t-test can handle data from same or different sized groups. Valid use of this test does require, however, that (*a*) data are interval or ratio in nature, (*b*) distributions of the two data sets are approximately normal; and (*c*) variances of the population comparison groups are approximately equal. For this example, let's assume that these requirements are met.

X_A	X_B
7	6
6	5
5	4
5	3
4	2
3	

Quick inspection reveals that the means of the groups are different. But is the difference statistically significant? This question can be answered by the t-test. The formula for calculation of the independent samples t-test:

$$t = \frac{|\overline{X}_A - \overline{X}_B|}{\sqrt{\left[\frac{\sum X_A^2 - \frac{\left(\sum X_A\right)^2}{n_A} + \sum X_B^2 - \frac{\left(\sum X_B\right)^2}{n_B}}{(n_A + n_B) - 2}\right]\left[\frac{1}{n_A} + \frac{1}{n_B}\right]}} \qquad \text{Formula 6-2}$$

where the subscripts A and B identify values for two independent groups on variable X.

Before you can work the formula, you need to find the following values for this example:

$$\sum X_A = \quad \sum X_B =$$

$$n_A = \quad n_B =$$

$$\overline{X}_A = \quad \overline{X}_B =$$

$$\sum X_A^2 = \quad \sum X_B^2 =$$

Once you've calculated these values, enter the values into Formula 6-2:

$$t = \frac{|5-4|}{\sqrt{\left[\dfrac{160 - \dfrac{(30)^2}{6} + 90 - \dfrac{(20)^2}{5}}{(6+5)-2}\right]\left[\dfrac{1}{6} + \dfrac{1}{5}\right]}}$$

Do you understand what each of these values represents? If so, carry out the operations, following the precedence rules for formulaic calculations. (Take a quick peek at Chapter 5 if you are unsure about the order for any of the calculations.)

When all is said and done, you should get a calculated t of 1.108. You're almost done. Hang in there!

Turn to Table 6-4 to find the critical value. To use this table, you need to know the preselected p and the df. Table 6-4 lists the critical values for probability levels of .10, .05, and .01. Assume you want to do a two-tailed test of significance using a p value of .05, so use the middle column in the table. The formula for degrees of freedom for an independent samples t-test is $df = n_A + n_B - 2$. For this example, $df = 6 + 5 - 2 = 9$. So for $p = .05$ and 9 df, the critical value is 2.262. If the calculated t equals or exceeds the critical t, you reject the null hypothesis; if the calculated t is less than the critical t, you accept the null hypothesis.

So what is the decision? Right! Since 1.108 is less than 2.262, you accept the null hypothesis. Alternatively, you *retain* the null hypothesis. Are the means of the two samples different? Yes. Are the means of the two samples significantly different? No. Then why is there a difference between the two sample means? Probably because of chance sampling variations. These samples may have been drawn from the same population.

Congratulations. You have just conducted a test of significance—an independent samples t-test. Ready for the next one?

Calculation of the Paired Samples t-Test

Assume the following test scores for variable *X for a sample group measured at two different times.* You want to know whether there is a significant difference between the mean performances from the first time to the second. Notice that the scores are paired; there are two scores for each person in the sample group. The paired samples t-test is appropriate for this situation.

TABLE 6-4	Table of Critical Values of *t*		
DEGREES OF FREEDOM[a]	p = .10 (.05 FOR 1-TAILED TEST)	p = .05 (.025 FOR 1-TAILED TEST)	p = .01 (.005 FOR 1-TAILED TEST)
1	6.314	12.706	63.657
2	2.920	4.303	9.925
3	2.353	3.182	5.841
4	2.132	2.776	4.604
5	2.015	2.571	4.032
6	1.943	2.447	3.707
7	1.895	2.365	3.499
8	1.860	2.306	3.355
9	1.833	2.262	3.250
10	1.812	2.228	3.169
11	1.796	2.201	3.106
12	1.782	2.179	3.055
13	1.771	2.160	3.012
14	1.761	2.145	2.977
15	1.753	2.131	2.947
16	1.746	2.120	2.921
17	1.740	2.110	2.898
18	1.734	2.101	2.878
19	1.729	2.093	2.861
20	1.725	2.086	2.845
21	1.721	2.080	2.831
22	1.717	2.074	2.819
23	1.714	2.069	2.807
24	1.711	2.064	2.797
25	1.708	2.060	2.787
26	1.706	2.056	2.779
27	1.703	2.052	2.771
28	1.701	2.048	2.763
29	1.699	2.045	2.756
30	1.697	2.042	2.750
40	1.684	2.021	2.704
60	1.671	2.000	2.660
120	1.658	1.980	2.617
∞	1.645	1.960	2.576

The observed difference between two group means is significant if the calculated *t* value equals or exceeds the tabled critical value.
[a]$(n_A + n_B) - 2$ for independent groups, where n_A and n_B are the number of subjects in groups A and B, respectively; $N - 1$ for paired groups, where N is the total number of paired data sets.
Adapted from Fisher, R.A.: Statistical Tables for Biological, Agricultural and Medical Research. New York, Longman, 1995.

	X_A	X_B
Ben	6	9
Hal	5	9
Bob	4	3
Joe	3	7
Abe	2	7

The formula for calculation of the paired samples t-test:

$$t = \frac{|\overline{X}_A - \overline{X}_B|}{\sqrt{\dfrac{\sum D^2 - \dfrac{\left(\sum D\right)^2}{N}}{N(N-1)}}}$$
Formula 6-3

where D is the difference between each pair of scores and N is the number of pairs of scores.

To find the values for D and D^2, it is helpful to create two new columns as shown below:

	X_A	X_B	D	D^2
Ben	6	9	+3	9
Hal	5	9	+4	16
Bob	4	3	−1	1
Joe	3	7	+4	16
Abe	2	7	+5	25

The next step is to calculate the following values that are needed in Formula 6-3:

$X_A =$ $\Sigma D =$
$X_B =$ $\Sigma D^2 =$
$N =$

Plug these values into the formula, then do the defined computations. Your equation should like this:

$$t = \frac{|4-7|}{\sqrt{\dfrac{67 - \dfrac{(15)^2}{5}}{5(5-1)}}}$$

The calculated *t* works out to be 2.860. Now you need the critical value from Table 6-1. Again use a *p* value of .05, but for this example there are only four degrees of freedom. This is because the formula for degrees of freedom for the paired samples t-test is *N−1*—or the number of pairs of scores minus 1. Therefore, the critical *t* is 2.776.

So what's the decision? Since 2.860 is greater than 2.776, you reject, or fail to support, the null hypothesis. You conclude that there *is* a significant difference between the means for variable *X* at points A and B. You also assume that the improvement (assuming a higher score is better) you observed in the sample will also hold true for the population.

Congratulations. You have now learned how to calculate and interpret both versions of the t-test.

SELF-TEST QUESTIONS: PART B

1. What is the null hypothesis for the value of the difference between means for a t-test? $H_o = $ _____

2. In Formula 6-2 for the independent samples t-test, what symbol indicates the size of the second group? _____

3. In Formula 6-3 for the paired samples t-test, what symbol indicates the difference between the raw scores for each pair of data? _____

4. Using *p* = .05, what is the critical *t* for a paired samples t-test based on 30 subjects?

5. A researcher hypothesizes that intercollegiate basketball team starters have a *better* vertical jump score than nonstarters. (He is concerned only with differences in a positive direction.) He randomly selects two groups of 15 starters and 30 nonstarters and tests them on their vertical jumps. To test his hypothesis, what type of t-test should he conduct?
   A. A one-tailed independent t-test
   B. A two-tailed independent t-test
   C. A one-tailed paired samples t-test
   D. A two-tailed paired samples t-test

6. How many degrees of freedom are there for this example?

   _____

ANSWERS

1. $H_o = 0$ 2. n_B 3. *D*
4. 2.045   5. A   6. 43

One-Way Analysis of Variance

What if you need to compare the means of three, four, five, or even more groups? The **one-way analysis of variance (ANOVA)** is used to determine whether there is a significant difference among several means. For example, an ANOVA can be used to compare the mean scores on a fitness test for samples of sixth-, seventh-, and eighth-graders. Compare the means of the three groups to determine whether the averages for the three populations are likely to differ. (The ANOVA can also serve as an alternative to the independent samples t-test for comparison of the means of two independent samples.)

> The ANOVA is a statistical test used to determine whether two or more means are significantly different at a preselected probability level.

The logic of ANOVA is similar to that of the t-test, but an *F* ratio is computed instead of a *t* ratio. The *F* ratio compares two sources of variability in the scores. The variability among the sample means, called **between-group variance,** is compared with the variability among individual scores within each of the samples, called **within-group variance.** The calculated *F* will be compared with a tabled critical *F*. As was true for the t-test, if the calculated value is less than the tabled critical value, you accept the null hypothesis. The null hypothesis for the ANOVA is a statement that the population means are identical. Reject the null hypothesis if the calculated *F* equals or exceeds the tabled critical value at the preselected probability level. Rejection of the null hypothesis means acceptance that the population averages differ.

> Between-group variance is the variability among the sample means.

> Within-group variance is the variability among individual scores within the samples.

Like the t-test, the ANOVA also assumes that (*a*) data are interval or ratio, (*b*) distributions of the data sets are approximately normal; and (*c*) variances of the population comparison groups are approximately equal. Marked violations of these assumptions may invalidate the results.

Calculation of One-Way ANOVA

These scores are for three *independently formed groups*. In this example all three groups are the same size, but this is not a requirement for ANOVA. Like the independent t-test, the ANOVA can be used for same or different sized groups. Scores on variable *X* for this example:

X_A	X_B	X_C
4	7	7
3	6	7
3	5	6
3	4	5
2	3	5

The means for the three groups are 3, 5, and 6. Are the three sample means different? Yes. Are they significantly different? A one-way ANOVA will answer this question. The first step is to find values for the variance terms that are needed for the ANOVA. The variance terms are the total sums of squares (SS_{total}), the between sums of squares (SS_{bt}) and the within sums of squares (SS_{wi}). To facilitate calculation of these terms, create new columns for X^2 for each of the groups. The original and the new columns:

X_A	X_A^2	X_B	X_B^2	X_C	X_C^2
4	16	7	49	7	49
3	9	6	36	7	49
3	9	5	25	6	36
3	9	4	16	5	25
2	4	3	9	5	25
$\Sigma = 15$	$\Sigma = 47$	$\Sigma = 25$	$\Sigma = 135$	$\Sigma = 30$	$\Sigma = 184$

The formula for calculation of SS_{total} is given in Formula 6-4:

$$SS_{total} = \sum X^2 - \frac{\left(\sum X\right)^2}{N}$$

Formula 6-4

where X is the variable of interest and N is the total number of subjects across all groups.

Do you see how to get SS_{total}? The ΣX^2 is found by adding the three X^2 columns: $47 + 135 + 184 = 366$. The ΣX is obtained by adding the three X columns: $15 + 25 + 30 = 70$. Follow through with the formula, using 15 for the value of N. The value of SS_{total} is 39.3. This number is the total amount of variance, that is, the sum of SS_{bt} and the SS_{wi}.

The formula for SS_{bt}, the variability among the sample means:

$$SS_{bt} = \frac{\left(\sum X_A\right)^2}{n_A} + \frac{\left(\sum X_B\right)^2}{n_B} + \frac{\left(\sum X_C\right)^2}{n_C} - \frac{\left(\sum X\right)^2}{N}$$

Formula 6-5

The value of SS_{bt} is $45 + 125 + 180 - 326.7 = 23.3$. The value of SS_{wi} can be determined by subtracting SS_{bt} from SS_{total}—$39.3 - 23.3 = 16$.

The next step is to construct an ANOVA summary table, filling in the values you just calculated:

SOURCE OF VARIATION	SUM OF SQUARES	FORMULA FOR df	df	MEAN SQUARES	F
Between	23.3	(K – 1)	2	11.65	8.76
Within	16.0	(N – K)	12	1.33	
Total	39.3	(N – 1)	14		

Notice the formulas for degrees of freedom. K refers to the number of groups, three for this example. *Mean squares (MS)* are calculated by dividing the *SS* values by the appropriate *df*. The *F* ratio is the ratio of MS_{bt} in the numerator and MS_{wi} in the denominator. The calculated *F*, therefore, is 8.76.

Can you guess what to do next? Determine the critical *F* by referring to Table 6-5. There are three sections to this table; select the section for your preselected *p*

TABLE 6-5A	Table of Critical Values of *F*

$p = .10$ (.05 FOR A 1-TAILED TEST)					
Degrees of Freedom for MS$_{wi}$[a]	**Degrees of Freedom for MS$_{bt}$**[b]				
	1	**2**	**3**	**4**	**5**
1	39.9	49.5	53.6	55.8	57.2
2	8.53	9.00	9.16	9.24	9.29
3	5.54	5.46	5.39	5.34	5.31
4	4.54	4.32	4.19	4.11	4.05
5	4.06	3.78	3.62	3.52	3.45
6	3.78	3.46	3.29	3.18	3.11
7	3.59	3.26	3.07	2.96	2.88
8	3.46	3.11	2.92	2.81	2.73
9	3.36	3.01	2.81	2.69	2.61
10	3.28	2.92	2.73	2.61	2.52
11	3.23	2.86	2.66	2.54	2.45
12	3.18	2.81	2.61	2.48	2.39
13	3.14	2.76	2.56	2.43	2.35
14	3.10	2.73	2.52	2.39	2.31
15	3.07	2.70	2.49	2.36	2.27
16	3.05	2.67	2.46	2.33	2.24
17	3.03	2.64	2.44	2.31	2.22
18	3.01	2.62	2.42	2.29	2.20
19	2.99	2.61	2.40	2.27	2.18
20	2.97	2.59	2.38	2.25	2.16
21	2.96	2.57	2.36	2.23	2.14
22	2.95	2.56	2.35	2.22	2.13
23	2.94	2.55	2.34	2.21	2.11
24	2.93	2.54	2.33	2.19	2.10
25	2.92	2.53	2.32	2.18	2.09
26	2.91	2.52	2.31	2.17	2.08
27	2.90	2.51	2.30	2.17	2.07
28	2.89	2.50	2.29	2.16	2.06
29	2.89	2.50	2.28	2.15	2.06
30	2.88	2.49	2.28	2.14	2.05
40	2.84	2.44	2.23	2.09	2.00
60	2.79	2.39	2.18	2.04	1.95
120	2.75	2.35	2.13	1.99	1.90
∞	2.71	2.30	2.08	1.94	1.85

There is a significant difference between at least two group means if the calculated *F* equals or exceeds the tabled critical value.
[a] $N - K$ for one-way ANOVA where *N* is the total number of subjects across all groups and *K* is the number of groups.
[b] $K-1$ for one-way ANOVA where *K* is the number of groups.
Adapted from Fisher, R.A.: Statistical Tables for Biological, Agricultural and Medical Research. New York, Longman, 1995.

TABLE 6-5B	Table of Critical Values of *F*

p = .05 (.025 FOR A 1-TAILED TEST)

Degrees of Freedom for MS_{wi}[a]	Degrees of Freedom for MS_{bt}[b]				
	1	2	3	4	5
1	161	200	216	225	230
2	18.5	19.0	19.2	19.2	19.3
3	10.1	9.55	9.28	9.12	9.01
4	7.71	6.94	6.59	6.39	6.26
5	6.61	5.79	5.41	5.19	5.05
6	5.99	5.14	4.76	4.53	4.39
7	5.59	4.74	4.35	4.12	3.97
8	5.32	4.46	4.07	3.84	3.69
9	5.12	4.26	3.86	3.63	3.48
10	4.96	4.10	3.71	3.48	3.33
11	4.84	3.98	3.59	3.36	3.20
12	4.75	3.88	3.49	3.26	3.11
13	4.67	3.80	3.41	3.18	3.02
14	4.60	3.74	3.34	3.11	2.96
15	4.54	3.68	3.29	3.06	2.90
16	4.49	3.63	3.24	3.01	2.85
17	4.45	3.59	3.20	2.96	2.81
18	4.41	3.55	3.16	2.93	2.77
19	4.38	3.52	3.13	2.90	2.74
20	4.35	3.49	3.10	2.87	2.71
21	4.32	3.47	3.07	2.84	2.68
22	4.30	3.44	3.05	2.82	2.66
23	4.28	3.42	3.03	2.80	2.64
24	4.26	3.40	3.01	2.78	2.62
25	4.24	3.38	2.99	2.76	2.60
26	4.22	3.37	2.98	2.74	2.59
27	4.21	3.35	2.96	2.73	2.57
28	4.20	3.34	2.95	2.71	2.56
29	4.18	3.33	2.93	2.70	2.54
30	4.17	3.32	2.92	2.69	2.53
40	4.08	3.23	2.84	2.61	2.45
60	4.00	3.15	2.76	2.52	2.37
120	3.92	3.07	2.68	2.45	2.29
∞	3.84	2.99	2.60	2.37	2.21

There is a significant difference between at least two group means if the calculated *F* equals or exceeds the tabled critical value.
[a] *N – K* for one-way ANOVA where *N* is the total number of subjects across all groups and *K* is the number of groups.
[b] *K–1* for one-way ANOVA where *K* is the number of groups.
Adapted from Fisher, R.A.: Statistical Tables for Biological, Agricultural and Medical Research. New York, Longman, 1995.

TABLE 6-5C	Table of Critical Values of *F*

$p = .01$ (.005 FOR A 1-TAILED TEST)

Degrees of Freedom for MS_{wi}[a]	Degrees of Freedom for MS_{bt}[b]				
	1	2	3	4	5
1	NR	NR	NR	NR	NR
2	98.5	99.0	99.2	99.2	99.3
3	34.1	30.8	29.5	28.7	28.2
4	21.20	18.00	16.69	15.98	15.52
5	16.26	13.27	12.06	11.39	10.97
6	13.74	10.92	9.78	9.15	8.75
7	12.25	9.55	8.45	7.85	7.46
8	11.26	8.65	7.59	7.01	6.63
9	10.56	8.02	6.99	6.42	6.06
10	10.04	7.56	6.55	5.99	5.64
11	9.65	7.20	6.22	5.67	5.32
12	9.33	6.93	5.95	5.41	5.06
13	9.07	6.70	5.74	5.20	4.86
14	8.86	6.51	5.56	5.03	4.69
15	8.68	6.36	5.42	4.89	4.56
16	8.53	6.23	5.29	4.77	4.44
17	8.40	6.11	5.18	4.67	4.34
18	8.28	6.01	5.09	4.58	4.25
19	8.18	5.93	5.01	4.50	4.17
20	8.10	5.85	4.94	4.43	4.10
21	8.02	5.78	4.87	4.37	4.04
22	7.94	5.72	4.82	4.31	3.99
23	7.88	5.66	4.76	4.26	3.94
24	7.82	5.61	4.72	4.22	3.90
25	7.77	5.57	4.68	4.18	3.86
26	7.72	5.53	4.64	4.14	3.82
27	7.68	5.49	4.60	4.11	3.78
28	7.64	5.45	4.57	4.07	3.75
29	7.60	5.42	4.54	4.04	3.73
30	7.56	5.39	4.51	4.02	3.70
40	7.31	5.18	4.31	3.83	3.51
60	7.08	4.98	4.13	3.65	3.34
120	6.85	4.79	3.95	3.48	3.17
∞	6.64	4.60	3.78	3.32	3.02

There is a significant difference between at least two group means if the calculated *F* equals or exceeds the tabled critical value.
[a] $N - K$ for one-way ANOVA where *N* is the total number of subjects across all groups and *K* is the number of groups.
[b] $K - 1$ for one-way ANOVA where *K* is the number of groups.
Adapted from Fisher, R.A.: *Statistical Tables for Biological, Agricultural and Medical Research.* New York, Longman, 1995.

value. For this example, assume that $p = .01$. (This more stringent p was chosen because the researcher or practitioner wanted to reduce the possibility of making a type I error.) Use the column for the degrees of freedom for MS_{bt} and the row for the degrees of freedom for MS_{wi}. The tabled critical value is 6.93. The calculated F is greater than the critical value.

So what is the decision? This ANOVA suggests that on the basis of the sample data, you should reject the null hypothesis. The sample means *are* significantly different, so you conclude that there is probably a difference in the population averages. To be more specific, the significant F ratio indicates that there is at least one significant difference among the three means. It does not, however, tell us which of the means is different from which of the other means.

Multiple Comparisons

An ANOVA tells us whether or not there is a significant difference among the sample means. If the F ratio for the ANOVA is nonsignificant, there is no need for any further testing. If, however, the F ratio for an ANOVA is significant, you must conduct **post hoc multiple comparisons** to determine where exactly the significant differences are. Don't be scared off by this technical language. *Post hoc* simply means that the test is a follow-up test done after the original ANOVA. *Multiple comparisons* means that you do a series of comparisons, one for each two-way comparison of interest.

> Post hoc multiple comparison is a procedure used after a significant ANOVA to determine which pair or pairs of means are significantly different.

Any of several multiple comparisons tests can be used. One of the easiest is the Scheffé test, which is very conservative. That means that the probability of making a type I error is never greater than the p value used in the original ANOVA. It also means that occasionally one has a significant ANOVA yet does not find a significant difference among any of the pairs of means on the Scheffé test.

The formula for the Scheffé test is given in Formula 6-6:

$$F = \frac{(\overline{X}_Y - \overline{X}_Z)^2}{MS_{wi}\left(\dfrac{1}{n_Y} + \dfrac{1}{n_Z}\right)(K-1)}$$
Formula 6-6

where $\overline{X}_Y$ and $\overline{X}_Z$ represent the two comparison means. For the ANOVA example, you have to compare the means of A versus B, B versus C, and A versus C.

Compare the means of groups A and C first. Group C performed better than group A, but are their means significantly different? Plugging the appropriate values into Formula 6-7 yields the following equation:

$$F_{A,C} = \frac{(3-6)^2}{1.33\left(\dfrac{1}{5} + \dfrac{1}{5}\right)(2)}$$

The value for $F_{A,C}$ is 8.46. This exceeds the critical F of 6.93, so the original conclusion appears to be correct. The mean of group C is significantly greater than the mean of group A. It is safe to conclude that the average for population C is greater than the average for population A.

What about the means for groups B and C? The mean of C is greater than that of B, but is the difference statistically significant? The equation for comparison of the means of these two groups:

$$F_{B,C} = \frac{(5-6)^2}{1.33\left(\dfrac{1}{5}+\dfrac{1}{5}\right)(2)}$$

The value for $F_{B,C}$ is 0.94. Since this is less than the critical F, the difference between the means of group B and group C is nonsignificant. The population averages of these two groups are likely to be essentially the same.

The equation for comparison of the means of group A and group B:

$$F_{A,B} = \frac{(3-5)^2}{1.33\left(\dfrac{1}{5}+\dfrac{1}{5}\right)(2)}$$

The value of $F_{A,B}$ is 3.76. This is also less than the critical F of 6.93. Conclusion: there is no significant difference between the means of groups A and B.

On the basis of the Scheffé test, it appears that the significance of the original ANOVA reflected the difference in the means of group A and C. The other group mean comparisons were nonsignificant.

SELF-TEST QUESTIONS: PART C

1. A basketball coach wants to know whether there is a significant difference in the mean agility scores for forwards, guards, and centers. Which of the following statistical procedures should be conducted?
   A. An independent samples t-test
   B. A one-way analysis of variance
   C. A three-way analysis of variance
   D. A Scheffé test

2. If one computes an ANOVA and finds a nonsignificant F value, what should be done next?
   A. Perform a post hoc multiple comparisons test, such as the Scheffé test, to determine which group means are significantly different from each other.
   B. Nothing; conclude that the observed differences in group means are probably due to sampling errors.
   Consider the following ANOVA summary table for questions 3 to 6:

SOURCE OF VARIATION	SUM OF SQUARES	df	MEAN SQUARES	F
Between	900	3	300	3.00
Within	2600	26	100	
Total	3500	29		

3. How many groups were compared? _____

4. How many total subjects were there across all groups? _____

5. What is the tabled critical value for $p = .10$? _____

6. Should a Scheffé test be conducted? _____

ANSWERS

1. B   2. B   3. 4 groups
4. 30 subjects   5. 2.31   6. Yes

Pearson Correlation: An Inferential Statistic

You are already familiar with this statistic. In Chapter 5 you learned to calculate and interpret the Pearson product moment correlation, also known as the Pearson r, as a descriptive statistic. When used as a descriptive statistic, Pearson r defines the strength and direction of the linear relationship between variable X and variable Y. (Variables X and Y are two different interval or ratio scores.) When Pearson r is used as an inferential statistic, it determines whether the relationship is significant. In other words, Pearson r tells whether the relationship found for the sample is likely to be true for the population. To determine statistical significance, compare the calculated r with a critical value. The significance rule is the same as for the t-test and ANOVA. If the calculated r equals or exceeds the tabled critical value, the relationship is significant. If the calculated r is less than the critical r, the relationship is nonsignificant.

Try an example. Table 5-9 calculated the relationship between the number of putts sunk at 5 feet and at 10 feet for a small group of beginning golfers. The raw data:

GOLFER	PUTTS AT 5 FEET	PUTTS AT 10 FEET
A	9	7
B	7	7
C	7	4
D	6	5
E	5	2

The value of r is +.79. The guidelines in Table 5-8 identify this as a strong correlation. If these golfers are a sample of a larger population, it is appropriate to ask whether the relationship is statistically significant. In other words, is the correlation found for the sample likely to exist in the population? Use Table 6-6 to find the critical value. You need df and p to use this table. Degrees of freedom for the Pearson r are determined by the formula $N-2$, that is, the number of subjects minus 2. In this example there are only three degrees of freedom. If you select a p value of .05, the tabled critical r value is .8783.

What is the decision? Since the calculated r of .79 is less than the critical r, the relationship is nonsignificant. In other words, even though there is a strong correlation in the five-person sample, it is unlikely that such a relationship exists in the population of beginning golfers. The null hypothesis assumed no correlation in the

TABLE 6-6	Table of Critical Values of *r*		
DEGREES OF FREEDOM[a] (N − 2)	*p* = .10 (.05 FOR 1-TAILED TEST)	*p* = .05 (.025 FOR 1-TAILED TEST)	*p* = .01 (.005 FOR 1-TAILED TEST)
1	.98769	.99692	.99988
2	.90000	.95000	.99000
3	.80540	.87830	.95873
4	.72930	.81140	.91720
5	.66940	.75450	.87450
6	.62150	.70670	.83430
7	.58220	.66640	.79770
8	.54940	.63190	.76460
9	.52140	.60210	.73480
10	.49730	.57600	.70790
11	.47620	.55290	.68350
12	.45750	.53240	.66140
13	.44090	.51390	.64110
14	.42590	.49730	.62260
15	.41240	.48210	.60550
16	.40000	.46830	.58970
17	.38870	.45550	.57510
18	.37830	.44380	.56140
19	.36870	.43290	.54870
20	.35980	.42270	.53680
25	.32330	.38090	.48690
30	.29600	.34940	.44870
35	.27460	.32460	.41820
40	.25730	.30440	.39320
45	.24280	.28750	.37210
50	.23060	.27320	.35410
60	.21080	.25000	.32480
70	.19540	.23190	.30170
80	.18290	.21720	.28300
90	.17260	.20500	.26730
100	.16380	.19460	.25400

There is a statistically significant relationship between variable *X* and variable *Y* if the calculated *r* equals or exceeds the tabled critical value.

[a]*N* is the total number of subjects for whom you have paired data on variable *X* and variable *Y*. Adapted from Fisher, R.A.: Statistical Tables for Biological, Agricultural and Medical Research. New York, Longman, 1995.

population; the null hypothesis is accepted. However, the decision for an r of $+.79$ would have been different with even a slightly larger sample; the critical r for a sample of 7 golfers ($df = 5$) is .7545. Furthermore, the decision regarding significance would be the same whether the r value was $+.79$ or $-.79$. Only the magnitude of the calculated value is considered in a two-tailed test of significance.

Simple Linear Prediction

Simple linear prediction is an extension of the Pearson r correlation. If two variables are found to be correlated, you can use the knowledge of their relationship to develop a **prediction** equation that will allow estimation from one variable to another. The stronger the linear correlation (i.e., the closer the data points fall to a straight line) in the sample, the better the prediction. Typical practice is to develop a prediction equation from a sample, then make predictions and apply them to the population from which the sample was drawn.

> Prediction is the process of estimating a score on one variable from knowledge of a score on another variable.

The general form of the equation for simple linear prediction:

$$Y' = bX + a$$

Formula 6-7

where Y' is the predicted Y value and X is the observed value. The b in this formula represents the slope of the line of best fit, that is, the straight line that minimizes the distances from the line for all data points in a scattergram. The Y intercept for the line of best fit is represented by a.

The values of b and a can be calculated from easy formulas. The formula for calculating b:

$$b = \frac{n\left(\sum XY\right) - \left(\sum X\right)\left(\sum Y\right)}{n\left(\sum X^2\right) - \left(\sum X\right)^2}$$

Formula 6-8

where n is the number of sample subjects (for whom we have paired data). The formula for calculating a:

$$a = \overline{Y} - b\overline{X}$$

Formula 6-9

Now apply these formulas to the example of the putting scores for the five beginning golfers. Calculating an r of $+.79$ (Table 5-9) produced intermediate values of $\Sigma X = 34$, $\Sigma Y = 25$, $\Sigma X^2 = 240$, and $\Sigma XY = 180$. The mean of X was 6.8 and the mean of Y was 5.0. Use these values in Formula 6-8 to find the value of b. The equation for this calculation:

$$b = \frac{5(180) - (34)(25)}{5(240) - (34)^2}$$

Rounding to three decimal places, b is 1.136. The value of a is found by solving the equation $a = \overline{Y} - b\overline{X}$. Thus a is -2.725.

You now have everything you need to define the linear prediction equation for this example:

$$Y' = 1.136 (X) - 2.725$$

This prediction equation can be used to find any value of X. Assume you wonder how a beginning golfer who sinks 8 putts from 5 feet will do from 10 feet. The answer is 6.4 putts.

Remember that Y' is an estimate. A strong and significant relationship between variables X and Y in the sample produces confidence that predictions are likely to be true for the population.

SELF-TEST QUESTIONS: PART D

1. An exercise physiologist wants to examine the nature of the relationship between isotonic and isometric measures of muscular endurance. Which of the following inferential statistical procedures should he or she use?
   A. An independent t-test
   B. A paired samples t-test
   C. A Pearson's product moment correlation
   D. A Spearman's ranked order correlation

2. For this example, 50 subjects are tested on both types of muscular endurance. How many degrees of freedom are there? _____

3. For this example, a p value of .05 is preselected and an r of +.84 is calculated. What is the tabled critical r? _____

4. Is the observed r statistically significant?

5. Is it *possible* that the observed correlation was obtained by chance?
   _____

6. Is it *likely* that the observed correlation was obtained by chance?
   _____

ANSWERS

1. C   2. 48   3. ≈.28
4. Yes   5. Yes   6. No

One-Way Chi Square

The final inferential statistic to be presented is the **chi square**, symbolized by χ^2. (I'm sure you'll be glad to know that we saved the easiest for last.) Chi square, which is used with nominal data, determines the significance of the pattern of the number of persons, objects, or responses that fall into two or more categories. The logic of this test is to compare the observed frequencies in each category with the frequencies that would be expected to occur by chance or according to a null hypothesis. If the observed and expected frequencies are similar in each category, the chi square test is nonsignificant. If the observed frequencies deviate considerably from the expected frequencies in one or more categories, the chi square test is significant. A significant chi square test suggests that there is likely to be a real difference across the categories in the population from which the sample was drawn.

> Chi square is a statistical test that determines the significance of the pattern of the number of persons, objects, or responses that fall into two or more categories.

Calculation of a One-Way Chi Square

Suppose a small college has decided to add one women's sport to its intercollegiate offerings. Which sport should it add? After considering cost, competition opportunities, and several other factors, the committee narrows the list of possible sports to three—say, lacrosse, fencing, and golf (Fig. 6-4). They ask 60 randomly selected women students to indicate which of the three sports they think should be added. If there is no difference among the preference for the sports, the same number will choose each sport, that is, 20 students would select each of the three sports. The hypothetical data:

	SPORT A	SPORT B	SPORT C
Observed	28	15	17
(Expected)	(20)	(20)	(20)

To determine whether the observed frequencies are significantly different from the expected frequencies, we calculate χ^2:

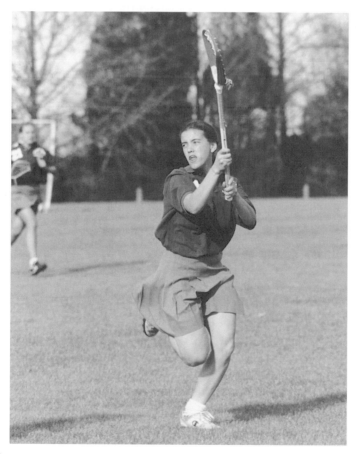

FIGURE 6-4

Should a small college add lacrosse to the intercollegiate sport offerings for women? (Photo by John Bell, Touch a Life Photography, Greensboro, NC.)

$$\chi^2 = \sum \frac{(O_i - E_i)^2}{E_i} \qquad \qquad \text{Formula 6-10}$$

where O_i represents the observed frequency for an individual category and E_i represents the expected frequency for that same category. The sum sign tells us to add all these values across all categories.

When we enter the values for this example into Formula 6-10, the equation is:

$$\chi^2 = \frac{(28 - 20)^2}{20} + \frac{(15 - 20)^2}{20} + \frac{(17 - 20)^2}{20}$$

The value of χ^2 is 4.90.

To decide about statistical significance, refer to Table 6-7, the table for critical values of χ^2. The *df* for a one-way χ^2 are determined by the formula $K - 1$, where K is the number of categories. In this example, K is 3, so *df* is 2. What is the critical value of χ^2 for a *p* value of .05 and 2 *dfs*? Yes, 5.991.

What's the decision? Since 4.90 is less than 5.991, there is no significant difference among the preferences for the three sports. Even though nearly half of the sample members preferred sport A, this pattern of responses is *not* significantly different from a pattern that could have occurred purely by chance.

SELF-TEST QUESTIONS: PART E

1. The inventor of a new sport drink wants to determine which of two flavors, mango kiwi or papaya coconut, is preferred by recreational runners. Can a one-way χ^2 test be used to study this question? _____

2. The inventor has 100 randomly selected runners test each of the flavors, then tell him which they prefer. What level of measurement are these data?

    _____

3. If there is really no clear preference among the population for one of the two flavors, what is the expected frequency among the 100 runners for mango kiwi and for papaya coconut? _____ and _____

4. For a one-way χ^2 test of significance, how many degrees of freedom are there?

    _____

5. Assume 60 runners expressed a preference for mango kiwi and 40 preferred papaya coconut. What is the calculated χ^2? _____

6. At the .05 level of significance ($p = .05$), is there a significant difference in these frequencies? _____ Assume the costs of making and marketing the wrong flavor of sport drink are very high. At the .01 level of significance ($p = .01$), is there a significant difference in these frequencies?

    _____

ANSWERS

1. Yes   2. Nominal   3. 50 and 50
4. $K - 1 = 1$ 5. $\chi^2 = 4.00$ 6. Yes; no

TABLE 6-7	Table of Critical Values of χ^2		

DEGREES OF FREEDOM[a]	$p = .10$	$p = .05$	$p = .01$
1	2.706	3.841	6.635
2	4.605	5.991	9.210
3	6.251	7.815	11.345
4	7.779	9.488	13.277
5	9.236	11.070	15.086
6	10.645	12.592	16.812
7	12.017	14.067	18.475
8	13.362	15.507	20.090
9	14.684	16.919	21.666
10	15.987	18.307	23.209
11	17.275	19.675	24.725
12	18.549	21.026	26.217
13	19.812	22.362	27.688
14	21.064	23.685	29.141
15	22.307	24.996	30.578
16	23.542	26.296	32.000
17	24.769	27.587	33.409
18	25.989	28.869	34.805
19	27.204	30.144	36.191
20	28.412	31.410	37.566
21	29.615	32.671	38.932
22	30.813	33.924	40.289
23	32.007	35.172	41.638
24	33.196	36.415	42.980
25	34.382	37.652	44.314
26	35.563	38.885	45.642
27	36.741	40.113	46.963
28	37.916	41.337	48.278
29	39.087	42.557	49.588
30	40.256	43.773	50.892

The observed pattern of frequencies is significant if the calculated chi square equals or exceeds the tabled critical value.
[a]$K - 1$ for one-way chi square where K is the number of categories (cells); $(R-1)(C-1)$ for factorial chi square where R is the number of rows and C is the number of columns.
Adapted from Fisher, R.A.: Statistical Tables for Biological, Agricultural and Medical Research. New York, Longman, 1995.

Use of Computers

Calculating more than just a few examples of inferential statistics by hand is not a good use of your time. (Wouldn't you rather see a good movie?) This section explores the use of computers for calculation of inferential statistics.

Chapter 5 identifies the options available to the person wanting to use a computer program for calculating descriptive statistics. It should come as no surprise to you that the options are essentially the same for inferential statistics. Many programs exist for mainframe computers (2–4). Many also exist for microcomputers. They vary considerably in cost and user friendliness.

Chapters 4 and 5 features the use of *Statistics on Software (S.O.S.)* for construction of frequency distributions and histograms and for calculation of several descriptive statistics (5). This easy-to-use shareware program for IBM-PCs is an excellent package for novices in statistics and computers. The next section demonstrates how to use *S.O.S.* for calculation of a number of inferential statistics. The ANOVA is demonstrated by means of a computer program called *MYSTAT* (6).

Calculation of the Independent Samples t-Test by *S.O.S.*

Earlier in this chapter you calculated an independent samples t-test for the following scores from two randomly formed samples:

X_A	X_B
7	6
6	5
5	4
5	3
4	2
3	

Hand calculations produced a *t* of 1.108. Since the calculated *t* was less than the critical value of 2.262 (Table 6-3, for 9 *df* and *p* = .05), you accepted the null hypothesis of no difference between the averages for the populations from which these samples were drawn. Now you will use these same data and conduct an independent samples t-test using the *S.O.S.* program. The steps:

Step 1. From the main menu, select 2 SAMPLE t-TEST FOR DIFF. IN MEANS. (This describes the function of the t-test for independent samples.)

Step 2. Respond to "ARE YOU WORKING WITH..." Select SAMPLE SETS. (This assumes that you will enter raw scores for the two samples.)

Step 3.   Respond to "Do you wish to restore a sample set from the data manage-ment file (Y/N)?" Select no if you have not yet entered the data, select yes if you have previously entered the data by means of the data management option.

Step 4.   Select 2-tailed test.

Step 5.   Select level of significance of .05.

Step 6.   Define hypothesized difference between means as 0.000.

Step 7.   Enter scores for sample #1 data: 7, 6, 5, 5, 4, 3. (Scores are entered by typing the score value, then hitting the Enter key. After all scores are entered, hit the Page Down key.)

Step 8.   Answer yes to the question, "Test for normality (Y/N)?" (This is a re-quirement for valid use of the t-test. The computer screen will display the distribu-tion of scores within 1, 2, 3, and 4 standard deviations of the mean. The data are considered to be normally distributed if approximately 68% of the scores fall within ± 1 standard deviations (s) of the mean, approximately 95% of the scores fall within ± 2 s of the mean, and 99% of the scores fall within ± 3 s of the mean.)

Step 9.   Enter scores for sample #2 data: 6, 5, 4, 3, 2.

Step 10.   Answer yes to "Test for normality?" Also answer yes to "Are popula-tion variances approximately equal (Y/N)?"

Step 11.   Inspect the screen for the results of the independent samples t-test (Fig. 6-5). Print the screen by hitting the Print Screen key on your computer if you wish to have a hard copy of the t-test results.

```
         TWO SAMPLE STUDENT'S t-TEST FOR DIFFERENCES BETWEEN MEANS

   TWO-TAILED TEST                     df  =    9

                SAMPLE 1                          SAMPLE 2
   n   =        6                      n   =      5

   X̄   =        5.00000               X̄   =      4.00000

   s   =        1.41421               s   =      1.58114

   s² =         2.00000               s² =       2.50000

   RETAIN THE NULL HYPOTHESIS AT THE .0500 LEVEL OF SIGNIFICANCE
   BECAUSE t OF 1.107823 IS < THE CRITICAL VALUE OF 2.262000.

   P Value is greater than .200

           EXAMPLE OF AN INDEPENDENT SAMPLES T-TEST BY S.O.S.
```

FIGURE 6-5

Results of an independent samples t-test by *S.O.S.* microcomputer program. (Reprinted with permission from Timko, J., and Downie, J.: Statistics on Software, Version 2.0. Or-ange, CA, Statistics for Management, 1992.)

The _S.O.S._ results state, "RETAIN THE NULL HYPOTHESIS AT THE .0500 LEVEL OF SIGNIFICANCE BECAUSE _t_ OF 1.107823 IS LESS THAN THE CRITICAL VALUE OF 2.262000." Yes, the results of the _S.O.S._ t-test and our hand calculations are identical.

Calculation of the Paired Samples t-Test by _S.O.S._

The steps for this calculation are similar to those for the independent samples t-test:

**Step 1.** From the main menu, select T-TEST FOR PAIRED DIFFERENCES.

**Step 2.** Respond to "Do you wish to restore a sample set from the data management file (Y/N)?" Select no if you have not yet entered the data.

**Step 3.** Select 2-TAILED TEST.

**Step 4.** Select LEVEL OF SIGNIFICANCE of .05.

**Step 5.** Define POPULATION MEAN DIFFERENCE as 0.000.

**Step 6.** Enter paired scores in columns 1 and 2: 6 and 9, 5 and 9, 4 and 3, 3 and 7, and 2 and 7. Hit Page Down after entering all data.

**Step 7.** Answer yes to "TEST FOR NORMALITY (Y/N)?"

**Step 8.** Answer yes to "ARE THE DIFFERENCES BETWEEN PAIRS NORMALLY DISTRIBUTED (Y/N)?"

**Step 9.** Inspect the screen for the results of the paired samples t-test (Fig. 6-6). The test results call for rejection of the null hypothesis at the .05 level of significance. This was the same conclusion reached via our hand calculations. Ta-dah!

```
   t   TEST    FOR    DIFFERENCES    BETWEEN    PAIRS


   TWO-TAILED TEST                 df   = 4

   n   = 5

   X̄(D) = -3.00000            µ(D) = 0.00000

   s(D) = 2.34521


   REJECT THE NULL HYPOTHESIS AT THE .0500 LEVEL OF SIGNIFICANCE
   BECAUSE t OF -2.860388 IS >= THE CRITICAL VALUE OF -2.776000.

   P Value is between .050 and .020


             EXAMPLE OF A PAIRED SAMPLES T-TEST BY S.O.S.
```

FIGURE 6-6

Results of a paired samples t-test by _S.O.S._ microcomputer program. (Reprinted with permission from Timko, J., and Downie, J.: Statistics on Software, Version 2.0. Orange, CA, Statistics for Management, 1992.)

Calculation of a One-Way ANOVA by *MYSTAT*

The *S.O.S.* statistical package does not include an option for a one-way ANOVA. So for this demonstration, we will use *MYSTAT* (6). *MYSTAT* is a commercially available statistics package that offers full-screen spreadsheet data entry for a wide variety of descriptive and inferential statistics. It can handle up to 50 variables and 32,000 cases. There are versions available for IBM-PC and for Macintosh.

These are the directions for using the IBM-PC version of *MYSTAT* to conduct a one-way ANOVA on the data presented earlier in this chapter:

Step 1. From the menu, select EDIT. (The function EDIT is used to enter, edit, and transform data.)

Step 2. Label two columns for data entry; enter "GROUP" and "SCORE". (Variable names must be in single or double quotation marks.) Press the Home key to move the cursor to the first blank cell under GROUP.

Step 3. Enter data as shown in Figure 6-7. After entering all data, press the Esc key to move the cursor to the prompt (>) under the worksheet.

Step 4. Save the data under a file name up to 8 characters long. Do this by typing SAVE <file name>.

Step 5. At the prompt, instruct the program to USE <file name>.

Step 6. Enter CATEGORY GROUP = 3.

Step 7. Enter ANOVA SCORE.

		GROUP	SCORE
CASE	1	1.000	4.000
CASE	2	1.000	3.000
CASE	3	1.000	3.000
CASE	4	1.000	3.000
CASE	5	1.000	2.000
CASE	6	2.000	7.000
CASE	7	2.000	6.000
CASE	8	2.000	5.000
CASE	9	2.000	4.000
CASE	10	2.000	3.000
CASE	11	3.000	7.000
CASE	12	3.000	7.000
CASE	13	3.000	6.000
CASE	14	3.000	5.000
CASE	15	3.000	5.000

FIGURE 6-7

Data entry for one-way ANOVA for comparison of three group means for *MYSTAT* microcomputer program. (Reprinted with permission from SYSTAT: MYSTAT, Version 2.1.)

```
                    ANALYSIS OF VARIANCE

SOURCE    SUM-OF-SQUARES    DF   MEAN-SQUARE    F-RATIO      P

 GROUP          23.333      2      11.667       8.750     0.005


 ERROR          16.000     12       1.333
```

FIGURE 6-8

Results of a one-way ANOVA by *MYSTAT* microcomputer program. (Reprinted with permission from SYSTAT: MYSTAT, Version 2.1.)

Step 8.   Enter ESTIMATE.

Step 9.   Inspect the screen for the results of the one-way ANOVA (Fig. 6-8). Except for minor differences due to rounding, the results match those found by hand calculation. *MYSTAT* does not state a decision for the user. It does, however, provide a p value associated with these calculations. If the printed p is equal to or less than the preselected probability level, the decision is to reject the null hypothesis.

Calculation of Pearson Correlation and Prediction by S.O.S.

To have *S.O.S.* calculate Pearson r for the correlation between putts of two distances for five beginning golfers, follow these steps:

Step 1.   From the main menu, select PEARSON'S CORRELATION & SIMPLE LINEAR REGRESSION ANALYSIS.

Step 2.   Respond to "DO YOU WISH TO RESTORE A SAMPLE SET FROM THE DATA MANAGEMENT FILE (Y/N)?" Select no if you have not yet entered the data.

Step 3.   Select 2-TAILED TEST.

Step 4.   Select LEVEL OF SIGNIFICANCE of .05.

Step 5.   Enter pairs of data into columns X and Y: 9 and 7, 7 and 7, 7 and 4, 6 and 5, 5 and 2. After all scores are entered, press the Page Down key.

Step 6.   Inspect the screen for the results of the Pearson correlation. Notice that the results provide r and a statement, "RETAIN THE NULL HYPOTHESIS AT THE .0500 LEVEL OF SIGNIFICANCE BECAUSE r OF 0.794552 IS LESS THAN THE CRITICAL VALUE OF 0.878000."

Step 7.   Respond yes to the question, "DO YOU WANT TO PREDICT A "Y" VALUE FROM AN "X" VALUE (Y/N)?". At the prompt, type in the X value, 8.

Step 8.   Inspect the results. Notice the values are given for Y', a, and b (Fig. 6-9).

```
ĕĕĕĕĕĕĕĕĕĕĕĕĕĕĕĕĕĕĕĕĕĕĕĕĕĕĕĕĕĕĕĕĕĕĕĕĕĕĕĕĕĕĕĕĕĕĕĕĕĕĕĕĕĕĕĕĕĕĕĕĕĕĕĕĕ£
¤  P E A R S O N ' S   P R O D U C T - M O M E N T   C O R R E L A T I O N   ¤
úááááááááááááááááááááááááááááaaaaaaaaaaaaaaaaaaaaaaaaaaaaaaaaaaaaaaaaaaaN
¤                                                                          ¤
¤                                                                          ¤
¤   TWO-TAILED TEST                              X VALUE =     8.000       ¤
¤                                                                          ¤
¤   n = 5                    X̄    = 6.80000      Y' = 6.364                ¤
¤                                                a  = -2.727               ¤
¤   r = 0.79455              s(x) = 1.32665      b  = 1.136                ¤
¤                                                                          ¤
¤   r² = 0.63131             Ȳ    = 5.00000                                ¤
¤                                                                          ¤
¤   k² = 0.36869             s(y) = 1.89737                                ¤
¤                                                                          ¤
¤   RETAIN THE NULL HYPOTHESIS AT THE .0500 LEVEL OF SIGNIFICANCE          ¤
¤   BECAUSE r OF 0.794552 IS < THE CRITICAL VALUE OF 0.878000.             ¤
¤                                                                          ¤
¤   P Value is greater than .100                                          ¤
¤                                                                          ¤
úáááááááááááááááááááááááááááááááááááááááááááááááááááááááááááááááááááááááÑ
¤       EXAMPLE OF PEARSON CORRELATION & LINEAR REGRESSION BY S.O.S.       ¤
ãĕĕĕĕĕĕĕĕĕĕĕĕĕĕĕĕĕĕĕĕĕĕĕĕĕĕĕĕĕĕĕĕĕĕĕĕĕĕĕĕĕĕĕĕĕĕĕĕĕĕĕĕĕĕĕĕĕĕĕĕĕĕĕĕĕ¥
```

FIGURE 6-9

Results of a Pearson correlation and prediction by *S.O.S.* microcomputer program. (Reprinted with permission from Timko, J., and Downie, J.: Statistics on Software, Version 2.0. Orange, CA, Statistics for Management, 1992.)

Calculation of One-Way Chi Square by *S.O.S.*

Procedures to calculate a one-way chi square by *S.O.S.* are given next. Data are as in the chi square example given earlier in this chapter.

Step 1. From the main menu, select GOODNESS-OF-FIT TEST.

Step 2. Enter 3 in response to "ENTER NUMBER OF CELLS".

Step 3. Select LEVEL OF SIGNIFICANCE as .05.

Step 4. For each cell, enter the observed frequencies [f (o)] and the expected frequencies [f (e)]: 28 and 20, 15 and 20, 17 and 20.

Step 5. Inspect the results. The decision: "RETAIN THE NULL HYPOTHESIS AT THE .0500 LEVEL OF SIGNIFICANCE BECAUSE CHI SQUARE IF 4.900000 IS LESS THAN THE CRITICAL VALUE OF 5.991000" (Fig. 6-10).

Chapter Summary

Inferential statistics are important tools for the ESS professional. They allow the professional to make informed decisions on the basis of sample data. Although there are hundreds of inferential statistics, some are commonly used by nearly all ESS professionals. These include t-tests, ANOVAs, Pearson correlations and predictions, and chi square tests. Each of these tests has a specific function for analyses of specific types of data.

Before you can fully appreciate the calculations and interpretations of individual inferential statistics, it is important to understand the concepts that underlie the use of all inferential statistics. One of the most important concepts is that the samples used to make inferences must be representative of their populations. Another impor-

```
GOODNESS   OF   FIT   TEST

   df =   2          α = 0.05        χ² >=   5.9910

   f(o)    f(e)
   28      20        3.20
   15      20        1.25
   17      20        0.45




   RETAIN THE NULL HYPOTHESIS AT THE .0500 LEVEL OF SIGNIFICANCE
   BECAUSE  χ² OF 4.900000 IS < THE CRITICAL VALUE OF 5.991000.

   P Value is between .100 and .050

              EXAMPLE OF A ONE-WAY CHI SQUARE TEST BY S.O.S.
```

FIGURE 6-10

Results of a one-way chi square test by *S.O.S.* microcomputer program. (Reprinted with permission from Timko, J., and Downie, J.: Statistics on Software, Version 2.0. Orange, CA, Statistics for Management, 1992.)

tant concept is that sampling errors, that is, the expected variations in statistical values within samples, are normally distributed. Statistical significance is the conclusion that the observed values (or differences or relationships) in the sample are real, that is, they are unlikely to be due to mere chance.

Inferential statistics can be calculated by hand or by computer. In either case, a decision is made by comparing the calculated statistic with the critical value associated with the appropriate degrees of freedom at a preselected level of significance.

DOING PROJECTS FOR FURTHER LEARNING

1. Go to the library and find a current issue of a research journal that publishes quantitative research in your area of interest. For example, an athletic trainer might select the *Journal of Athletic Training*; an aspiring sport manager might select the *Journal of Sport Management*; a physical education major might select the *Journal of Teaching in Physical Education*. Skim the Results section of several articles and select one article that used at least one of the inferential statistics discussed in this chapter. Then do the following:

    A. List all of the statistics that are reported in the Results section of the research report. How many of the statistics are familiar to you? How many are unfamiliar?
    B. Review the descriptive statistics that were calculated for the sample or samples. In your own words, describe the central tendency and the variability of the sample data.
    C. Review at least one of the inferential statistics reported in the Results. What level of probability was used? How do you know? How many subjects were in the sample? How do you know? Was statistical significance found? How do you know?

2. Make an appointment with an ESS professional (a professor or a practitioner) who is an active researcher. Ask him or her to explain how inferential statistics are used in his or her research. What computer programs does he or she use for statistical analyses?

3. Create several small sets (no more than 10 cases) of hypothetical data, using the examples in this chapter as a guide. Practice calculating inferential statistics by hand and by computer. Compare the results.

REFERENCES

1. Gay, L.R.: Educational Research: Competencies for Analysis and Applications. 5th ed. Paramus, NJ, Prentice Hall, 1995.
2. Statistical Package for the Social Sciences Staff: SPSS Base 7.5 for Windows: User's Guide. Paramus, NJ, Prentice Hall, 1996.
3. Statistical Analysis System Institute: SAS/ETS User's Guide, Version 6. Cary, NC, Statistical Analysis System Institute, 1998.
4. Minitab Staff: Stat 101: Software for Statistics Instruction. Reading, MA, Addison Wesley Longman, 1993.
5. Timko, J., and Downie, J.: Statistics on Software, Version 2.0. Orange, CA: Statistics for Management, 1992.
6. Aczel, A.D.: Complete Business Statistics MYSTAT Software with QC Tools. Burr Ridge, IL, McGraw-Hill Higher Education, 1994.

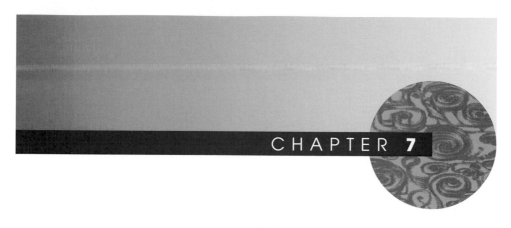

CHAPTER **7**

Using Assessment Data for Grading

At their best grades are informative and positively reinforcing. However, grades are often vague and demotivating, even to some students who are good at physical education (1, 2). Anyone who aspires to be a good educator must learn to grade so as to produce positive outcomes. Chapter 7 examines common grading practices and offers suggestions for improving grading practices.

The original of this chapter was written by Rosemary McGee for the fourth edition of this textbook (3). Her chapter received high praise from readers and reviewers, so it is included here with only minor modifications. Information on computer-assisted grading has been updated, some references have been updated, and a few changes were made to achieve greater consistency with the layout of other chapters in this text.

As you read this chapter, watch for the following keywords:

Change score
  (improvement score)
Contract grading
Criterion-referenced
  grading

Discrimination
Gender-fair grading
Grades
Grade inflation

Grade point
  (grade point average)
Multiple grades
Weighting

Common Frustrations in Grading

Grading probably causes more consternation than any other aspect of education. Doubtless, **grades** are often a chore to teachers and an enigma to students. Several reasons emerge to account for frustrations with grading. Among them are (*a*) vagueness in defining levels of excellence, (*b*) use of varying grading scales, (*c*) problems converting performances to a 100-point scale, (*d*) indecision about where to make cutoffs, (*e*) difficulty with grading small classes fairly, and (*f*) confusion about what to include in the grade and how to weight each factor.

What Do YOU Think?

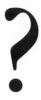

Imagine the case of Jessica, an 18-year-old high school senior. The dean of students has just informed her that she will graduate second in her class. Jessica is disappointed. She hoped that her hard work over the past 4 years would place her at the very top of her class, not in second place. After all, she earned all A's—except for two B's in required first-year physical education.

It does not seem fair to Jessica that physical education is her undoing. It's true that she wasn't very good in any of the activities they did—volleyball, archery, tennis, and track. In fact, she really was quite awful, but she had good attendance, had a positive attitude, got A's on all the written tests, and actually improved her performances a little during each of the instructional units. Jessica thinks the B's were probably fair grades. What she thinks is unfair is that physical education grades should figure into her overall grade point average in the same way as grades from "real" classes.

What do YOU think? Were the B's that Jessica received in physical education fair grades? Do you think it is right that physical education grades are counted in a student's overall grade point average? Is there a better way to handle physical education grades? Is physical education a "real" subject that is just as important as other subjects (4)?

> Grades are symbols used to denote an estimate of students' status, progress, and/or achievement.

Two recent additions to the long list of frustrations are **grade inflation** and diversity of factors included in grades. The interpretation of grades is so varied that some educators believe grades are becoming nearly meaningless. An A is no longer a symbol of excellence; it may be the result of no more than above-average work. C traditionally represented average work, but B is now the most frequently occurring grade. Grade inflation has eroded commonly held interpretations of letter grades. Once upon a time, if a student received a B in a beginning tennis class, one could expect that student to play a better-than-average game for a beginner and to know something about the rules, strategy, and techniques of the game. Today that same B may mean that the student tried hard, improved greatly, and/or attended regularly. The grade does not necessarily reflect the student's level of performance. The more sensitive atmosphere in education is to be applauded, but the realities of accountability and credibility must still be faced.

> Grade inflation is a systematic increase in grades given for work of a constant quality or quantity.

Special Grading Concerns

Several measurement practices have the potential to make grading more effective and efficient. To address these concerns, criterion-referenced grading, gender-fair grading, ability grouping, multiple grades, improvement scores, and computer-assisted grading are topics discussed in this chapter.

Criterion-Referenced Grading

Traditionally grades were norm-referenced. Students were compared with others of their peer group and often made to feel that they were competing for achievement. Kleinsasser called the traditional approach to grading an academic economy in which the currency is the number of A's, B's, C's, D's, and F's distributed (5). The underlying theory of the academic economy is that there must be fewer A's than B's or C's. However, **criterion-referenced grading** is becoming more prevalent. This is the result of task-referenced or mastery learning, that is, the practice of holding students, teachers, and school systems accountable by setting specific standards of achievement. Tasks are set by the teacher, sometimes in conjunction with students, and are designed to reflect the learning requirements for a course, unit, or lesson. Students are then assessed in relation to their achievement in accomplishing the set tasks. Because they are not assessed in relation to each other, students understand that they are not competing for a limited number of high grades.

> Criterion-referenced grading is the practice of assigning grades to students' performance in accordance with a specific standard of achievement.

The implication may seem to be that criterion-referenced assessment has become the only acceptable way to measure achievement. This is not intended. Sometimes norm-referenced assessment is meaningful and helpful to the student, just as sometimes self-referenced assessment is appropriate. What is intended is that criterion-referenced assessment be given more consideration. In the past, norm-referenced evaluation was almost the sole basis of assigning grades and consequently contributed to problems such as how to arrive at grades for small groups. Criterion-referenced assessment demands a more precise statement of objectives and clarification of learning expectations. This type of assessment is prevalent in school systems with systemwide or statewide competency-based curricula. Competency levels are determined with norm-referenced information, and subsequent testing for students' achievement uses a criterion-referenced orientation.

Often mastery learning can be assessed periodically within a unit, reflecting formative evaluation. Even at these times the teacher must use some norm-based frame of reference to establish reasonable levels of mastery at various stages in the unit. The summary measure may be either criterion-referenced or norm-referenced, depending on how the grade is to be used and on the levels of achievement that have been set. It seems reasonable to expect a criterion-referenced measure used for summate purposes to be somewhat congruent with the norm expectations of the group. This may not be true, however, in school systems that use competency-based curricula and that are trying to upgrade students' performance by expecting more of both teachers and students.

Gender-Fair Grading

Since the advent of Title IX legislation requiring coeducational enrollment in physical education classes, there has been concern about **gender-fair grading.** For performance evaluation when size, strength, and/or speed are involved, separate standards are usually needed for the genders. Knowledge, participation, and effort, aspects often included in physical education grades, do not and should not require separate standards.

Deutsch (6) explained the challenge of gender-fair grading: "The dilemma which must be addressed is if the same standard is used for both boys and girls, the result may be [that] lower grades occur for one sex. On the other hand, if one uses a double standard, this may serve to perpetuate sex differences. It would seem that, if a grade is based solely upon innate factors which favor one sex (for example, upper body strength for males), different standards should be used. If a grading plan encompasses a balance in skill factors and includes a process and product orientation, a single standard is in order thereby facilitating the equity orientation (6)".

> Gender-fair grading is the practice of assigning grades in such a way that grade distributions for both genders are approximately the same.

McGonagle and Stevens (7) submitted to the Illinois State Board of Education an approach to gender-fair grading. Their plan placed more emphasis on the quality of movement than on results of the movement, especially for results of movements in which there was a distinct strength advantage. Skills were scored on a range of 0 to 3, the total score being incorporated into the unit grade. In this way students could be evaluated on their skill performance using the same criteria without regard to gender. Figure 7-1 illustrates the system McGonagle and Stevens recommended for grading a volleyball skill.

In the McGonagle and Stevens system some of the skill assessment is objective, but most is subjective. The teacher can select the aspects of the activity to be evaluated and the methods of assessing them. The figure further shows the role of skill assessment in the overall physical education grades in the Evanston system. These weightings could be adjusted to fit the grading philosophy of the individual teacher, school, or system. The figure shows one way to accommodate gender-fair grading in the skill area.

Ability Grouping

Ability grouping is advocated within classes if enrollments are not homogeneous. If 9th- to 12th-graders with diverse skill levels are enrolled in the same class, subgroupings help with instruction as well as with grading. Groupings do require a little extra administrative time at the beginning of a unit. Nonetheless, the potential to enhance the learning environment and fairness in grading seems to justify the time. Ability grouping is one of the primary ways of meeting Title IX legislative requirements and assigning gender-fair grades.

When a disability places a restriction on the degree of proficiency a mainstreamed student can attain in fitness or sports skills, some adjustment should be made. The special student should receive a fair and encouraging grade within the limits of his or her abilities.

Multiple Grades

Often confronted with large classes of many different skill levels that meet 2 to 5 times a week, many physical educators resort to computing grades based on behaviors that are unrelated to performance or knowledge objectives, for example, partici-

VOLLEYBALL SKILL EVALUATION	
Scoring: Each area of evaluation is scored from 0 to 3 points.	
	Example
Serve	
Successful serves in 3 tries	2
Toss	2
Strike	3
Follow-through	2
Bump (forearm pass)	
Successful passes in 3 tries	2
Legs	3
Arms	2
Hands	2
Overhead set	
Successful sets in 3 tries	3
Legs	3
Arms	2
Hands	2
TOTAL SKILL TEST POINTS (36 maximum)	28

POINTS TO GRADE CONVERSION	
30–36	A
24–29	B (in example, 28 points = B)
17–23	C
14–16	D
13 or fewer	No credit

EXAMPLE AS APPLIED TO EVANSTON TOWNSHIP HIGH SCHOOL GRADING SYSTEM		
Participation	40%	A
Effort	30	A
Skill	20	B
Written test	10	B
	Unit grade = A–	

FIGURE 7-1

Gender-Fair Grading for Volleyball Skill Used at Evanston Township High School in Evanston, Illinois

pation, effort, and discipline (8). Some teachers also include improvement as a component of the grade. This is inconsistent with other subject fields and tends to distort the meaning of the grade. For this reason there is merit in considering a physical education grading plan that shows **multiple grades.** One grade may represent achievement in motor performance and knowledge; this is the "real" grade comparable with grades received in other subjects. Participation, effort, discipline, and improvement grades may be reported separately for physical education just as for other subjects. Adding or averaging these grades makes the overall physical education grade less informative than the use of multiple grades. An example later in the chapter shows use of multiple grades.

> Multiple grades refers to the practice in which two or more grades are reported to represent a student's status in different areas of concern within a teaching unit. For example, one grade is reported for motor skill, another for participation, effort, and discipline, and a third for improvement.

Lashuk (9) recommended a different approach to multiple grades. He argued that traditional techniques of classroom grading are seldom applicable to physical education classes because other subject areas report grades related solely to cognitive learning. Since physical education has objectives in several domains, we should report grades of achievement in each of the areas that constitute its mandate. Lashuk advocated a grading system and report card unique to physical education. This multiple grading plan would accommodate the uniqueness of physical education.

Improvement Scores

It is difficult to evaluate improvement because the increment of gain varies in qualitative value. It becomes increasingly difficult to improve as one becomes more skilled. For example, it is easier for a golfer to cut his or her score from 120 to 110 than to reduce the score from 80 to 70. The **change score (improvement score)** traditionally has been treated as a valid component in the grading formula. It is now commonly acknowledged that there should be adjustments in change scores to address the inequity of scores along an improvement continuum. The improvement grade also provides another opportunity for a two- to a three-track multiple grading system. If such information is deemed important enough to be reported, improvement can be assessed and reported separately from the grade that reflects actual achievement.

> A change score (improvement score) is a numerical value that represents the gain or loss between measures taken at two different times.

 ## Computer-Assisted Grading

Computer software makes grading more efficient. In addition, once established, the printed results provide more information for students and parents than do traditional grades. Computer programs such as Aeius Gradebook, Class Recorder & Grader, Darn Good Grade Book, Gradebook For Windows, and Making the Grade are all available to review from SOFTSHARE for a minimal initial cost (10). These programs are worth the attention of every physical educator. They can average, weigh, convert to standard or norm scales, give means, standard deviations, scale, and convert scores to letter grades. If a grading program is unavailable, grade reports can also be created with a spreadsheet program such as Excel or Quatro Pro.

Purposes of Grading

Physical education is a part of total education. To achieve this portion of education, objectives have been established to serve as guides and to indicate direction. It has been suggested that grades be used to indicate students' achievement in terms of stated objectives. Such grades have several purposes and are useful for the following groups.

Students

Grades are useful to students. Grades may indicate standing within the group with respect to established objectives. They may show standing in relation to the mastery level of predetermined content. They may motivate the student to greater efforts. In addition, students' attitudes toward physical education and their feelings about themselves may be positively influenced.

There is, however, a major danger inherent in grades. Since the grades themselves are frequently more tangible than the goals they represent, they sometimes become ends rather than means. Grades are often the primary object that the student seeks. Of course, the student should be more interested in the degree of progress toward the objectives and the outcomes they represent. This preferred attitude is most likely to occur when the grades are fair representations of the achievement of objectives.

Parents and Guardians

Grades enable parents and guardians to follow the progress and achievements of their children. Parents and guardians can be informed about the overall objectives of physical education and of objectives for specific units and can be furnished the facts about their child's progress toward the objectives. Grades probably provide one of the most important links between the parent and the school. Expanded report cards and conferences between students, teachers, and parents can be beneficial.

Teachers

Grades serve many purposes for the teacher. First, they encourage the teacher to make a competent evaluation of each student, providing a comprehensive understanding of the student. Second, they furnish information to assist in the teacher's role of helping students to learn. In addition, the teacher is provided with data that can be used to evaluate the effectiveness of the program and the quality of the teaching. Grades indirectly reflect a teacher's philosophy of education, professional attitudes, and goals.

Administrators

Grades are absolutely necessary data for the school administrator. Both educational accountability and administrative decisions frequently stem from interpretations of the performance records of students. Grades are used as a basis for graduation and promotion, for academic honors, for college entrance, and for guidance. Physical education grades should be considered in conjunction with other academic grades whenever academic decisions are made about students. If they represent pupils' progress and achievement, they should become a part of the permanent records of the school.

Measurable Factors

There is no single best method of grading, although all good systems have certain characteristics and are based on definite well-established criteria. The system of grading selected by a teacher should reflect his or her basic beliefs and philosophy of grading. The kind of grades (or whether or not there are grades at all in physical education) depends on the instructor's philosophy, modified by the policies of a particular school system. Also, students' achievement in physical education classes reflects the focus of the evaluation system (11, 12). Students graded heavily on skills demonstrate more on-task behaviors and perform better at the conclusion of the instructional unit than do those who are graded on other standards.

In general, if a program is to accomplish the recognized, well-rounded objectives of physical education, grades must reflect several factors. Procedures for evaluating each factor must be determined. Certainly a large proportion of a student's grade should be based on the results of assessments of skills acquired, fitness developed, and knowledge learned (Fig. 7-2).

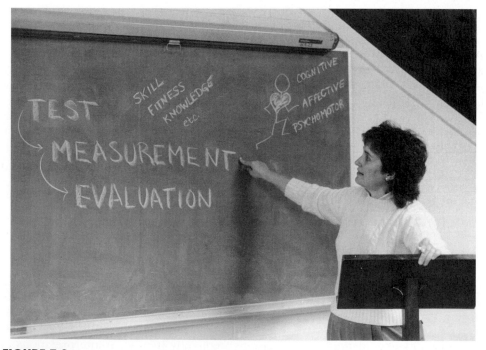

FIGURE 7-2

Grades in physical education are often a composite of factors such as skill, fitness, and knowledge. (Photo by Dr. Karen Uhlendorf, University of Vermont, Burlington, VT.)

Psychomotor Factors

Probably the most commonly used factors for grading in physical education are skill in the activity, game performance, and fitness. These factors should be weighted as logic dictates and should usually be consistent with the time allotted to each. In the skills area the grade for each sport or activity area might be determined with several measures, for example a skill test or rating scale, performance on a team, tournament standing in individual sports, and a subjective analysis of the student's ability to play the sport. While skill tests can play an important role, they are not the only way by which to determine students' abilities in the various skills of the sport.

Cognitive Factors

A portion of the grade should reflect the cognitive domain based on understanding, application, and analysis of the activity. Usually included on tests are questions about rules, performance, strategy, techniques, history, and information concerning physiology, fitness, and conditioning. Knowledge tests for fitness, sports, and other activities are generally objective but may come in any format. Standardized tests may be employed, but usually a well-constructed homemade test is better for local use.

Affective Factors

The affective assessment may include evaluation of such factors as attitude, appreciation, sportsmanship, cooperation, helpfulness, and leadership. A liberal definition of the affective domain includes social qualities, although there is some thought that the social area should be identified by a domain of its own. The student should be evaluated on the affective area but probably not graded in the sense of an official recording. If it is a matter of record, the affective grade should be separated from the grade representing achievement in the motor and cognitive objectives. Such a multiple grade system is practiced in many schools. This practice isolates the affective assessment. The affective grade submitted by the teacher should be free of personal bias and have no bearing on cognitive and motor assessments.

Affective and social qualities are best assessed on the basis of observation and ratings by both the teacher and students themselves. Self-appraisal records must be used judiciously, however, since some students tend to rate themselves too severely and some too leniently. Numerous checklists and rating scales are available. These tools are valuable for assessing such subjective factors as responsibility, behavior, and self-concept (Fig. 7-3).

Questionable Factors

Items such as showers, absences, dress, and punctuality have been used in grading. These administrative concerns seem out of place and are questionable factors in grading. They should be addressed by departmental policies but should not be part of the grade. Grades based on showers and dress are held by many to be inconsistent with modern philosophies of physical education. These factors are important and should be emphasized, but they should not be used as factors in grades. When

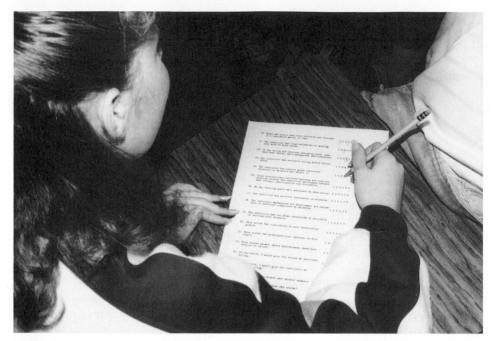

FIGURE 7-3

A student's affective development can be evaluated by means of a self-report rating scale. (Photo by Dr. Karen Uhlendorf, University of Vermont, Burlington, VT.)

included, they are viewed as a weapon to enforce desired student behavior. Grades based on these items mislead both parents and administrators.

The practice of grading partly on participation or attendance is fairly common. Those who would lower a grade because of excessive excuses from participation argue that the student who does not participate cannot hope to achieve the course objectives. More logically, a participation grade may be justified as a supplement to imperfect and incomplete skill assessments. Nevertheless, those who are opposed to grading directly on participation contend that absences from class are reflected in the achievement of the student anyway, and thus participation is an inconsequential factor. It is probably true that the final status of any student in well-organized programs of physical education is somewhat lower if participation is poor.

Effort is another factor mentioned frequently in any discussion of grading. Effort is used as a factor of grading because it is believed by some to motivate students. Effort is similar to improvement in that it is difficult to evaluate. In the early stages of learning, it is easy to identify the effort being put forth by the learner. The learner often must expend a great amount of effort to accomplish a little. As the student becomes more proficient, however, accomplishment is possible with less effort. The record breaker in a mile run usually comes in with knees high and in full stride, whereas the last-place runner plods along, struggling to keep moving. It is virtually impossible to attach a value to levels of effort. It does make sense, however, to grade on level of achievement. Achievement can be evaluated and definitely is related to effort.

Criteria for Grades

Relation to Objectives

Grades must be determined in relation to stated objectives. It is necessary to determine what each student should be able to achieve in each unit of instruction. The grade should then indicate the student's degree of proficiency in the established objectives of the program. The final grade usually reflects a combination of the psychomotor and cognitive achievements of the student in relation to the unit objectives.

Validity

Validity in respect to grading simply means that grades truthfully measure the qualities or factors intended. Grades should honestly represent the achievements for which they are purportedly a symbol. The validity of most grading systems is lessened somewhat by the fact that if grades are to be related to objectives, the physical educator must measure the immeasurable or the hard-to-measure. Frequently, the intangibles are more valuable than the measurable qualities in the quest for good living. For example, such qualities as team spirit and willingness to sacrifice oneself for the good of the group are important in team games and sports, but it is difficult to assign a degree of achievement to them. Validity can never be as high as desired. When the intangibles are objectified, something is inevitably lost in the process, in the same manner that something is lost when a circle is squared or when a poem is translated.

The validity of the grading system is enhanced when there is congruency among the values, objectives, procedures, and evaluation. For example, if a program emphasizes the motor development of the student, the values, objectives, procedures, and evaluation should be consistent with that emphasis. The orientation in modern education has put a renewed emphasis on self-concept and self-direction, on helpful caring interpersonal relationships, and on aesthetic sensibilities. This emphasis may be stressed more than the psychomotor and intellectual growth of the student. If this is the case, certain values, objectives, and procedures accrue, and the evaluation procedures must be congruent with that curricular philosophy. The same is true of curricula that emphasize the fitness objective of physical activity; evaluative procedures must be consistent with that thrust.

Reliability

The system must report consistently whatever it does report. The reliability of the grading system may be determined by asking, "Will the system be apt to generate the same grades for students if their performances are reassessed?" An affirmative answer means the system has reliability.

Objectivity

Objectivity in grading means the degree to which different instructors arrive at the same grade for the same student when they have access to the same information. In other words, an objective grading system generates the same grade for each student regardless of who does the grading. This implies, of course, that to eliminate bias and subjective opinion, objective tests should be used when available. However, not all important objectives of physical education can be measured in quantitative terms. When no objective tests are available to measure a particular factor, subjective methods must be used. Even when objective tests are used, the subjective is not entirely eliminated, since levels of achievement are arbitrarily set by the instructor.

When the instructor grades subjectively, he or she must take care that they are not based on vague factors or carelessly awarded. The subjective can be made more reliable only when it is objectified, and this is best done through the prudent use of rating scales and checklists.

Understandability

Grades must be understandable to the student and to parents and should be easily interpreted by the teacher. Students must know the basis on which the grades are given, and they must understand how the system operates. The student should have a feeling for what the grade will be before it is assigned. Time should be devoted to the explanation of grades. Interpretation is best accomplished through the results of objective tests in relation to levels on a scale or to preset criterion standards. Such tests and accompanying interpretation leave little doubt about what a grade means.

Weightings

Since factors in grading are not all equally important, it is common to weight the measurable elements according to their relative importance. The final answer in **weighting** the various factors must be determined logically by the teacher. In some cases it is appropriate for the students to be involved in this process.

> Weighting refers to the comparative valuing of various components of a grade.

There is no broad agreement about how the three domains, the psychomotor, cognitive, and affective, should be weighted. For reasons of logic, psychomotor achievement is generally weighted heaviest, cognitive assessment next, and the affective usually lightest if it is considered at all. Not only does the teacher have to weigh the three domains of learning according to their relative importance but must also weight the factors within each domain according to emphasis. Several skill measures may have to be weighted according to their contributions to the student's overall physical performance. It is impossible for a grade to reflect everything in the unit, but it should represent an adequate sampling of the entire course or unit. Properly weighted factors result in a meaningful achievement grade for each student.

Discrimination

Whether norm-referenced or criterion-referenced, grades should **discriminate** between levels of achievement (Fig. 7-4). Norm-referenced grades reflect a continuum of performance levels in relation to how other students performed. They are reported by letters, numbers, or descriptive statements indicating a broad range of performance.

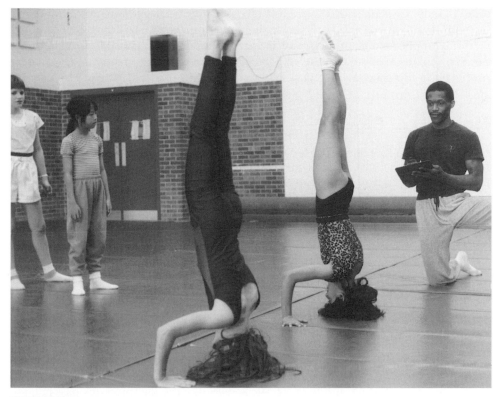

FIGURE 7-4

The grading system used by this gymnastics instructor must be able to discriminate between the different levels of headstand skill demonstrated by these two girls. (Photo by Dr. Karen Uhlendorf, University of Vermont, Burlington, VT.)

> Discrimination refers to the ability of a grade or score to differentiate among students who are truly different in levels of attainment.

Criterion-referenced grades must also discriminate, but they do it in terms of those who pass or fail at an established level of attainment. A cutting point may be set at a high mastery level equivalent to an A or B normative grade, or it may be set at D to indicate the line between passing and failing. The criterion-referenced grade must be somewhat influenced by the logical application of the cutting point decided by the teacher and partially determined by what the teacher knows students can reasonably be expected to attain. In any case, the discrimination is based on whether the student does or does not meet the criterion standard regardless of how the student's performance compares with those of other students.

Administrative Economy

The grading system must operate within the framework of time, cost, and personnel efficiency. The most important consideration is time. Because a teacher's first duty is to teach, no undue amount of time should be spent on a complicated grading system. A grading system should work as a tool to improve instruction, not to hinder it. Objectives to be used as a basis for grading must be kept to a minimum. Too many factors complicate the process and make grades incomprehensible. Several computer programs are listed in the references in the hope that teachers will become proficient in this time-saving technology.

Methods of Grading

A method of grading that is based on a sound philosophy and well-established criteria is appropriate. One of the essential requirements of any grading system is that the instructor can justify the grade. Although it is necessary to adhere to certain criteria and principles in grading, there is no standard method or technique; this is probably appropriate. Many difficulties must be overcome in designing a grading system, but when a system is set up on some rational basis that is consistent with the local program and philosophy, many of these difficulties resolve themselves.

Dissatisfaction with traditional grading systems has given rise to many plans. Several have merit, and even if not adequate alone, they can be used in combination with other systems or for special purposes. Two points seem evident: First, the student is becoming a more active participant in the process and is no longer simply the recipient; and, second, the system can be flexible so as to adapt to ability groups, age levels, and units, and consequently may change from time to time and from unit to unit. There are numerous methods of grading, but in general they all end up similar to one of these three types: (*a*) the conventional letter or numerical grade such as A, B, C, D, and F, or 82, 96, and 75; (*b*) the dichotomous pass-fail, satisfactory-unsatisfactory method; and (*c*) the written or oral descriptive type. Regardless of the format, however, these systems place varying amounts of emphasis on the role of the student in the process. The teacher's role has always been assumed. Increasing the involvement of students in determining grades seems a worthy goal.

Letter Grades and Number Grades

Letter grades expressed as A, B, C, D, and F and number grades expressed as 5, 4, 3, 2, and 1 or 97, 86, 72, 65, and 45 are essentially the same. Although number grades are not used as extensively as letter grades, letter grades frequently must be converted to numbers when **grade points** are computed.

> A grade point (grade point average) is a numerical evaluation of scholastic achievement based upon a formula of equivalents that assigns varying credit with the grade attained, for example, 4 points for an A, 3 for a B, and zero or negative points for failure.

Letters and numbers represent gradations in the quality of work performed by students. Table 7-1 shows further translations of the gradations into words and numbers. The exact symbol system to be used is often a school policy.

Numerical grades based on a scale of 100 are computed as percentages. The percentage score is obtained by dividing the attained score by the highest possible score and multiplying by 100. For example, if Jerry scores 34 on a test and 40 is the

TABLE 7-1 Various Grade Symbols

GRADE	GRADE	GRADE	GRADE	GRADE	GRADE (T-SCORE)	GRADE (T-SCORE)	GRADE (PERCENTAGE)	GRADE (PERCENTAGE)	GRADE (PERCENTILE)
5	4	1	A	E–Excellent Superior	70–80	65 & above	95–100	90–100	80–100
4	3	2	B	G–Good Above average	60–69	55–64	88–94	80–89	60–79
3	2	3	C	A–Average Satisfactory	40–59	45–54	80–87	70–79	40–59
2	1	4	D	I–Inferior Below average	30–39	35–44	70–79	60–69	20–39
1	0	5	F	F–Failure Unsatisfactory	20–29	34 or below	Below 70	Below 60	0–19

highest possible score, the score of 34 is divided by 40 and multiplied by 100 to yield 85%. This is the system used for most knowledge testing.

One problem concerning letter grades is arriving at an average for the single final mark. The student's letter grades are converted into numerical scores, sometimes weighted, and summed for a numerical total. This total may be averaged by dividing by the number of grade weightings. A system of converting letter grades to numerical values is shown in Table 7-2. This conversion table is used in the examples that follow in this chapter.

The convenience of this conversion system is that a multiple of 3 represents all of the plain grades. Some question a weighting of 1 for an F, but it is difficult to imagine that a student would not absorb some learning if present in a class. This point is not as important as the 12, 9, 6, and 3 weightings for A's, B's, C's, and D's, respectively.

Self-Evaluation

Self-evaluations are usually used in conjunction with other methods of grading. They can be made on each assignment or test and on the unit as a whole. Self-assessments are viewed as important means by which students assume more responsibility for their own learning. LaPoint (13) indicated several disadvantages and advantages of self-grading. Among disadvantages: "administrators need to be kept more closely informed of the class activities, some students may lack the honesty needed for self-grading, and students may become less accurate as the process continues throughout the year." Among the advantages: increased personal responsibility and increased awareness of results on the part of the student.

Research findings are mixed. Some found students prone to evaluate themselves higher than justified, especially at first. Others reported self-ratings worthy of consideration when guidelines are established and when individual conferences are conducted to discuss the self-assigned grades.

Students need to be taught to use self-evaluation wisely. This type of involvement in evaluation seems especially appropriate when the students have set their own goals and determined the means to achieve them. Once these criteria are established in writing and/or in conference, students evaluate their progress toward their goals. Self-evaluation is not effective if sprung on the students on a one-shot basis. Responsibility for self-evaluation has to be a regular part of instruction throughout the course. Students soon become accustomed to the procedures and achieve some objectivity and consistency in assessing the worth of their own work.

TABLE 7-2	Numerical Conversion Table for Letter Grades		
A = 12	B− = 8	D+ = 4	
A− = 11	C+ = 7	D = 3	
B+ = 10	C = 6	D− = 2	
B = 9	C− = 5	F = 1	

Contract Grading

Contract grading can be applied to an entire class or to individual students. The class contract establishes the type, quantity, and quality of work to be accomplished to achieve various grades. These decisions can be made by the teacher but are usually more effective if jointly planned by the students and the teacher. Individual contracts designed by each student include setting the goals, methods for realizing them, and grading procedures. Since each contract is different, each grading system is tailored to fit the contract. It is essential that the methods of evaluation are agreed upon jointly by the teacher and each student and specifically stated in the written contract.

> Contract grading is the practice of agreement between teacher and students at the beginning of an instructional unit regarding goals and standards for grades.

Peer Evaluations

Subjective ratings by classmates of skill performance, contributions to the team, sportsmanship, helpfulness, and other such factors involve students in the evaluation process. Guidelines must cover such topics as impartiality, analysis of skills to be observed, and the use of rating scales. Probably several students should be involved in the ratings for each student. Both the peer raters and the students being rated can learn from these experiences. Ratings identify important factors and inform the student of his or her status in each. The ratings can lead to important discussions between the raters and the rated and between the teacher, the raters, and the rated. Some evidence suggests that peer ratings can have a high degree of consistency and can show good agreement with instructors' ratings (14).

With adequate training, high school and college students are capable of conducting valid and reliable peer evaluations. In the lower grades peer evaluations give students experience and understanding but probably should not be part of the final grade. Use of this process at any educational level involves students in the instructional strategy.

Pass-Fail

In the pass-fail system criteria for a passing grade are established at the beginning of the course and ideally should be decided together by the students and teacher. Students who meet the criteria pass; students who do not, fail. Often failing students are allowed to continue working until a passing standard can be achieved. Some educators prefer this plan because it increases the motivation to learn and decreases the motivation just to earn grades. The biggest criticism of pass-fail grading is that it fails to discriminate between excellent and adequate students. The pass-fail plan is based on mastery learning. A standard is set, and if it is achieved, mastery is claimed. In this case passing is analogous to mastery. Often, however, mastery is set at a higher standard than just passing. If the pass-fail system is used, it probably should be supplemented by individual conferences to discuss achievement in various objectives of physical education.

Credit–no record is a variation of the pass-fail plan. This system credits students only if their work is at least passing quality. If it is not passing work, no official record is kept to indicate that the student took the course. This is similar to the pass-fail option except that there is no record of failure. Students are free to elect challenging and exploratory courses with no fear of tarnishing their academic records. Students are informed of their status by the usual appraisal methods.

Descriptive Statements

Written statements are frequently more meaningful to parents and students than the more traditional letter or number grades. Phrases or words commonly used are *excellent*, *fair*, *unsatisfactory*, *improving*, *needs to*, *applying*, *seems unable*, and *showing progress*. These words or phrases may be in the form of a checklist or rating scale, and evaluation may be made in an objective or a subjective manner. This method can become more elaborate and take the form of a short anecdotal written analysis of the student's status and achievement. There is no doubt of the value of this scheme, but for the instructor with a large number of students, such reports are prohibitively time consuming. In addition, it is relatively easy to describe the good performer and the poor performer, but it becomes increasingly difficult to describe the many who are in the average group. In these many instances the descriptive method can become a perfunctory and meaningless device.

Descriptive statements, narrative comments, and written evaluations are all terms for a prose account of the results of evaluative procedures. These are done periodically to summarize students' strengths and weaknesses. They are criticized as being too subjective and too time consuming. If carefully constructed, they are beneficial, however, because they describe each student's unique performance.

 Computerized Descriptions

Pools of descriptive statements are available on computer evaluation programs. Teachers can select the appropriate descriptive phrases, and the computer composes a narrative evaluation statement. This is a significant aid to the teacher who has limited time but wants to use descriptive statements for grading.

Rating Scales

Descriptive statements can be modified and organized into a rating scale that enumerates the crucial components of the unit. The student is evaluated on a series of components related to the stated objectives. This replaces the single symbolic grade with a profile. Such a system gives more information than the five levels of traditional letter grades and is more convenient to use than descriptive statements. It has special merit for physical education because it can accommodate the myriad factors that are included in the physical education grade. In addition to achievement in skills and understandings, a rating scale can include factors such as effort, improvement, and cooperation without having to transform them into a single grade.

Individual Conferences

Conferences may follow testing sessions in skill and understandings and can be used for analytical remarks. The testing results are not used for determining grades translated into A, B, C, D, and F or perhaps even pass-fail but are used to help each student understand personal achievements. Individual conferences can be used in conjunction with descriptive statements serving as report cards. However, students are still likely to want to know their grades.

Parents and guardians can also be included in conferences. This practice used to be considered appropriate only when a disciplinary action was indicated, but today it is viewed as a more thorough involvement of students, teachers, and family in the education process. Individual and parent conferences are often used for special cases with unique problems and to help to clarify school policies. They should be used routinely so that students do not view them as indicated only when something is wrong. Parental involvement in conferences is increasingly difficult because of working schedules, but such meetings are considered worthwhile in spite of the extra effort needed to arrange them. Teachers may have to schedule conferences in the evening and/or on weekends.

Sample System of Grading

A grading system should meet most of the criteria discussed earlier in the chapter. At the same time, it must be flexible enough to meet the needs of the local situation. It is best for individual teachers and schools to develop grading systems that fit their procedures and reflect their own philosophies and curricula. It is essential that all teachers in a physical education department adopt a grading plan that is implemented consistently among teachers. Otherwise students will compare the different plans and think they are being treated unfairly.

Converting Raw Scores

Before it is possible to arrive at a final grade, it is necessary to convert raw scores to scale scores or grades. Table 7-3 illustrates this procedure by depicting scores for 22 students who took a badminton wall test of skill using the forehand. The six grading plans can be considered in light of a teacher's grading philosophy. Since grading is arbitrary, the plan most congruent with the grading philosophy of the teacher and/or the school can be selected. The plans are related to the grading symbols in Table 7-1. Table 7-3 shows that the beginning badminton students scored 22 to 40 on a timed wall test. An important concept is that no maximum score related to the examples in Table 7-3.

Plan 1 uses natural breaks in the distribution to assist with the designation of letter grades. This is helpful when assigning grades for small groups. It is not as feasible with large groups because there are likely to be no natural breaks and the distribution will look normal.

T-scores were used for plans 2 and 3. These T-scores were computed for this skill test using 496 beginning badminton players who were tested previously. The grade conversion from T-score to letter grade for plan 2 is stricter than that for plan 3. It also follows the cutoff levels for the first T-score equivalencies given on Table 7-2. For ex-

TABLE 7-3 Alternative Ways of Converting Badminton Wall Test Scores

RAW SCORES	NO. OF STUDENTS	NATURAL BREAKS PLAN 1	T-SCORES COMPUTED ON PREVIOUS CLASSES N=496	#1 PLAN 2	#2 PLAN 3	T-SCORES COMPUTED ON THIS CLASS N=22	#1 PLAN 4	#2 PLAN 5	% OF BEST SCORE	PLAN 6
40	1	A	88	A	A	70	A	A	100	A
39			84			68			98	
38	1	A−	80	A	A−	66	B	A−	95	A
37	1	A−	76	A	A−	64	B	A−	93	A
36	1	A−	72	A	A−	62	B	A−	90	A
35			68			60			88	
34	1	B+	64	B	B+	58	C	B+	85	B
33	1	B	60	B	B	56	C	B	83	B
32	4	B	56	C	B	54	C	B	80	B
31	2	B	52	C	B	52	C	B	78	C
30			48			50			75	
29	2	C+	44	C	C+	48	D	C+	73	C
28	1	C	40	C	C	46	D	C	70	C
27	1	C	36	D	C	44	D	C	68	D
26	1	C	32	D	C	42	D	C	65	D
25	1	D	28	F	D	40	D	C	63	D
24	1	D	24	F	D	38	F	D	60	D
23	1	D	20	F	D	36	F	D	58	F
22	2 / 22	D	16	F	D	34	F	D	55	F

ample, a player who scored 32 on the skill test would receive a T-score of 56; that is equivalent to a C using the first T-score cutoffs in Table 7-1. If a more generous conversion scale is desired, the second T-scale equivalency on Table 7-1 can be used. In this case the student who scored a 32 would still have a T-score of 56 but would be assigned a B. The different T-score conversions to grades shown in Table 7-1 illustrate only two options to implement a philosophical position on grading; one is fairly strict and the other one more generous. Many other variations are possible.

Then T-scores were computed for just the 22 students in this beginning badminton class. Because of the small number, the distribution of scores is not normal, and the T-scale reflects that. The natural breaks and the strict or liberal orientation of the teacher are reflected in the grades assigned in plans 4 and 5.

Another alternative to converting raw scores to grades is to use a percentage procedure such as is shown in plan 6. In this case the highest score made on the skill test by these 22 students, that is, 40, is assumed to be the maximum score, and all other scores are converted to a percentage of this score. Then the numerical percentage is converted to a letter grade using the 10-point scale shown in the second to last column of Table 7-1.

Table 7-4 shows the scores made by the same 22 students on a knowledge test covering the content of the badminton unit. It was possible to make 50 points on the test. In this case the maximum score possible is known. Obviously, the test did not discriminate very well and therefore probably was not too valid or reliable. Giving the students the benefit of doubt that the test was not a particularly good one, the teacher might use plan 1 to assign grades. However, if the student with the highest score knew only 86% of the content on the test, a grade of B might be appropriate, as shown in plan 2. There are natural breaks in the distribution, and the teacher should use them rather than force grade levels at every 5, 7 or 10 points, for example. In plan 3, assume that the criterion-referenced level for mastery is set at 70%. All of the 22 students met this standard and therefore passed the knowledge test.

In the previous examples two sets of scores have been presented along with several alternative ways to assign a letter grade to the performance of each of the 22

TABLE 7-4	Grades Assigned for a Badminton Knowledge Test				
NO. OF ITEMS CORRECT	**NO. OF STUDENTS**	**% OF 50 PTS.**	**PLAN 1**	**PLAN 2**	**PLAN 3**
43	4	86	A	B	P
42	1	84	A	B	P
41		82			
40	7	80	B+	C	P
39	5	78	B	C	P
38	4	76	B–	C	P
37		74			
36		72			
35	1	70	C	D	P
	$\overline{22}$				

students. These examples should help to illustrate the point made earlier that there is no single best procedure for assigning grades. Perhaps the arbitrary nature of grading and the importance of the teacher having an established plan and a firm philosophy of grading now seems even more evident!

Letter Grade Example

Table 7-5 shows the assessment of one student on a beginning badminton unit. Some evaluated factors are not counted in determining the final single grade. Even so, the student has a report on these factors and is better informed about his or her performance in all facets of the unit objectives.

Notice also that the grades in the five motor factors are not averaged to get one motor grade to be weighted seven times. Each factor has kept its own identity and integrity in the total. In addition, the teacher has avoided two additional computational steps that are unnecessary and would distort the total grade. The conversions from letter grades to points are made by referring to Table 7-2. If the student receives an A on all weighted factors, the total points can be 108, that is, 9×12. All of the totals of weighted points for the class can be placed in a frequency distribution so they are organized conveniently for grade decisions: (*a*) various grade levels, (*b*) pass-fail cutoff point or other criterion-related levels, or (*c*) qualitative levels expressed in good, fair, excellent, and so forth. The teacher has several ways to convert the 89 points into a final grade:

Determine the percentage: $89 \div 108 = 82\%$. Record the numerical grade of 82. Divide the total points by the number of weightings: $89 \div 9 = 9.9$. Table 7-2 shows 9.9 equals a grade of B+. Compare the 82% with a predetermined standard of accomplishment that would indicate mastery, for example, 80%. Record a pass because the student has exceeded the cutoff point, indicating sufficient proficiency in badminton to continue to the intermediate level of instruction.

Descriptive Statement Example

Statements must be based on information, and a summary of performance similar to the one in Table 7-5 is still necessary. It serves, however, only as a basis for the descriptive statement and is not usually transmitted to the parent. An example of what is communicated:

"Jerry learned the importance of a good serve in badminton. His skill in serving helped him perform well in the tournament play, but he needs to work on his other strokes. His score on the knowledge test covering skills, strategy, and rules of badminton showed good comprehension which he was able to apply in game play. His classmates considered his helpfulness to them in class very valuable."

Evaluation of a Grading System

Eble refers to grades as one of the "grubby stuff and dirty work" aspects of teaching (15). This cannot be refuted. Some unpleasant dimensions of grading are tedium, lack of confidence, misinterpretations, and short deadlines. These unpleasantries can be minimized by establishing a grading philosophy, developing an efficient scheme to implement it, involving students in the process, reducing the red tape,

TABLE 7-5   Summary of Unit Evaluations

STUDENT _____ UNIT _____ DATE _____

AREAS	WEIGHTING OF AREA	FACTORS	WEIGHTING OF FACTORS		GRADE ON FACTOR	POINTS
Psychomotor	7	Self-rating of skill	1	X	B (9)	9
		Peer rating of skill	1	X	A– (11)	11
		Teacher rating of skill	1	X	B (9)	9
		Tournament standing	2	X	B (9)	13
		Skill test, serve	2	X	A (12)	24
		Improvement	0		A	0
Cognitive	2	Knowledge test	2	X	B (9)	18
Affective	0	Peer rating on helpfulness	0		A	0
		Self-rating on helpfulness	0		B	0
		Teacher rating on helpfulness	0		B	0
Totals	9		9			85

Comments: Grade:

THE GRADING SYSTEM	NONE	POOR	FAIR	GOOD	EXCELLENT
1. Is based on performance objectives for the course	___	___	___	___	___
2. Samples performance from all areas of the course	___	___	___	___	___
3. Weights the contribution of each type of performance on the basis of its relative importance	___	___	___	___	___
4. Provides a consistent method for assigning grades to various levels of performance	___	___	___	___	___
5. Conforms to schoolwide grading policy	___	___	___	___	___
6. Is compatible with the grading system used by other teachers in related areas	___	___	___	___	___
7. Provides a well-organized, convenient way of recording grades	___	___	___	___	___
8. Informs students of the basis and system for determining their grades	___	___	___	___	___
9. Maintains accurate and complete records of performance	___	___	___	___	___
10. Is consistent with the grading system	___	___	___	___	___
11. Provides students with regular appraisals of their achievement	___	___	___	___	___
12. Provides useful information about students' achievements to administrators and other teachers	___	___	___	___	___
13. Provides useful information to parents and guardians	___	___	___	___	___

FIGURE 7-5

Checklist for Evaluating a Grading System. (Adapted from the Professional Teacher Education Module Series, Module D-5, Determine Student Grades, developed at The National Center for Research in Vocational Education at The Ohio State University.)

and closely tying the evaluation process to the learning process. The checklist in Figure 7-5 can help you evaluate a personal grading system. It can also help the in-service teacher assess the system in use (16).

Chapter Summary

Grades are symbols used to denote an estimate of students' status, progress, and/or achievement. They serve many purposes and can be useful to students, parents or guardians, teachers, and school administrators. The student and the in-service teacher are encouraged to make their grading more effective and efficient by using criterion-referenced grading, gender-fair grading, and ability grouping. They are also encouraged to report multiple grades and improvement scores. And, of course, whenever possible, a computer should be used to reduce the tedium of grading.

Discussed in this chapter are negative practices, such as grade inflation, that make grades increasingly difficult to interpret. An undesirable practice common to physical education is including factors such as showers, absences, dress, and punctuality. Physical education grades more appropriately should be based on students' performance related to stated objectives in the psychomotor, cognitive, and affective domains. The grades themselves must be valid, reliable, objective, and understandable to all parties. Furthermore, the grading factors must be weighted in a way that is consistent with the emphasis placed on these factors in the learning environment. Finally, grades must discriminate among levels of achievement by various students.

There is no single best method of grading. Many grading systems have been promoted by educators, but essentially all systems can be categorized as (*a*) conventional letter or numerical, (*b*) pass-fail, or (*c*) written or oral. This chapter concludes with a 13-item checklist that can be used to evaluate the strengths and weaknesses of any particular grading system.

SELF-TEST QUESTIONS

1. A girl who scores 28 of a possible 40 points on a badminton skills test receives a B+. The next year, another girl scores 28 points on the same test and is assigned an A−. What may this example demonstrate?
   A. Criterion-referenced grading
   B. Gender-fair grading
   C. Grade inflation
   D. Multiple grades

2. In which of the following classes should separate standards be established for grading the physical performances of high school boys and girls?
   A. Weight training
   B. Jazz dance
   C. Softball
   D. A, C
   E. A, B, and C

3. Which of the following can be a positive outcome of ability grouping?
   A. Administrative economy
   B. Resistance to grade inflation
   C. Fairer grading of both genders
   D. More meaningful grades

4. This is a student's end-of-semester grades for a weight training class:
   Strength (from maximum lift tests)   C+
   Improvement (strength gains)   A
   Knowledge of weight training principles   A−

This is an example of _____.
A. Ability grouping
B. Criterion-referenced grading
C. Grade inflation
D. Multiple grades

5. Which of the following is *least* justifiable as a factor in grading in physical education?
    A. Effort
    B. Participation
    C. Personal hygiene
    D. Knowledge

6. Although one student has performed considerably better than another in a physical education class, both students receive the same grade. Which of the following can be said about the grading system?
    A. It is too subjective.
    B. It is too objective.
    C. It is low in reliability.
    D. It does not discriminate well.

7. Using the conversions given in Table 7-2, what is the final letter grade for a student who receives an A−, a D+, and a B on three examinations that are all weighted equally?
    A. B
    B. B−
    C. C+
    D. C

8. A student receives grades of A−, a D+, and a B on three equally weighted unit examinations and a D on the final examination. If the final examination grade is weighted twice as heavily as any one of the unit examination grades, what is the final letter grade for this student?
    A. C
    B. C−
    C. D+
    D. D

9. In which of the following grading practices do students play a major role in the grading?
    A. Self-evaluation
    B. Contract grading
    C. Peer evaluation
    D. A and C
    E. A, B, and C

10. Refer to Table 7-5. How many grade points does this student earn if the teacher rating is changed to a weight of 2, and the tournament standing is given a weight of 3? All other grading factors stay the same. _____
    points

11. What percentage of the total points possible did the same student earn?
    _____%

ANSWERS

1. C   2. D   3. C   4. D   5. C   6. D
7. B   8. A   9. E   10. 107   11. 80%

DOING PROJECTS FOR FURTHER LEARNING

1. Contact AAHPERD and request a copy of the SOFTSHARE catalog. Order a grading program.

2. It is very common for the interviewer to ask the applicant for a physical education teaching job, "What is your philosophy of grading?" Write out a sample answer to this question. Identify what you believe to be the purpose of grading and the most important factors in physical education grading. Also expound on common problems associated with some grading practices.

3. Select a sport that you know well and assume you have been hired to teach a unit in it at your local high school. What are your objectives for the students? Describe the procedures you will use for grading. What factors will contribute to the grade? How will they be weighted? Will your students participate in the grading process? How will you communicate the meanings of grades to students, parents, and administrators?

REFERENCES

1. Morey, R.S., and Karp, G.G.: Why do some students who are good at physical education dislike it so much? Physical Educator, 55(2):89, 1998.
2. Carlson, T.B.: We hate gym: student alienation from physical education. Journal of Teaching in Physical Education, 14:467, 1995.
3. Barrow, H.M., McGee, R.M., and Tritschler, K.A.: Measurement and Evaluation in Sport and Physical Education. 4th ed. Baltimore, Williams and Wilkins, 1989.
4. Carlson, T.B.: A study of the relationship between student attitudes and student expectations toward physical education. Presented at the American Educational Research Association, San Francisco, April, 1995.
5. Kleinsasser, A.M.: Assessment culture and national testing. Clearing House, 68:205, 1995.
6. Deutsch, H.: Sex fair grading in physical education. Physical Educator, 41:137, October 1984.
7. McGonagle, K., and Stevens, A.: A practical approach to sex fair performance evaluation in secondary physical education. Illinois State Board of Education, Springfield, 13, 1981.
8. Imwold, C.H., Rider, R.A., and Johnson, D.J.: The use of evaluation in public school physical education programs. Journal of Teaching in Physical Education, 2:13, 1982.
9. Lashuk, M.: A percentile method of grading physical education. Canadian Journal of Health, Physical Education, and Recreation, March-April, p. 8, 1984.
10. Department of Kinesiology, California State University at Fresno: SOFTSHARE Catalog. Available from American Alliance of Health, Physical Education, Recreation, and Dance Bookstore, Reston, VA, AAHPERD, 1999.
11. Lund, J.: Assessment and accountability in secondary physical education. Quest, 44:352, 1992.

12. Mao, Y., and Youxiang-Zakrajsek, D.: Effects of grading on achievement in college physical education. Physical Educator, 50:201, 1993.
13. LaPoint, J.D.: Developing student responsibility through self-grading and peer cooperation. Kansas Association for Health, Physical Education, and Recreation, 9–11, October 1981.
14. Hill, G.M., and Miller, T.A.: A comparison of peer and teacher assessment of students' physical fitness performance. Physical Educator, 54:40, 1997.
15. Eble, K.E.: The Craft of Teaching: A Guide to Mastering the Professor's Art. 2nd ed. San Francisco, Jossey-Bass, 1994.
16. National Center for Research in Vocational Education, Ohio State University: Determine Student Grades. 2nd ed. Module D-5, Instructional Evaluation. Professional Teacher Education Module Series. (Report ISBN 0-89606-148-5).

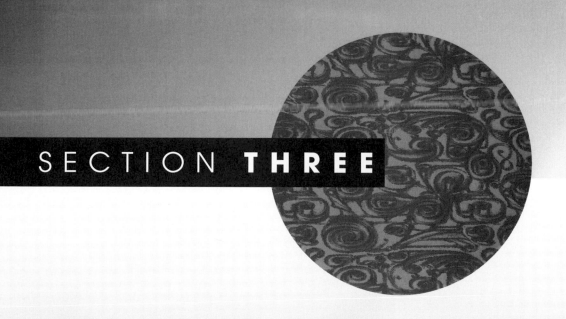

Assessment of Physical Fitness and Motor Skills

CHAPTER 8

Assessing Body Composition

To serve our clients well, clinicians and practitioners working in sports medicine and physical education must perform valid and reliable body composition assessments. Research has substantiated the relation between desirable body composition and overall health and well-being. We are now all too aware that excessive body fat increases one's risk of developing a number of serious diseases, including coronary heart disease, hypertension, stroke, chronic obstructive pulmonary disease, diabetes, arthritis, and some forms of cancer. We also know that undesirable body compositions detract from many types of athletic performances. For example, excessive body fat reduces aerobic fitness and impairs whole-body movements such as jumping and dodging. This chapter critically reviews the methods by which body composition can be assessed. It also instructs you in techniques for accurate body composition assessment that can be employed in field and clinical settings.

As you read this chapter, watch for the following keywords:

Bioelectrical analysis	Caliper	Obesity
Bod Pod	Creeping obesity	Skinfold
Body composition	Essential body fat	Wasit-to-hip ratio
Body mass index	Morphological fitness	

Defining Body Composition

Morphological fitness, one of three broad components of health-related physical fitness (HRPF), is assessed by measuring bone density and body composition. A person who is morphologically fit has positive bone density and body composition profiles. At present there are no simple field measures of bone density. Since the focus of this text is on practical field assessments, only body composition is discussed in this chapter.

> Bone density and body composition together constitute morphological fitness.

Body composition assessment involves quantification of the relative contributions of the major structures of the human body. Our bodies are composed of a variety of structures, including muscle mass, bone, fat, blood, and other types of fluids and tissues. Most theoretical models of body composition are two-factor models based on the premise that a person's total body weight (TBW) is the sum of his or her fat weight (FW) plus lean body weight (LBW). Percent body fat (%BF) is calculated by Formula 8-1:

$$\%BF = (FW \div TBW) \times 100 \qquad\qquad \text{Formula 8-1}$$

Percent body fat therefore is the proportion of one's total body weight that is contributed by fat weight. Consider, for example, a person who weighs 150 lb and is assessed as having 20% body fat. According to the two-factor model of **body composition,** 30 lb (20% of 150 lb) is contributed by fatty tissues and 120 lb (150 lb − 30 lb) is in the form of muscle, bones, water, and other residual fluids and tissues. How do these values change if the person is assessed as having only 10% body fat? What if he or she were 180 lb?

> Body composition comprises the relative contributions of fat and lean body tissues to the overall weight of the body.

Why Assess Body Composition?

There is clearly a need to assess body composition for a number of client populations. Here are some of the reasons practitioners, clinicians, and researchers conduct body composition assessments:

As Part of a Comprehensive Health-Related Physical Fitness Assessment.   Desirable body composition is deemed important for the health and well-being of all children and adults. The Centers for Disease Control and Prevention began regular tracking of obesity in the American population in the 1960s.

As Part of a Comprehensive Physical Examination or Cardiovascular Risk Factor Assessment.   As already noted, excessive body fat is related to increased risk of cardiovascular and other diseases.

To Monitor Changes in Body Components in Response to Weight Loss or Gain Programs.   Modifications in diet and exercise regimens can be made to accommodate observed changes. Objective information about changes in body fat and lean tissues can motivate clients to adhere to their programs.

To Monitor the Effectiveness of Physical Training Regimens for Athletes.   A competitive edge may be gained by the athlete who can achieve the optimal balance between *fat weight* and *lean body weight* for his or her particular sport. This varies considerably by sport and by gender. Elite male marathoners may carry only about 5% body fat, while one of the best long-distance open-water swimmers in the world is a woman who competes best at 33% body fat.

To Monitor Nutrition.   Skinfolds and circumferences can provide indices of nutritional status and fat patterning among children and adults.

To Identify the Potential Effectiveness of Fitness Professionals.   Research has shown that a fitness professional who is obviously *overfat* is perceived by

What Do YOU Think?

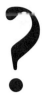

The admission committee for a university physical education department is troubled over the application of a particular candidate for the program. The candidate under consideration has an outstanding academic record, has demonstrated leadership in community service organizations, and is very popular among her peers and teachers. Furthermore, she was a star fullback on the women's field hockey team during her first 2 years at the university. However, she's 5 feet 2 inches and weighs more than 200 lb; her body fat percentage is measured at 40%.

If you were a member of the admission committee, how would you vote on this young woman's application? If you do admit her to the physical education program, can you require her to lose weight before she is allowed to graduate from the program? What if she fails to comply with the weight loss requirement? Is it ethical and/or legal to deny her a physical education degree because of her obesity? If she is granted her degree, is it ethical and/or legal for a public school system to deny her a job teaching physical education because of her obesity? What do YOU think?

P. S. You may want to do a legal search to determine what the U.S. courts have said in cases similar to this. Look under civil rights laws.

---

clients as being less knowledgeable and less motivational than a fitness professional whose weight is near the ideal (1).

To Advance Research on the Relations Between Body Composition and Other Physical and Psychological Phenomena. Researchers are studying body composition as it relates to arthritis, osteoporosis, lupus, breast cancer, colon cancer, acquired immunodeficiency syndrome (AIDS), and so on. Other researchers are studying the role of body composition in pregnancy, aging, menopause, and other aspects of women's health. Still others are examining body composition as a factor in psychological traits, such as self-concept, depression, aggression, and leadership.

For Use in Product Design and Setting of Safety Standards. Designers and builders of a wide array of products (e.g., clothing, automobiles, elevators, stadium seats) need accurate information about the sizes and weights of the adults and children who are potential consumers of their products. Data revealing ranges and averages for measurements of height, weight, trunk and abdominal girths, and center of gravity are particularly useful. The U.S. Consumer Product Safety Commission maintains and periodically updates its data bank of measurements of adults and children in the United States. It uses these data in the setting of safety standards for products and facilities (2).

Methods of Body Composition Assessment

Archimedes studied body composition assessment in Greece more than 22 centuries ago. However, like many other areas of physical assessment, major research interest and concomitant technological advances have occurred only within the past few decades. Dozens of methods are being used to assess body composition. They vary considerably in their accuracy, required instruments, and practicality. There are distinct pros and cons associated with the various methods, and in general there is a tradeoff between accuracy and practicality. The most accurate of all methods requires boiling the body parts of a cadaver—not particularly practical. The following is a selected review of methods that can be used with *living* human beings.

Hydrostatic Weighing

When performed correctly, hydrostatic weighing is a highly accurate method of assessing body composition. Hydrostatic weighing, also known as underwater weighing, is based on Archimedes' principle for measuring the density of an object. By this method, a nude or swimming suit–clad client sits in a special chair that is submerged in a 1000-gallon tank of water. While submerged, the person exhales as completely as possible and is weighed on a hanging scale while the volume of water displaced by his or her body is recorded. This procedure is repeated 7 to 10 times, and the consistently heaviest underwater weight is recorded.

According to Archimedes' original calculations, the weight of the displaced water is equal to the difference between the body's weight on dry land and the underwater weight. When determining body density, this method assumes that the submerged body is composed of varying proportions of fat, lean tissue, and air. Residual lung air, air in the gastrointestinal tract, and air trapped in hair or clothing is assumed to have a density of zero. Although the density of lean tissue varies among individuals, largely because of varying bone densities, the calculations for hydrostatic weighing assume the average density of lean tissues to be 1.1 g/mL. The density of fat is assumed to be 0.9 g/mL. These values are used to calculate overall body density from prediction formulas. Body density is then converted to percent body fat by a simple mathematical equation (3, 4).

Limitations of Hydrostatic Weighing

Under ideal testing conditions, hydrostatically determined percent body fat is considered the gold standard against which other body composition estimates are validated. There are, however, distinct limitations in the use of hydrostatic body composition. Clearly, it is inappropriate for settings that cannot house a 1000-gallon tank. The tank must be cleaned and disinfected regularly, and the tank water must be maintained within a range of acceptable temperatures, because the density of water varies with temperature. The testing procedures and calculations are relatively simple except for the determination of residual lung volume. Because the density of air is zero, even a small error in the estimate of air volume can significantly affect the calculation of body density. Residual lung volume, that is, the volume of air left in the lungs at the end of complete expiration, should be measured by use of a body box. Body boxes are expensive, however, so alternatively researchers employ either a helium dilution or a nitrogen washout technique. A final limitation associated with hydrostatic weighing is that this method cannot be used with persons who are afraid of total immersion in water. Neither is it an appropriate method for persons with certain medical challenges such as asthma and emphysema. Furthermore, special adjustments must be made for morbidly obese persons, who tend to float in water; they must wear weights to keep them under water.

Accuracy of Hydrostatic Weighing

Although it is the gold standard, hydrostatic weighing is not error free. The standard error of estimate for hydrostatic weighing is believed to be in the range of ±0.8% and ±1.2% of the estimate (5, 6). This is relatively small, so estimates of body composition by hydrostatic weighing are quite precise. (You may want to turn back to Chapter 6 to review how to interpret the standard error of estimate.) The two major sources of error for hydrostatic weighing are caused by mismeasurement of air and by averaging the densities of lean tissues.

A modified hydrostatic weighing procedure employs a plastic frame and chair that are used in the diving area of a swimming pool. Some people erroneously assume that this procedure has the same accuracy attributed to the laboratory tank procedures. But because residual lung volume is estimated rather than measured directly, the accuracy of the modified hydrostatic weighing procedure is significantly lower. The standard error of estimate for this procedure is estimated to be ±3.9% (6).

The Bod Pod

While hydrostatic weighing has been the gold standard for body composition assessment for about 3 decades, a new procedure, the **Bod Pod,** may soon replace it. The Bod Pod was developed with funding from the National Institutes of Health (NIH). Considerable testing is under way to determine its feasibility and psychometric qualities in various settings and with various populations. The Bod Pod's computer estimates overall body density from a measure of air displacement rather than water displacement. This is seen as a major advantage over hydrostatic weighing because nearly everyone can be comfortable sitting quietly in the Bod Pod's air chamber for the 5 minutes of data collection.

> The Bod Pod is a body composition procedure for estimating body density from a measure of air displacement.

At $35,000, the Bod Pod is not for everyone. It is, however, being tried out in university laboratories across the country and by the U.S. Air Force Academy and the Army Reserve (7). Because these military organizations may invest as much as $100,000 in a new trainee, they consider $35,000 reasonable if it allows them to retain even a single person who might be dismissed by their current body composition estimation that uses neck and waist circumferences.

Stay tuned for more news about the Bod Pod. It will be interesting to see how this new technology will affect the exercise and sport sciences. (Also watch for news of the new version of the Bod Pod for infants, aptly labeled the Pea Pod. NIH is funding this project.)

Skinfold Thickness Measurement

Skinfold body composition is based on the assumption that approximately half of an adult's body fat is in the subcutaneous tissues, that is, the tissues immediately beneath the skin. Overall body composition is estimated from skinfold thickness measurements taken at selected sites on the body. A **skinfold** is a double fold of skin and the immediate layer of subcutaneous fat, the width or thickness of which is measured in millimeters by a special tool called a **caliper.**

> A skinfold is a double fold of skin and the immediate layer of subcutaneous fat.

> A caliper is a tool used to measure the thickness of a skinfold to estimate body fat.

Type of Caliper

Accuracy and precision of skinfold measurements are affected by the type of caliper used. Harpenden and Lange calipers, which cost several hundred dollars, are precision measuring tools that yield reasonably reliable skinfold measurements (8). Across the entire range of skinfold thickness, these calipers exert a constant pressure of 10 g/mm^2 (that is, 10 g pressure for each square millimeter of caliper jaw surface). Inexpensive plastic calipers are available from a number of sources. Measurements taken with plastic calipers correlate moderately well with measurements from high-quality calipers, especially if the person measuring the skinfolds is experienced (9). However, the plastic calipers tend to be most accurate through the middle ranges of percent body fat; the measurements of very thin and thick skinfolds are more likely to be inaccurate. *Whenever possible, it is best to use the type and brand of caliper that was used in developing the selected skinfold procedure* (5, 10). Appendix B lists organizations and companies that sell calipers.

There are more than 100 equations to estimate percent body fat from skinfold thickness (11). The equations differ by number and location of skinfold sites. In research settings a seven-site procedure is most often employed, with measurements taken by Harpenden or Lange calipers. In clinical and field settings, four-site, three-site, two-site, and even single-site procedures conducted with a variety of caliper types are popular. In these settings the loss in accuracy to use of fewer skinfold sites is largely compensated for by the gain in practicality. Jackson and Pollock have estimated that the sum of three and seven skinfolds are highly correlated, that is, $r \geq .97$ (12). So the moral for ESS practitioners is that they do not have to feel compelled to use the full seven-site procedure if time constraints make it difficult.

How to Measure a Skinfold

The technique to measure a skinfold is the same regardless of the particular equations being used to assess body composition (13). The examiner should use the thumb and forefinger of the left hand to lift a fold of skin and subcutaneous adipose tissue. The thumb and forefinger should be placed about 1 cm *above* the site where the skinfold is to be measured by the calipers. The skinfold is lifted by placing the thumb and forefinger on the skin about 8 cm apart and perpendicular to the desired skinfold, then drawing the digits together to get a firm grasp of a fold of skin. *The amount of tissue that is lifted should be sufficient to form a skinfold with approximately parallel sides*. If the layer of subcutaneous fat is particularly thick, the starting separation between the thumb and forefinger must be greater than 8 cm. It is important to lift only skin and fat, not underlying muscle. If you think muscle tissue may be included in the skinfold, simply ask the client to tense his or her underlying muscle. When tensed, the muscle will pull away from the skinfold.

The skinfold is held firmly while the caliper jaws are slipped over the fold exactly at the site where the measurement is to be taken. *The caliper jaws are placed perpendicular to the long axis of the skinfold and about midway between the base and the crest of the skinfold. At this point the sides of the skinfold are approximately parallel to each other.* As the thumb and forefinger continue to hold the skinfold, caliper pressure is applied to the measurement site, either by releasing the lever of the high-quality caliper or by pressing to align the arrows on the plastic caliper. The measurement is read about 2 seconds after the caliper pressure is applied. Read Harpenden calipers to the nearest 0.1 mm, Lange calipers to 0.5 mm, and plastic calipers to the nearest 1 mm.

The measurement should be repeated after a brief rest. If measures vary by more than 1 mm, additional measurements should be taken. An average skinfold value is recorded for each skinfold site. It is important, however, that some time pass between successive measurements at the same site. Subcutaneous fat compresses as pressure is applied to it, so successive measurements progressively get smaller. Fat compressibility varies with age, amount of fat, and state of hydration.

Skinfolds should always be taken when the client's skin is dry and lotion free. Accuracy is nearly impossible if skinfolds are measured through clothing; *only bare skin measures are recommended.* Avoid taking skinfolds immediately after the client has exercised, because increased blood flow to the skin surface may raise the reading.

Location of Skinfold Sites

It is important to practice precise location of sites. Low interexaminer reliability is most commonly due to improper site location (12). It is recommended that beginners in skinfold measurements use a tape measure to find maximal circumferences and midpoints between anatomical landmarks. It is also recommended that beginners mark sites with a washable marker before taking the actual measurement. And last but not least, beginners must practice, practice, practice! Before undertaking an official measurement assignment, examiners should practice on 50 to 100 subjects (9). Supervision of practice sessions by someone experienced in skinfold measurements can also be helpful.

Although all skinfold sites are on the right side of the body, there unfortunately is no unanimity in locations of skinfold sites. For example, one procedure describes the abdominal skinfold as a vertical fold 2 cm to the right of the umbilicus, while another measures a horizontal fold immediately to the right of the umbilicus. *It is important to use the same site locations that were used by the test developers in creation of their formulas.* If you are ever in doubt about the site to be used, refer to the *Anthropometric Standardization Reference Manual* (13). Table 8-1 describes locations of skinfold sites used by Jackson and Pollock and described in the next two sections of this chapter (12). Figures 8-1 to 8-4 illustrate several common skinfold site locations.

Jackson and Pollock Percent Body Fat Assessment for Women

Purpose

This procedure is a valid and practical field assessment of body composition for women. Test results estimate percent body fat for women aged 18 to more than 57 years who have body fat percentages between about 9% and 45%.

TABLE 8-1	Jackson and Pollock Skinfold Site Locations		
SKINFOLD SITE	**DIRECTION OF FOLD**	**ANATOMICAL LOCATION**	**LOCATION PROCEDURES**
Abdomen (women)	Vertical	Approximately 2 cm to right of umbilicus	
Chest (men)	Diagonal	Midway between right nipple and anterior axillary line (imaginary line dropping straight down from front of armpit)	Client may rest right arm across your shoulders.
Subscapular (men)	Diagonal	1 to 2 cm from inferior angle of right scapula on diagonal line from vertebral border	Ask client to place back of right hand against small of back; in this position inferior angle of scapula becomes prominent. After locating skinfold site, have client return arm to a relaxed position at side.
Suprailium (women)	Diagonal	Just above crest of right ilium where imaginary line comes down from anterior axillary line	
Triceps (men and women)	Vertical	Posterior midline of right upper arm over triceps midway between acromion (tip of shoulder) and olecranon (tip of elbow)	Position client with elbow flexed 90°. Use tape measure to locate midpoint between acromion and inferior margin of elbow along side of arm. Mark this point, first on side, then on back of arm over triceps. After locating skinfold site, have client extend elbow and return arm to a relaxed position at side.

Psychometric Information

This three-site skinfold procedure was validated on 283 women. Body densities from hydrostatic weighing were compared with body densities derived from a generalized regression equation using the sum of the triceps, suprailium, and abdominal skinfolds. In this equation age was treated as an independent variable. A multiple correlation value of .83 was obtained. It was also demonstrated that the three-site method was highly correlated ($r \geq +.97$) with a seven-site skinfold method. Reliability data were not provided, but other studies have reported test-retest reliability coefficients for skinfolds as high as .95. Ease of measurement was considered in the recommendation of the sites. An alternative three-site procedure using the thigh rather than the abdominal site yielded a slightly higher multiple correlation, but the procedure was not recommended because technicians found the thigh skinfold difficult to measure on many women.

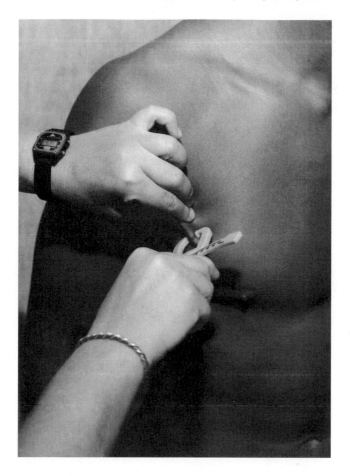

FIGURE 8-1

The chest skinfold on a male client is measured by a diagonal fold taken midway between the right nipple and the anterior axillary line. (Photo by Marvin Arrington, Heritage Photography, Greensboro, NC.)

Procedures

1. Using suggested techniques, measure the triceps, abdomen, and suprailium skinfolds. Jackson and Pollock recommend use of a Lange caliper for these measurements; if another brand of caliper is used, it should yield results consistent with those of the Lange. Read the caliper dial to the nearest 0.5 mm approximately 1 to 2 seconds after applying pressure. Jackson and Pollock also specify that a minimum of two measurements should be taken at each site. If the repeated measurements vary by more than 1 mm, a third measurement should be taken. The two most representative measurements are averaged, and this average value is recorded. Usually the tester completes a measurement at one site before going on to the next. The exception is when consecutive measurements become smaller and smaller, indicating fat compression. In this case it is best to go on to another site and later return to the troublesome site.

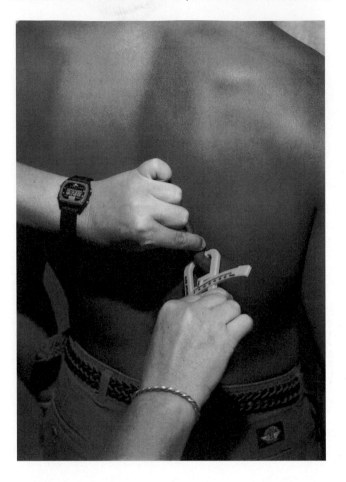

FIGURE 8-2

The subscapular skinfold is measured 1 to 2 cm from the inferior angle of the right scapula on a diagonal line coming from the vertebral border. (Photo by Marvin Arrington, Heritage Photography, Greensboro, NC.)

2. Sum the three skinfold measures; then read the estimated percent body fat from Table 8-2. Alternatively, you may calculate percent body fat according to the formulas that Jackson and Pollock used to construct Table 8-2. Body density (BD) is calculated by Formula 8-2, where X is the sum of the three skinfolds and Y is age in years. Percent body fat is calculated from body density by an equation developed by Siri. This is given in Formula 8-3:

$$BD_{women} = 1.089733 - 0.0009245 \ (X) + 0.0000025 \ (X)^2 \\ - 0.0000979 \ (Y)$$ Formula 8-2

$$\%BF = (495 \div BD) - 450$$ Formula 8-3

Comment
The Siri equation given above for converting body density to percent body fat works well for most healthy young to middle-aged adult women. Alternative formu-

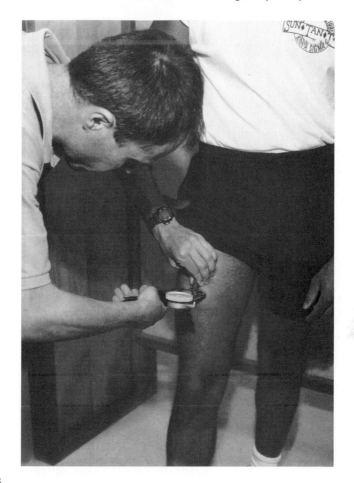

FIGURE 8-3

The thigh skinfold is measured by a vertical fold on the front of the thigh midway between the hip and knee joints. (Photo by Marvin Arrington, Heritage Photography, Greensboro, NC.)

las have been developed for children, elderly adults, the infirm, and athletes in training (14).

Jackson and Pollock Percent Body Fat Assessment for Men

Purpose

This procedure is a valid and practical field assessment of body composition for men. Test results estimate percent body fat for men aged 18 to more than 57 years who have body fat percentages between about 2% and 35%.

Psychometric Information

This three-site skinfold procedure was validated on 402 men. Hydrostatically determined body densities were compared with body densities calculated from a general regression equation using the sum of the triceps, chest, and subscapular skinfolds. In this equation, age was treated as an independent variable. A multiple correlation value of .89 was obtained. Reliability data were not provided, but other

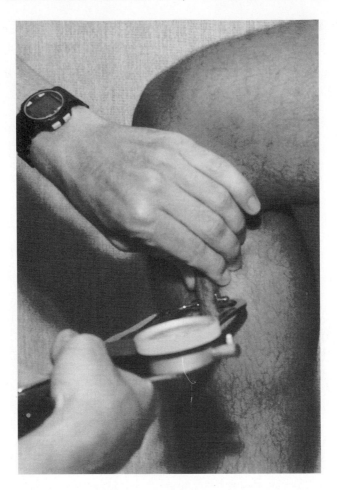

FIGURE 8-4

The calf skinfold is measured by a vertical fold on the inside of the right lower leg at the level of the greatest girth. (Photo by Marvin Arrington, Heritage Photography, Greensboro, NC.)

studies have reported test-retest reliability coefficients as high as .95. Ease of measurement was considered in the recommendation of the skinfold sites. An alternative procedure using the abdominal, thigh, and chest skinfolds yielded a slightly higher multiple correlation, but the procedure was not recommended because technicians found the abdominal skinfold difficult to measure on many men.

Procedures
1. Using suggested techniques, measure the chest, triceps, and subscapular skinfolds. Lange calipers should be used, and a minimum of two measurements should be taken at each site.
2. Sum the three measures; then read the estimated percent body fat from Table 8-3. Alternatively, you may calculate percent body fat according to the formulas that Jackson and Pollock used to construct Table 8-3. Body density is calculated by Formula 8-4, where X is the sum of the three skinfolds and Y

| TABLE 8-2 | Jackson and Pollock Percent Body Fat Estimate for Women from Sum of Triceps, Abdomen, and Suprailium Skinfolds |

SUM OF SKINFOLDS (mm)	AGE TO LAST YEAR								
	18-22	23-27	28-32	33-37	38-42	43-47	48-52	53-57	OVER 57
8-12	8.8	9.0	9.2	9.4	9.5	9.7	9.9	10.1	10.3
13-17	10.8	10.9	11.1	11.3	11.5	11.7	11.8	12.0	12.2
18-22	12.6	12.8	13.0	13.2	13.4	13.5	13.7	13.9	14.1
23-27	14.5	14.6	14.8	15.0	15.2	15.4	15.6	15.7	15.9
28-32	16.2	16.4	16.6	16.8	17.0	17.1	17.3	17.5	17.7
33-37	17.9	18.1	18.3	18.5	18.7	18.9	19.0	19.2	19.4
38-42	19.6	19.8	20.0	20.2	20.3	20.5	20.7	20.9	21.1
43-47	21.2	21.4	21.6	21.8	21.9	22.1	22.3	22.5	22.7
48-52	22.8	22.9	23.1	23.3	23.5	23.7	23.8	24.0	24.2
53-57	24.2	24.4	24.6	24.8	25.0	25.2	25.3	25.5	25.7
58-62	25.7	25.9	26.0	26.2	26.4	26.6	26.8	27.0	27.1
63-67	27.1	27.2	27.4	27.6	27.8	28.0	28.2	28.3	28.5
68-72	28.4	28.6	28.7	28.9	29.1	29.3	29.5	29.7	29.8
73-77	29.6	29.8	30.0	30.2	30.4	30.6	30.7	30.9	31.1
78-82	30.9	31.0	31.2	31.4	31.6	31.8	31.9	32.1	32.3
83-87	32.0	32.2	32.4	32.6	32.7	32.9	33.1	33.3	33.5
88-92	33.1	33.3	33.5	33.7	33.8	34.0	34.2	34.4	34.6
93-97	34.1	34.3	34.5	34.7	34.9	35.1	35.2	35.4	35.6
98-102	35.1	35.3	35.5	35.7	35.9	36.0	36.2	36.4	36.6
103-107	36.1	36.2	36.4	36.6	36.8	37.0	37.2	37.3	37.5
108-112	36.9	37.1	37.3	37.5	37.7	37.9	38.0	38.2	38.4
113-117	37.8	37.9	38.1	38.3	39.2	39.4	39.6	39.8	39.2
118-122	38.5	38.7	38.9	39.1	39.4	39.6	39.8	40.0	40.0
123-127	39.2	39.4	39.6	39.8	40.0	40.1	40.3	40.5	40.7
128-132	39.9	40.1	40.2	40.4	40.6	40.8	41.0	41.2	41.3
133-137	40.5	40.7	40.8	41.0	41.2	41.4	41.6	41.7	41.9
138-142	41.0	41.2	41.4	41.6	41.7	41.9	42.1	42.3	42.5
143-147	41.5	41.7	41.9	42.0	42.2	42.4	42.6	42.8	43.0
148-152	41.9	42.1	42.3	42.8	42.6	42.8	43.0	43.2	43.4
153-157	42.3	42.5	42.6	42.8	43.0	43.2	43.4	43.6	43.7
158-162	42.6	42.8	43.0	43.1	43.3	43.5	43.7	43.9	44.1
163-167	42.9	43.0	43.2	43.4	43.6	43.8	44.0	44.1	44.3
168-172	43.1	43.2	43.4	43.6	43.8	44.0	44.2	44.3	44.5
173-177	43.2	43.4	43.6	43.8	43.9	44.1	44.3	44.5	44.7
178-182	43.3	43.5	43.7	43.8	44.0	44.2	44.4	44.6	44.8

Reprinted with permission from Jackson, A.S., and Pollock, M.L.: Practical assessment of body composition. Physician and Sportsmedicine, 13(5), 1985, p. 88.

TABLE 8-3	Jackson and Pollock Percent Body Fat Estimate for Men from Sum of Triceps, Chest, and Subscapular Skinfolds

SUM OF SKINFOLDS (mm)	AGE TO LAST YEAR								
	UNDER 22	23–27	28–32	33–37	38–42	43–47	48–52	53–57	OVER 57
8–10	1.5	2.0	2.5	3.1	3.6	4.1	4.6	5.1	5.6
11–13	3.0	3.5	4.0	4.5	5.1	5.6	6.1	6.6	7.1
14–16	4.5	5.0	5.5	6.0	6.5	7.0	7.6	8.1	8.6
17–19	5.9	6.4	6.9	7.4	8.0	8.5	9.0	9.5	10.0
20–22	7.3	7.8	8.3	8.8	9.4	9.9	10.4	10.9	11.4
23–25	8.6	9.2	9.7	10.2	10.7	11.2	11.8	12.3	12.8
26–28	10.0	10.5	11.0	11.5	12.1	12.6	13.1	13.6	14.2
29–31	11.2	11.8	12.3	12.8	13.4	13.9	14.4	14.9	15.5
32–34	12.5	13.0	13.5	14.1	14.6	15.1	15.7	16.2	16.7
35–37	13.7	14.2	14.8	15.3	15.8	16.4	16.9	17.4	18.0
38–40	14.9	15.4	15.9	16.5	17.0	17.6	18.1	18.6	19.2
41–43	16.0	16.6	17.1	17.6	18.2	18.7	19.3	19.8	20.3
44–46	17.1	17.7	18.2	18.7	19.3	19.8	20.4	20.9	21.5
47–49	18.2	18.7	19.3	19.8	20.4	20.9	21.4	22.0	22.5
50–52	19.2	19.7	20.3	20.8	21.4	21.9	22.5	23.0	23.6
53–55	20.2	20.7	21.3	21.8	22.4	22.9	23.5	24.0	24.6
56–58	21.1	21.7	22.2	22.8	23.3	23.9	24.4	25.0	25.5
59–61	22.0	22.6	23.1	23.7	24.2	24.8	25.3	25.9	26.5
62–64	22.9	23.4	24.0	24.5	25.1	25.7	26.2	26.8	27.3
65–67	23.7	24.3	24.8	25.4	25.9	26.5	27.1	27.6	28.2
68–70	24.5	25.0	25.6	26.2	26.7	27.3	27.8	28.4	29.0
71–73	25.2	25.8	26.3	26.9	27.5	28.0	28.6	29.1	29.7
74–76	25.9	26.5	27.0	27.6	28.2	28.7	29.3	29.9	30.4
77–79	26.6	27.1	27.7	28.2	28.8	29.4	29.9	30.5	31.1
80–82	27.2	27.7	28.3	28.9	29.4	30.0	30.6	31.1	31.7
83–85	27.7	28.3	28.8	29.4	30.0	30.5	31.1	31.7	32.3
86–88	28.2	28.8	29.4	29.9	30.5	31.1	31.6	32.2	32.8
89–91	28.7	29.3	29.8	30.4	31.0	31.5	32.1	32.7	33.3
92–94	29.1	29.7	30.3	30.8	31.4	32.0	32.6	33.1	33.4
95–97	29.5	30.1	30.6	31.2	31.8	32.4	32.9	33.5	34.1
98–100	29.8	30.4	31.0	31.6	32.1	32.7	33.3	33.9	34.4
101–103	30.1	30.7	31.3	31.8	32.4	33.0	33.6	34.1	34.7
104–106	30.4	30.9	31.5	32.1	32.7	33.2	33.8	34.4	35.0
107–109	30.6	31.1	31.7	32.3	32.9	33.4	34.0	34.6	35.2
110–112	30.7	31.3	31.9	32.4	33.0	33.6	34.2	34.7	35.3
113–115	30.8	31.4	32.0	32.5	33.1	33.7	34.3	34.9	35.4
116–118	30.9	31.5	32.0	32.6	33.2	33.8	34.3	34.9	35.5

Reprinted with permission from Jackson, A.S., and Pollock, M.L.: Practical assessment of body composition. Physician and Sportsmedicine, 13(5), 1985, p. 87.

is age in years. Percent body fat is calculated from body density by the same Siri equation given in Formula 8-3.

$$BD_{men} = 1.1125025 - 0.0013125\ (X) + 0.0000055\ (X)^2$$
$$- 0.0002440\ (Y) \qquad\qquad \text{Formula 8-4}$$

$$\%BF = (495 \div BD) - 450 \qquad\qquad \text{Formula 8-3}$$

Comment

The Siri equation for converting body density to percent body fat works well for most healthy young to middle-aged adult men. Alternative formulas have been developed for children, elderly adults, the infirm, and athletes in training (14).

Circumference Measurements

Body composition can also be estimated from circumference, or girth, measurements with a simple tape measure. Girth measurements are most useful for (*a*) determining patterns of fat distribution in a person, (*b*) identifying changes in a person's fat pattern over time, and (*c*) ranking individuals within a group according to fatness. This method is based on the understanding that fat is most likely to be found at body sites such as the abdomen, hips, and thighs, while muscle tissue is most likely to be found at sites such as the forearms, calves, and over the biceps on the upper arm. Estimates of percent body fat are based on ratios of girth measurements.

Frank Katch and William McArdle are the leading researchers in circumference measurements for body composition assessment. Presented here are their procedures for estimation of percent body fat from circumferences for young women and men aged 17 to 26. Katch and McArdle have developed similar procedures for adults aged 27 to 50 years (15).

Accuracy of Circumference Estimates

Katch and McArdle (15) have determined that their circumference methods have standard errors of ±2.5 to ±4%. This suggests that their circumference estimates of percent body fat are generally comparable with those from skinfold measurements. Lohman and associates (5) rate circumferences as a "good" method of body composition. Katch and McArdle caution, however, that the equations to predict percent body fat from circumferences are population specific and should not be used for persons who have participated for years in weight training and/or strenuous sports. There may also be problems with the Katch and McArdle equations for persons who are very thin or very fat.

If the measurer takes care to locate the tape properly and to apply the recommended amount of tension to the tape, circumference measurements can be highly reliable and objective (15). Test-retest reliability of limb measures may be as high as .99. Trunk area circumferences are a little less reliable, probably because of variations due to breathing. Intermeasurer and intrameasurer objectivity coefficients are generally in the upper .90s (13).

How to Measure a Circumference

The tape measure should be flexible but inelastic and fairly narrow; 0.7 cm is recommended (13). It is desirable to use a tape measure with a spring-retraction mechanism so that constant tension can be applied during measurements. The examiner should hold the zero end of the tape in the left hand, just above or below the remaining tape held by the right hand. The tape should be snug around the body part without indenting the skin or compressing subcutaneous adipose tissue. Duplicate measurements should be taken, and the girth measurement should be recorded to the quarter inch (13, 15). Figure 8-5 shows proper technique for measurement of the thigh girth.

Location of Circumference Sites

Incorrect positioning of the tape measure reduces validity and reliability. Unless otherwise specified, *tape location is perpendicular to the long axis of the body part and parallel to the floor*. Table 8-4 describes the proper locations for the circumference measurements employed by Katch and McArdle for the methods described in the next two sections of this chapter (15).

Katch and McArdle Percent Body Fat Assessment for Young Women

Purpose

This procedure estimates percent body fat from selected circumference measurements of women 17 to 26 years of age.

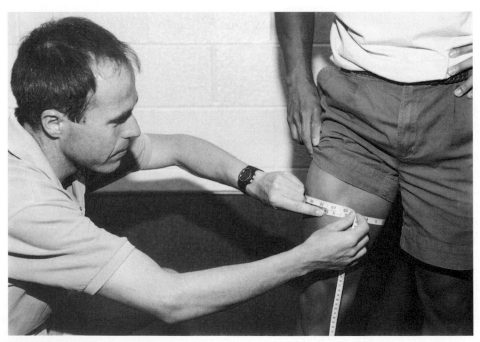

FIGURE 8-5

For an accurate girth measurement, the tape should be snug around the body part without indenting the skin or compressing the underlying fat tissue. (Photo by Marvin Arrington, Heritage Photography, Greensboro, NC.)

TABLE 8-4	McArdle, Katch, and Katch Circumference Measurement Locations	

CIRCUMFERENCE SITE	ANATOMICAL LOCATION
Abdomen	1 inch above umbilicus
Right thigh	Upper thigh just below buttocks
Right upper arm	Arm straight, palm up, extended in front of body; measure at midpoint between shoulder and elbow
Right forearm	Maximal circumference with arm extended in front of body and palm up

Psychometric Information

Using criteria of body density and percent body fat determined by hydrostatic weighing, prediction equations were developed to estimate percent body fat from a combination of three circumferences.

Procedures

1. Using recommended techniques, measure the abdomen, right thigh, and right forearm. Duplicate measurements should be taken, and values should be recorded to the nearest quarter inch.
2. Use Table 8-5 to determine the value of constants A, B, and C.
3. If the subject is *not* a regular participant in a vigorous exercise program (minimum of 240 minutes per week), calculate her percent body fat by Formula 8-5:

   %BF = constant A + constant B − constant C − 19.6   Formula 8-5

4. If the subject is a regular exerciser, calculate her percent body fat by Formula 8-6:

   %BF = constant A + constant B − constant C − 22.6   Formula 8-6

Katch and McArdle Percent Body Fat Assessment for Young Men

Purpose

This procedure estimates percent body fat from selected circumference measurements of men 17 to 26 years of age.

Psychometric Information

Using criteria of body density and percent body fat determined by hydrostatic weighing, prediction equations were developed to estimate percent body fat from a combination of three circumferences.

Procedures

1. Using recommended techniques, measure the abdomen, right upper arm, and right forearm. Duplicate measurements should be taken, and values should be recorded to the nearest quarter inch.

(*text continues on page 222*)

TABLE 8-5	McArdle, Katch, and Katch Conversion Constants to Predict %BF for Young Women From Abdomen, Thigh, and Forearm Circumferences				
ABDOMEN		THIGH		FOREARM	
INCHES	CONSTANT A	INCHES	CONSTANT B	INCHES	CONSTANT C
20.00	26.74	14.00	29.13	6.00	25.86
20.25	27.07	14.25	29.65	6.25	26.94
20.50	27.41	14.50	30.17	6.50	28.02
20.75	27.74	14.75	30.69	6.75	29.10
21.00	28.07	15.00	31.21	7.00	30.17
21.25	28.41	15.25	31.73	7.25	31.25
21.50	28.74	15.50	32.25	7.50	32.33
21.75	29.08	15.75	32.77	7.75	33.41
22.00	29.41	16.00	33.29	8.00	34.48
22.25	29.74	16.25	33.61	8.25	35.56
22.50	30.08	16.50	34.33	8.50	36.64
22.75	30.41	16.75	34.85	8.75	37.72
23.00	30.75	17.00	35.37	9.00	38.79
23.25	31.08	17.25	35.89	9.25	39.87
23.50	31.42	17.50	36.41	9.50	40.95
23.75	31.75	17.75	36.93	9.75	42.03
24.00	32.08	18.00	37.45	10.00	43.10
24.25	32.42	18.25	37.97	10.25	44.18
24.50	32.75	18.50	38.49	10.50	45.26
24.75	33.09	18.75	39.01	10.75	46.34
25.00	33.42	19.00	39.53	11.00	47.41
25.25	33.76	19.25	40.05	11.25	48.49
25.50	34.09	19.50	40.57	11.50	49.57
25.75	34.42	19.75	41.09	11.75	50.65
26.00	34.76	20.00	41.61	12.00	51.73
26.25	35.09	20.25	42.13	12.25	52.80
26.50	35.43	20.50	42.65	12.50	53.88
26.75	35.76	20.75	43.17	12.75	54.96
27.00	36.10	21.00	43.69	13.00	56.04
27.25	36.43	21.25	44.21	13.25	57.11
27.50	36.76	21.50	44.73	13.50	58.19
27.75	37.10	21.75	45.25	13.75	59.27
28.00	37.43	22.00	45.77	14.00	60.35
28.25	37.77	22.25	46.29	14.25	61.42
28.50	38.10	22.50	46.81	14.50	62.50
28.75	38.43	22.75	47.33	14.75	63.58
29.00	38.77	23.00	47.85	15.00	64.66
29.25	39.10	23.25	48.37	15.25	65.73
29.50	39.44	23.50	48.89	15.50	66.81
29.75	39.77	23.75	49.41	15.75	67.89
30.00	40.11	24.00	49.93	16.00	68.97
30.25	40.44	24.25	50.45	16.25	70.04

TABLE 8-5		*(Continued)*			

ABDOMEN		THIGH		FOREARM	
INCHES	CONSTANT A	INCHES	CONSTANT B	INCHES	CONSTANT C
30.50	40.77	24.50	50.97	16.50	71.12
30.75	41.11	24.75	51.49	16.75	72.20
31.00	41.44	25.00	52.01	17.00	73.28
31.25	41.78	25.25	52.53	17.25	74.36
31.50	42.11	25.50	53.05	17.50	75.43
31.75	42.45	25.75	53.57	17.75	76.51
32.00	42.78	26.00	54.09	18.00	77.59
32.25	43.11	26.25	54.61	18.25	78.67
32.50	43.45	26.50	55.13	18.50	79.74
32.75	43.78	26.75	55.65	18.75	80.82
33.00	44.12	27.00	56.17	19.00	81.90
33.25	44.45	27.25	56.69	19.25	82.98
33.50	44.78	27.50	57.21	19.50	84.05
33.75	45.12	27.75	57.73	19.75	85.13
34.00	45.45	28.00	58.26	20.00	86.21
34.25	45.79	28.25	58.78		
34.50	46.12	28.50	59.30		
34.75	46.46	28.75	59.82		
35.00	46.79	29.00	60.34		
35.25	47.12	29.25	60.86		
35.50	47.46	29.50	61.38		
35.75	47.79	29.75	61.90		
36.00	48.13	30.00	62.42		
36.25	48.46	30.25	62.94		
36.50	48.80	30.50	63.45		
36.75	49.13	30.75	63.98		
37.00	49.46	31.00	64.50		
37.25	49.80	31.25	65.02		
37.50	50.16	31.50	65.54		
37.75	50.47	31.75	66.06		
38.00	50.80	32.00	66.58		
38.25	51.13	32.25	67.10		
38.50	51.47	32.50	67.62		
38.75	51.80	32.75	68.14		
39.00	52.14	33.00	68.66		
39.25	52.47	33.25	69.18		
39.50	52.81	33.50	69.70		
39.75	53.14	33.75	70.22		
40.00	53.47	34.00	70.74		

Adapted from McArdle, W.D., Katch, F.I., and Katch, V.L.: Exercise Physiology: Energy, Nutrition and Human Performance. 4th ed. Baltimore, Williams & Wilkins, 1996, pp. 549–550.

2. Use Table 8-6 to determine the value of constants A, B, and C.
3. If the subject is *not* a regular participant in a vigorous exercise program (minimum of 240 minutes a week), calculate his percent body fat by Formula 8-7:

%BF = constant A + constant B − constant C − 10.2   Formula 8-7

4. If the subject is a regular exerciser, calculate his percent body fat by Formula 8-8:

%BF = constant A + constant B − constant C − 14.2   Formula 8-8

Bioelectrical Analysis of Body Composition

Bioelectrical analysis is a relatively new technique for assessing body composition. It has been documented as a safe, convenient, and potentially accurate procedure. Bioelectrical analysis is based on the understanding that lean tissue, because of its higher water content, is a much better conductor of electricity than is fat tissue. The method is simple. The client lies on his or her back on a nonconducting surface. Electrodes are placed on the client's wrist and ankle, and a low-level single-frequency electrical current is introduced. A meter measures the resistance and feeds this information directly into a computer. Body composition is calculated from a prediction equation that includes the measure of resistance plus the square value of the client's height. Today's computer programs print attractive, colorful, individualized analyses for each client.

Despite the price tag of several thousand dollars per unit, many fitness clubs, employee fitness centers, and universities have purchased bioelectrical analysis equipment. Why? Clients appreciate the individualized feedback about this aspect of their fitness. But why spend thousands of dollars for bioelectrical analysis equipment instead of a couple of hundred dollars for a good skinfold caliper? First, the training for use of the bioelectrical analysis equipment is minimal. Second, clients appreciate the noninvasiveness of this technique. A wrist and an ankle are the only body parts that must be bared; there is no need to disrobe in front of a stranger. Third, the technique is very fast, taking only a couple of minutes per client. This makes it very practical for use with large groups.

> Bioelectrical analysis is a method for determining body composition calculated from the measure of resistance to electrical current plus the square value of the client's height.

Accuracy of Bioelectrical Analysis

Only a few years ago the standard error for bioelectrical analysis technology was ±6%, a value considered by most people to be too large to justify the expense of the machine. Recent technological advances have lowered the standard error to about ±3.5%, or about the same as for skinfold assessments (5, 16). Early instruments measured bioelectrical impedance, which is composed of a resistive component and a reactive component. Newer instruments measure only bioelectrical resistance (16). This change, along with enhanced calibration, has improved the predictive ability of equations based on bioelectrical resistance.

TABLE 8-6	McArdle, Katch, and Katch Conversion Constants to Predict %BF for Young Men From Upper Arm, Abdomen, and Forearm Circumferences				

UPPER ARM		ABDOMEN		FOREARM	
INCHES	CONSTANT A	INCHES	CONSTANT B	INCHES	CONSTANT C
7.00	25.91	21.00	27.56	7.00	38.01
7.25	26.83	21.25	27.88	7.25	39.37
7.50	27.76	21.50	28.21	7.50	40.72
7.75	28.68	21.75	28.54	7.75	42.08
8.00	29.61	22.00	28.87	8.00	43.44
8.25	30.53	22.25	29.20	8.25	44.80
8.50	31.46	22.50	29.52	8.50	46.15
8.75	32.38	22.75	29.85	8.75	47.51
9.00	33.31	23.00	30.18	9.00	48.87
9.25	34.24	23.25	30.51	9.25	50.23
9.50	35.16	23.50	30.84	9.50	51.58
9.75	36.09	23.75	31.16	9.75	52.94
10.00	37.01	24.00	31.49	10.00	54.30
10.25	37.94	24.25	31.82	10.25	55.65
10.50	38.86	24.50	32.15	10.50	57.01
10.75	39.79	24.75	32.48	10.75	58.37
11.00	40.71	25.00	32.80	11.00	59.73
11.25	41.64	25.25	33.13	11.25	61.08
11.50	42.56	25.50	33.46	11.50	62.44
11.75	43.49	25.75	33.79	11.75	63.80
12.00	44.41	26.00	34.12	12.00	65.16
12.25	45.34	26.25	34.44	12.25	66.51
12.50	46.26	26.50	34.77	12.50	67.87
12.75	47.19	26.75	35.10	12.75	69.23
13.00	48.11	27.00	35.43	13.00	70.59
13.25	49.04	27.25	35.76	13.25	71.94
13.50	49.96	27.50	36.09	13.50	73.30
13.75	50.89	27.75	36.41	13.75	74.66
14.00	51.82	28.00	36.74	14.00	76.02
14.25	52.74	28.25	37.07	14.25	77.37
14.50	53.67	28.50	37.40	14.50	78.73
14.75	54.59	28.75	37.73	14.75	80.09
15.00	55.52	29.00	38.05	15.00	81.45
15.25	56.44	29.25	38.38	15.25	82.80
15.50	57.37	29.50	38.71	15.50	84.16
15.75	58.29	29.75	39.04	15.75	85.52
16.00	59.22	30.00	39.37	16.00	86.88
16.25	60.14	30.25	39.69	16.25	88.23
16.50	61.07	30.50	40.02	16.50	89.59
16.75	61.99	30.75	40.35	16.75	90.95
17.00	62.92	31.00	40.68	17.00	92.31
17.25	63.84	31.25	41.01	17.25	93.66
17.50	64.77	31.50	41.33	17.50	95.02

(continued)

TABLE 8-6	McArdle, Katch, and Katch Conversion Constants to Predict %BF for Young Men From Upper Arm, Abdomen, and Forearm Circumferences (*Continued*)

UPPER ARM		ABDOMEN		FOREARM	
INCHES	CONSTANT A	INCHES	CONSTANT B	INCHES	CONSTANT C
17.75	65.69	31.75	41.66	17.75	96.38
18.00	66.62	32.00	41.99	18.00	97.74
18.25	67.54	32.25	42.32	18.25	99.09
18.50	68.47	32.50	42.65	18.50	100.45
18.75	69.40	32.75	42.97	18.75	101.81
19.00	70.32	33.00	43.30	19.00	103.17
19.25	71.25	33.25	43.63	19.25	104.52
19.50	72.17	33.50	43.95	19.50	105.88
19.75	73.10	33.75	44.29	19.75	107.24
20.00	74.02	34.00	44.61	20.00	108.60
20.25	74.95	34.25	44.94	20.25	109.95
20.50	75.87	34.50	45.27	20.50	111.31
20.75	76.80	34.75	45.60	20.75	112.67
21.00	77.72	35.00	45.93	21.00	114.02
21.25	78.65	35.25	46.25	21.25	115.38
21.50	79.57	35.50	46.58	21.50	116.74
21.75	80.50	35.75	46.91	21.75	118.10
22.00	81.42	36.00	47.24	22.00	119.45
		36.25	47.57		
		36.50	47.89		
		36.75	48.22		
		37.00	48.55		
		37.25	48.88		
		37.50	49.21		
		37.75	49.54		
		38.00	49.86		
		38.25	50.19		
		38.50	50.52		
		38.75	50.85		
		39.00	51.18		
		39.25	51.50		
		39.50	51.83		
		39.75	52.16		
		40.00	52.49		
		40.25	52.82		
		40.50	53.14		
		40.75	53.47		
		41.00	53.80		
		41.25	54.13		
		41.50	54.46		
		41.75	54.78		
		42.00	55.11		

Adapted from McArdle, W.D., Katch, F.I., and Katch, V.L.: Exercise Physiology: Energy, Nutrition and Human Performance. 4th ed. Baltimore, Williams & Wilkins, 1996, pp. 546–547.

Accuracy of bioelectrical analysis also depends on use of standard measurement procedures, that is, use of a nonconducting surface, correct placement of electrodes, moderate temperatures, normal hydration of the client, and restriction of exercise and food for 4 hours prior to the measurement. It has also been found that fluid retention associated with a woman's menstrual cycle can reduce the accuracy of this method (11).

Near-Infrared Interactance

Used commercially to measure the fat content of meats, near-infrared interactance has been found useful to assess body composition in human beings. In this method a small instrument is held over the biceps and a reading is taken. This is a very fast, noninvasive method of body composition. However, standard errors are greater than ±4.0%, that is, a little larger than for skinfolds, circumferences, and bioelectrical analysis (5). Near-infrared interactance is therefore not so far a preferred procedure.

Dual Energy X-ray Absorptiometry

Dual energy x-ray absorptiometry (DXA) is a new and promising technique for assessment of body composition (17). Because of equipment costs, however, it is not considered a practical method for most field settings. DXA is based on a three-component model of body composition, that is, bone, fat, and lean soft tissue. The client lies on his or her back while an x-ray unit scans the body. A single scan produces regional and whole-body estimates of bone mineral density, fat, and lean tissue. By comparing regional estimates for the trunk area with fat on the extremities, clinicians and researchers can get a very good idea of the client's risk of contracting several chronic diseases. The DXA scan is quick and noninvasive, and it can be used on adults, children, and special populations.

Evaluation of Body Fat Percentages

What do these body fat percentages mean? How much fat is too much? The U.S. Department of Health and Human Services has defined **obesity** as an excess of fat at which point health risks begin to increase (18). Health officials and researchers are not in agreement about where that point lies. This is no doubt because most studies of body composition and health use convenience samples. Lohman and associates (5) used epidemiology data from the National Health and Nutrition Examination Survey (NHANES) to develop new fat standards for healthy adult men and women (5). Because these standards are based on data from a very large, nationally representative sample of men and women, it is believed that they are more accurate than standards developed from convenience sample data. They offer separate standards for men and women by age categories. Table 8-7 shows the new fat health standards, that is, the levels of body fat that best support health and well-being. It is assumed that obesity and the concomitant health risks begin at the upper limits of these recommendations.

Obesity is the level of excess fat at which fat-related health risks begin to increase.

TABLE 8-7	New Percent Fat Health Standards for Men and Women				
	RECOMMENDED BODY FAT (%BF) LEVELS				
	Not Recommended	Low	Mid	Upper	Obesity
MEN					
Young adult	<8	8	13	22	→
Middle age	<10	10	18	25	→
Elderly	<10	10	16	23	→
WOMEN					
Young adult	<20	20	28	35	→
Middle age	<25	25	32	38	→
Elderly	<25	25	30	35	→

Adapted from Lohman, T.G., Houtkooper, L., and Going, S.B.: Body fat measurement goes high-tech: not all are created equal. ACSM's Health & Fitness Journal, 1(1): p. 32, 1997.

What can you conclude from analysis of Table 8-7? First, it is clear that women are expected to carry considerably more body fat than men. Second, there appears to be a fairly large range of acceptable body fatness. It is likely that these values are affected by genetics and vary from one person to another (19).

Epidemiological research has demonstrated that mortality rates are J-shaped. This means that death rates are higher for both overfat and too-thin persons than for persons in the middle range. In other words, health risks are associated with extremes on both ends of the body fatness continuum. As already noted, overfatness is associated with high risks of cardiovascular and other serious diseases. Underfatness may impair the body's ability to function normally, to regulate temperatures, and to protect internal organs from trauma. Biologists believe that the level of **essential body fat** for women is about 12%; the level for men is about 3% (15). For optimal health, no one, not even an elite athlete, should carry less than these levels of body fat.

> Essential body fat is the minimal level of fat necessary for maintenance of normal functions of the body.

Effect of Aging on Evaluation of Body Composition

With aging, less of a person's body fat lies in subcutaneous storage and more surrounds the internal organs. Furthermore, skeletal bones demineralize and become increasingly porous. These phenomena explain why age must be considered in percent body fat calculations. However, neither of these facts directly addresses how body fat evaluations are affected by age. It is common for both women and men to gain *fat weight* as they age. In fact, the median percent body fat goes from 11 and 27% for young adult men and women, respectively, to 17 and 35% for elderly men and women (5). While relatively few health risks seem to be associated with modest increases, it is unclear whether there are any advantages. **Creeping obesity** is most likely the result of adaptations to sedentary living. Thus, some experts maintain that optimal body fat standards should remain constant throughout adulthood.

> Creeping obesity is the tendency for aging adults to accumulate gradually greater amounts of body fat.

Body Fat for Optimal Wellness and Athletic Performance

What if someone is concerned with more than just preventing illness and maintaining normal body functions? What about fitness and wellness? What if athletic excellence is one's goal? Obviously, evaluations of percent body fat are affected by many types of concerns.

On the average, athletes and other physically active persons have less body fat than their peers. Women athletes have an average of 12 to 22% body fat; men athletes have average values of 5 to 13% (19). Optimal body fat percentages vary greatly from one sport to another (20). They also vary from person to person within a single sport. Athletes must work carefully with their coaches and trainers to determine their personal optimal competitive fat weight.

For nonathletic persons who are concerned with general fitness, that is, those who desire an active lifestyle to optimize the physical dimension of their wellness, standards probably fall somewhere between the recommendations for general health and the averages for athletes. Table 8-8 provides fat fitness standards for active men and women of varying ages. Like the fat health standards, they were developed from the NHANES data.

TABLE 8-8	New Percent Fat Fitness Standards for Active Men and Women		
RECOMMENDED %BF LEVELS			
	Low	Mid	Upper
MEN			
Young adult	5	10	15
Middle age	7	11	18
Elderly	9	12	18
WOMEN			
Young adult	16	23	28
Middle age	20	27	33
Elderly	20	27	33

Adapted from Lohman, T.G., Houtkooper, L., and Going, S.B.: Body fat measurement goes high-tech: Not all are created equal. ACSM's Health & Fitness Journal, 1(1): p. 33, 1997.

Body Fat for Aesthetics

What about the person who just wants to feel good about the way he or she looks? What is the responsibility of exercise and sport practitioners to this person? We must not underestimate the importance of physical looks to many of the people we are charged to assist. Social messages about thinness and muscularity are powerful; they inundate us daily. As a culture, although we are getting fatter, our body shape preferences are now thinner than they were only a couple of decades ago (21). While being careful to honor each client's feelings, we must also do whatever we can to encourage a broader definition of body beauty. We must not let beauty be defined for us and for our clients by the fashion industry and electronic media. Body beauty, thinness, and muscularity are not synonymous with worth as a human being (22). When working with clients, we should reinforce the health benefits of the broad middle range of body fatness. As we do so, we should assist our clients to accept their own body. As suggested in Figure 8-6, it is important to learn to be more accepting of your body. After all, there is a large range of acceptable body fatness.

Calculating Desirable Body Weight From Percent Body Fat

If a client's percent body fat estimate does not match the percent body fat that is deemed desirable, a simple series of calculations can reveal what she or he should weigh at the desired percent body fat. The difference between present and desired body weight is the amount of fat that should be lost or gained by a monitored program of diet and exercise. (This is oversimplified. When body fat is lost, the lean mass that was developed to support the extra fat is also considered excessive. Nonetheless, these calculations provide a starting point to understand the goals of a weight control program.)

The steps for these calculations:

1. Determine present body composition status, including *present percent body fat* and *present total body weight*.
2. Calculate *present fat weight* and *lean body weight*. (FW = %BF × TBW and LBW = TBW − FW.)

SALLY FORTH

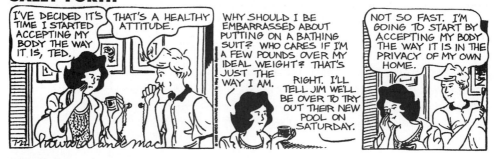

FIGURE 8-6

Like many others of us, Sally is trying to learn to be more accepting of her body. (Reprinted with permission from *Sally Forth*, by Greg Howard, distributed by King Features Syndicate, July 22, 1983.)

3. Determine *desired percent body fat*. (Hint: Use a conservative figure.)
4. Determine *desired lean body percentage*. (1 − desired %BF = desired LB%.)
5. Calculate *desired body weight* by dividing LBW by desired LB%.
6. Calculate *fat weight to be lost or gained*. (TBW − desired BW = FW to be lost or gained.)

EXAMPLE

Client: Jane Doe, aged 20

Present %BF = 32% (determined by three-site skinfolds) ; present TBW = 150 lb
Present FW = .32 × 150 = 48 lb; present LBW = 150 − 48 = 102 lb
Desired %BF = 25% (top limit for optimal fitness)
Desired LB% = 1 − 25% = 75% = 0.75
Desired BW = 102 lb ÷ 0.75 = 136 lb
FW to be Lost = 150 lb − 136 lb = 14 lb

Screening Techniques for Body Composition

Discussed thus far are "true" methods of body composition assessment. They are true in the sense that they quantify the relative contributions of lean and fat tissues to the overall weight of the human body. Neither of the following methods does this. Instead they use anthropometric measures of height, weight, and selected circumferences to assess body composition indirectly. For this reason they are considered to be screening tools for body composition. These methods are highly practical and can be extremely useful in many clinical and field settings.

Body Mass Index

In 1953 the Metropolitan Life Insurance Company developed the first tables of "desirable" body weights for women and men according to height. These tables and subsequent revisions of them were based on actuarial data from insured persons; the data did not represent all ages, races, and socioeconomic groups. Despite their ease of interpretation and appropriateness for some persons, height-weight tables are insufficient for body composition assessment. Their use may lead to invalid conclusions, particularly for two types of persons. A heavily muscled person may be *overweight* according to the tables but may actually have an appropriate percent body fat. Similarly, an undermuscled person with excessive body fat may register as desirable in weight or perhaps even underweight.

Body mass index (BMI) is an improvement over height-weight tables, although height and weight are the only factors used in the calculation of the index. BMI is defined as the ratio of total body weight in kilograms (1 kg = 2.2 lb) to the square of height (Ht) expressed in meters (1 m = 39.4 inches). It is calculated by Formula 8-9:

BMI = TBW in kg ÷ (Ht in m) ^{2} Formula 8-9

For example, a person who is 5 feet 8 inches (1.73 m) and weighs 150 lb (68.2 kg) has a BMI of 22.8 [68.2 ÷(1.73) ^{2}]. An alternative computationally equivalent calculation is to multiply weight in pounds by 700, then divide the result by the square of height in inches. (If you're a typical American, the chances are that you'll find this second calculation easier.)

In June 1998 the National Heart, Lung, and Blood Institute (NHLBI) released the first federal guidelines on the identification, evaluation, and treatment of overweight and obesity among adults (23). Until the release of these guidelines, researchers and practitioners did not agree on the definitions of normal, overweight, and obesity levels of BMI. The new federal standards for classification of overweight and obesity by BMI values are given in Table 8-9. The NHLBI has estimated that about 97 million American adults are overweight or obese according to the report's criteria. This is approximately 55% of the adult population.

> Body mass index is defined as the ratio of total body weight in kilograms to the square of height expressed in meters.

Accuracy of the BMI

The BMI is widely used in large health studies and is very informative, but its standard error is quite large. It is especially prone to errors for children and the elderly, whose muscle and bone weights in relationship to their heights are changing rapidly. But even for young and middle-aged adults, the relationship between BMI and percent body fat is imprecise. A woman with a BMI of 23 may have a percent body fat anywhere between 24.0 and 34.4%; a man with a BMI of 23 may range in percent body fat from 9.3 to 21.3% (24). Since the BMI fails to distinguish between fat weight and lean body weight, it has limited value as a method of assessing body composition. It is therefore recommended that exercise and sport studies (ESS) practitioners use and interpret the BMI with caution. BMI can be a valuable screening tool to identify persons who *may* have problematic body composition profiles. The screening can be followed up with a true body composition assessment for individuals whose BMI values are 25 and higher.

How to Measure Height and Weight for BMI Calculations

In many situations subjects or clients can be asked to provide their weight and height for calculations of BMI, but some give inaccurate values. Sometimes this is purposeful, but often it is inadvertent. If more precision and/or confidence is needed, height and weight can be measured directly.

TABLE 8-9	Federal Guidelines for Classifying Overweight and Obesity in Adults by BMI	
OVERWEIGHT CLASSIFICATION	**OBESITY CLASS**	**BMI (kg/m^2)**
Underweight		<18.5
Normal		18.5–24.9
Overweight		25.0–29.9
Obesity	I	30.0–34.9
	II	35.0–39.9
Extreme obesity	III	≥40

Reprinted with permission from National Heart, Lung, and Blood Institute: Clinical Guidelines on the Identification, Evaluation, and Treatment of Overweight and Obesity in Adults. Washington, National Institutes of Health, 1998.

The following are the recommended techniques for height and weight measurements (12). Height should be measured from a fully erect position with arms at the sides and hands facing the thighs. Feet should be bare (thin socks are permissible), heels touching, and weight evenly distributed on both feet. Ask the client to inhale deeply and hold his or her breath as the measurement is taken. Weight should be measured on a level platform scale. Light clothing can be worn, but shoes should be removed. Figure 8-7 shows proper measurement of height.

Waist-to-Hip Ratio

In terms of overall health risks, *where* one carries excessive body fat matters. "Apples" have greater health risks than "pears." Excessive fat carried in the abdominal region (the apple shape) is more dangerous than excessive fat carried in the gluteofemoral region (the pear shape). Excessive abdominal fat is associated with elevated risks of coronary heart disease, hypertension, and diabetes (25, 26).

The **waist-to-hip ratio** (WHR) is a quick and easy screening tool that is very effective in identifying persons with elevated health risks due to abdominal fat. The

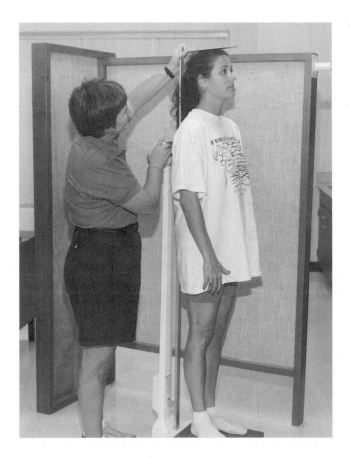

FIGURE 8-7

Height is measured with the client fully erect with arms at the sides and hands facing the thighs. (Photo by Marvin Arrington, Heritage Photography, Greensboro, NC.)

WHR is simply the waist circumference divided by the hip circumference, as expressed in Formula 8-10:

$$WHR = \text{waist circumference} \div \text{hip circumference} \qquad \text{Formula 8-10}$$

The developer of the waist-to-hip ratio, Ahmed Kissebah, suggested that women should have a WHR of .85 or less and men should have a WHR of .95 or less (27). At or below these values the risks of many fat-related chronic diseases may be lower.

For WHR calculations, the waist circumference is defined as the minimum circumference measurement between the rib cage and the pelvis. This measurement should be taken directly on the skin without clothing. The hip measurement is the maximum girth below the pelvic rim. The measurements may be taken in any units, such as inches or centimeters.

Waist Circumference

There is mounting evidence that waist measurement may be an independent risk factor for fat-related diseases and morbidity (23, 28). As such, it may replace the WHR as a predictor of risk. The NHLBI proposed gender-specific cutoff standards for waist circumferences. The cutoff value for women is 35 inches; the value for men is 40 inches (23). So for women whose BMI values are above the "normal" value of 25, a waist measurement larger than 35 inches is thought to add to the risk of heart disease and diabetes. The same is true for men who have a BMI over 25; a waist measurement larger than 40 inches adds to the heart and diabetes risk.

When assessing a client for health risks or to evaluate candidacy for weight loss therapy, the NHLBI recommended consideration of a combination of BMI, waist circumference, and overall risk status related to disease conditions and other obesity-associated diseases (23). Thus, ESS professionals must be knowledgeable and skilled in BMI and waist circumference measurements, calculations, and interpretations.

Body Composition and Children

Should the body composition of children be assessed? YES! It has been determined that 80 to 86% of obesity in adulthood is rooted in childhood overfatness (29). The really bad news is that American children are getting fatter with every passing decade.

Skinfold Assessment of Children

To develop procedures to assess the body composition of children, it was necessary to develop new body density equations for hydrostatic weighing. Equations for adults are not valid for children because children have more water and less bone mineral content in their lean tissues than do adults. Timothy Lohman has conducted extensive research with children and has proposed two highly practical, valid, and reliable skinfold procedures. Each of these procedures employs measurements from only two sites, either the triceps plus subscapular or the triceps plus calf skinfolds. The triceps plus calf procedure is especially useful for mass testing of children because the sites on the extremities are easy to locate and measure. These locations are described in Table 8-10. The triceps plus calf skinfold method is described in the next section (30).

TABLE 8-10	Lohman Tricep and Calf Skinfold Site Locations and Recommended Procedures for Accurate Location		
SKINFOLD SITE	**DIRECTION OF FOLD**	**ANATOMICAL LOCATION**	**LOCATION PROCEDURES**
Triceps	Vertical	Midway between acromion and olecranon on posterior of right arm	Position client with elbow flexed 90°. Use tape measure to locate midpoint between acromion and inferior margin of elbow along side of arm. Mark this point, first on side, then on back of the arm over triceps. After locating skinfold site, have client extend elbow and return arm to a relaxed position at side.
Calf	Vertical	Medial aspect of right calf at greatest girth	Position client with right foot on bench and knee flexed 90°. Use tape measure to locate greatest girth. Mark site on inside of lower leg in line with medial malleolus.

Lohman's Percent Body Fat Assessment for Children and Youth

Purpose

The purpose of assessing body fat in children and youth is to provide a valid and reliable estimate of percent body fat from triceps and calf skinfolds.

Psychometric Information

Skinfold estimates of percent body fat were validated by comparing them with estimates obtained by hydrostatic weighing. In several studies the correlations between skinfolds and hydrostatically determined body fat estimates for children approximated values obtained for adults, that is, from .70 to .90. Test-retest reliability coefficients have exceeded .95 when examiners were properly trained.

Procedures

1. Locate and mark the triceps and calf skinfolds, using procedures described in Table 8-10.
2. At each of the skinfold sites, take three measurements and record the median measurement (i.e., the middle value).
3. Sum the triceps and calf measurements and convert to percent body fat according to the nomograms in Figure 8-8. Standards for evaluation are also provided.

Comment

Please exercise extreme caution when advising weight loss or gain for children and adolescents. These populations can be oversensitive to suggestions that they are overweight, and this type of feedback from a teacher has the potential to contribute

Skinfolds, mm

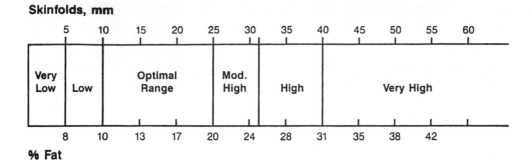

% Fat

Skinfolds, mm

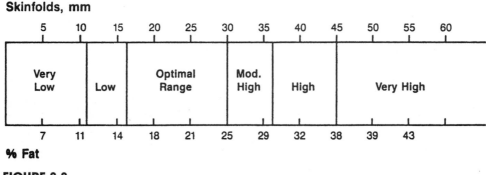

% Fat

FIGURE 8-8

Body composition nomograms for boys (*top*) and girls (*bottom*) for the triceps plus calf skinfolds. (Reprinted with permission from Lohman, T.G.: The use of skinfolds to estimate body fatness on children and youth. Journal of Physical Education, Recreation and Dance, 58(9):67, 69, 1987.)

to development of an eating disorder. The best course of action is to involve parents or guardians in decisions and programs related to weight control.

Body Mass Index for Children

BMI is sometimes calculated as an alternative body composition method for children. As noted earlier, however, it is more prone to errors when used with children than with adults. The index is calculated the same as for adults, but the evaluation differs. BMI values for the FITNESSGRAM "healthy zone" for children from ages 5 to 17+ are given in Tables A-1 and A-2 in Appendix A (31). (The FITNESSGRAM test is described in detail in Appendix A.)

Administrative Suggestions for Body Composition Assessment

Body composition is one of the most sensitive areas of assessment engaged in by exercise and sport practitioners. When performed well, however, it has the potential to provide information that can benefit the client. This should always be our goal.

The conscientious professional should consider the following when performing body composition assessments:

Explain the Assessment. Before taking any measurements, discuss the purpose of the assessment and explain how it will benefit the client. Also explain the actual assessment procedures in detail, including location of measurement sites, proper dress, preassessment exercise and diet restrictions, and so on. Emphasize to the client that he or she may stop the procedure at any time. You *must* explain these matters to parents or guardians before you assess the body composition of a child. For research studies, you may also need a signed human subjects permission form.

Guard the Privacy of the Client. Arrange the environment to allow the client privacy during measurements. A dressing screen can provide a visual barrier to separate the client being measured from those waiting. Record measurements without comments that others could overhear. Depending upon the perceived intimacy of the procedure, consider use of an examiner who is the same gender as the client. You may also wish to have a recorder of the same gender as the client.

Conduct the Evaluation in a Setting Different From That of the Measurements. Allow the client to dress, then sit down together in a quiet area to discuss the assessment. During mass testing, separating the evaluation from the taking of measurements produces best use of time.

Do NOT Overemphasize Thinness. Recognize ranges of acceptable body fat, especially the large ranges for optimal health. Remind your clients about the positive functions of body fat. Never use language or gestures that communicate anything but respect for the client.

Recognize the Limitations of Body Composition Assessment. Explain to clients that the percent body fat estimate is just that—an estimate, *not* a precise measurement. The estimate merely names the midpoint in the range of values that are likely to include the true body fat percentage. Using whatever words you think will be clearest to the client, explain the concept of the standard error of measurement. You might say something like, "The standard error for the three-site skinfold assessment is ±3.5%. This means that for most people, their true body fat percentage may actually be larger or smaller than the value we estimated from the skinfold measurements we took. Your own true body fat percentage is probably somewhere between X and Y%. Let's talk and explore what this may mean for you."

What Do YOU Think?

At its 1994 annual conference, the National Education Association (NEA) issued a warning to teachers to refrain from touching students so as to prevent sexual harassment charges. In light of this warning from the NEA, what should the public school physical education teacher do about body composition assessment? What do YOU think?

Encourage Clients to Ask Questions and Express Their Feelings About the Assessment. Clients will undoubtedly have questions that you can answer for them. Don't rush through the evaluation. Clients who understand and appreciate the original body composition assessment are much more likely to follow diet and exercise regimens than those who do not.

Follow Assessment With Appropriate Diet and Exercise Recommendations. Assessment is only half of your responsibility to your clients. If the client desires your help, work with the client and possibly the parents, medical doctor, coach, and so on to plan and execute a healthy strategy for fat loss or gain and/or muscle mass increases.

Maintain Confidentiality of Body Composition Records. In research studies it is common practice to use numerical codes to identify subjects on data records. Although this degree of secrecy may not be necessary in other settings, it is important to limit access to body composition records. Do not violate your original agreement with the client.

Computers and Body Composition Assessment

Computers can play an important part in assessment of body composition. They are particularly valuable in the evaluation of measurement scores. Numerous commercial programs convert skinfold and/or other anthropometric measurements to percent body fat estimates and present exercise recommendations based on these estimates. In most cases these programs include body composition evaluation as part of a comprehensive fitness assessment. Such programs are advertised widely in journals such as *Fitness Management* and *ACSM's Health & Fitness Journal*.

If you are working within a limited budget, there are at least two viable options. One is to locate an appropriate freeware or shareware program. One of the most affordable and versatile freeware packages includes six Apple programs available on a single diskette, aptly titled Body Composition Programs. These programs were created by Rose M. Rummel and Jean Dalton. The package of programs may be ordered from SOFTSHARE (32). The SOFTSHARE catalog is available from AAHPERD (American Alliance of Health, Physical Education, Recreation, and Dance) Publications. Another economical option is to write your own program. In most cases this is a straightforward process easily done by someone who knows BASIC. For example, a simple program can do the calculations in Formulas 8-2 and 8-3. These will give you an estimate of percent body fat from skinfold measurements and age data.

Computers are quickly transforming the world we live in, in some cases providing sophistication beyond our wildest dreams. Some of today's body composition instruments are truly remarkable. Earlier in this chapter we discussed bioelectrical analysis equipment. The computerization of this equipment has made bioelectrical analysis feasible for use by the practitioner in fitness clubs, corporate wellness centers, and so on. Similarly, small computerized units have been built into other types of body composition equipment. The Skyndex caliper by Cramer Products has an internal computer that can be programmed for various skinfold site equations. The examiner simply takes the skinfolds in the prescribed order, and the caliper displays the percent body fat estimate. There is no manual recording and no charts or formulas to follow. It is not difficult to foresee that many more computerized body composition tools will be developed in the near future.

Chapter Summary

This chapter discusses several methods of valid and reliable body composition assessment. These methods are categorized as either true or screening methods. The chapter recommends ways to evaluate body composition data that these methods produce. This chapter also addresses how and why exercise and sport practitioners may want to undertake body composition assessment for the benefit of their clients. The chapter concludes with a discussion of how body composition assessment can be conducted in a professional manner.

SELF-TEST QUESTIONS

1. Which of the following diseases is *not* commonly associated with overfatness?
   A. Cancer
   B. Coronary heart disease
   C. Diabetes
   D. Epilepsy

2. Using the two-factor model for body composition, what is the fat weight of a 200-lb man whose percent body fat is 22%? _____

3. In this example what is the man's lean body weight? _____

4. Hydrostatic weighing is used to obtain an estimate of body density, which is then used to estimate _____.
   A. Body circumference
   B. Bone density
   C. Percent body fat
   D. Total body weight

5. What is the 68% confidence interval for a person who is estimated to have 20% body fat? (Assume this client was measured in a laboratory using hydrostatic weighing with direct measurement of gases, so use an average standard error of ±1.0%.) _____ to _____

6. Approximately what percent of an adult's total body fat is subcutaneous?
   A. 25%
   B. 50%
   C. 75%
   D. Virtually all, or 100%

7. When using a plastic caliper, which one of the following skinfold measurements is likely to be most accurate?
   A. A triceps measurement of 4 mm
   B. A triceps measurement of 24 mm
   C. A triceps measurement of 44 mm

8. If skinfold measures are taken after aerobic exercise when the client is overheated, the measure will probably be _____.
   A. Smaller than the true measure

    B. Larger than the true measure

    C. Unpredictable in the nature of the error

    D. Accurate but difficult to take due to sweat

9. Poor agreement between skinfold measurements taken by two different examiners is most commonly caused by _____.

    A. Errors in site location

    B. Errors in reading the caliper scale

    C. Poor technique for lifting the skinfold

    D. Erroneous placement of the calipers on skinfold

10. According to Jackson and Pollock, the suprailium skinfold site should be a diagonal fold taken at the level of the iliac crest at a point in line with the

    _____.

    A. Anterior axillary line

    B. Midaxillary line

    C. Posterior axillary line

11. Percent body fat is predicted using an equation that includes two variables, the sum of the skinfold sites and _____.

    A. Age in years

    B. Height in meters

    C. Weight in kilograms

    D. All of the above

12. As men and women age, what generally happens to their patterns of fat deposits?

    A. A greater percentage of total body fat is deposited subcutaneously.

    B. A greater percentage of total body fat is deposited around the trunk organs.

    C. Overall body fat increases, but the pattern of deposits remains constant.

13. According to Table 8-3, what is the percent body fat of a 50-year-old man whose sum of triceps, chest, and subscapular skinfolds is 108 mm?

    _____

14. If the man in question 13 weighs 200 lb, how much fat weight should he lose? Use 25% as desired percent body fat. _____lb

15. According to Katch and McArdle, at which one of the following girth measurement sites is fat most likely to be deposited?

    A. Calf

    B. Forearm

    C. Thigh

    D. Upper arm over biceps

16. Which one of the following body composition methods has the *largest* standard error?

    A. Bioelectrical analysis

    B. Circumferences

    C. Seven-site skinfolds using Lange calipers

    D. Near-infrared interactance

17. BMI is calculated by _____.

    A. Dividing weight in pounds by the square of height in inches

    B. Dividing height in inches by the square of weight in pounds

C. Dividing weight in kilograms by the square of height in meters

D. Dividing height in meters by the square of weight in kilograms

18. If a 5-foot 8-inch woman weighs 160 lb, is her BMI in the normal range?

_____

19. Men should have a WHR equal to or less than

A. 1.05

B. .95

C. .85

D. .75

20. If a woman has a waist circumference of 30 inches and a hip circumference of 40 inches, is her WHR at the desirable level? _____

ANSWERS

1. D	2. 44 lb	3. 156 lb	4. C	5. 19.8–20.2%
6. B	7. B	8. B	9. A	10. A
11. A	12. B	13. 34%	14. 24 lb	15. C
16. D	17. C	18. Yes	19. B	20. Yes

DOING PROJECTS FOR FURTHER LEARNING

1. Visit a local fitness club, a university athletic training facility, or other facility where body composition assessments are done. Ask either to observe or to be measured yourself. Discuss the procedures with the practitioner. In particular, ask about the pros and cons of the procedure used. Also ask about how he or she learned to do body composition assessment.

2. Begin your skinfold practice. Follow the directions in this chapter as closely as you can. Work with a partner and compare the measurements that each of you obtains for each volunteer subject. When differences greater than 1 mm are noted, discuss the procedures used and try to discern the cause of the difference.

3. If you have access to a personal computer and know BASIC computer language, write a program that will perform the calculations in Formulas 8-2 and 8-3. If you do not know computer programming, try to locate a student who does and enlist his or her help.

REFERENCES

1. Melville, D.S., and Cardinal, B.J.: The problem: body fatness within our profession. Journal of Physical Education, Recreation and Dance, 57(7):85, 1988.

2. Kid size: Measurements could use an update. Greensboro, NC: News & Record, August 4, 1997.

3. Siri, W.E.: Body composition from fluid space and density. In J. Brozek and A. Hanschel (eds.). Techniques for Measuring Body Composition. Washington, National Academy of Science, 1961.

4. Brozek, J., et al.: Densiometric analysis of body composition: revision of some quantitative assumptions. Annals of the New York Academy of Science, 110:113, 1963.

5. Lohman, T.G., Houtkooper, L., and Going, S.B.: Body fat measurement goes high-tech: not all are created equal. ACSM's Health & Fitness Journal, 1(1):30, 1997.

6. Baumgartner, T.A., and Jackson, A.S.: Measurement for Evaluation in Physical Education and Exercise Science. 5th ed. Madison, WI, Brown & Benchmark, 1995.

7. Smith, N.: Measuring fat no problem with the mod Bod Pod. Birmingham, AL, Birmingham Business Journal, 15(35), p. 8, 1998.

8. Pollock, M.L., and Jackson, A.S.: Research progress in validation of clinical methods of assessing body composition. Medicine and Science in Sports and Exercise, 16:606, 1984.

9. Lohman, T.G., and Pollock, M.L.: Which caliper? How much training? Journal of Physical Education, Recreation and Dance, 52(1):27, 1981.

10. Gruber, J.J., et al.: Comparison of Harpenden and Lange calipers in predicting body composition. Research Quarterly for Exercise and Sport, 61:184, 1990.

11. Heyward, V.H.: Advanced Fitness Assessment and Exercise Prescription. 3rd ed. Champaign, IL, Human Kinetics, 1997.

12. Jackson, A.S., and Pollock, M.L.: Practical assessment of body composition. Physician and Sportsmedicine, 13(5): 76, 1985.

13. Lohman, T.G., Roche, A.F., and Martorell, R. (eds.): Anthropometric Standardization Reference Manual. Abridged ed. Champaign, IL, Human Kinetics, 1991.

14. Lohman, T.G.: Advances in Body Composition Assessment. Champaign, IL, Human Kinetics, 1992.

15. McArdle, W.D., Katch, F.I., and Katch, V.L.: Exercise Physiology: Energy, Nutrition and Human Performance. 4th ed. Baltimore, Williams & Wilkins, 1996.

16. Lohman, T.G.: The Valhalla study: evaluation of bioelectrical resistance as a measure of body composition. San Diego, Valhalla Scientific, 1991.

17. Lohman, T.G.: Dual energy x-ray absorptiometry. In A.F. Roche, S.B. Heymsfield, and T.G. Lohman (eds.). Human Body Composition. Champaign, IL, Human Kinetics, 1996.

18. U.S. Department of Health and Human Services: Surgeon General's Report on Nutrition and Health. Washington, U.S. Government Printing Office, Publication 88-50210, 1988.

19. Wilmore, J.H., Buskirk, E.R., DiGirolamo, M., and Lohman, T.G.: Body composition: a round table. Physician and Sportsmedicine, 14(3):144, 1986.

20. American College of Sports Medicine: Resource Manual for Guidelines for Exercise Testing and Prescription. 7th ed. Baltimore, Williams & Wilkins, 1998.

21. Garner, D.M.: The 1997 body image survey results. Psychology Today, 30(2):30, 1997.

22. Tritschler, K.A.: Battling a double-edged sword: threats of mind-body dualism and body devaluation. Proceedings of the 1993 Conference of the Southern Association of Physical Education for College Women. Mobile, AL, SAPECW, 1994.

23. National Heart, Lung, and Blood Institute: Clinical Guidelines on the Identification, Evaluation, and Treatment of Overweight and Obesity in Adults. Washington, National Institutes of Health, 1998.

24. Ross, R.M, and Jackson, A.S.: Exercise Concepts, Calculations, and Computer Applications. Madison, WI, Brown & Benchmark, 1990.

25. National Research Council: Diet and Health: Implications for Reducing Chronic Disease Risk. Washington, U.S. Government Printing Office, 1989.

26. Kaplan, N.M.: The deadly quartet: upper-body obesity, glucose intolerance, hypertriglyceridemia, and hypertension. Archives of Internal Medicine, 149:1514, 1989.

27. Avery, C.S.: Abdominal obesity: scaling down this deadly risk. Physician and Sportsmedicine, 9(10):137, 1991.

28. Lean, M.E.J., and Han, T.S.: Waist circumference as a measure for indicating need for weight management. British Medical Journal, 311(6998):158, 1995.

29. National Children and Youth Fitness Study: Summary of findings from national children and youth fitness study. Journal of Physical Education, Recreation and Dance, 56(9):43, 1985.

30. Lohman, T.G.: The use of skinfolds to estimate body fatness on children and youth. Journal of Physical Education, Recreation and Dance, 58(9):67, 1987.

31. Cooper Institute for Aerobics Research: The FITNESSGRAM Test Administration Manual. Champaign, IL, Human Kinetics for the American Fitness Alliance, 1999.

32. Department of Kinesiology, California State University at Fresno: SOFTSHARE Catalog. Available from American Alliance of Health, Physical Education, Recreation, and Dance Bookstore, Reston, VA, AAHPERD, 1999.

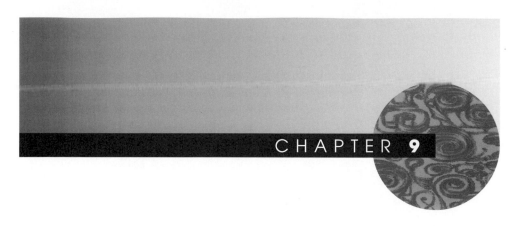

CHAPTER 9

Assessing Cardiorespiratory Fitness

Good cardiorespiratory fitness is essential to humans from the perspectives of both health and performance. High levels of cardiorespiratory fitness are associated with reduced risk of dying of the leading killer of Americans—cardiovascular disease. Largely because of this relationship, *cardiorespiratory fitness is acknowledged as the single most important contributor to overall health-related fitness* And if that is not reason enough to pay attention to this area of fitness, good cardiorespiratory fitness also makes it possible for humans to participate in many of the daily living, occupational, and recreational activities that give our lives meaning and joy (Fig. 9-1). To say that exercise and sport professionals must be knowledgeable about this area of assessment is to state the obvious.

The many physical fitness batteries vary considerably in terms of focus, intended test population, and specific tests. Common to every fitness battery, however, is at least one test of cardiorespiratory fitness. There are also many stand-alone tests of cardiorespiratory fitness; some were developed for use in the laboratory and some, for use in the field. This chapter presents a number of stand-alone field assessments of cardiorespiratory fitness for adults of varying ages. Appendix A has physical fitness batteries for children and for adults.

As you read this chapter, watch for the following keywords:

Blood pressure	Maximal oxygen	Systolic blood
Bradycardia	consumption (VO$_2$max)	pressure
Cardiorespiratory fitness	MET	Tachycardia
Diastolic blood pressure	PAR-Q	Test specificity
Hypertension	Submaximal exercise	
Maximal aerobic power	endurance (stamina)	

Defining Cardiorespiratory Fitness

Cardiorespiratory fitness is a multifactorial construct that is best defined in terms of its components. According to the medical, health, and exercise researchers and practitioners who congregated for the Second International Consensus Symposium,

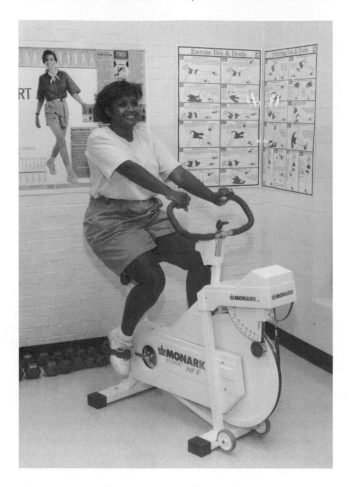

FIGURE 9-1

Good cardiorespiratory fitness makes it possible for adults to participate in daily living, occupational, and recreational activities that give our lives meaning and joy. (Photo by Marvin Arrington, Heritage Photography, Greensboro, NC.)

cardiorespiratory fitness is composed of (*a*) submaximal exercise endurance, (*b*) maximal aerobic power, (*c*) heart and lung function, and (*d*) blood pressure (1).

> Cardiorespiratory fitness consists of submaximal exercise endurance, maximal aerobic power, heart and lung functions, and blood pressure.

Submaximal exercise endurance is defined as a person's level of tolerance to low-intensity exercise demands for long periods. In lay terms it is called **stamina.** Persons with poor submaximal exercise endurance are unable to maintain even low levels of exertion for extended periods. Submaximal exercise endurance is determined by several physiological and metabolic factors, but the primary factor is the efficiency of the body's oxygen delivery system. Also important to submaximal exercise endurance are effective temperature regulation, regeneration of adenosine triphosphate (ATP), and substrate mobilization and use.

> Submaximal exercise endurance (stamina) is the level of tolerance to low-intensity exercise demands for long periods.

Maximal aerobic power is assessed by measuring **maximal oxygen consumption (VO_2max),** that is, the greatest rate at which oxygen can be taken in, distributed, and used during exercise (2). Because it is impossible to maintain an activity at an intensity that requires more oxygen than one's body can provide, the measure of VO_2max defines the upper limit of aerobic exercise. Maximal aerobic power is also positively correlated with health status (3). Maximal aerobic power is determined primarily by the functioning of the cardiovascular and respiratory systems; it is also influenced by the musculoskeletal system.

> Maximal aerobic power, measured by maximal oxygen consumption (VO_2max), refers to the upper limit or maximal rate at which oxygen can be taken in, distributed, and used by the body during exercise.

Heart and lung functions are assessed by a number of indicators that are typically measured both at rest and during exercise. Simple field measurements of heart and lung functions include heart rate and respiration rate. Normal resting heart rates (RHRs) for adults range between 60 and 100, although the RHRs of highly conditioned athletes may be considerably lower. The normal respiration rate during rest is 12 to 15 breaths per minute. Laboratory tests measure stroke volume and cardiac output of the heart and various lung volumes, such as total lung capacity and forced expiratory volume in one second.

Blood pressure is the force or pressure exerted by the blood against the interior walls of the arteries. Two blood pressure phases are special concerns. **Systolic blood pressure** is the measure of greatest force. It occurs at systole, that is, when the heart contracts and pumps a large volume of blood into the arteries. **Diastolic blood pressure,** the measure of lowest force, occurs when the heart is refilling between contractions. Blood pressure is usually recorded as if it were a fraction, that is, systolic pressure/diastolic pressure. The unit of measurement is millimeters of mercury (mm Hg). An average adult blood pressure measurement is 120/80 mm Hg. Normal systolic pressure is less than 130 mm Hg, and normal diastolic pressure is less than 85 mm Hg (2).

> Blood pressure is a measure of the force or pressure exerted by the blood against the interior walls of the arteries.

> Systolic blood pressure is the measure of force of blood at systole (when the heart muscle is contracting and pumping blood into the aorta and pulmonary artery); diastolic blood pressure is the measure of force of blood at diastole (when the heart muscle is relaxed and chambers are filling with blood).

Both systolic and diastolic pressures are typically measured during rest with the subject supine and then sitting or standing. Systolic and diastolic blood pressures are also monitored during exercise testing (Fig. 9-2). Chronically elevated blood pressure, that is, systolic pressure over 140 mm Hg and/or diastolic pressure over 90 mm Hg, is defined as **hypertension.** Hypertension is believed to be a causal factor in death from ischemic heart disease, cardiac failure, stroke, and renal failure. Ex-

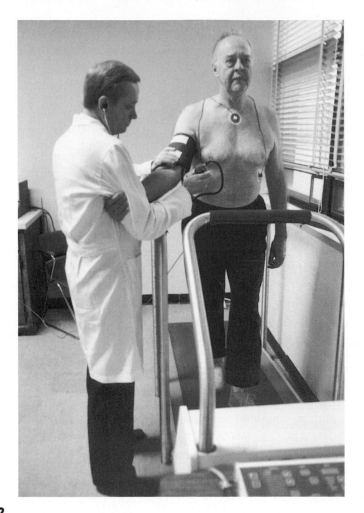

FIGURE 9-2

Systolic and diastolic blood pressures are monitored during exercise testing. (Photo by Dr. Karen Uhlendorf, University of Vermont, Burlington, VT.)

tremely low blood pressure, or *hypotension*, can also be a health and performance concern because a person with very low blood pressure cannot make quick postural changes without becoming dizzy and risking a fall.

> Hypertension is a disease characterized by chronically elevated blood pressure, that is, systolic blood pressure above 140 mm Hg and/or diastolic blood pressure above 90 mm Hg.

Why Assess Cardiorespiratory Fitness?

There are many reasons to assess cardiorespiratory fitness. Here is a sampling:

As Part of a Comprehensive Health-Related Physical Fitness Assessment. Cardiorespiratory fitness, morphological fitness, musculoskeletal fitness, motor fitness, and metabolic fitness are essential components of health-related physical fitness. These qualities are deemed important for the health and well-being of all adults and children. A comprehensive health-related physical fitness assessment includes assessments of all of these components.

As Part of a Comprehensive Physical Examination or Cardiovascular Risk Factor Assessment. Just as good cardiorespiratory function is associated with reduced risks associated with cardiovascular diseases, it is also associated with a low incidence of non–insulin-dependent diabetes mellitus and obesity. A recent study by Lee and associates (4) determined that cardiorespiratory fitness may be more important to overall health than maintaining a normal body weight, that is, BMI less than 25. In their study unfit men had higher all-cause and cardiovascular disease mortality than fit men. The health benefits of normal weights appear to be limited to men who have moderate or high levels of cardiorespiratory fitness.

To Monitor Changes in Cardiorespiratory Functioning in Response to Health-Related Exercise Programs. All-cause mortality rates are lower for persons who expend as few as 2000 kcal of energy per week in walking, stair climbing, and recreational activities, and modest health benefits can accrue from energy expenditures as low as 150 kcal per day or 1000 kcal per week (5, 6). The Centers for Disease Control and Prevention (CDC) and the American College of Sports Medicine (ACSM) have gone on record with a recommendation that every adult accumulate 30 minutes of moderate-intensity physical activity on "most, preferably all, days of the week" (6, 7). For significant improvement in the cardiorespiratory fitness of healthy adults, ACSM recommends *20 to 60 minutes of continuous or intermittent (minimum of 10-minute bouts) of aerobic activity*, at an *intensity of 55 or 65 to 90% of the maximum theoretical exercise heart rate* (i.e., HRmax = 220 − client's age in years), *3 to 5 days per week* (8). A cardiorespiratory fitness assessment can give objective information about the effectiveness of a particular training regimen. This feedback may motivate clients to adhere to aerobic exercise programs.

To Monitor the Effectiveness of Aerobic Training Programs for Athletes and Employees. Training programs must achieve the desired results; regular assessments are essential to the evaluation of training programs.

To Identify Potential in Sports and Areas of Employment With High Aerobic Demands. Cardiorespiratory fitness can assist in the identification of those who are most likely to excel in sports that have high aerobic demands, such as cross-country skiing, running, speed skating, cycling, the biathlon, orienteering, the pentathlon, rowing, and swimming (9) (Fig. 9-3). Similarly, cardiorespiratory assessments can help identify workers who are fit enough to withstand the high aerobic demands of fire fighting, logging, fitness instruction, and military combat.

Does Cardiorespiratory Testing Replace a Medical Examination?

Neither field nor laboratory assessment of cardiorespiratory fitness can substitute for a medical examination. A comprehensive medical examination, especially one that includes a graded exercise test (GXT), is the best way to assess a client's general health and risk of degenerative and chronic diseases and disorders. Cardiorespira-

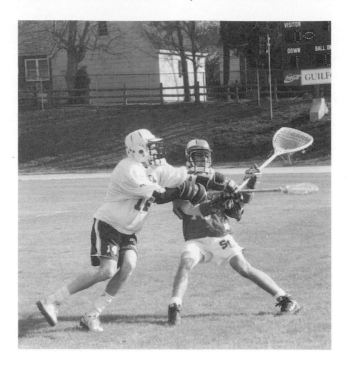

FIGURE 9-3

A cardiorespiratory assessment may identify potential in a sport, such as lacrosse, that has high aerobic demands. (Photo by John Bell, Touch a Life Photography, Greensboro, NC.)

tory fitness assessments described in this chapter should be considered supplemental to regular physician administered medical examinations. They do *not* take the place of medical examinations!

Health Risk Screening Procedures

Is cardiorespiratory fitness assessment safe? Yes! Laboratory and field assessments of cardiorespiratory fitness are very safe for nearly everyone (2). There are, however, considerable, even life threatening, risks for some small numbers of persons. Therefore, before conducting any type of exercise testing, you as the test administrator must conscientiously and carefully screen out all those for whom exercise testing is medically contraindicated. The following health screening procedures are recommended.

ACSM Exercise Testing Guidelines

The ACSM has published guidelines for exercise testing that should be adhered to by researchers, clinicians, and practitioners (2). The ACSM guidelines are summarized here.

Prior to engaging in *submaximal* exercise testing, the following persons should be referred to a physician for a medical examination and clinical exercise testing, and a physician should be present during their test:

Those with known cardiac, pulmonary, or metabolic disease
Those with symptoms or signs suggesting possible cardiopulmonary or meta-
bolic disease (Table 9-1)

Similarly, these persons should obtain medical clearance before beginning an exercise program that requires exercise of moderate intensity. Moderate exercise is defined as requiring an intensity that is well within the person's current capacity, that is, exercise that can be sustained comfortably for as much as an hour. Moderate exercise should also have a gradual warm-up and progression, and it is generally not competitive.

Prior to engaging in *maximal* exercise testing, ACSM recommends that the following persons be referred to a physician for a medical examination and clinical exercise testing, and that a physician be present during their testing:

Those with known cardiac, pulmonary, or metabolic disease
Those with symptoms or signs suggesting possible cardiopulmonary or meta-
bolic disease as given in Table 9-1
Asymptomatic persons with two or more major coronary risk factors (Table
9-2)
Apparently healthy men over age 40 and apparently healthy women over
age 50

Similarly, these persons should obtain medical clearance before engaging in an exercise program that requires vigorous exercise. ACSM defines vigorous exercise as that which requires a "substantial cardiorespiratory challenge" or "that results in fatigue within 20 minutes."

The test administrator is responsible for obtaining information necessary to ascertain a client's status relative to the ACSM exercise testing guidelines. The test ad-

TABLE 9-1	**Major Symptoms or Signs Suggestive of Cardiopulmonary Disease**

1. Pain, discomfort (or other anginal equivalent) in the chest, neck, jaw, arms, or other areas that may be ischemic in nature
2. Shortness of breath at rest or with mild exertion
3. Dizziness or syncope
4. Orthopnea or paroxysmal nocturnal dyspnea
5. Ankle edema
6. Palpitations or tachycardia
7. Intermittent claudication
8. Known heart murmur
9. Unusual fatigue or shortness of breath with usual activities

These symptoms must be interpreted in the clinical context in which they appear, since they are not all specific for cardiopulmonary or metabolic disease.
Reprinted with permission from American College of Sports Medicine: ACSM's Guidelines for Exercise Testing and Prescription. 5th Ed. Baltimore: Williams & Wilkins, 1995, p. 17.

TABLE 9-2	Coronary Artery Disease Risk Factors

POSITIVE RISK FACTORS

Age. Men who are more than 45 years of age; women who are more than 55 years of age or who have premature menopause without estrogen replacement therapy

Family history. Myocardial infarction (heart attack) or sudden death before age 55 in father or other male first-degree relative or before age 65 in mother or other female first-degree relative

Current cigarette smoking.

Hypertension. Blood pressure ≥ 140/90 mm Hg, confirmed on at least two separate occasions, or taking antihypertensive medication

Hypercholesterolemia. Total serum cholesterol ≥ 200 mg/dL (5.2 mmol/L) if lipoprotein profile is unavailable or HDL < 35 mg/dL (0.9 mmol/L)

Diabetes mellitus. Persons with IDDM who are more than 30 years of age or have had IDDM for more than 15 years and persons with NIDDM who are over 35 years of age should be classified as patients with disease

Sedentary lifestyle or physical inactivity. Persons in the least active 25% of the population, as defined by the combination of jobs involving sitting for a large part of the day and no regular exercise or active recreational pursuits

NEGATIVE RISK FACTOR

High Serum HDL Cholesterol. HDL > 60 mg/dL (1.6 mmol/L)

HDL, high-density lipoprotein; IDDM, insulin-dependent diabetes mellitus; NIDDM, non–insulin-dependent diabetes mellitus.

It is common to sum risk factors in making clinical judgments. If HDL is high, subtract one risk factor from the positive risk factors, since high HDL decreases risk of coronary artery disease.

Obesity is not listed as an independent positive risk factor because its effects are exerted through other risk factors (e.g., hypertension, hyperlipidemia, diabetes). Obesity should be considered as an independent target for intervention.

Adapted from American College of Sports Medicine: ACSM's Guidelines for Exercise Testing and Prescription. 5th ed. Baltimore, Williams & Wilkins, 1995, p. 18.

ministrator should also guarantee that all site personnel are trained in test protocols and are certified in cardiopulmonary resuscitation (CPR).

Physical Activity Readiness Questionnaire

The Physical Activity Readiness Questionnaire (PAR-Q) has been used successfully as a screening tool for exercise testing (10). After eliminating candidates according to the ACSM guidelines, a test administrator can use the PAR-Q to identify any remaining candidates for whom exercise testing may be risky. In 1998 ACSM and the American Heart Association issued a joint position statement recommending use of the PAR-Q (along with another one-page screening questionnaire) for screening before participation in all public and private health or fitness facilities (11).

The **PAR-Q** is a brief set of straightforward questions that may be administered orally or in writing. *A candidate who answers yes to any of the questions is advised to consult with his or her personal physician before undergoing exercise testing. A candidate who is pregnant or temporarily ill is directed to delay exercise until after the pregnancy or until he or she is feeling better.* The 1994 revision of the PAR-Q is shown in Figure 9-4.

Physical Activity Readiness
Questionnaire - PAR-Q
(revised 1994)

PAR - Q & YOU

(A Questionnaire for People Aged 15 to 69)

Regular physical activity is fun and healthy, and increasingly more people are starting to become more active every day. Being more active is very safe for most people. However, some people should check with their doctor before they start becoming much more physically active.

If you are planning to become much more physically active than you are now, start by answering the seven questions in the box below. If you are between the ages of 15 and 69, the PAR-Q will tell you if you should check with your doctor before you start. If you are over 69 years of age, and you are not used to being very active, check with your doctor.

Common sense is your best guide when you answer these questions. Please read the questions carefully and answer each one honestly: check YES or NO.

YES	NO		
☐	☐	1.	Has your doctor ever said that you have a heart condition <u>and</u> that you should only do physical activity recommended by a doctor?
☐	☐	2.	Do you feel pain in your chest when you do physical activity?
☐	☐	3.	In the past month, have you had chest pain when you were not doing physical activity?
☐	☐	4.	Do you lose your balance because of dizziness or do you ever lose consciousness?
☐	☐	5.	Do you have a bone or joint problem that could be made worse by a change in your physical activity?
☐	☐	6.	Is your doctor currently prescribing drugs (for example, water pills) for your blood pressure or heart condition?
☐	☐	7.	Do you know of <u>any other reason</u> why you should not do physical activity?

If
you
answered

YES to one or more questions

Talk with your doctor by phone or in person BEFORE you start becoming much more physically active or BEFORE you have a fitness appraisal. Tell your doctor about the PAR-Q and which questions you answered YES.

- You may be able to do any activity you want—as long as you start slowly and build up gradually. Or, you may need to restrict your activities to those which are safe for you. Talk with your doctor about the kinds of activities you wish to participate in and follow his/her advice.
- Find out which community programs are safe and helpful for you.

NO to all questions

If you answered NO honestly to <u>all</u> PAR-Q questions, you can be reasonably sure that you can:

- start becoming much more physically active—begin slowly and build up gradually. This is the safest and easiest way to go.
- take part in a fitness appraisal—this is an excellent way to determine your basic fitness so that you can plan the best way for you to live actively.

DELAY BECOMING MUCH MORE ACTIVE:

- if you are not feeling well because of a temporary illness such as a cold or a fever—wait until you feel better; or
- if you are or may be pregnant—talk to your doctor before you start becoming more active.

Please note: If your health changes so that you then answer YES to any of the above questions, tell your fitness or health professional. Ask whether you should change your physical activity plan.

<u>Informed Use of the PAR-Q</u>: The Canadian Society for Exercise Physiology, Health Canada, and their agents assume no liability for persons who undertake physical activity, and if in doubt after completing this questionnaire, consult your doctor prior to physical activity.

You are encouraged to copy the PAR-Q but only if you use the entire form

NOTE: If the PAR-Q is being given to a person before he or she participates in a physical activity program or a fitness appraisal, this section may be used for legal or administrative purposes.

I have read, understood and completed this questionnaire. Any questions I had were answered to my full satisfaction.

NAME _____

SIGNATURE _____ DATE _____

SIGNATURE OF PARENT _____ WITNESS _____
or GUARDIAN (for participants under the age of majority)

© *Canadian Society for Exercise Physiology*
Société canadienne de physiologie de l'exercice

Supported by: 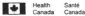 Health   Santé
Canada   Canada

FIGURE 9-4

The PAR-Q can be used to identify adults for whom physical activity might be inappropriate. (Reprinted with permission from the Canadian Society for Exercise Physiology.)

The PAR-Q is a brief, self-administered questionnaire used to identify adults for whom physical activity might be inappropriate.

Resting Evaluation

Before administering an exercise test, it is often useful to conduct a resting evaluation of selected cardiac functions. In field and clinical settings, a resting evaluation usually includes RHR and resting blood pressure (RBP). In laboratories and medical settings an electrocardiogram may also be given. The resting evaluation is actually the beginning of the cardiorespiratory fitness assessment, because the testing provides information about cardiorespiratory function and establishes baseline values for exercise measures. The resting evaluation also serves as one final safety net to catch someone for whom exercise testing is contraindicated.

The following resting measures should be taken in a quiet room with moderate temperature and humidity. The examinee should sit and rest quietly for at least 5 minutes before measurements are taken. The RHR should be taken before the RBP. The examinee should be well rested, well hydrated, and dressed in loose, comfortable clothing. He or she should not have smoked, eaten, or ingested caffeine within the past 3 hours. In anticipation of exercise testing, he or she should not have exercised that day or consumed alcohol or drugs other than prescription drugs for the past 24 hours.

Field Measurement of Resting Heart Rate

RHR can be measured either by *auscultation* using a stethoscope or by palpation of the radial or carotid arteries.

Procedure for Auscultation
1. Place the bell of the stethoscope to the left of the sternum just above the level of the nipples.
2. Count the lub-dubs for 30 seconds, then double to get RHR per minute.

Procedure for Palpation
1. Find the pulse at either the radial or carotid artery. The radial pulse is on the inside of the lower arm just above the wrist and in line with the thumb. The carotid pulse can be found in the neck on either side of the larynx.
2. Use the index and middle fingers to apply firm but light pressure at the site of the pulse.
3. Start a stopwatch simultaneously with a pulse. Count that pulse as zero, then continue counting pulses for 30 seconds. Double the 30-second value to estimate RHR.

Evaluation
RHRs decline from childhood to adulthood. For example, the average RHR is 140 beats per minute (bpm) for a newborn infant, 115 bpm for a 1-year old, and 100 bpm for an 8-year old. The average RHR for adults is 72 bpm. However, the RHR is somewhat difficult to interpret. The range of normal RHRs for adult women and men is very large, that is, 60 to 100 bpm. A RHR higher than 100 (**tachycardia**) or lower than 60 (**bradycardia**) may indicate a disease or disorder; however, it *may not*. The RHRs of endurance sport athletes are often as low as 30 to 40 bpm. Their low RHRs indicate

conditioned heart muscles that don't have to beat very often because each contraction pumps a large volume of blood. On the other hand, an abnormally low RHR can also indicate a pathologically diseased heart. A higher-than-normal RHR may indicate a poorly conditioned, sedentary person who has the beginnings of cardiovascular problems. Or it may be a normal response to emotion, pain, exertion, digestion of food, excessive heat, or other factors. Therefore, the RHR must be evaluated for each person within a context of knowledge about his or her background. This information can be obtained from a series of lifestyle questions. The RHR is generally responsive to aerobic conditioning, dropping as training progresses. However, it is not a highly valid or reliable measure of cardiorespiratory fitness.

> Tachycardia is a resting heart rate higher than 100 bpm; bradycardia is a resting heart rate lower than 60 bpm.

Field Measurement of Resting Blood Pressure

RBP is measured indirectly by auscultation using a stethoscope and a sphygmomanometer. The sphygmomanometer consists of an inflatable blood pressure cuff, an inflating bulb, a deflation valve, and an aneroid manometer or a mercury column pressure gauge. It is important to use a cuff of the correct size. Cuffs come sized for children, regular-sized adults, and larger adults (Fig. 9-5). The rubber bladder of the cuff should encircle at least two-thirds of the upper arm. A cuff that is too small overestimates the true blood pressure and vice versa.

Procedure

1. Rest the examinee's forearm on a surface so that the forearm is supported at the level of the heart. The arm should be relaxed, with the palm up and the elbow slightly flexed.
2. Wrap the cuff firmly around the upper arm with the lower edge of the cuff about 1 inch above the inner elbow crease (antecubital space). Align the cuff with the brachial artery.
3. Place the bell of the stethoscope lightly over the brachial artery about half an inch below the antecubital space. Do not let the stethoscope touch the cuff or clothing.
4. Quickly inflate the cuff either to 200 mm Hg or about 20 mm Hg above the estimated systolic blood pressure.
5. Listen as you release the pressure slowly, at 2 to 3 mm Hg per second. (You may release the pressure even more slowly if the heart rate is very low.)
6. Note the systolic blood pressure value at the point where the first sound is heard as blood rushes into the artery (the phase I Korotkoff sound).
7. As you continue to deflate the cuff, you will hear sharp tapping sounds that correspond to the contractions of the heart. Listen for the point at which these sounds become muffled (phase IV Korotkoff sound) and for the point at which they disappear (phase V Korotkoff sound). For an adult you should record the diastolic blood pressure as the value at which the sounds disappeared.
8. Release all pressure from the cuff. Wait for at least 30 seconds, then repeat the measurement another time or two until consistent systolic and diastolic values are obtained.

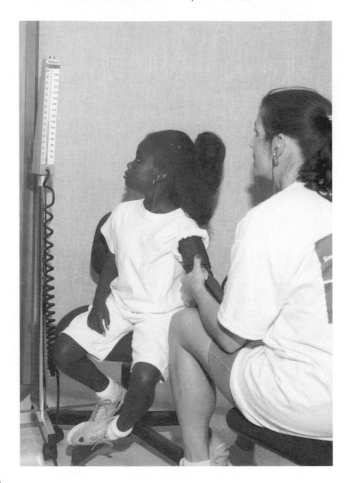

FIGURE 9-5

Blood pressure cuffs are available in sizes for children, regular-sized adults, and larger adults. (Photo by Marvin Arrington, Heritage Photography, Greensboro, NC.)

Evaluation

Blood pressure rises from childhood to adulthood. For example, systolic blood pressure averages about 70 mm Hg for newborn infants, 90 mm Hg for 1-year-olds, and 100 for 8-year olds. Table 9-3 interprets RBP for adults aged 18 years or older (12). However, resting blood pressures fluctuate widely because of many of the same sorts of influences that affect RHR, such as emotion, pain, exertion, digestion of food, and other factors. It is fairly common for blood pressure to increase by as much as 10 mm Hg when taken in a doctor's office instead of in one's home. Therefore, diagnosis of hypertension is based on an average of two or more readings on two or more occasions.

General Exercise Testing Guidelines

After screening according to the ACSM guidelines, administration of the PAR-Q, and administration of the resting evaluation, you may generally proceed with exercise testing. Explain the testing procedures, potential benefits, and risks in detail. Allow

TABLE 9-3	Classification of Resting Blood Pressure for Adults			
BLOOD PRESSURE CATEGORY	**SYSTOLIC BP (mm Hg)**		**DIASTOLIC BP (mm Hg)**	**RECOMMENDED FOLLOW-UP**
Optimal[a]	less than 120	and	less than 80	Recheck in 2 years
Normal	less than 130	and	less than 85	Recheck in 2 years
High normal	130–139	or	85–89	Recheck in 1 year
Hypertension				
Stage 1 (mild)	140–159	or	90–99	Confirm within 2 mo
Stage 2 (moderate)	160–179	or	100–109	Evaluate within 1 month
Stage 3 (severe)	180 or higher	or	110 or higher	Evaluate immediately or within 1 week, per clinical situation

BP, blood pressure.
[a]Unusually low readings should be evaluated for clinical significance.
Reprinted with permission from Joint National Committee: The sixth report of the Joint National Committee on Detection, Evaluation, and Treatment of High Blood Pressure. Archives of Internal Medicine, 157:2413, 1997.

the examinee time to ask questions. Remind the examinee that it is his or her right to discontinue a test at any time.

Monitor the examinee closely at all times during testing. Do not hesitate to stop the testing if you have any concerns about how the examinee is adjusting to the physiological demands of the test. Obvious stop signs include angina, nausea, pallor, light-headedness, and motor coordination problems.

Laboratory Assessment of Maximal Aerobic Capacity

In the exercise physiology laboratory, maximal aerobic capacity is assessed by direct measurement of maximal oxygen consumption (VO_2max) from administration of a GXT. The typical GXT is a maximal exertion, multistage test that is performed on a treadmill or a bicycle ergometer. The examinee either runs or pedals at higher and higher work loads until exhaustion occurs. Gas analysis equipment is used to measure the amount of oxygen consumed by the examinee; this is determined by comparing the oxygen content of inspired and expired air. VO_2max is recorded when oxygen consumption has either peaked or reached a plateau. If a true maximal value has been reached, further increases in the work load will not raise the oxygen consumption.

The measurement of VO_2max varies somewhat according to the testing mode; this attributed to **test specificity.** For the same examinee, a treadmill GXT generally yields a higher VO_2max score than a bicycle ergometer GXT. This appears to be a reflection of the quantity of muscle mass taxed by the mode of exercise.

Test specificity is a term used to explain measurement differences caused by differences in the nature or demands of various tests.

Many protocols for GXTs have been developed. Some of the more popular GXTs for the treadmill are the Bruce, modified Bruce, and Balke protocols. Popular bicycle ergometer GXTs are the Astrand, Fox, and McArdle et al. protocols. All of these tests are time consuming and require expensive equipment and highly trained test administrators. Additionally, examinees must be highly motivated and in good health to perform a test requiring maximal exertion.

Also performed in the laboratory are treadmill and bicycle ergometer tests that are *submaximal,* that is, tests requiring less than maximal exertion on the part of the examinee. Submaximal tests predict VO_2max from exercise heart rates or work performance data. The basis for these predictions is a theoretical positive linear relation of heart rate, work load, and oxygen consumption. Heart rate increases proportionally to the work load and to the amount of oxygen being consumed, up to VO_2max. Therefore, researchers can extrapolate to a VO_2max that will occur at the theoretical maximum exercise heart rate. (Neat, huh?) The maximum exercise heart rate (HRmax) is assumed to be 220 minus the examinee's age in years. However, there is a large variation in this value from person to person; the standard deviation for HRmax has been reported as ±12 bpm (13). Therefore, submaximal exercise tests tend to be less accurate than maximal exercise tests. Predictions from submaximal tests tend to overpredict actual VO_2max for aerobically conditioned persons and underestimate these values for sedentary ones (14).

Evaluation of VO_2max

Absolute comparisons of VO_2max measured in liters of oxygen consumed per minute do not adequately explain differences in exercise performances. Therefore, VO_2max is most commonly reported in relative terms, that is, as milliliters of oxygen consumed by the examinee per kilogram of body weight per minute of exercise. The factoring in of body weight allows aerobic power comparisons between persons of different sizes. An alternative unit for reporting oxygen consumption is the **MET.** One MET is defined as the oxygen consumption required at rest for a "reference man." A MET is equivalent to 3.5 $mL \cdot kg^{-1} \cdot min^{-1}$, so METs can be converted to $mL \cdot kg^{-1} \cdot min^{-1}$ simply by multiplying METs by a factor of 3.5.

> A MET is a measure of energy expenditure; one MET is equivalent to 3.5 $mL \cdot kg^{-1} \cdot min^{-1}$, or the basal metabolic rate of a subject at rest.

The higher one's maximal oxygen consumption, the greater the amount and intensity of aerobic work he or she can perform. Although there are theoretical maximal values for VO_2max and METs, we can look to elite athletes in endurance sports to learn about practical limits. It is generally agreed that the highest aerobic power measures are recorded by elite international competitors in cross-country skiing. This is a sport in which competitors' bodies must be able to distribute oxygen to the working muscles of the legs, arms, and back for up to 3 hours at a time. A top international woman cross-country skier may have a VO_2max of about 63 $mL \cdot kg^{-1} \cdot min^{-1}$, or 18 METs. A top male skier may have a VO_2max of about 84 $mL \cdot kg^{-1} \cdot min^{-1}$, or 24 METs.

Table 9-4 shows normal values and standard deviations for VO_2max for adults of both genders (15). The standards given are for each decade of life from age 20 to 79.

Factors That Affect VO₂max

Exercise physiologists have studied the extent to which one's maxim___ power is determined by gender, age, and genetic background. These fac___ special interest because they are givens, that is, out of the control of the ___ Researchers have concluded that all three of these factors significantly influence maximal aerobic power.

Even when body mass differences are accounted for by reporting VO_2max in $mL \cdot kg^{-1} \cdot min^{-1}$, men generally have VO_2max values that are 15 to 30% higher than those of women (16). The male advantage is explained in terms of body composition and hemoglobin content. Men can generate more aerobic energy because of greater muscle mass and less body fat and because they can carry more oxygen because of the higher concentration of hemoglobin in their blood. Gender differences in VO_2max are somewhat less for trained athletes, but men still maintain an advantage. However, that individual variation is considerable. This means that not all men have VO_2max values higher than those of all women. This is true particularly for trained women athletes and sedentary men.

The amount of oxygen that can be consumed, measured in absolute terms, increases rapidly throughout childhood, peaking at puberty for both genders. If, however, VO_2max is measured as $mL \cdot kg^{-1} \cdot min^{-1}$, boys' values remain constant between ages 6 and 16 (16). Girls' values decline across these same years as body fat increases. As men and women age beyond about age 25, VO_2max declines about 1% per year (Fig 9-6). Remaining active slows but does not prevent this decline.

Heredity has been studied by comparing VO_2max values of brothers, fraternal twins, and identical twins. It is estimated that genetic variability may account for

TABLE 9-4	Normal Values of Maximal Oxygen Uptake in Milliliters per Kilogram per Minute ± Standard Deviation	
AGE (yr)	**MEN**	**WOMEN**
20–29	43 ± 7.2 12 METs	36 ± 6.9 10 METs
30–39	42 ± 7.0 12 METs	34 ± 6.2 10 METs
40–49	40 ± 7.2 11 METs	32 ± 6.2 9 METs
50–59	36 ± 7.1 10 METs	29 ± 5.4 8 METs
60–69	33 ± 7.3 9 METs	27 ± 4.7 8 METs
70–79	29 ± 7.3 8 METs	27 ± 5.8 8 METs

Reprinted with permission from American Heart Association: Medical/Scientific Statement on Exercise: benefits and recommendations for physical activity programs for all Americans. Circulation, 94:857, 1996.

about 40% or perhaps even more of observed differences in VO₂max (16). There may be a great deal of truth to the belief that great endurance sport athletes are born, not made. But regardless of one's genetic potential, aerobic training can have a marked positive effect on maximal aerobic power, possibly increasing one's VO₂max by as much as 50% (8).

Is VO₂max the Best Measure of Cardiorespiratory Fitness?

To many people, maximal aerobic power is synonymous with cardiorespiratory fitness. VO₂max has been the focus of cardiorespiratory fitness assessment for decades. Only recently has its appropriateness been seriously questioned (14, 17). VO₂max is an unambiguous measure, but is it the best indicator of cardiorespiratory fitness? The answer may depend upon your perspective. From the perspective of performance, perhaps VO₂max is the best measure of cardiorespiratory fitness, but a focus on maximal aerobic power may not be appropriate from a health perspective (14). Perhaps it would be better to assess one's ability to tolerate submaximal levels of work for extended periods, that is, submaximal exercise endurance. Perhaps we should attempt to measure cardiorespiratory responses to standard work loads that are at least moderate in intensity, that is, at a level at which one must exercise to im-

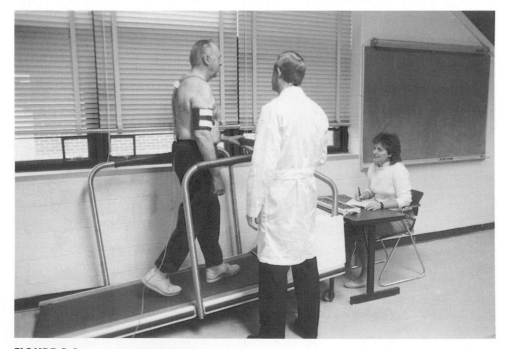

FIGURE 9-6

Measures of VO₂max decline about 1% per year after age 25. (Photo by Dr. Karen Uhlendorf, University of Vermont, Burlington, VT.)

prove the respiratory and cardiovascular systems. In the next few years we are likely to witness the development of new laboratory and field tests that will assess sub maximal exercise endurance with or without maximal aerobic power. In the meantime, practitioners and clinicians should continue to assess cardiorespiratory fitness by administration of field tests of maximal aerobic power.

Field Tests of Maximal Aerobic Power

Popular field assessments of maximal aerobic power include distance run tests, walk tests, and step tests. Several other testing procedures also exist.

Maximal-Effort Distance Runs

Distance runs are amazingly popular as field tests of maximal aerobic power. To tell the truth, they are generally more popular with test administrators than with the examinees themselves, but no one can deny that distance runs are easy to administer, inexpensive, and easy to score. These qualities no doubt explain the popularity of distance run tests with test administrators.

Unfortunately, distance run tests also have a number of serious concerns that cannot be ignored. Examinees' motivation markedly affects test scores, yet motivation is virtually impossible to control. Anyone who has ever observed or taken part in the administration of a distance run test to high-school students can attest to the nature of motivation problems. Test-associated orthopaedic injuries and coronary incidents are infrequent, but they do happen, because most distance run tests require examinees to perform at maximal levels of exertion. Injuries and accidents are concerns especially for untrained, elderly, and obese examinees. Furthermore, on any given day the weather may impair performances. Few people run their best on hot and humid days or when bundled up to prevent frostbite. Less-than-best performances produce an underestimation of VO_2max. Despite these problems, distance runs have many times been used successfully to assess maximal aerobic power.

Administratively the most practical and popular distance run test is the 1-mile run. Distance run tests shorter than a mile are generally questionable in terms of validity. A valid run test must be long enough to tax the cardiorespiratory functions of the examinee. Other common test distances are 1.5 and 2 miles. Also popular but more difficult to score is the 12-Minute Walk/Run Test developed by Kenneth Cooper in the late 1960s (18). All of these tests require the examinee to run, or runwalk, at a pace that either minimizes the time to cover a prescribed distance or maximizes distance traveled during the prescribed time. For highly motivated examinees who are experienced or trained in running, distance run times correlate highly with graded exercise tests on a treadmill.

In the late 1980s researchers developed equations to predict VO_2max from measures of running speeds for various distances (19). These equations assume that the examinee has run the distance at maximum speed. The average running speed is calculated in kilometers per hour, and this value is used in the appropriate equation. There follows a recommended protocol for a 1-mile run test and instructions for calculating VO_2max from the 1-mile test score.

Mile Run Protocol and Calculation of VO₂max

Purpose

The purpose of the mile run protocol and calculation of VO_2max is to assess maximal aerobic power from a field run test or a competitive race of 1 mile.

Psychometric Information

Some 41 male runners completed a series of runs at distances ranging from 200 m to 42.2 km (the distance of a marathon). They also performed a maximal multistage aerobic track test to determine VO_2max; this test had been validated against treadmill measures of VO_2max. Regression equations were developed to predict VO_2max from running performances for each distance. For the mile run the correlation between the calculated VO_2max and the measured VO_2max was r = +.95. The standard error of the estimate of VO_2max was ±2.3%.

Gender and Level

This test is appropriate for adults of both genders who are experienced in running or who have trained for at least several weeks.

Facilities

An indoor or outdoor track or other relatively flat course of 1 mile.

Equipment

This test requires a stopwatch.

Administrative Concerns

Weather should be moderate.

Procedure

1. Ask examinees to warm up with a few minutes of slow jogging and proper stretching.
2. Instruct examinees to run the mile as fast as possible, using a pace that can be maintained through most of the distance. They should refrain from walking if possible and should sprint as they near the finish line.
3. Examinees are started on a signal. A timer starts a stopwatch as the runner crosses the starting line; the stopwatch is stopped when the first part of the examinee's body crosses the finish line.
4. Runners should cool down with several minutes of walking, followed by stretching.

Scoring

1. Record mile run time (MRT) as a fraction of an hour (to the nearest 0.0001 hour). (*Calculation tip*: Convert time in minutes and seconds to total seconds, then divide total seconds by 3600 to obtain MRT as a fraction of an hour. For example, 10:20 equals 620 seconds; 620 divided by 3600 equals 0.1722 hour.)
2. Calculate average speed in kilometers per hour. This is done by dividing 1.6093 km (1 mile expressed in kilometers) by MRT. (For example, 1.6093 km divided by 0.1722 hour equals 9.3456 kph.)
3. Calculate METs by the following equation:

METs = 2.5043 + (0.8400 × kph)   Formula 9-1

4. Convert METs to VO₂max in milliliters per kilogram per minute by multiplying METs by 3.5.

Sample Calculation
This calculation is for a person whose MRT is 10:20.

MRT = 620 sec
MRT = 620 sec ÷ 3600 sec/hr = 0.1722 hr
Average run speed = 1.6093 km ÷ 0.1722 hr = 9.3456 kph
METs = 2.5043 + (0.8400 × 9.3456) = 10.3546 METs
$VO_2max \; mL \cdot kg^{-1} \cdot min^{-1}$ = 10.3546 × 3.5 = *36.2 mL·kg⁻¹·min⁻¹*

Comments
Races sponsored in your local area are excellent opportunities to obtain maximal run performances. Races of 5 and 10 km are now common in the United States. Also common is the marathon run of 26.2 miles, or 42.2 km. Tokmakidis and associates (19) also developed equations to predict VO₂max from average running speeds at these distances (Table 9-5).

Table 9-6 presents equivalent performances for maximal runs of varying distances. This is interesting information. For example, if you have the aerobic power to run a mile in 8:33, you should, after practicing at each specific distance, be able to run a 5-km race in 31:04, a 10-km race in 1:11:43, and a marathon in 6:49:3. If you cannot run the longer distances at the equivalent times, you need further endurance work. The researchers who did this work suggest that this table can help a runner set realistic goals for training and competition that do not overestimate or underestimate one's actual physiological potential.

Submaximal Track Jog

An alternative run test, a submaximal mile track jog, has recently been developed. This test has several advantages over traditional distance run tests (20). Because it requires submaximal rather than maximal exertion, it is both more enjoyable and safer

| TABLE 9-5 | Equations to Predict Maximal Oxygen Consumption in METs From Average Running Speed in Kilometers per Hour for Various Race Distances |

DISTANCE (km)	VO₂max (METs) PREDICTION EQUATION	CORRELATION WITH MEASURED VO₂max	STANDARD ERROR OF VO₂max PREDICTION
1.6093 (mile)	METs = 2.5043 + (0.8400 × kph)	.95	±2.3%
5	METs = 3.1747 + (0.9139 × kph)	.98	±2.3
10	METs = 4.7226 + (0.8698 × kph)	.88	±4.8
42.195 (marathon)	METs = 6.9021 + (0.8246 × kph)	.85	±5.6

Adapted from Tokmakidis, S.P., et al.: New approaches to predict VO₂max and endurance from running performances. Journal of Sports Medicine, 27:402, 1987.

TABLE 9-6	Equivalent Running Performances at Various Distances

METs	VO₂ max mL·kg⁻¹·min⁻¹	TIME FOR 1.6093 km	TIME FOR 5 km	TIME FOR 10 km	TIME FOR 42.195 km
>8	28.0	14:46	56:49	2:39:14	31:41:25
9	31.5	12:29	47:04	2:02:00	16:35:05
10	35.0	10:49	40:10	1:38:53	11:13:52
11	38.5	9:33	35:02	1:23:08	8:29:26
12	42.0	8:33	31:04	1:11:43	6:49:30
13	45.5	7:44	27:54	1:03:03	5:42:21
14	49.0	7:03	25:20	0:56:15	4:54:07
15	52.5	6:29	23:11	0:50:47	4:17:48
16	56.0	6:01	21:23	0:46:17	3:49:28
17	59.5	5:36	19:50	0:42:30	3:26:44
18	63.0	5:14	18:30	0:39:18	3:08:06
19	66.5	4:55	17:20	0:36:33	2:52:34
20	70.0	4:38	16:18	0:34:10	2:39:23
21	73.5	4:23	15:23	0:32:04	2:28:05
22	77.0	4:09	14:34	0:30:12	2:18:16
23	80.5	3:57	13:50	0:28:33	2:09:41
24	84.0	3:46	13:10	0:27:04	2:02:06
25	87.5	3:36	12:34	0:25:44	1:55:21

Adapted from Tokmakidis, S.P., et al.: New approaches to predict VO₂max and endurance from running performances. Journal of Sports Medicine, 27:404, 1987.

for examinees. Cardiovascular incidents and injuries to knees, ankles, and feet are less likely during submaximal than maximal exercise (8). Furthermore, the test itself models healthy aerobic exercise.

Submaximal Mile Track Jog

Purpose

The purpose of this test is to estimate the VO_2max of relatively fit young adults from a submaximal mile track jog.

Gender and Age

This test is appropriate for adults of both genders who are aged 18 to 29.

Psychometric Information

A total of 106 subjects performed both the mile track jog and a maximal treadmill graded exercise test. Multiple regression analysis was used to develop an equation to predict VO_2max for 31 men and 23 women from variables of gender, body mass, elapsed mile jog time (MJT), and exercise heart rate. The regression equation was cross-validated for the predicted and observed scores of an additional 32 men and 20 women. The standard error was estimated to be ±3.1 mL·kg⁻¹·min⁻¹. The track jog test was deemed valid for young adults with adequate to good cardiorespiratory fitness, that is, those with VO_2max values between approximately 35 and 60 $mL \cdot kg^{-1} \cdot min^{-1}$.

Facility Needs
This test requires a measured outdoor or indoor track; a 440-yard track is ideal.

Equipment
This test requires a stopwatch for the partner of each examinee and an electronic heart rate monitor for each examinee. (If this is not possible, manual heart rate palpation may be used.)

Administrative Concerns
Weather should be moderate.

Procedure
1. Weigh each examinee, who should be wearing light jogging clothes and no shoes. Record body weight in kilograms (pounds divided by 2.2).
2. Pair each examinee with a partner who will time each lap and MJT.
3. Instruct examinees to jog the mile at a steady, submaximal pace. *Men may not run the mile in less than 8 minutes; women may not run the mile in less than 9 minutes. Final exercise heart rates must not exceed 180 bpm.* Perceived exertion should be about 11 (or fairly light exercise intensity) on the 15-point Rate of Perceived Exertion Scale (21). *A steady pace should be maintained throughout the jog, with no sprinting at the end.*
4. Have examinees warm up for 2 to 3 minutes, practicing the proper submaximal jogging pace. *Men should not run a 440-yard lap faster than 2 minutes; women should not run a 440-yard lap faster than 2.25 minutes.*
5. Examinees may be tested as a group. Each examinee's partner is responsible for reporting lap times to the runner and reporting the elapsed time for the mile jog in minutes and seconds to the recorder.
6. *Immediately upon finishing the mile jog*, each examinee's exercise heart rate (EHR) should be determined and recorded. This value can be read directly from the electronic monitor. Alternatively, the EHR may be determined manually by taking a 10-second carotid artery count immediately upon finishing the run, beginning the count no more than 5 seconds after the examinee crosses the finish line, then multiplying this value by 6 to convert the 10-second heart rate to beats per minute. The partner can assist by timing the 10-second period while either the examinee or the partner counts the heartbeats during this period.

Scoring
Calculate VO_2max from these gender-specific prediction equations:

$$\text{Women: } VO_2\text{max} = 100.5 - 0.1636 \text{ (BW)} - 1.438 \text{ (MJT)}$$
$$- 0.1928 \text{ (EHR)} \qquad \text{Formula 9-2}$$

$$\text{Men: } VO_2\text{max} = 108.844 - 0.1636 \text{ (BW)} - 1.438 \text{ (MJT)}$$
$$- 0.1928 \text{ (EHR)} \qquad \text{Formula 9-3}$$

where BW is body weight in kilograms (nearest 0.1 kg) and MJT is in minutes (nearest 0.01 minute).

Comments

What a concept! Although I enjoy recreational jogging immensely, I dislike taking maximal run tests. This submaximal test is actually fun. One hopes this test will soon be modified and validated for use with younger and older populations. Although the instructions may sound a bit difficult because of the time limitations to ensure submaximal levels of exertion, examinees very quickly discover appropriate paces. Most people can use their recreational jogging pace.

Walking Tests

To address the problems associated with maximal exertion run tests, a number of walking tests have been developed for use in field settings. The Rockport Fitness Walking Test (RFWT) is an easy-to-administer submaximal test for estimating VO₂max (22). The RFWT requires the examinee to walk as fast as possible over a measured mile. At the end of the walk the examinee's exercise heart rate is measured by an electronic heart rate monitor. VO₂max is estimated from a prediction equation, using variables of body weight, age, walk time, and EHR.

Rockport Fitness Walking Test

Purpose

The purpose of the RFWT is to assess cardiorespiratory fitness by estimating VO₂max for men and women from a 1-mile walk.

Gender and Age

This test is appropriate for adults of both genders who are 30 to 69 years of age.

Psychometric Information

A standard treadmill protocol was used to measure VO₂max for 165 healthy men and 178 healthy women. A general equation was developed to estimate VO₂max in mL/(kg·min) using body weight, age, mile walk time (MWT), and exercise heart rate. The multiple correlation was .88, and the standard error of the estimate was ±5.0 $mL \cdot kg^{-1} \cdot min^{-1}$. Cross-validation data supported the conclusion that the RFWT yields a valid estimate of maximal oxygen consumption for adults aged 30 to 69.

Facility Needs

A measured flat course of 1 mile.

Equipment

This test requires a stopwatch and an electronic heart rate monitor for each examinee.

Administrative Concerns

Weather should be moderate.

Procedure

1. Measure body weight to the nearest pound.
2. Record age in years.
3. Instruct examinees to walk the course as fast as possible but at a steady pace. As each examinee crosses the finish line, the EHR is read from the heart rate monitor and recorded.

4. Record elapsed MWT to the nearest 0.01 minute. (Calculation tip: divide seconds by 60 to convert to fractional minutes. For example, 15 seconds equals 0.25 minutes.)

Scoring

Calculate VO_2max from these gender-specific equations:

Women: VO_2max = 132.853 − 0.0769 (BW) − 0.3877 (age)

       − 3.2649 (MWT) − 0.1565 (EHR)   Formula 9-4

Men: VO_2max = 139.168 − 0.0769 (BW) − 0.3877 (age)

      − 3.2649 (MWT) − 0.1565 (EHR)   Formula 9-5

where age is recorded in years and MWT is taken to the nearest 0.01 minute.

Sample Calculation

The following demonstrates calculation of VO_2max using Formula 9-5.

Gender, male
Body weight, 170 lb
Age, 60 years
MWT, 15:30 (15.5 min)
EHR, 132 bpm

  VO_2max = 139.168 − 0.0769 (170) − 0.3877 (60) − 3.2649 (15.50)

     − 0.1565 (132)

  $= 31.6 \ mL\cdot kg^{-1}\cdot min^{-1}$

Comments

In a separate study the RFWT was validated for women aged 65 to 79 (23). Therefore, it may be used to assess the cardiorespiratory fitness of older women. The RFWT does not, however, appear to be a valid assessment for adults under age 30 or for mentally retarded adults (24, 25). The original RFWT prediction equations overpredicted VO_2max for both of these populations.

Electronic monitoring is recommended for measurement of exercise heart rate. If no electronic heart rate monitor is available, the exercise heart rate may be determined by palpation of either the carotid or radial artery. If a group is being examined, each examinee should be paired with a partner who will time the 10-second period for the determination of exercise heart rate while either the examinee or the partner counts the beats. Teach examinees and their partners to take an accurate exercise heart rate before administering the test.

Step Tests

There are several step tests for field assessment of cardiorespiratory fitness. They are all based on the same principle, that is, that cardiorespiratory fitness can be estimated by observing the examinee's heart rate response to a measured workload. The work is a rhythmic stepping up and down at a prescribed cadence, from a bench of a prescribed height, for a prescribed time. Available tests vary in the stepping rate, height of the step, and stepping time. Described next is the Queens College Step Test (26).

Queens College Step Test

Purpose

The purpose of the Queens College Step Test is to predict VO_2max for college-age men and women from an easily administered field test of bench stepping.

Psychometric Information

This test was developed and normed on data from thousands of students at Queens College in New York. Using a treadmill measure of VO_2max as the criterion, concurrent validity was estimated at −.75 for women and −.72 for men. (The validity coefficient is negative because low heart rates on the step test tended to be associated with high VO_2max values from the treadmill test.) Test-retest reliability was estimated at .92 for women and .89 for men. The standard error of the estimate was ±16% of the actual VO_2max.

Gender and Age

This test is appropriate for adults of both genders of traditional college age.

Equipment

This test requires a bench 16.25 inches high, metronome to establish stepping pace, and a stopwatch.

Procedure

1. Demonstrate and instruct examinees in the four-count stepping pattern: up with the left foot, up with the right foot, down with the left foot, down with the right foot. In the up position, the examinee's knee and hip joints should be fully extended.
2. Set metronome at 88 counts per minute (22 complete step cycles) for women or 96 counts per minute (24 complete step cycles) for men.
3. After 15 seconds of practice or until pattern and cadence are learned, have examinees begin stepping and continue for 3 minutes.
4. Stop examinees at the end of 3 minutes and have them remain standing. Allow 5 seconds to locate the carotid artery pulse; then count the pulse for 15 seconds. Multiply this value by 4 to obtain the recovery heart rate (HR_{rec}).

Scoring

The RHR is used with Table 9-7 to determine the predicted VO_2max. Table 9-7 also gives the corresponding norm values expressed in percentile ranks. Alternatively, you may calculate the predicted VO_2max by one of the following equations:

Women: VO_2max = 65.81 − 0.1847 (RHR)   Formula 9-6

Men: VO_2max = 11.33 − 0.42 (RHR)   Formula 9-7

Comments

The step height used for this test was the height of the bleacher steps in the gymnasium at Queens College. The bleachers in your local athletic facility may also be 16.25 inches high. If so, this is a superb opportunity for mass testing. Each examinee can be paired with a partner who monitors the step pattern and assists with taking the RHR. It works well to have the partner sit on the second or third row of the bleachers directly in front of the examinee. It also helps to amplify the cadence ("up, up, down, down") with a microphone so the cadence can be discerned over

TABLE 9-7	Queens College Step Test: Percentile Rankings for Recovery Heart Rate and Predicted Maximal Oxygen Consumption for College Students			
PERCENTILE RANKING	RECOVERY HEART RATE, WOMEN	PREDICTED VO$_2$max (mL·kg^{-1}·min^{-1})	RECOVERY HEART RATE, MEN	PREDICTED VO$_2$max (mL·kg^{-1}·min^{-1})
100	128	42.2	120	60.9
95	140	40.0	124	59.3
90	148	38.5	128	57.6
85	152	37.7	136	54.2
80	156	37.0	140	52.5
75	158	36.6	144	50.9
70	160	36.3	148	49.2
65	162	35.9	149	48.8
60	163	35.7	152	47.5
55	164	35.5	154	46.7
50	166	35.1	156	45.8
45	168	34.8	160	44.1
40	170	34.4	162	43.3
35	171	34.2	164	42.5
30	172	34.0	166	41.6
25	176	33.3	168	40.8
20	180	32.6	172	39.1
15	182	32.2	176	37.4
10	184	31.8	178	36.6
5	196	29.6	184	34.1

Reprinted with permission from Katch, F.I., Katch, V.L., and McArdle, W.D.: Nutrition, Weight Control, and Exercise. 3rd ed. Philadelphia, Lea & Febiger, 1988.

the noise of bleacher stepping. You may also try tape-recording test instructions and cadence chanting.

The published norms were determined for Queens College students during the 1980s. This may not be an appropriate comparison for your group. If not, you may wish to collect data and develop local norms.

Nonexercise Tests

Sometimes an estimate of maximal oxygen consumption is desired, but for some reason an exercise test cannot or should not be administered. The University of Houston Non-Exercise Test requires no physical exercise (27). The VO$_2$max is predicted, with a reasonable amount of accuracy, from an activity code, age, and body composition measure. The rationale for this assessment comes from research substantiating that VO$_2$max is negatively related to age and to body composition but is positively related to exercise habits. Two versions of the Houston Non-Exercise Test have been developed. One uses percent body fat from skinfolds as the body composition measure; the other uses the body mass index (BMI) described in Chapter 8. The BMI version is included here because of its high feasibility. The test authors justified this procedure by noting that even if an examinee reported a body weight in error by as much as 10 pounds, the predicted VO$_2$max would in most cases be affected by less than 1.5 mL·kg^{-1}·min^{-1} (27).

University of Houston Non-Exercise Test (BMI Version)

Purpose

The purpose of the University of Houston Non-Exercise Test is to estimate VO$_2$max without a physical response on the part of the examinee.

Psychometric Information

As part of their annual health examination, 2009 employees from the NASA/Johnson Space Center in Houston, Texas, had VO$_2$max measured by a standard treadmill GXT; 1543 of them constituted the original validation sample for development of a prediction equation to estimate VO$_2$max from an activity code, age, and BMI. The multiple correlation was .794, and the standard error of the estimate was ±5.55 mL·kg^{-1}·min^{-1}. The prediction equation was cross-validated on 466 persons from the original pool of subjects. Additional cross-validation samples consisted of 59 men who were on antihypertensive medication and 71 men who had abnormal exercise electrocardiograms "positive" for potential heart disease.

Gender and Age

The Houston Non-Exercise Test is reported to be valid for adults of both genders who have VO$_2$max values less than 55 mL·kg^{-1}·min^{-1}.

Procedure

1. Determine an activity code for each examinee by administering the Code for Physical Activity (Fig. 9-7). This instrument was validated by demonstrating a significant correlation to measured VO$_2$max.
2. Record age in years of each subject.
3. Obtain measures of height and weight for each examinee. Ideally these measures should be taken according to the procedures described in Chapter 8. If this is not feasible, examinees may self-report height and weight. Convert height to meters by dividing height in inches by 39.4. Convert weight to kilograms by dividing weight in pounds by 2.2.
4. Calculate BMI from Formula 9-8 for each examinee.

$$BMI = (\text{weight in kilograms}) \div (\text{height in meters})^2 \qquad \text{Formula 9-8}$$

Scoring

Calculate VO$_2$max from the appropriate prediction equation for women or men.

$$\text{Women: VO}_2\text{max} = 56.363 + 1.921(AC) - 0.381(\text{age})$$
$$- 0.754\ (BMI) \qquad \text{Formula 9-9}$$

$$\text{Men: VO}_2\text{max} = 67.350 + 1.921(AC) - 0.381(\text{age})$$
$$- 0.754\ (BMI) \qquad \text{Formula 9-10}$$

where AC is the activity code (1–7), age is reported in years, and BMI is given to the nearest hundredth.

CODE FOR PHYSICAL ACTIVITY

Select the one value that best represents your
general ACTIVITY LEVEL for the PREVIOUS MONTH.

DO NOT PARTICIPATE REGULARLY IN PROGRAMMED
RECREATION SPORT OR HEAVY PHYSICAL ACTIVITY.

0 = Avoid walking or exertion, e.g., always use elevator, drive
whenever possible instead of walking.

1 = Walk for pleasure, routinely use stairs, occasionally exercise
sufficiently to cause heavy breathing or perspiration.

PARTICIPATE REGULARLY IN RECREATION OR WORK
REQUIRING MODEST PHYSICAL ACTIVITY, SUCH AS GOLF, HORSEBACK
RIDING, CALISTHENICS, GYMNASTICS,
TABLE TENNIS, BOWLING, WEIGHT LIFTING, YARD WORK.

2 = 10 to 60 minutes per week.

3 = Over 1 hour per week.

PARTICIPATE REGULARLY IN HEAVY PHYSICAL EXERCISE SUCH
AS RUNNING OR JOGGING, SWIMMING, CYCLING, ROWING,
SKIPPING ROPE, RUNNING IN PLACE, OR ENGAGING
IN VIGOROUS AEROBIC ACTIVITY-TYPE EXERCISE
SUCH AS TENNIS, BASKETBALL, OR HANDBALL.

4 = Run less than 1 mile per week or spend less than 30 minutes
per week in comparable physical activity.

5 = Run 1 to 5 miles per week or spend 30 to 60 minutes per
week in comparable physical activity.

6 = Run 5 to 10 miles per week or spend 1 to 3 hours per week in
comparable physical activity.

7 = Run over 10 miles per week or spend over 3 hours per week
in comparable physical activity.

FIGURE 9-7

The Rating Scale for Exercise Habits is used to determine the activity code for the University of Houston Non-Exercise Test. (Reprinted with permission from Ross, R.M., and Jackson, A.S.: Exercise Concepts, Calculations, & Computer Applications. Madison, WI, Brown & Benchmark, 1990, p. 109.)

Sample Calculation

This calculation uses Formula 9-9.

Gender, female
Activity code, 7
Age in years, 42
Body weight, 132 lb ÷ 2.2 = 60 kg
Height, 5 feet 6 inches = 66 inches ÷ 39.4 = 1.675 m
BMI, $60/(1.675)^2 = 21.40$

$$VO_2max = 56.363 + 1.921(7) - 0.381(42) - 0.754\,(21.40) = 37.7\ mL{\cdot}kg^{-1}{\cdot}min^{-1}$$

Comments

This nonexercise test is very useful as a quick and easy classification tool when high accuracy of predicted aerobic power or cardiorespiratory fitness is not needed. It can also be used to identify persons who may benefit from a follow-up test that is more psychometrically sound.

There is some question whether the University of Houston Non-Exercise Test has the broad applicability to adult populations that was reported by the test developers. Recent research attempted to cross-validate this test on a university student population. It was found that it significantly underpredicted actual measured VO_2max values (28). Further research is needed to clarify this apparent contradiction. The problem may lie in the nature of the test populations. Of the original NASA/Johnson Space Center subjects, 90% were men who had an average VO_2max of 39.7 and average values of 4.3 for the activity code, 43.7 years for age, and 25.50 for the BMI. Further testing should include more women and subjects of both genders who are heterogeneous in the relevant variables.

Other Cardiorespiratory Fitness Assessments

Researchers have developed several novel approaches for field assessments of cardiorespiratory fitness. Besides his famous 12-Minute Walk/Run Test, Kenneth Cooper, the father of aerobics, also developed the 12-Minute Swim Test and the 12-Minute Cycle Test (29). Neither has particularly high validity, but these tests can be useful in classification of those who use swimming or cycling as their primary mode of cardiorespiratory exercise (30, 31). Described below is another creative classification field test that can be used with clients who enrolled in a water aerobics course (32).

Ball State 500-Yard Water Run

Purpose

The purpose of the Ball State 500-Yard Water Run is to classify examinees according to cardiorespiratory fitness based upon performance data for a walk or run conducted in a swimming pool.

Psychometric Information

This test was developed and normed on undergraduate students enrolled in water aerobics classes to fulfill a general studies fitness and wellness requirement at Ball State University in Muncie, Indiana. There were 15 men and 28 women in the validation study. Concurrent validity, assessed by correlating water run times with treadmill measures of VO₂max, was =.796.

Gender and Age
This test is appropriate for adults of both genders who are under age 30.

Facility Needs
The Ball State 500-Yard Water Run may be performed on the long axis of a swimming pool of constant depth or across the shallow end of a variable-depth pool.

Equipment
This test requires a stopwatch.

Procedure
1. Measure pool and calculate lengths or widths to cover 500 yards.
2. Ask examinees to warm up with a couple of minutes of easy jogging in the water.
3. For each examinee, select a starting point along the pool edge where the water comes to a midpoint between the examinee's navel and nipples.
4. Instruct examinees in the proper mode of movement for the test. Runners should use their arms to pull as they run through the water but must stay vertical. Tell examinees, "Carve your own path through the water and avoid drafting in the wake of another runner."
5. Time each examinee for 500 yards. If mass testing, a partner can count completed laps. Record time to run 500 yards in water in minutes and seconds to the nearest whole second.
6. Ask examinee to cool down and then stretch.

Scoring
Gender-appropriate fitness classifications are based on the norms given in Table 9-8.

Comments
The developers of this instrument recommend that examinees practice before the test. Their research suggests that practice eliminates the undue influence of initial skill learning as one learns to run more efficiently in water. The Ball State 500-

TABLE 9-8	Norms for the Ball State 500-Yard Water Run Test	
CLASSIFICATION	**MEN**	**WOMEN**
Excellent	≤ 6:53	≤ 7:47
Good	6:54–7:22	7:48–8:29
Average	7:23–7:50	8:30–9:10
Poor	7:51–8:19	9:11–9:52
Very poor	≤ 8:20	≤ 9:53

Reprinted with permission from Robbins, G., and Powers, D.: The Ball State 500-Yard Water Run: a new fitness field test for non swimming water exercisers. Journal of the International Council for Health, Physical Education, and Recreation, 29:11, summer 1993.

Yard Water Run is extremely valuable for use in aerobic exercise classes. It can provide data for use in formative and summative evaluations. Because of test specificity, distance runs, step tests, and other field assessments may not adequately demonstrate improved cardiorespiratory fitness associated with water exercise.

Chapter Summary

This chapter explains why and how to conduct safe and informative cardiorespiratory fitness assessments. It discusses how to screen exercise testing candidates using the American College of Sports Medicine guidelines, the PAR-Q screening questionnaire, and resting evaluations of heart rate and blood pressure. It also examines some of the many field assessments that can be used to predict an examinee's maximal oxygen consumption. These include maximal run, jogging, walking, water run, and step tests. Also examined is a nonexercise test that can be used to estimate cardiorespiratory fitness.

SELF-TEST QUESTIONS

1. If performed at the correct intensity, time, and frequency, which of the following activities is *least* likely to cause an improvement in cardiorespiratory fitness?
   A. Bicycling
   B. Bowling
   C. Dancing
   D. Walking

2. According to ACSM guidelines, which of the following persons should have a medical examination before participating in a *maximal* exertion exercise test?
   A. Woman, aged 46, asymptomatic
   B. Woman, aged 36, smoker with no symptoms
   C. Woman, aged 26, smoker with diagnosed hypertension
   D. All of the above

3. Using ACSM guidelines, which of the following persons should have a medical examination before a *submaximal* exertion exercise test?
   A. Man, aged 22, asthma
   B. Man, aged 22, diabetes
   C. Man, aged 22, heart murmur
   D. All of the above

4. Using the PAR-Q, should an otherwise healthy woman who has a common cold and low fever take part in a fitness appraisal?
   A. No.
   B. Yes.
   C. Yes, but she may want delay the test until feeling better.
   D. The PAR-Q does not address this issue.

5. Which of the following RHRs is the threshold for tachycardia?
   A. Heart rate greater than 80 bpm
   B. Heart rate greater than 90 bpm
   C. Heart rate greater than 100 bpm
   D. Heart rate greater than 110 bpm

6. Which of the following procedures is *not* consistent with recommended procedures for a sitting blood pressure measurement by auscultation? (Identify *all* incorrect procedures.)
   A. Have client sit quietly for 2 minutes before taking the measurement.
   B. Allow client to rest arm on a table at heart level.
   C. Place deflated cuff around bare arm with the cuff 1 inch above elbow crease.
   D. Place bell of the stethoscope over brachial artery about half an inch below elbow crease.
   E. Quickly inflate cuff pressure to 240 mm Hg or about 40 mm Hg above estimated systolic pressure.
   F. Slowly release cuff pressure at 2 to 3 mm Hg per second while listening for the first Korotkoff sound.

7. Which of the following describes the phase V Korotkoff sound?
   A. Strong tapping
   B. Muffled tapping
   C. Swoosh
   D. Cessation of sound

8. The upper limit of normal *systolic* blood pressure for an adult is
   A. 129 mm Hg
   B. 139 mm Hg
   C. 149 mm Hg
   D. 159 mm Hg

9. What is the theoretical exercise HRmax for a 20-year old man?
   _____

10. Which of the following exercise intensities is recommended to improve the cardiorespiratory fitness of a 20-year old man?
    A. Exercise HR 120 to 180 bpm
    B. Exercise HR 100 to 160 bpm
    C. Exercise HR 90 to 140 bpm
    D. Exercise HR more than 180 bpm

11. What are the units for measurement of maximal oxygen consumption (VO_2max)?
    A. L·min
    B. METs
    C. mL·kg^{-1}·min^{-1}
    D. All of the above

12. If a particular exercise requires 12 METs, can this exercise be performed aerobically by a person with a VO_2max of 37 mL·kg^{-1}·min^{-1}? _____

13. Calculate the VO_2max in mL·kg^{-1}·min^{-1} for a man who runs a mile in 7:03 minutes during a maximal effort run test. _____

14. Using Table 9-4, evaluate the same score for a 20-year-old man.
    A. Below average
    B. Average
    C. Above average

15. If the young man in the previous problem were trained for long distance running, what would his marathon time be? ___:___:___

16. What is the normal value of VO_2max for a college-age woman?

    _____

17. What is the estimated VO_2max for a 20-year old woman who weighs 154 lb, has a MJT score of 9:18, and has an EHR of 126 for the submaximal 1-mile jog test?

    _____

18. When a step test is used to assess cardiorespiratory fitness, the examinee's test score is derived from
    A. Recovery heart rate
    B. Exercise respiration rate
    C. Stepping cadence
    D. VO_2max

19. Using reported standard errors, which of the following tests is the *most* accurate predictor of VO_2max?
    A. Submaximal 1-mile jog test
    B. RFWT
    C. University of Houston Non-Exercise Test
    D. All are approximately equal in accuracy of estimating VO_2max

20. Using the reported standard error of ± 5.0 mL·kg^{-1}·min^{-1}, what is the 68% confidence interval for an examinee who scores 37 on the RFWT? (In other words, 68 out of 100 times it is likely that this examinee's true VO_2max is likely to fall between these values.) _____ to _____

ANSWERS

1. B	2. C	3. D	4. C
5. C	6. A, E	7. D	8. B
9. 200	10. A	11. D	12. No
13. 49.0	14. C	15. 4:54:07	16. 36
17. 51.4	18. A	19. A	20. 32 to 42

DOING PROJECTS FOR FURTHER LEARNING

1. Self-administer two or more of the field tests in this chapter that require some form of exercise.
   A. Compare the VO_2max predictions. How similar or different are the predicted values?
   B. Add or subtract one standard error to each of the estimates to create a 68% confidence band around each of the estimates. Now compare the confidence bands for each of the VO_2max predictions. Do they overlap?
   C. Analyze the nature of the exercise required by each of the field tests. What body parts were most taxed? How long was the period of exercise for each test? How intensive was the exercise? Given what you know about specificity of exercise, are you surprised by your test results? Explain.

2. Administer an appropriate cardiorespiratory fitness field test to someone such as a friend, teacher, or relative. Interpret his or her score and explain the test results to the examinee. Assuming your subject is interested in improving cardiorespiratory fitness,

what mode and dosage (i.e., frequency, intensity, and duration) of exercise do you recommend?

3. Make an appointment with the manager of a local fitness facility. Ask whether the facility offers any kind of cardiorespiratory fitness assessment.
    A. If it does, why? What test or tests does it offer? How and why was this test or tests chosen? Who administers the test? How were the examiners trained? What medical clearance is required prior to exercise testing? How are the test scores interpreted? Do they use national and/or local norms?
    B. If the facility does not do cardiorespiratory fitness testing, why not? In your opinion, are these valid reasons? Explain.

REFERENCES

1. Bouchard, C., and Shephard, R.J.: Physical activity, fitness, and health: The model and key concepts. In C. Bouchard, R.J. Shephard, and T. Stephens (eds.), *Physical Activity, Fitness, and Health: International Proceedings and Consensus Statement*. Champaign, IL, Human Kinetics, 1994, pp. 77–88.
2. Mahler, D.A., et al.: ACSM's Guidelines for Exercise Testing and Prescription. 5th ed. Baltimore, Williams & Wilkins, 1995.
3. Blair, S.N., et al.: Physical fitness and all-causes mortality: a prospective study of healthy men and women. Journal of the American Medical Association, 262:2395, 1989.
4. Lee, C.D., Jackson, A.S., and Blair, S.N.: U.S. weight guidelines: is it also important to consider cardiorespiratory fitness? International Journal of Obesity and Related Metabolic Disorders, 22 (Suppl 2):S2, 1998.
5. Paffenbarger, R.S., Hude, R.T., Hseih, C.C., and Wing, A.L.: Chronic disease in former college students: physical fitness and all-causes mortality, and longevity of college alumni. New England Journal of Medicine, 314:605, 1986.
6. U.S. Department of Health and Human Services: Physical activity and health: a report of the Surgeon General at a glance. Atlanta: U.S. Department of Health and Human Services, Centers for Disease Control and Prevention, National Center for Chronic Disease Prevention and Health Promotion, 1996.
7. Pate, R.R., et al.: Physical activity and public health: a recommendation from the Centers for Disease Control and Prevention and the American College of Sports Medicine. Journal of the American Medical Association, 273:402, 1995.
8. American College of Sports Medicine: ACSM position stand on the recommended quantity and quality of exercise for developing and maintaining cardiorespiratory and muscular fitness, and flexibility in healthy adults. Medicine and Science in Sports and Exercise, 30:975, 1998.
9. Shephard, R.J.: Aerobic Fitness and Health. 2nd ed. Champaign, IL, Human Kinetics, 1998.
10. Thomas, S., Reading, J., and Shephard, R.J.: Revision of the Physical Activity Readiness Questionnaire (PAR-Q). Canadian Journal of Sport Science, 17:338, 1992.
11. American College of Sports Medicine and American Heart Association: Joint position statement recommendations for cardiovascular screening, staffing, and emergency policies at health/fitness facilities. Medicine and Science in Sports and Exercise, 30:1009, 1998.
12. Joint National Committee: The sixth report of the Joint National Committee on Prevention, Detection, Evaluation, and Treatment of High Blood Pressure. Archives of Internal Medicine, 157:2413, 1997.
13. Nieman, D.C.: Fitness and Sports Medicine: A Health-Related Approach. 3rd ed. Menlo Park, CA, Bull, 1995.

14. Skinner, J.S., and Oja, P.: Laboratory and field tests for assessing health-related fitness. In C. Bouchard, R.J. Shephard, and T. Stephens (eds.), Physical Activity, Fitness, and Health: International Proceedings and Consensus Statement. Champaign, IL, Human Kinetics, 1994, pp. 160–179.

15. American Heart Association: Medical/scientific statement on exercise: benefits and recommendations for physical activity programs for all Americans. Circulation 94:857, 1996.

16. McArdle, W.D., Katch, F.I., and Katch, V.L.: Exercise Physiology: Energy, Nutrition, and Human Performance. 4th ed. Baltimore, Williams & Wilkins, 1996.

17. Sharkey, B.J.: New Dimensions in Aerobic Fitness: Current Issues in Exercise Science. Monograph 1. Champaign, IL, Human Kinetics, 1991.

18. Cooper, K.H.: A means of assessing maximal oxygen intake. Journal of the American Medical Association, 203:201, 1968.

19. Tokmakidis, S.P., et al.: New approaches to predict VO_2max and endurance from running performance. Journal of Sports Medicine, 27:401, 1987.

20. George, J.D., et al.: VO_2max estimation from a submaximal 1-mile track jog for fit college-age individuals. Medicine and Science in Sports and Exercise, 25:401, 1993.

21. Borg, G.A.V.: Psychological basis of perceived exertion. Medicine and Science in Sports and Exercise, 14:377, 1982.

22. Kline, G.M., et al.: Estimation of VO_2max from a one-mile track walk, gender, age, and body weight. Medicine and Science in Sports and Exercise, 19:253, 1987.

23. Fenstermaker, K.L., Plowman, S.A., and Looney, M.A.: Validation of the Rockport Fitness Walking Test in females 65 years and older. Medicine and Science in Sports and Exercise, 24:322, 1992.

24. Dolgener, F.A., Hensley, L.D., Marsh, J.J., and Fjelstul, J.K.: Validation of the Rockport Fitness Walking Test in college males and females. Research Quarterly for Exercise and Sport, 65:152, 1994.

25. Kittredge, J.M., Rimmer, J.H., and Looney, M.A.: Validation of the Rockport Fitness Walking Test for adults with mental retardation. Medicine and Science in Sports and Exercise, 26:95, 1994.

26. Katch, F.I., Katch, V.L., and McArdle, W.D.: Nutrition, Weight Control, and Exercise. 3rd ed. Baltimore, Williams & Wilkins, 1991.

27. Jackson, A.S., et al.: Prediction of functional aerobic capacity without exercise testing. Medicine and Science in Sports and Exercise, 22:863, 1990.

28. Kolkhorst, F.W., and Dolgener, F.A.: Nonexercise model fails to predict aerobic capacity in college students with high VO_2 peak. Research Quarterly for Exercise and Sport, 65:78, 1994.

29. Cooper, K.H.: The Aerobics Program for Total Well-Being. New York, Bantam, 1982.

30. Conley, D.S., Cureton, K.J., Dengel, D.R., and Weyand, P.G.: Validation of the 12-minute swim as a field test of maximal aerobic power in young men. Medicine and Science in Sports and Exercise, 23:766, 1991.

31. Conley, D.S., et al.: Validation of the 12-minute swim as a field test of maximal aerobic power in young women. Research Quarterly for Exercise and Sport, 63:153, 1992.

32. Robbins, G., and Powers, D.: The Ball State 500-yard water run: a new field test for nonswimming water exercisers. Journal of the International Council for Health, Physical Education, and Recreation, 29:9, 1993.

CHAPTER 10

Assessing Musculoskeletal and Motor Fitness

The fitness of skeletal muscles is a well-recognized component of physical fitness. Responsible for all voluntary movement, the 660 skeletal muscles of the human body contribute approximately 40% to our total body mass (1). Although there is no definitive evidence that muscular fitness directly increases longevity, no one would argue that it is unimportant. Muscular fitness enables human beings to perform the daily living activities that allow for independent living throughout life. In fact, the progressive loss of lean tissue that occurs with aging is responsible for a large percentage of the commitments to nursing homes. But even earlier in life, as we seek to provide the potential for a higher quality of life, we want more than mere minimal levels of skeletal muscle strength, endurance, and flexibility. We also want muscles that function in organized patterns to exhibit the motor fitness qualities of agility, balance, coordination, power, and speed of movement. This chapter explores assessments of musculoskeletal and motor fitness as they are conducted by exercise and sport practitioners and clinicians.

As you read this chapter, watch for the following keywords:

Concentric muscular contraction	Flexibility	One-repetition maximum (1 RM)
Eccentric muscular contraction	Goniometer	Valsalva maneuver
	Motor fitness	
	Musculoskeletal fitness	

Defining Musculoskeletal Fitness

Musculoskeletal fitness has to do with the physiological status of skeletal muscles. Recognized components of musculoskeletal fitness are strength, endurance, and flexibility. *Muscular strength* is measured as the maximal single-effort force that can be generated by a muscle or muscle group against a resistance. *Muscular endurance* is the ability of a muscle or muscle group to maintain application of a submaximal force. *Flexibility* is the functional capacity of a joint to move through its full range of movement.

> Musculoskeletal fitness results from the optimal development of muscular strength, muscular endurance, and flexibility.

Relationship to Health

Unlike body composition and cardiorespiratory fitness, there is no direct relationship between skeletal muscle status and longevity. Musculoskeletal fitness is, however, positively related to functional health and well-being for both genders and for persons of all ages. In a series of position papers, the American College of Sports Medicine (ACSM) has addressed the musculoskeletal needs of adults, the elderly, and adolescents.

For the average healthy adult, ACSM advocates resistance training to enhance strength and muscular endurance and for the maintenance of optimal fat-free mass (2) (Fig. 10-1). Those guidelines specify a *minimum of 8 to 10 exercises* involving all major muscle groups to be performed *2 to 3 days per week*. Most persons should *complete 8 to 12 (near exhaustion) repetitions* of each exercise. For those who have more time to invest in resistance training, ACSM suggests multiple-set regimens. Healthy adults should also engage in regular flexibility training to develop and maintain range of motion (ROM). Static and dynamic flexibility exercises that stretch all major muscle groups should be performed 2 to 3 days per week.

The older adult should also engage in resistance training and flexibility training (2, 3). Like the younger adults, the older adult should do a *minimum of 8 to 10 ex-*

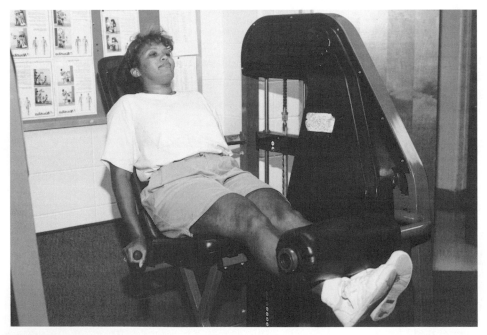

FIGURE 10-1

The American College of Sports Medicine recommends resistance training for all healthy adults. (Photo by Marvin Arrington, Heritage Photography, Greensboro, NC.)

ercises involving all major muscle groups to be performed *2 to 3 days per week*. They may, however, do better with 10 to 15 repetitions instead of 8 to 12 repetitions. ACSM strongly endorses strength and flexibility training to help the older person maintain functional capacity and postural stability. ACSM also suggests that strength training may be an important intervention to counteract weight loss among the elderly.

Younger persons should also engage in activities that develop and maintain good strength, muscular endurance, and flexibility. Young athletes of both genders should, according to ACSM, have musculoskeletal testing as part of their examinations in preparation for participation in sport (4). Such testing should assess the strength, relative symmetry, and flexibility of all major muscle groups and the stability, symmetry, and ROM of all major joints. Strength and flexibility deficits can identify conditions that require special protection, treatment, or referral for a special training program.

What are the advantages of strong and flexible muscles? Strong muscles increase joint stability and reduce the wear and tear on joint surfaces. They also allow a greater perfusion of active fibers for any muscular contraction, so a strong, flexible person can exercise with smaller increases in blood pressure and is less likely to incur local ischemia than a weak and inflexible person (5). Because of the insulin sensitivity of active skeletal muscles, muscular strength that is achieved through regular physical activity may be necessary for normal metabolic function. Furthermore, flexible muscles are critically important to prevent joint injuries during falls or accidental collisions.

Many health officials believe that musculoskeletal fitness plays an important role in the prevention of back pain, an exceedingly common disorder among adults who live in industrial societies. It is not known whether poor muscle fitness is the cause or the consequence of back pain, but it has been observed that back, neck, and shoulder pain and poor muscle fitness appear together in many persons. The traditional approach to predicting low back pain was to assess both trunk flexion strength and lower back and hamstring flexibility. It was hypothesized that the combination of weak abdominal muscles with tight hamstring and tight lower back muscles caused a forward tilting of the pelvis that stressed the lower back. However, it has since been suggested that weak trunk extensors may actually be a better predictor of low back pain than weak trunk flexors (6). It has also been suggested that back pain is particularly likely to occur with an imbalance between the strength of trunk extensors and trunk flexors (7). Other researchers have noted the important roles of supporting muscles, such as the abdominal oblique muscles and the large muscles of the arms and legs, in the prevention of back pain. Similarly, researchers studying the causes of back pain are focusing on general spine mobility rather than just low back mobility and hamstring flexibility.

Defining Motor Fitness

Motor fitness is the quality that allows organized patterns of muscular contractions and relaxations. It defines readiness for effective and efficient movements requiring the large muscles of the body. Components of motor fitness include agility, balance, coordination, power, and speed of movement. *Agility* is the ability to change positions and directions of the whole body rapidly and accurately. *Balance* is the ability to maintain postural equilibrium while in static positions and while moving. *Coordination* is the ability to integrate movements into repeatable patterns that are effective and efficient. *Muscular power* is the ability to apply maximal strength in a rapid, explosive movement. *Speed* is the ability to change the location of a body part or to move the whole body in a single direction quickly.

> Motor fitness is the result of optimal development of agility, balance, coordination, muscular power, and speed.

Relationship to Health

Agility, balance, coordination, power, and speed are often taken for granted by persons in their middle years, but these abilities are central to the lives of children. Many of a child's movement explorations test the developing limits of his or her motor fitness (Fig. 10-2). The elderly are also much concerned with aspects of motor

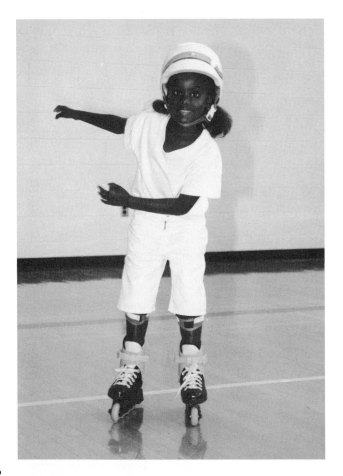

FIGURE 10-2

This young roller blader tests the limits of her agility, balance, coordination, power, and speed. (Photo by Marvin Arrington, Heritage Photography, Greensboro, NC.)

fitness, especially balance and coordination. Poor gait and poor balance predispose both children and older persons to falls. Falls can, of course, cause serious injuries to children, but they are an even greater concern among the elderly, especially post-menopausal women with osteoporosis. All too often a fall precipitates a disastrous train of events: a bone fracture, followed by hospitalization, followed by pneumonia, followed by premature death.

Why Assess Musculoskeletal and Motor Fitness?

Physical education teachers, coaches, fitness professionals, athletic trainers, physical therapists, occupational therapists, and other practitioners and clinicians have many reasons for conducting musculoskeletal and motor fitness assessments. The following are some of these reasons:

To Identify Individuals at Risk for the Development of Back Pain. If high-risk persons can be identified, they may be counseled about exercises to remediate their weakness. They may also be taught lifting techniques to minimize back strain.

To Identify Elderly Persons Who Are at Risk for Falls Because of Poor Balance. Balance testing may help to identify persons at risk, so attempts can be made to reduce risks before a fall occurs. Muscular strength testing may also be helpful in this regard, because muscle strength, even in younger adults, has been found to be an independent predictor of bone mineral density (8). Therefore, strong persons, if they do fall, are less likely to incur fractures than weak ones.

To Assess the Adequacy of the Habitual Levels of Physical Activity Among Younger Adults. A sedentary young adult may be motivated to increase his or her level of activity because of an objective comparison of his or her muscular strength to normative values for older adults. "It is precisely at this time, with the organism still at its full functional peak and with the prospect of impaired functioning psychologically remote in the 'distant future,' that an objective indicator could prove useful in prodding, when needed, for the assumption of a physically more active life-style" (9, p. 1380).

To Assess the Nature and Severity of Orthopaedic Injuries. Sports medicine practitioners assess orthopaedic injuries by measuring strength and flexibility. A common approach is to compare strength and flexibility measures of the involved limb with those of the contralateral limb (see Chapter 15.).

To Identify Athletes Whose Risk of Injury Is Higher Than Normal. Preseason examinations of athletes often include comprehensive flexibility and muscular strength assessments. Athletic trainers identify joints that have a restricted range of motion or hypermobility. They also test for imbalances in strength between contralateral limbs and between agonist and antagonist muscle groups. Despite little supportive research evidence, it is believed that remediating these problems during the preseason reduces the likelihood of an injury during the competitive season (10).

To Monitor Rehabilitation From an Injury.   Sports medicine personnel use flexibility, strength, and endurance measures to assess progress in rehabilitation. Reliable measurement is essential, as is good record keeping.

To Monitor the Effectiveness of a Weight Training Program.   Weight training is no longer just for athletes. Private and public fitness facilities feature an array of weight training equipment and have trained personnel to assist clients in their muscular development. Periodic assessments of strength, endurance, and flexibility are important aspects of weight training. Feedback from periodic tests also keeps clients motivated and attending the gym on a regular basis.

As Part of the Evaluation for a Course of Instruction in Fitness, Weight Training, Gymnastics, Dance, and so on.   Formative and summative evaluations in a variety of physical activity courses can include the results of formal assessments of strength, endurance, and/or flexibility.

To Assess a Person's Potential for Success in a Sport With High Musculoskeletal Fitness and/or Motor Fitness Demands.   Coaches in all sports use tests for a variety of reasons, but preseason cuts are a common reason. Football coaches employ a battery of tests to help identify general potential and potential for success at specific positions. Popular football tests include measures of strength (e.g., dead lift), muscular power (e.g., vertical jump test), speed (e.g., 40-yard sprint), and agility (e.g., rope ladder test). Coaches in other sports also use such testing.

To Assess Potential Success in Employment That Has High Musculoskeletal Fitness and/or Motor Fitness Demands.   Some workers, such as firefighters, police, nurses, and aides on orthopaedic wards, must be able to carry or lift people or objects. Applicants for these positions are often required to take strength and/or endurance tests. Tests of agility, balance, coordination, power, and speed may be used in preemployment testing for jobs with high demands for motor fitness.

General Guidelines for Muscular Testing

The conscientious test administrator screens potential candidates much as he or she did prior to cardiorespiratory exercise testing. In addition to formal screening, good judgment must be followed at all times. In no case should any form of testing that might cause an injury or aggravate an existing injury or illness be used. In addition, the test administrator should take heed of the following commonsense recommendations:

Make liberal use of mats, towels, or other padding materials.
Use trained spotters or other assistants.
Be cautious about encouraging all-out efforts among elderly and unconditioned clients.
Do not allow bouncing during flexibility tests.
Perform balance tests close to a wall or other support that can be touched to regain balance.
Perform agility tests on nonskid surfaces.

Some tests have greater inherent risks than others. Strength tests are particularly risky because by definition the examinee is asked to exert a maximal force. Many people tend to hold their breath during strength testing, so the test administrator must encourage the correct pattern of breathing. *During strength testing the examinee should breathe out during the active lifting or pressing phase and breathe in during the release or return phase.* This pattern of breathing helps to prevent the **Valsalva maneuver,** a condition commonly associated with a heart attack. A Valsalva maneuver refers to an increase in intrathoracic pressure that then in turn causes a slowing of the pulse, decreased return of blood to the heart, and increased venous pressure.

> Valsalva maneuver, which entails holding one's breath during physical exertion, causes an increase in intrathoracic pressure that slows the pulse, decreases return of blood to the heart, and increases venous pressure.

Types of Muscle Contractions

Skeletal muscles can contract in several ways. In *isometric (static) contractions* (e.g., flexed arm hang), there is no visible movement during the contraction because the resistance is greater than the force of the contraction. In *isotonic (dynamic) contractions* there is movement, but the contractions can be concentric, eccentric, or isokinetic. During a **concentric contraction** (e.g., the lifting phase of a pull-up) the resistance is less than the force of contraction, so the muscle shortens as the bony levers are drawn together. During an **eccentric contraction** (e.g., the lowering phase of a pull-up) the muscle lengthens while exerting force against resistance. The amount of resistance that can be applied in concentric and eccentric contractions is limited by the strength of the muscle group at its weakest joint angle. An *isokinetic contraction* (e.g., an arm curl on a Nautilus machine) is a contraction against a resistance that moves at a constant speed through the range of movement at the associated joint. This results in a maximal contraction at every joint angle through the entire range of movement. These contraction types are summarized in Table 10-1.

> A concentric muscular contraction occurs when the muscle shortens as bony levers are drawn together.

> An eccentric muscular contraction occurs when the muscle lengthens during exertion of force against resistance.

Laboratory Assessment of Strength and Endurance

In the laboratory, specialized equipment can be used to measure isometric contractions and all three types of isotonic contractions. Laboratory equipment for strength and endurance measurement include dynamometers, cable tensiometers, electromechanical and hydraulic devices such as force platforms, and constant- and variable-resistance exercise machines such as the Cybex, Orthotron, and Kin-Com.

TABLE 10-1	**Types of Muscle Contractions**
TYPE OF CONTRACTION	**MOVEMENT EXAMPLES**
Isometric (static): no visible movement during contraction because resistance is greater than force of contraction	Flexed arm hang, V-sit, wall sit, 90° stationary push-up
Isotonic (dynamic): movement during contraction because force of contraction is greater than resistance	Lift phase of pull-up, lift phase of arm curl, lift phase of dip
Concentric: muscle shortens	
Eccentric: muscle lengthens	Lowering of pull-up, lowering of arm curl, lowering of dip
Isokinetic: maximal contraction through entire ROM	Nautilus arm curl, Cybex leg extension

On these machines the speed of contraction is mechanically controlled so the resistance varies to match the muscular force produced at each joint angle through the ROM. Some models have a computer and printer that plot an accurate and reliable strength curve over the full ROM at the involved joint. These computerized machines are expensive, and their operation and interpretation of results require intensive training. They are, however, remarkable. Physical therapists have found variable-resistance machines to be invaluable as they work with clients in rehabilitation of orthopaedic injuries.

Field Assessment of Strength and Endurance

Practitioners who work in schools and public or private fitness centers are unlikely to have much specialized muscle testing equipment. They may have a grip dynamometer and perhaps even a cable tensiometer, but they are less likely to have access to force platforms and variable-resistance machines. Instead, field assessment procedures use the equipment found in most gymnasiums, such as bars and free weights. Unfortunately, a comprehensive muscle assessment cannot be performed without some of the specialized equipment. For example, isokinetic contractions cannot be measured without variable-resistance machinery. Therefore, all field assessments of muscle strength and endurance are limited to isometric and to concentric and eccentric dynamic contractions.

Field Testing of Muscular Strength

In the field the strength of isotonic contractions is commonly measured by having the examinee perform a **one-repetition maximum (1 RM, or one rep max)** test. The 1-RM test uses either free weights or an appropriate setting on a Universal machine. *The objective of a 1-RM test is to determine the maximum amount of weight that the examinee can lift only one time.* The strength of all major muscle groups can be assessed using a 1-RM protocol. For example, a 1-RM arm curl test can assess the strength of the elbow flexors; a 1-RM squat test can assess the strength of the leg extensors; and a 1-RM leg curl can assess the strength of the knee flexors (Fig. 10-3). All 1-RM tests are conducted according to the same basic protocol. The protocol described next is for a 1-RM bench press test using free weights:

> 1 RM, or one rep max, refers to the maximum weight that can be lifted only one time (i.e., one repetition).

1-RM Bench Press Test Protocol for Free Weights

Purpose

The purpose of the 1-RM Bench Press Test Protocol is to assess the dynamic muscular strength of the upper arm and shoulder girdle muscles, specifically, the triceps, pectoralis major, and anterior deltoid muscles.

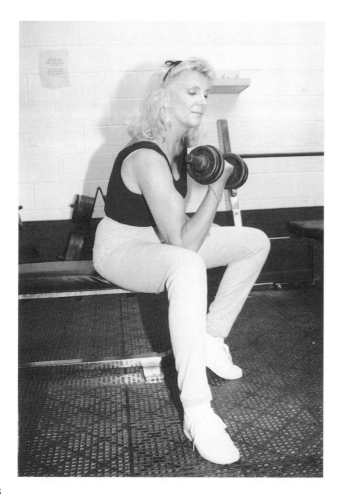

FIGURE 10-3

A 1-RM arm curl test can assess the strength of the elbow flexors. (Photo by Marvin Arrington, Heritage Photography, Greensboro, NC.)

Psychometric Information

Face validity is claimed because of the consistency between the test objective and the theoretical definition of muscular strength. Test-retest reliability was assessed by correlating scores recorded on separate days; the r value was .93 (11).

Gender and Age

This test is appropriate for both genders and for most adults. Lifting of maximal weights by prepubescent persons is *not* recommended (12).

Equipment

This test requires a weight bench, bar, and a range of free-weight plates.

Administrative Concerns

The examinee should be familiar with correct bench press techniques, including the motion and the breathing pattern. If the examinee is a novice to the bench press, it is likely that this test will underestimate his or her true strength.

Procedure

1. Allow the examinee to warm up with a light load.
2. The maximal weight is determined by trial and error. A beginning weight *that is less than the anticipated maximal weight* is put on the bar. An experienced lifter can give you an idea where to start, but some general guidelines may be helpful for an examinee who is new to 1-RM strength testing. A good starting place for the bench press for young, active men is about 70 to 80% of their body weight; young, active women can begin at about 50 to 60% of their body weight.
3. The examinee lies supine on the bench with feet on the floor on either side of the bench. Hands should grip the bar at about shoulder width, with thumbs in line with the armpits (Fig. 10-4).
4. A spotter helps lower the bar to the examinee's chest. The examinee takes a breath, then exhales while pushing the bar straight up until the elbows are locked. The spotter should help the examinee replace the bar on the rack.
5. Before attempting to lift a greater weight, allow a recovery period of at least 3 minutes to allow for restoration of muscle stores of ATP (adenosine triphosphate) and CP (creatine phosphate).
6. Increase the weight by 5 to 10 pounds and repeat. Allow as many trials as necessary to achieve a maximum, always allowing a full rest between trials. Record the score as the weight lifted just prior to an unsuccessful lift.

Scoring

1. Since absolute strength is largely determined by one's body mass, scores are best interpreted by calculating the relative strength. **Relative strength** is found by dividing the maximal lift by the examinee's body weight, as in Formula 10-1:

   Relative strength = maximal lift ÷ body weight   Formula 10-1

   Maximal lift and body weight must be in the same units (pounds or kilograms).
2. Interpret relative strength for young adults by comparing the relative strength score with optimal relative-strength values in Table 10-2 (13). Optimal strength scores for older adults are approximately 10% lower per decade

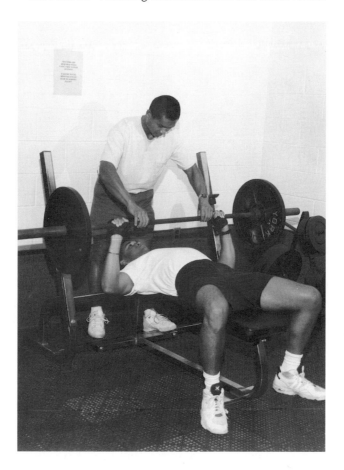

FIGURE 10-4

The examinee for a 1-RM bench press uses a shoulder-width grip with thumbs in line with the armpits. (Photo by Marvin Arrington, Heritage Photography, Greensboro, NC.)

(14). For persons who are overfat, you may wish to use an optimal body weight value for calculations of optimal relative strength.

Comments

Strength assessment is specific to the muscle groups being tested, so it is difficult to generalize about overall strength from the score for one muscle group. Some believe, however, that the 1-RM bench press test is the best single test for predicting overall dynamic strength (15). If two tests are used to assess dynamic strength, the bench press should be used for upper-body strength and the leg press should be used for lower-body strength (16).

Heyward (14) developed a battery of six free-weight and Universal machine tests that collectively assess overall dynamic strength for college age men and women. In Heyward's battery points are awarded for each of the six tests according to the relative strength score for each 1-RM test (Table 10-3). For example, a 120-lb woman who bench-presses a maximum of 60 lb has a relative strength score of 0.50, so she receives 3 points for the bench press test. Overall dynamic strength is evalu-

TABLE 10-2	Optimal Relative Strength Values for Selected 1-RM Tests			
	BENCH PRESS	**LEG PRESS**	**ARM CURL**	**MILITARY PRESS**
Men	1.00	2.00	0.50	0.67
Women	0.70	1.40	0.35	0.47

Values were determined using Universal weight apparatus. Values may differ somewhat for free weight testing.
Adapted from Pollock, M.L., Wilmore, J.H., and Fox, S.M.: Health and Fitness Through Physical Activity. New York, John Wiley & Sons, 1978, p. 106.

ated by totaling the scores for the six tests. Heyward developed her scoring scheme from data for 250 college-age men and women.

Predicting 1 RM From Submaximal Repetitions

Despite its conceptual appeal for assessing muscular strength, 1-RM testing has several distinct drawbacks. Besides being quite time consuming, especially in mass testing, the 1-RM test is not recommended for the inexperienced or prepubescent lifter. Furthermore, for any lifter, regardless of experience or age, there is a risk of injury whenever the tensile strength of the anatomical structural components is exceeded by the stress of the weight being lifted. For some lifters there is also concern about increased blood pressure.

Fortunately, researchers have discovered that the 1-RM value can be estimated with a fair degree of accuracy from maximal repetitions of a submaximal weight. (This is similar to the process of predicting VO_2max from a submaximal work load.) The rationale for this prediction is the approximately linear relation between the 1-RM value and maximal repetitions performed at relatively high intensities (17, 18). At least three equations have been proposed for the estimation of the 1-RM value from maximal repetitions of submaximal lifts. One is based on 2 to 10 repetitions, one on 2 to 20 repetitions, and another on maximal repetitions in 1 minute (19–21). All three equations yield similar 1-RM values. The 2-to-10 procedure is described here.

Prediction of 1 RM From 2 to 10 Repetitions-to-Fatigue (19)

Purpose
The purpose of this test is to estimate 1 RM from 2 to 10 repetitions-to-fatigue of a submaximal weight. This protocol can be used to test a variety of muscle groups with standard free weights or Universal machinery.

Psychometric Information
This procedure is based on the theoretical relation between muscular strength and muscular endurance. Face validity is claimed. Another study reported test-retest reliabilities for various lifts at submaximal intensities that ranged from .79 to .98 (22).

| TABLE 10-3 | Strength-to-Body Weight Ratios for Selected Dynamic Strength Tests for College-Aged Men and Women | | | | | |

BENCH PRESS	ARM CURL	LATERAL PULL-DOWN	LEG PRESS	LEG EXTENSION	LEG CURL	POINTS
MEN						
1.50	0.70	1.20	3.00	0.80	0.70	10
1.40	0.65	1.15	2.80	0.75	0.65	9
1.30	0.60	1.10	2.60	0.70	0.60	8
1.20	0.55	1.05	2.40	0.65	0.55	7
1.10	0.50	1.00	2.20	0.60	0.50	6
1.00	0.45	0.95	2.00	0.55	0.45	5
0.90	0.40	0.90	1.80	0.50	0.40	4
0.80	0.35	0.85	1.60	0.45	0.35	3
0.70	0.30	0.80	1.40	0.40	0.30	2
0.60	0.25	0.75	1.20	0.35	0.25	1
WOMEN						
0.90	0.50	0.85	2.70	0.70	0.60	10
0.85	0.45	0.80	2.50	0.65	0.55	9
0.80	0.42	0.75	2.30	0.60	0.52	8
0.70	0.38	0.73	2.10	0.55	0.50	7
0.65	0.35	0.70	2.00	0.52	0.45	6
0.60	0.32	0.65	1.80	0.50	0.40	5
0.55	0.28	0.63	1.60	0.45	0.35	4
0.50	0.25	0.60	1.40	0.40	0.30	3
0.45	0.21	0.55	1.20	0.35	0.25	2
0.35	0.18	0.50	1.00	0.30	0.20	1

Total Points	Strength Fitness Category
48–60	Excellent
37–47	Good
25–36	Average
13–24	Fair
0–12	Poor

Reprinted with permission from Heyward V.H.: Advanced Fitness Assessment and Exercise Prescription. 3rd ed. Champaign, IL, Human Kinetics, 1997, p. 112.

Gender and Age

This test is appropriate for both genders and a wide variety of ages, including adolescents and older adults.

Administrative Concerns

The examinee should receive basic instruction on weight lifting and breathing techniques.

Procedure
1. Allow the examinee to warm up with a light load.
2. Select a submaximal weight that the examinee can lift at least twice but no more than 10 times before fatiguing. If an approximate 1-RM value is known, select a weight about 75% of this value. If an approximate 1-RM value is not known, refer to Table 10-2 for guidance in selection of a submaximal weight.
3. Instruct the examinee to perform repeated lifts until he or she can do no more with good technique. Count the repetitions.
4. If more than 10 repetitions are performed, stop the examinee. Repeat the test with a heavier weight after a rest period or preferably the next day.

Scoring
Calculate the predicted 1-RM by the following equation:

Predicted 1 RM = weight lifted ÷ [1.0278 − 0.0278 (number of reps)]

Formula 10-2

Sample Calculation
A person lifts or presses 90 lb a total of 8 times.
Predicted 1 RM = 90 lb ÷ [1.0278 − 0.0278 (8)] = *112 lb*

Comments
For mass testing the administrator may choose to use the same weight for all examinees of the same gender whose body weights fall within a certain range.

Field Testing of Muscular Endurance

Field assessments of static and dynamic muscular endurance are either relative or absolute. *Relative muscular endurance* tests come in two basic formats. These tests require the examinee to work a muscle group against a submaximal resistance that is either (*a*) proportional to the examinee's own body weight or (*b*) proportional to the maximum strength of the same muscle group. *Absolute muscular endurance* tests require all examinees to perform work against the same resistance. Testing entails exercising the muscle group to exhaustion or completing as many repetitions as possible within a certain time. Examples of both formats are presented here.

YMCA Bench Press Test (23)

Purpose
The purpose of this test is to assess the absolute dynamic endurance of the upper arm and shoulder girdle muscles, specifically the triceps, pectoralis major, and anterior deltoid muscles.

Psychometric Information
No psychometric information has been reported.

Gender and Age
This test is suitable for adults of both genders. It is appropriate for younger persons, but no norms are available except for adults.

Equipment
This test requires a standard weight bench, a 35-lb barbell for women, an 80-lb barbell for men, and a metronome.

Procedure
1. The examinee lies supine on the bench with feet on the floor on either side of the bench. The examinee flexes the elbows and prepares to receive the barbell with the palms facing upward. The tester or spotter hands the barbell to the examinee, who grips the bar with hands a shoulder-width apart.
2. He or she presses the barbell upward to a position with full elbow extension. From full extension the barbell is returned to the original down position. Repeat. These up-and-down movements are performed in rhythm to a metronome set at 60 beats per second; each click signals either an up or down movement.
3. The examinee should be reminded to exhale with each upward movement and inhale during each downward movement.
4. Count each completed up position. The test is terminated when the examinee cannot fully extend the elbows or keep the cadence.

Evaluation
Table 10-4 has age-adjusted norms.

Comments
The YMCA bench press is a test of absolute dynamic muscular endurance. It allows a head-to-head comparison among men and among women for three age groupings. No consideration is given to body weight or maximal strength. Because of this

TABLE 10-4	Age Norms for the YMCA Bench Press Test						
RATING	% RANK	18–25	26–35	36–45	46–55	56–65	OVER 65
MEN							
Excellent	95	42	40	34	28	24	20
Good	80	32	29	25	21	18	12
Above average	65	26	24	21	16	12	10
Average	50	22	20	17	12	8	6
Below average	35	17	14	13	9	6	4
Poor	20	12	10	9	5	2	2
Very poor	5	2	2	2	1	0	0
WOMEN							
Excellent	95	42	40	32	30	30	22
Good	80	29	26	22	21	18	13
Above average	65	24	21	18	14	14	10
Average	50	20	17	13	11	9	6
Below average	35	14	13	10	8	6	3
Poor	20	9	8	6	4	2	1
Very poor	5	2	1	1	0	0	0

Adapted from Golding, L.A., Myers, C.R., and Sinning, W.E. (eds.): Y's Way to Physical Fitness: The Complete Guide to Fitness Testing and Instruction. 3rd ed. Champaign, IL, Human Kinetics for the YMCA, 1989, pp. 113–124.

the YMCA bench press test may not be a good measure of health-related muscular endurance. It can, however, be very useful as a preemployment test for certain work in which persistence with submaximal weights is important (e.g., construction, fire fighting, warehouse loading dock). This test may also be used by an occupational therapist to assess an injured employee's readiness to return to one of these lines of work.

70% of Maximum Strength Testing Protocol

Purpose
The puppies of this test is to assess the relative, dynamic muscular endurance of a muscle group.

Psychometric Information
No psychometric information has been reported.

Gender and Age
This test is suitable for both genders, adolescents to adults.

Equipment
This test requires free weights or Universal machinery.

Procedure
1. For each muscle group to be tested, ascertain a 1-RM value, then calculate 70% of this maximal value.
2. Have examinee perform repeated lifts to exhaustion. Count successful repetitions.

Evaluation
It has been suggested that recreational athletes or the health-seeking exerciser should be able to perform 12 to 15 repetitions; the competitive athlete should be able to perform 20 to 25 repetitions for each muscle group (13).

Comments
No norms for relative dynamic muscular endurance for this testing protocol have been developed. The standards suggested herein are just that—suggested standards. However, the logic is good. The success of this testing obviously depends on an accurate 1-RM value.

You may wonder how this assessment is different from the test that predicts a 1 RM from 2 to 10 repetitions-to-fatigue. The repetitions-to-fatigue test provides a simultaneous assessment of muscular strength and endurance. However, the percent of maximum strength can be determined only post hoc, that is, after the test. When one begins the repetitions-to-fatigue test, it is not clear what percent load the examinee is lifting. If it happens to be 70%, the results should be consistent with the evaluation provided earlier.

Traditional Push-up Test

Purpose
The purpose of this test is to assess the relative dynamic muscular endurance of muscles active in elbow extension and shoulder lateral flexion.

Psychometric Information
Face validity is claimed. Reliability and objectivity are reported to be high (11).

Gender and Age

This test is appropriate for adults of both genders. Standards for younger persons are not available.

Equipment

This test requires a mat.

Administrative Concerns

If the examinee feels pain at the shoulder joint during the push-up motion, discontinue the test.

Procedure

1. Boys and men perform a full-body push-up. Beginning position is body straight with weight supported on balls of feet and hands. Girls and women perform a modified push-up. Beginning position is upper body straight, with weight supported on knees and hands. For both types of push-ups, hands are directly under the shoulders, and elbows are fully extended in the starting position.
2. The tester places his or her fist on the mat directly beneath the examinee's chest. The examinee flexes at the elbows and lowers the body until the chest touches the tester's fist. He or she then pushes upward to return to the starting position. The body is kept straight at all times. Perform repeatedly.
3. Count repetitions until muscle fatigue.

Evaluation

Table 10-5 has age-adjusted norms.

TABLE 10-5	Push-up Muscular Endurance Standards				
RATING	20–29	30–39	40–49	50–59	60–69
MEN					
Excellent	55 and above	45 and above	40 and above	35 and above	30 and above
Good	45–54	35–44	30–39	25–34	20–29
Average	35–44	25–34	20–29	15–24	10–19
Fair	20–34	15–24	12–19	8–14	5–9
Poor	0–19	0–14	0–11	0–7	0–4
WOMEN					
Excellent	49 and above	40 and above	35 and above	30 and above	20 and above
Good	34–48	25–39	20–34	15–29	5–19
Average	17–33	12–24	8–19	6–14	3–4
Fair	6–16	4–11	3–7	2–5	1–2
Poor	0–5	0–3	0–2	0–1	0

Values are approximations, since actual norms are not available.
Reprinted with permission from Pollock, M.L., Wilmore, J.H., and Fox, S.M.: Health and Fitness Through Physical Activity. New York, Wiley, 1978, p. 109.

Comments

The traditional push-up test is a relative test of dynamic muscular endurance. The load lifted is relative to one's body weight, but not everyone works at the same percent of body weight. One's body fatness, trunk length, and limb lengths prevent equal comparisons. Evaluations by norms ignores this problem. No doubt criterion-referenced standards should be developed for this and for other calisthenic muscular endurance tests.

Flexed Arm Hang for Boys and Girls

Purpose
To assess the static muscular endurance of the elbow and shoulder flexors.

Psychometric Information
No psychometric information has been reported.

Gender and Age
This test is suitable for both genders, ages 6 to 17 and above and for college-age women.

Equipment
This test requires a pull-up bar and a stopwatch.

Procedure
1. Lift or assist examinee up to a 1-inch-diameter bar. Examinee should grasp bar with an overhand grasp, palms away and hands shoulder-width apart. Chin should be above the bar. Legs should be extended and stationary.
2. Begin timing immediately. Stop the watch when the examinee's chin falls below the level of the bar. Record time to the nearest 0.1 second.

Evaluation
Norms (Tables 10-6 and 10-7) for boys and girls are based on the 1985 School Population Fitness Survey conducted for the President's Council (24). (Also see Tables A-1 and A-2 in Appendix A for the FITNESSGRAM Healthy Fitness Zone standards for the flexed arm hang.)

The contrasting groups procedure was used to classify untrained and trained college women. Trained women in this study had participated in a 12-week training program for lower-body strength and endurance. A criterion standard of 5 seconds was established for trained women (25).

Robertson Modified Curl-up Test (26)

Purpose
The purpose of this test is to assess the dynamic muscular endurance of the abdominal muscles.

Psychometric Information
Validity was demonstrated by electromyograph (EMG) analysis showing electrical activity in the abdominal muscles without activity in the hip flexors. Reliability was demonstrated by high consistency between trials; that is, $R = .93$ and $.94$ for men and women, respectively (27). Further evidence of validity was provided by a study that used item response theory to identify the modified curl-up as an appropri-

TABLE 10-6	Norms for Flexed Arm Hang for Boys

| PERCEN- | AGE | | | | | | | | | | | | PER- |
TILE	6	7	8	9	10	11	12	13	14	15	16	17+	CENT
100	55	95	63	101	120	101	111	127	117	130	125	116	10
95	23	60	34	40	48	52	47	48	68	79	71	64	9
90	16	23	28	28	38	37	36	37	61	62	61	56	9
85	14	20	23	24	31	31	30	33	47	58	51	49	8
80	12	17	18	20	25	26	25	29	40	49	46	45	8
75	10	15	17	18	22	22	21	25	35	44	42	41	7
70	9	13	15	16	20	19	19	22	31	40	39	39	7
65	9	11	14	14	17	17	16	20	28	37	36	37	6
60	8	10	12	12	15	15	15	18	25	35	33	35	6
55	7	9	11	11	14	13	13	16	22	33	30	33	5
50	6	8	10	10	12	11	12	14	20	30	28	30	5
45	5	7	9	8	10	10	10	12	17	28	25	29	4
40	5	6	8	8	8	9	9	10	15	25	22	26	4
35	4	5	6	7	7	7	8	9	13	22	20	23	3
30	3	4	5	5	6	6	6	8	11	20	18	20	3
25	2	4	4	5	5	5	5	6	10	18	15	17	2
20	2	3	3	3	3	4	4	5	8	14	12	15	2
15	1	2	2	3	2	3	2	4	5	10	10	11	1
10	1	1	1	2	1	1	1	2	3	8	7	8	1
5	0	0	0	0	0	0	0	0	1	3	3	5	
0	0	0	0	0	0	0	0	0	0	0	0	0	

Reprinted from President's Council on Physical Fitness: 1985 PCPFS Youth Fitness Survey. Washington, U.S. Printing Office, 1986.

ate test for persons of average and low fitness (28). Preliminary norms were developed from 151 undergraduate physical education majors.

Equipment

This test requires a nonslip mat or padded carpet, a stopwatch, and a measuring strip 3 inches wide and approximately 1 yard long.

Procedure

1. The examinee lies supine on a mat with knees bent to 90° and head resting on the mat. The shoulder girdle is depressed, and arms are straight at the sides, with fingers reaching toward the heels. The lower back is flattened to the mat by a posterior pelvic tilt, achieved by contraction of the abdominal muscles.

TTABLE 10-7	Norms for Flexed Arm Hang for Girls

PERCEN-TILE	6	7	8	9	10	11	12	13	14	15	16	17+	PER-CENT
100	55	72	97	78	152	150	99	68	100	125	131	127	100
95	22	29	26	35	38	33	37	35	38	41	40	37	95
90	15	21	21	23	29	25	27	28	31	34	30	29	90
85	13	17	17	20	22	20	21	21	25	28	24	24	85
80	11	14	15	16	19	16	16	19	21	23	21	20	80
75	10	12	13	14	16	14	14	16	18	18	18	18	75
70	9	11	11	12	14	13	13	14	16	15	16	15	70
65	8	9	10	11	12	11	11	12	13	12	13	12	65
60	6	8	10	10	11	9	10	10	11	10	10	11	60
55	6	7	9	9	9	8	8	9	10	9	9	10	55
50	5	6	8	8	8	7	7	8	9	7	7	7	50
45	5	5	7	7	7	6	6	6	7	6	6	6	45
40	4	5	6	6	6	5	5	5	6	5	5	5	40
35	3	5	5	5	5	4	4	5	5	4	4	5	35
30	3	4	4	4	4	4	3	4	4	4	3	4	30
25	2	3	3	3	3	3	2	3	3	3	2	2	25
20	1	2	3	2	2	2	1	1	2	2	2	2	20
15	1	1	1	1	1	1	1	1	1	1	1	1	15
10	0	0	0	0	0	0	0	0	0	1	0	1	10
5	0	0	0	0	0	0	0	0	0	0	0	0	5
0	0	0	0	0	0	0	0	0	0	0	0	0	0

Reprinted from President's Council on Physical Fitness: 1985 PCPFS Youth Fitness Survey. Washington, U.S. Printing Office, 1986.

2. The measuring strip is positioned so that the longest finger just touches the front edge of the strip. The strip is then stabilized by a partner.
3. Allow the examinee five trial curl-ups to practice the correct form. The neck is to be flexed (chin to chest position) throughout the test. The shoulders and then the upper back are progressively curled off the mat, while the fingertips of both hands slide across the measuring strip. The curling continues until the fingertips simultaneously touch the far edge of the 3-inch-wide measuring strip. The examinee then uncurls until his or her scapulae touch the mat. The examinee should be reminded to exhale with each curl and inhale with each uncurl.
4. The examinee completes as many correct curl-ups as possible in 1 minute. The tester or partner counts aloud for each correct curl-up. If incorrect technique is used, the partner simply repeats the previous number.

5. At the end of the test the examinee returns to the starting position and the fingertip distance is checked to ensure that the examinee did not move during the test. If movement did occur, the test is to be repeated after an appropriate rest period.

6. The examinee should stretch leg and abdominal muscles.

Evaluation
Compare score with the preliminary norms presented in Table 10-8.

Comments
For the assessment of abdominal muscle endurance, this test is preferred to the traditional bent-leg or straight-leg sit-up. The sit-up has several problems. The final stage of the sit-up motion requires strong contraction of the hip flexors, so it is not considered a highly valid measure of abdominal muscle endurance. Furthermore, there is a marked risk of back injury because of lumbar hyperextension during sit-ups. The Robertson modified curl-up addresses both of these concerns.

Research using the Robertson modified curl-up is likely to provide us with norms and/or criterion-referenced standards for various age groups in the near future. If low back pain is associated with abdominal muscle weakness, it will be very important to know the levels of muscular strength and endurance that will provide protection against this disorder.

Couch Test (29)

Purpose
The purpose of this test is to assess the static muscular endurance of the trunk extensor muscles.

Psychometric Information
The couch test was administered to 53 men aged 27 to 60 and to 23 women aged 22 to 61. The coefficient of variation was .19; the 2-week test-retest correlation was r = .89.

TABLE 10-8	Preliminary Norms for the Robertson Modified Curl-up Test	
	SCORE	
PERFORMANCE	**Men**	**Women**
Excellent	103–118	98–115
Good	87–102	80–97
Average	69–86	60–79
Below Average	53–68	42–59
Poor	37–52	23–41

Based on scores of 79 men and 72 women undergraduate physical education majors at Northern Illinois University.
Reprinted with permission from MacFarlane, P.A.: Out with the sit-up, in with the curl-up! Journal of Physical Education, Recreation and Dance, 64(6), 1993, p. 66.

Gender and Age
This test is suitable for adults of both genders.

Equipment
This test requires a couch or padded table and a stopwatch.

Procedure
1. The examinee lies prone with the upper body hanging over the edge of a couch or padded table. The buttocks and legs are fixed by a strap, padded bar, or by an assistant; examinee's arms are crossed and held tight against the chest.
2. The examinee raises the upper body to the horizontal, then holds this position until exhaustion or to a maximum of 240 seconds. The stopwatch is stopped when the upper body falls below or is lifted above the horizontal.

Evaluation
A long time score is considered better than a short one, but no norms or criterion-referenced standards have yet been developed.

Comments
The test developers suggested that those with poor endurance of the back muscles are likely to suffer postural stresses that may cause low back pain. The couch test is suggested as one of a battery of tests to examine potential for low back pain.

Flexibility Assessment

Flexibility is relatively easy to assess. There are two basic approaches to the measurement of ROM at a joint. Flexibility can be assessed by a rotary measure, in which degrees of rotation around a 360° arc are determined by protractor instruments. Flexibility can also be assessed using a linear measure, in which scores are given in inches or centimeters. Both angular and linear flexibility measures can be static or dynamic. *Static flexibility* refers to the degree to which a joint can be passively moved by the tester. *Dynamic flexibility* is the degree to which a joint can be moved as a result of active muscular contraction by the examinee. Most flexibility tests assess a single joint, but some, primarily field tests, assess more than one joint.

> Flexibility refers to the ability of a joint to move through an optimal range of movement.

Devices used in precise laboratory assessments of flexibility include *elgons* (electrogoniometers), radiogoniometers, and photogoniometers. The elgon operates by a potentiometer that creates an electrical current. The current increases proportionally with increases in the ROM at a joint. In field and clinical settings instruments generally include a hand-held goniometer or a Leighton Flexometer. Simple tape measures, rulers, and yardsticks are used for linear measures of flexibility. **Goniometers** are essentially protractors with two long arms. The movable arm is aligned with the longitudinal axis of a moving body part, and the ROM is read from the protractor in the center of the goniometer. The Leighton Flexometer has a weighted 360° dial and a weighted pointer. The device is strapped onto the body segment being measured and the dial is locked at 0°. The full movement is performed; then the dial is locked at the other extreme. The ROM in degrees is read from the dial. Described later in this section are field assessment procedures that make use of goniometers, tape measures, and yardsticks.

> A goniometer is a protractorlike instrument that measures joint ROM in degrees.

Factors That Affect Flexibility

Flexibility is related to age, gender, and habitual physical activity. In general, we become less flexible as we age, and men and boys are commonly less flexible than women and girls (Fig. 10-5). Sedentary persons are generally less flexible than active persons. We also find restricted ROM among the obese at nearly all joints. However, flexibility is highly modifiable for nearly all persons of any age. The significant exceptions are those with painful orthopaedic or neuromuscular diseases. Most people's flexibility can be improved by increasing appropriate activity levels and reducing body fat. It has been found that approximately 41% of the total resistance at joints is explained by the inelasticity of muscles and their fascia (30). Even the elderly, whose muscles become less elastic with age, can improve flexibility with exercises. And even persons with large, hypertrophied muscles can improve. Muscles and fascia can be stretched and can become more elastic. Factors that are not modifiable include the bony structure of the joint itself and collagen structures, such as the joint capsule, tendons, and ligaments.

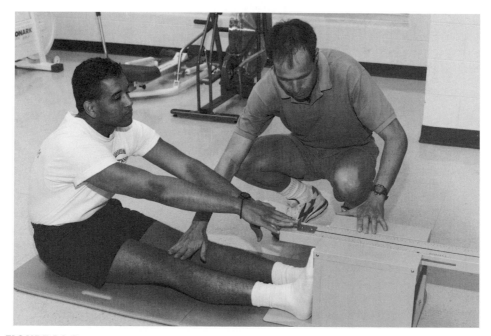

FIGURE 10-5

Men are commonly less flexible than women. (Photo by Marvin Arrington, Heritage Photography, Greensboro, NC.)

Issues Associated With Flexibility Assessment

Flexibility is highly specific to each joint. In terms of assessment this means we cannot measure the ROM at one joint and easily generalize to all joints of the body. Some people regularly exercise certain joints of the body while ignoring others. For example, the swimmer who regularly does the front crawl may have excellent flexibility at the shoulder joint but limited flexibility of the hip joint. The right-footed football punter may have a more flexible right than left hip (Fig. 10-6). For the past half-century, however, when a single measure of flexibility is taken, it has usually been a measure of trunk flexion. This is no doubt due to the relationship of low back and/or hamstring inflexibility to back pain.

Another assessment concern is the effect of warm-up on flexibility. Warm-up prior to flexibility assessment is essential for valid measurements because warm muscles stretch better than cold ones. Recommended prior to flexibility measurement is a general body warm-up of several minutes of light jogging followed by easy stretching of the muscles active at the joint to be measured.

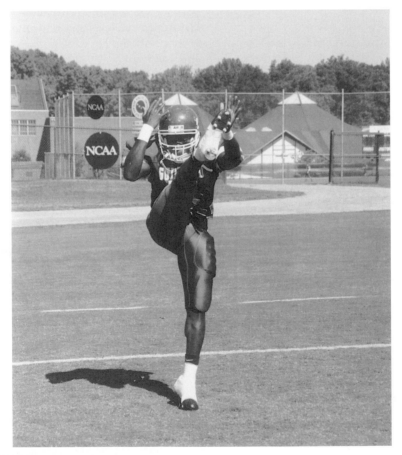

FIGURE 10-6

The right hip of this punter may be more flexible than his left hip.
(Photo by Marvin Arrington, Heritage Photography, Greensboro, NC.)

Field Testing of Flexibility

Because of the specificity of flexibility, there are almost as many flexibility tests as there are joints. It is impossible to review all of them, but here is a sampling of field tests of flexibility.

YMCA Trunk Flexion Test (23)

Purpose
The purpose of this test is to assess trunk flexion, especially to assess the flexibility of the hamstring muscles.

Psychometric Information
Validity is discussed in the Comments section. Reliability of the best of three trials has been reported as high, r = .94. Intertester objectivity was reported at .99 (11).

Gender and Age
Both genders, ages 18 to 65 and above.

Equipment
This test requires a yardstick or tape measure and a line drawn or taped on the floor at right angles to the 15-inch mark with the zero end toward the examinee.

Procedure
1. Allow the examinee to warm up before testing.
2. Examinee removes shoes, then sits on the floor with the yardstick between the legs. He or she sits with heels 10 to 12 inches apart and aligned at the 15-inch line.
3. Examinee slowly reaches forward and downward and slides the fingertips of both hands along the yardstick. Hands should stay aligned, with one on top of the other. Knees should stay fully extended; the tester should rest a hand lightly on top of the legs to ensure this position.
4. Examinee is to hold the final reach position momentarily, while the tester reads the linear measure from the yardstick. The examinee should be encouraged to exhale and drop the head between the arms for a maximal score.
5. Allow the examinee to relax, then repeat twice. The score is the farthest distance reached during the three trials, recorded to the nearest quarter inch.

Evaluation
Table 10-9 has norms for adults.

Comments
For many years after it was developed, the traditional sit-and-reach test was assumed to assess both hamstring flexibility and flexibility of the muscles of the lower back. Research has demonstrated that the sit-and-reach is moderately correlated (r = .60 to .73) with hamstring flexibility but weakly correlated (r = .27 to .30) with low back flexibility (31). Thus, the sit-and-reach is not a highly valid test of low back flexibility. This doesn't mean, however, that it is worthless. It is still a valuable field assessment of hamstring flexibility, one of the muscle groups that may be related to back problems. These comments can also be applied to the trunk flexion test.

TABLE 10-9	Age Norms for the YMCA Trunk Flexion Test						
RATING	% RANK	18–25	26–35	36–45	46–55	56–65	OVER 65
MEN							
Excellent	95	22	22	21	20	19	18
Good	80	19	18	17	17	15	14
Above average	65	17	17	15	15	13	12
Average	50	16	15	14	12	11	10
Below average	35	14	13	11	10	9	8
Poor	20	12	11	9	8	7	6
Very poor	5	7	7	5	4	3	3
WOMEN							
Excellent	95	25	24	23	22	21	21
Good	80	22	21	20	19	18	18
Above average	65	20	19	18	17	17	17
Average	50	19	18	16	16	15	15
Below average	35	17	16	15	14	13	13
Poor	20	15	14	12	12	11	10
Very poor	5	12	11	9	8	7	6

Adapted from Golding, L.A., Myers, C.R., and Sinning, W.E. (eds.): Y's Way to Physical Fitness: The Complete Guide to Fitness Testing and Instruction. 3rd ed. Champaign, IL, Human Kinetics for the YMCA, 1989, pp. 113–124.

President's Council V-Sit Reach

The President's Council V-Sit Reach (24) is essentially the same as the trunk flexion test with a few relatively minor procedural differences.

Gender and Age
Children and youth of both genders, ages 6 and under to 17 and above.

Procedure
1. The examinee sits with heels 8 to 12 inches apart and ankles flexed so toes point at the ceiling.
2. Heels are aligned with the measuring tape so that the heel line is at 0 inches. Stretches beyond the heel line are recorded as positive value numbers; stretches short of the heel line are recorded as negative values.
3. Three practice trials are allowed; the fourth reach is held for 3 seconds while that distance is measured and recorded. Scores are recorded to the nearest half inch.

Evaluation
Tables 10-10 and 10-11 have norms for children and youths.

Comment
Also see the FITNESSGRAM Back-Saver Sit-and-Reach Test described in Appendix A.

TABLE 10-10	Norms for V-Sit Reach for Boys

PER-CEN-TILE	6	7	8	9	10	11	12	13	14	15	16	17+	PER-CEN-TILE
100	7.0	9.0	7.0	13.0	14.5	14.5	13.5	11.0	12.0	12.0	13.0	12.5	100
95	5.0	5.0	4.0	5.0	7.0	6.5	5.5	5.0	6.5	7.0	8.0	8.5	95
90	4.0	4.0	3.5	4.0	5.0	5.0	5.0	4.0	5.0	6.0	7.0	8.0	90
85	3.5	3.5	3.0	3.0	4.0	4.0	4.0	3.5	4.5	5.0	6.0	7.0	85
80	3.0	3.0	2.5	3.0	3.0	4.0	3.0	3.0	4.0	5.0	5.5	6.0	80
75	2.0	2.0	2.0	2.0	3.0	3.0	3.0	2.5	3.5	4.0	5.0	5.5	75
70	2.0	2.0	2.0	2.0	2.0	2.5	2.0	2.0	3.0	4.0	4.5	5.0	70
65	1.5	2.0	1.0	1.5	2.0	2.0	2.0	1.5	2.5	3.0	4.0	4.5	65
60	1.0	1.5	1.0	1.0	1.5	2.0	1.5	1.0	2.0	3.0	3.5	4.0	60
55	1.0	1.0	1.0	1.0	1.0	1.0	1.0	1.0	2.0	2.5	3.0	3.5	55
50	1.0	1.0	0.5	1.0	1.0	1.0	1.0	0.5	1.0	2.0	3.0	3.0	50
45	0.5	0.5	0.0	0.0	0.5	1.0	0.0	0.0	1.0	2.0	2.0	3.0	45
40	0.0	0.0	0.0	0.0	0.0	0.0	0.0	0.0	1.0	1.0	2.0	2.0	40
35	0.0	0.0	−1.0	−0.5	0.0	0.0	−0.5	−1.0	0.0	1.0	1.5	1.5	35
30	0.0	−0.5	−1.0	−1.0	0.0	−1.0	−1.0	−1.0	0.0	0.0	1.0	1.0	30
25	−1.0	−1.0	−1.5	−1.5	−1.0	−1.0	−2.0	−2.0	−1.0	0.0	0.5	1.0	25
20	−1.5	−1.0	−2.0	−2.0	−2.0	−2.0	−2.0	−2.5	−2.0	−1.0	0.0	0.0	20
15	−2.0	−2.0	−3.0	−2.5	−2.5	−3.0	−3.0	−3.0	−2.0	−2.0	−1.0	−1.0	15
10	−3.0	−3.0	−3.0	−3.0	−3.5	−3.5	−4.5	−4.0	−4.0	−3.0	−3.0	−2.0	10
5	−4.5	−4.0	−4.0	−5.0	−5.0	−5.0	−6.0	−6.0	−5.0	−5.0	−4.0	−4.0	5
0	−10.0	−9.0	−10.0	−13.0	−12.0	−10.0	−12.0	−12.5	−12.0	−10.0	−12.0	−10.0	0

Reprinted from President's Council on Physical Fitness: 1985 PCPFS Youth Fitness Survey. Washington, U.S. Government Printing Office, 1986.

Modified Schober Test (32)

Purpose

The purpose of this test is to assess spinal flexion, especially the flexibility of the lower back muscles.

Psychometric Information

Validity of the modified Schober was demonstrated by a significant correlation with the fingertip-to-floor test and a nonsignificant correlation with the length of hamstrings test (33). Intratester and intertester objectivity estimates were .88 and .87, respectively (34).

Gender and Age

Both genders, children through the elderly.

TABLE 10-11	Norms for V-Sit Reach for Girls

PER-CEN-TILE	AGE 6	7	8	9	10	11	12	13	14	15	16	17+	PER-CEN-TILE
100	9.5	9.0	12.0	14.0	13.0	15.0	14.5	14.5	14.0	15.0	15.0	15.0	100
95	7.0	6.5	6.0	8.0	8.0	10.0	9.0	9.0	10.0	10.0	10.5	10.5	95
90	6.0	5.5	5.0	6.0	7.0	8.0	8.0	8.0	8.5	9.0	9.5	9.0	90
85	5.5	5.0	4.5	5.5	6.0	6.5	7.0	7.0	8.0	8.0	9.0	8.0	85
80	5.0	4.5	4.0	5.0	5.0	6.0	6.0	6.0	7.0	7.5	8.0	7.5	80
75	5.0	4.0	4.0	4.0	5.0	5.0	6.0	6.0	6.5	7.0	8.0	7.0	75
70	4.0	4.0	3.5	4.0	4.0	5.0	5.0	5.0	6.0	6.5	7.0	6.0	70
65	3.5	3.0	3.0	3.5	4.0	4.5	5.0	5.0	6.0	6.0	7.0	6.0	65
60	3.0	3.0	3.0	3.0	3.0	4.0	4.5	4.5	5.0	6.0	6.0	5.5	60
55	3.0	3.0	2.5	3.0	3.0	4.0	4.0	4.0	5.0	5.0	6.0	5.0	55
50	2.5	2.0	2.0	2.0	3.0	3.0	3.5	3.5	4.5	5.0	5.5	4.5	50
45	2.0	2.0	2.0	2.0	2.5	3.0	3.0	3.0	4.0	4.5	5.0	4.0	45
40	1.5	2.0	1.5	2.0	2.0	2.5	3.0	3.0	4.0	4.0	4.5	4.0	40
35	1.0	1.5	1.0	1.0	2.0	2.0	2.5	2.5	3.5	3.5	4.0	3.5	35
30	1.0	1.0	1.0	1.0	1.0	1.5	2.0	2.0	3.0	3.0	4.0	3.0	30
25	1.0	1.0	0.5	0.0	1.0	1.0	2.0	2.0	2.5	2.0	3.0	2.5	25
20	0.0	0.0	0.0	0.0	0.5	1.0	1.0	1.0	2.0	2.0	2.5	2.0	20
15	0.0	0.0	0.0	−0.5	0.0	0.0	0.5	0.5	1.0	1.0	2.0	1.5	15
10	−1.0	−1.0	−1.0	−1.0	−1.0	−0.5	0.0	0.0	0.0	0.5	1.0	1.0	10
5	−2.5	−3.0	−2.5	−3.0	−2.5	−3.0	−2.5	−2.5	−1.5	1.0	−0.5	−1.0	5
0	−9.0	−9.0	−6.0	−11.0	−17.0	−11.0	−11.0	−11.0	−10.0	−10.0	−6.0	−13.0	0

Reprinted from President's Council on Physical Fitness: 1985 PCPFS Youth Fitness Survey. Washington, U.S. Government Printing Office, 1986.

Equipment
This test requires a cloth centimeter tape measure and a washable marking pen.

Procedure
1. Allow a warm-up of easy stretching and spinal bending.
2. Examinee stands with feet a shoulder-width apart. Locate the spinous process of the S2 vertebra at the midpoint of a line drawn between the posterior superior iliac spinous (PSIS) processes. Mark a short horizontal line at this point. Use a tape measure to find a point on the spine that is 10 cm above the S2 point. Mark another short horizontal line.
3. The examinee lets arms hang while he or she flexes the trunk forward to the full limit of motion; knees are kept straight.
4. Measure the distance between the two marks while the examinee is in full trunk flexion. Record to the nearest 0.5 centimeter.

Evaluation

Compare the full flexion measurement with the original 10 cm measure. Greater flexibility is demonstrated by a larger difference. No norms are as yet available.

Comments

The modified Schober test is a widely used clinical test of spinal flexion. There is no reason fitness professionals in other settings cannot learn to use this test to assess low back flexibility. The only possible drawback is the issue of privacy; some examinees may not be comfortable with palpation of the PSIS and markings and measurements along the lower spine.

Shoulder Rotation Test (11)

Purpose

The purpose of this test is to assess shoulder rotation.

Psychometric Information

Face validity is claimed. Test-retest reliability for the best of three trials was reported as $r = .97$. Intertester objectivity was $r = .99$.

Gender and Age

This test is appropriate for both genders and many ages, but norms are available only for college-age persons.

Equipment

This test requires a rope approximately 60 inches long or an anthropometer.

Procedure

1. Allow examinee to warm up, especially stretching the upper body and shoulders.
2. The examinee grasps the rope with the left hand at one end and with the right a few inches away. The person extends both hands in front of the chest with thumbs together and slowly and smoothly rotates the rope over the head. As shoulder resistance begins, the examinee should allow the rope to slide through the right-hand grip. This allows the arms to spread and lower the rope until it rests across the back. Keeping the arms locked, the examinee retraces the path of shoulder rotation, returning the arms to the starting position.
3. Measure the rope between the thumbs in inches. Repeat twice and record the best of the three trials—that is, the shortest distance—to the nearest quarter inch.
4. The shoulder width from deltoid to deltoid (bisacromial width) is measured with the anthropometer from behind the examinee. Record to the nearest quarter inch.
5. The score is the difference between the best trial rope length and the shoulder width. (For example, 30.25 inches of rope − 19 inches of shoulder width = *11.25 inches*.)

Evaluation

The lower the score, the greater the shoulders' flexibility. Norms for college men and women are given in Table 10-12.

TABLE 10-12	Norms in Inches for Shoulder Rotation Test	
PERFORMANCE	**MEN**	**WOMEN**
Advanced	7 or less	5 or less
Advanced intermediate	11.5–7.25	9.75–5.25
Intermediate	14.5–11.75	13–10
Advanced beginner	19.75–14.75	17.75–13.25
Beginner	20 and above	18 and above

Based on the scores of 100 men and 100 women at Corpus Christi (Texas) State University, 1977. Reprinted with permission from Johnson, B.L., and Nelson, J.K.: Practical Measurement for Evaluation in Physical Education. 4th ed. Edina, MN, Burgess, 1986, p. 97.

Comments

From a sport performance viewpoint, a full range of shoulder flexibility in both glenohumeral joints is important in sports such as gymnastics (still rings, parallel bars, uneven bars) and swimming (butterfly, front crawl, back crawl). One-sided shoulder flexibility is important in a number of sports (tennis, lacrosse). The shoulder rotation test does not distinguish between flexibility of the right and left shoulders. Goniometric measurement can be used to assess a specific shoulder.

From a health viewpoint, limited ROM in one or both glenohumeral joints restricts many daily living motions that those with a full ROM may take for granted. Examples include reaching to get an object from a high shelf, combing one's hair, and fastening a bra that closes at the back.

Motor Fitness Assessment

Generally coaches are more interested in motor fitness assessment than are fitness professionals. However, this is not to say that motor fitness is unimportant to any exercise and sport professional. Human beings were made to move, and being able to move with good agility, balance, coordination, power, and speed are part of what makes us human. While these qualities were a matter of life and death to the cave person, modern humans can generally live a disease-free, meaningful life without well-developed motor fitness. However, agility, balance, coordination, power, and speed can protect us in accidents, and these qualities give us access to activities that are sources of joy and satisfaction.

Field Testing of Motor Fitness

Described in this next section are a few motor fitness tests that practitioners may find useful. There is no attempt to do a comprehensive review of motor fitness field tests here. The interested reader should consult the excellent coverage of motor fitness in *Practical Measurements for Evaluation in Physical Education* by Johnson and Nelson (11).

Stork Stand (11)

Purpose

The purpose of this test is to assess static balance.

Psychometric Information

This test has face validity. Test-retest reliability for two test days was r = .87. Objectivity was reported as .99.

Gender and Age

This test is appropriate for both genders, children through the elderly, but norms are provided only for college-age men and women.

Equipment

This test requires a stopwatch.

Procedure

1. Examinee stands on the dominant foot and places other foot on the inside of the supporting knee. Hands are on hips.
2. A signal is given, and examinee raises the heel of the supporting foot off the floor. Balance is maintained as long as possible without moving the ball of the support foot from its initial position or letting the heel touch the floor.
3. Balance time is recorded to the nearest whole second. Three trials are given; the score is the time of the longest balance.

Evaluation

Norms for college-age men and women are provided in Table 10-13.

Comments

There are several common variations to the stork stand: foot flat, eyes open or closed. The eyes-open, foot-flat test validly distinguishes elderly fallers from nonfallers (35). The eyes-closed version of this test is said to assess kinesthetic static balance, a quality that may be important, for example, when getting out of bed in a dark room at night. This is a common fall time for the elderly.

TABLE 10-13	Norms in Seconds for Stork Stand	
PERFORMANCE LEVEL	**MEN**	**WOMEN**
Advanced	51 and above	28 and above
Advanced intermediate	37–50	23–27
Intermediate	15–36	8–22
Advanced beginner	5–14	3–7
Beginner	0–4	0–2

Based on the scores of 50 men and 50 women at Corpus Christi (Texas) State University, 1976. Reprinted with permission from Johnson, B.L., and Nelson, J.K.: Practical Measurement for Evaluation in Physical Education. 4th ed. Edina, MN, Burgess, 1986, p. 238.

Vertical Power Jump (36)

Purpose
The purpose of this test is to assess power of the leg extensor muscles.

Psychometric Information
This test has demonstrated concurrent validity (r = .989) with the vertical power jump (horse power) for college men. Test-retest reliability is .977; objectivity is .99.

Gender and Age
This test is appropriate for both genders, children through adults. Norms are provided only for college-age men and women and high-school girls.

Equipment and Materials
This test requires a jump board or stick marked off in half-inch increments and anchored to a wall at a height appropriate for the examinee, chalk dust, and a weight scale.

Procedure
1. Required dress is specified as shorts, light shirt, and no shoes.
2. Examinee is weighed; body weight is recorded in pounds.
3. Examinee is allowed to warm up, especially preparing the leg extensors for a maximal jumping effort.
4. Examinee stands with side to the jump board with the *dominant* arm behind the small of the back and the hand grasping the waistband of the shorts. The other arm is raised straight up with the hand facing the wall and fingers extended. The examinee stands as tall as possible on the balls of the feet so the reaching height of the middle finger can be measured to the nearest half inch.
5. Chalk dust is placed on the middle finger of the reaching hand. The examinee squats with head and back erect. Then, using only the legs, the examinee jumps as high as possible and touches the jump board at the top of the jump. The tester records the height of the chalk mark to the nearest half inch.
6. Three trials are allowed. On the last trial, the tester is to say, "This is your last jump. Try to beat your other two jumps." Any trial in which the examinee loses balance or fails to maintain the defined position is repeated.
7. The leg power score is calculated in foot-pounds, according to the following formula:

Leg power score (in foot-pounds) =

[Distance jumped (inches) × body weight (pounds)] ÷ 12   Formula 10-3

where distance jumped is calculated as the difference between the best jump height and the reaching height.

Sample Calculation
Body weight, 140 lb
Reaching height, 9.5-inch mark
Best jump height, 19.5-inch mark
Distance jumped = 19.5 − 9.5 = 10 inches
Leg power score, 10 × 140 ÷ 12 = *117 foot-pounds*

Evaluation

Table 10-14 presents norms for college men, college women, and high-school girls.

Comments

Athletic power is assessed by measuring the output only, without regard for the resistance that was applied to achieve this result. An example is a vertical jump test that measures only the actual inches jumped by examinees. The vertical power jump test measures *work power.* This approach to power assessment allows meaningful comparisons between performers. It is also a useful approach for assessing the effectiveness of a power training program for a person whose body weight might increase during the course of training. Coaches are likely to find this test very informative.

Coaches may also want to consider a couple of minor administrative modifications to the vertical power jump test. They may allow gym shoes to be worn for the entire test, that is, for body weight, reach height, and jumping. They may also choose to allow an arm swing for added power. This introduces an aspect of coordination to the test but may yield results that are more applicable to sport settings. Of course, these changes invalidate the established norms, but coaches may wish to establish local norms for their own teams.

LSU Agility Obstacle Course (11)

Purpose

The purpose of this test is to assess overall agility by including various agility tasks in one test.

Psychometric Information

Face and construct validity are assumed. Intraclass correlation estimate of reliability for two trials was reported as r = .91. Intertester objectivity was reported as .98.

Gender and Age

This test is appropriate for both genders, children through adults.

TABLE 10-14	Norms in Foot-Pounds^a for Vertical Power Jump^b		
PERFORMANCE	**COLLEGE MEN**	**COLLEGE WOMEN**	**HIGH-SCHOOL GIRLS**
Advanced	301 and above	134 and above	119 and above
Advanced intermediate	240–300	108–133	98–118
Intermediate	115–239	55–107	51–97
Advanced beginner	54–114	30–54	29–50
Beginner	0–53	0–29	0–28

^{a}(Distance jumped × body weight) ÷ 12 = score in foot-pounds
^{b}Based on the scores of 125 college men, 100 college women, and 100 high-school girls.
Reprinted with permission from Johnson, B.L., and Nelson, J.K.: Practical Measurement for Evaluation in Physical Education. 4th ed. Edina, MN, Burgess, 1986, p. 233.

Facilities and Equipment

This test requires a badminton court with no net, seven cones, and a stopwatch.

Procedure

1. Cones are placed on the badminton court as shown in Figure 10-7.
2. Examinee is allowed to warm up.
3. Examinee lies supine just outside the sideline of the court with feet behind the end line. When ready, the examinee scrambles up and runs to left to cone 1, where he or she makes a complete circle around the cone. Examinee then does one squat thrust (four counts of squat, extend legs, squat, stand). He or she then runs to the left of cone 2, the right of cone 3, and so on, as shown in the figure. After passing cone 7, examinee performs two squat thrusts, then runs to the opposite sideline and touches the floor just beyond the sideline. Examinee then shuttles back and forth between the sidelines, touching the floor twice more (total of three hand touches). Examinee then races to the finish line.
4. Test administrator starts the stopwatch when examinee begins to get up; the watch is stopped as the examinee crosses the finish line. Time is recorded to the nearest 0.1 second.
5. The agility score is the elapsed time plus a 0.5-second penalty if any of the squat thrusts are not performed in a four-count pattern. No penalties are given for accidental cone touches.

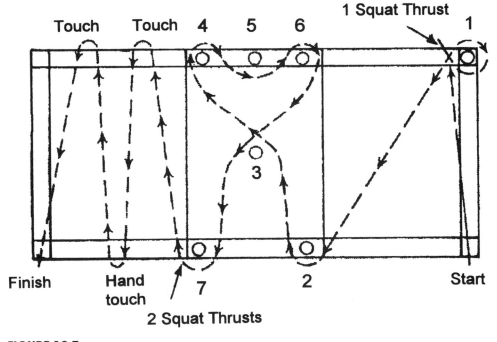

FIGURE 10-7

Floor plan for the LSU Agility Test. (Reprinted with permission from Johnson, B.L., and Nelson, J.K.: Practical Measurement for Evaluation in Physical Education. 4th ed. Edina, MN, Burgess, 1986, p. 233.)

TABLE 10-15	Norms in Seconds for LSU Agility Obstacle Course	
PERFORMANCE	**MEN**	**WOMEN**
Advanced	21.1 and below	23.0 and below
Advanced intermediate	22.3–21.2	25.1–23.1
Intermediate	23.6–22.4	27.4–25.2
Advanced beginner	24.8–23.7	29.5–27.5
Beginner	24.9 and above	29.6 and above

Based on the scores of 65 men and 84 women physical education majors at Louisiana State University, Baton Rouge, 1972.
Reprinted with permission from Johnson, B.L., and Nelson, J.K.: Practical Measurement for Evaluation in Physical Education. 4th ed. Edina, MN, Burgess, 1986, p. 233.

Evaluation
Norms for college men and women are found in Table 10-15.

Comments
The developers of this test believe that it assesses overall agility because it demands many forms of agility: zigzagging, dodging, shuttling, and whole-body changes in level. Most other agility tests focus on a single type of task.

Agility is an interesting motor quality. For a long time it was associated with athletic abilities in a variety of sports. Most agility assessments, however, fail to differentiate among agility, dynamic balance, and speed. Perhaps, as was suggested many years ago by Helen Eckert (37), agility is a combination of speed and dynamic balance that allows for rapid changes of direction. Certainly the LSU Agility Obstacle Course test requires all three of these qualities and perhaps even coordination.

Chapter Summary

I hope there is something for everybody in this chapter, which describes many field tests for the assessment of musculoskeletal and motor fitness. Collectively these tests apply to a wide variety of settings in exercise and sports. The chapter describes the components of musculoskeletal fitness and motor fitness and discusses their relations to health and well-being. The reader may now better appreciate the contributions of muscular strength, endurance, flexibility, and agility, balance, coordination, power, and movement speed to the lives of both athletes and others.

SELF-TEST QUESTIONS

1. Which of the following is *not* a component of musculoskeletal fitness?
   A. Flexibility
   B. Muscular strength
   C. Muscular endurance
   D. Muscular power

2. Which of the following is *not* an advantage of strong muscles?
   A. Increased joint stability
   B. Increased local ischemia
   C. Decreased wear and tear on joints
   D. Relatively small increases in blood pressure during exercise

3. Which of the following is probably the best predictor of low back pain?
   A. Weak trunk extensors
   B. Weak trunk flexors
   C. Tight hamstring muscles
   D. Tight lower back muscles

4. Which of the following is positively related to bone mineral density?
   A. Flexibility
   B. Muscular strength
   C. Muscular endurance
   D. Muscular power

5. Which of the following does *not* occur during a Valsalva maneuver?
   A. Increased heart rate
   B. Increased intrathoracic pressure
   C. Increased venous blood pressure
   D. Decreased venous blood return

6. What type of muscle contraction occurs in the *up phase* of a bench press?
   A. Isometric contraction of elbow extensors
   B. Concentric contraction of elbow extensors
   C. Eccentric contraction of elbow extensors
   D. Isokinetic contraction of elbow extensors

7. Which of the following machines *cannot* be used to measure isokinetic strength?
   A. Cybex
   B. Kin-Com
   C. Orthotron
   D. Universal

8. Which of the following is probably the best starting weight to use in a 1-RM bench press test for a 180-lb man?
   A. 100 lb
   B. 130 lb
   C. 160 lb
   D. 190 lb

9. Calculate the relative strength score for a 180-lb man whose maximal lift in an arm curl is 100 lb. _____

10. Evaluate the relative strength score calculated in question 9 for the arm curl.
    A. Poor
    B. Fair
    C. Good
    D. Excellent

11. Calculate the predicted 1 RM for a woman who bench-presses 60 lb a total of 6 times._____

12. The traditional push-up test is _____ dynamic test of muscular endurance.
    A. An absolute
    B. A relative

13. The couch test is a relative _____ test of muscular endurance.
    A. Dynamic
    B. Static

14. The Modified Schober Test assesses the flexibility of the _____ muscles.
    A. Abdominal
    B. Hamstring
    C. Lower back
    D. Upper back

15. Calculate the leg power score for a 150-lb person whose vertical jump distance is 8 inches. _____

ANSWERS

1. D	2. B	3. A	4. B	5. A
6. B	7. D	8. B	9. 0.56	10. C
11. 70 lb	12. B	13. B	14. C	15. 100 foot-pounds

DOING PROJECTS FOR FURTHER LEARNING

1. Identify several people who are similar in age to the persons you are most interested in working with. Select one or more age-appropriate tests from this chapter and administer the tests to these examinees. Interpret and explain the scores to the examinees. Discuss both health and performance concerns.

2. Set up an appointment to visit a physical therapy clinic. Discuss how they assess muscular strength, endurance, power, and flexibility. If they will permit it, ask them to demonstrate each of these measurements with you as the examinee.

3. Administer both a 1-RM leg press test and the vertical power jump test to a group of high-school or collegiate football, basketball, or volleyball players. Rank order the players on each of these measures. Compare. (*Hint:* You could calculate Spearman's rank order correlation coefficient.) How do you explain the relationship between leg strength and leg power for these scores?

REFERENCES

1. Faulkner, J.A., Green, H.J., and White, T.P.: Response and adaptation of skeletal muscle to changes in physical activity. In C. Bouchard, R.J. Shephard, & T. Stephens (eds.): Physical Activity, Fitness, and Health: International Proceedings and Consensus Statement. Champaign, IL, Human Kinetics, 1994.

2. American College of Sports Medicine: ACSM position stand on the recommended quantity and quality of exercise for developing and maintaining cardiorespiratory and muscu-

lar fitness, and flexibility in healthy adults. Medicine and Science in Sports and Exercise, 30:975, 1998.

3. American College of Sports Medicine: ACSM position stand on exercise and physical activity for older adults. Medicine and Science in Sports and Exercise, 30:992, 1998.

4. American College of Sports Medicine: Position stand on the prevention of sport injuries of children and adolescents. Medicine and Science in Sports and Exercise, 25: supplement, 1993.

5. Bouchard, C., and Shephard, R.J.: Physical activity, fitness, and health: the model and key concepts. In C. Bouchard, R.J. Shephard, & T. Stephens (eds.): Physical Activity, Fitness, and Health: International Proceedings and Consensus Statement. Champaign, IL, Human Kinetics, 1994.

6. Langrana, N., and Lee, C.: Isokinetic evaluation of trunk muscles. Spine, 9:171, 1984.

7. Beimborn, D., and Morrissey, M.: A review of the literature related to trunk muscle performance. Spine, 13:655, 1988.

8. Snow-Harter, C., et al.: Muscle strength as a predictor of bone mineral density in young women. Journal of Bone Mineral Research, 5:589, 1990.

9. Sandler, R.B., et al.: Muscle strength as an indicator of the habitual level of physical activity. Medicine and Science in Sports and Exercise, 23:1375, 1991.

10. Knapik, J.J., Jones, B.H., Bauman, C.L., and Harris, J.M.: Strength, flexibility and athletic injuries. Sports Medicine, 14(5):277, 1992.

11. Johnson, B.L., and Nelson, J. K.: Practical Measurement for Evaluation in Physical Education. 4th ed. Edina, MN, Burgess, 1986.

12. National Strength and Conditioning Association: Position paper on prepubescent strength training. National Strength Coaches Association Journal, 7:27, 1985.

13. Pollock, M.L., Wilmore, J.H., and Fox, S.M.: Health and Fitness Through Physical Activity. New York, Wiley, 1978.

14. Heyward, V.H.: Advanced Fitness Assessment and Exercise Prescription. 3rd ed. Champaign, IL, Human Kinetics, 1997.

15. Berger, R.A.: Applied Exercise Physiology. Ann Arbor, MI, Books on Demand, 1982.

16. Gettman, L.R.: Fitness testing. In S. Blair et al. (eds.): Resource Manual for Guidelines for Exercise Testing and Prescription. Philadelphia, Lea & Febiger, 1988.

17. Landers, J.: Maximum based on reps. National Strength and Conditioning Association Journal, 6(1):60, 1985.

18. Sale, D.G., and MacDougall, D.: Specificity in strength training: a review for the coach and athlete. Canadian Journal of Applied Sport Sciences, 6(2):87, 1981.

19. Bryzycki, M.: Strength testing: predicting a one-rep max from reps-to-fatigue. Journal of Physical Education, Recreation and Dance, 64(1):88, 1993.

20. Adams, G.M.: Isotonic strength test. In G.M. Adams (ed.): Exercise Physiology: Laboratory Manual. Madison, WI, Brown & Benchmark, 1994.

21. Mayhew, J.L., Ball, T.E., Arnold, M.D., and Bowen, J.C.: Relative muscular endurance as a predictor of bench press strength in college men and women. Journal of Applied Sport Science Research, 6:200, 1992.

22. Hoeger, W.W.K., Hopkins, D.R., Barette, S.L., and Hale, D.F.: Relationship between repetitions and selected percentages on one repetition maximum: a comparison between untrained and trained males and females. Journal of Applied Sport Science Research, 4(2):47, 1990.

23. Golding, L.A., Myers, C.R., and Sinning, W.E. (eds.): Y's Way to Physical Fitness: The Complete Guide to Fitness Testing and Instruction. 3rd ed. Champaign, IL, Human Kinetics for the YMCA, 1989.

24. President's Council on Physical Fitness: 1985 PCPFS Youth Fitness Survey. Washington, U.S. Government Printing Office.

25. Rutherford, W.J., and Corbin, C.B.: Validation of criterion-referenced standards for tests of arm and shoulder girdle strength and endurance. Research Quarterly for Exercise and Sport, 65:110, 1994.
26. MacFarlane, P.: Out with the sit-up, in with the curl-up. Journal of Physical Education, Recreation and Dance, 64(6):62, 1993.
27. Robertson, L.D., and Magnusdottir, H.: Evaluation of criteria associated with abdominal fitness testing. Research Quarterly for Exercise and Sport, 58:355, 1987.
28. Safrit, M.J., Zhu, W., Costa, M.G., and Zhang, L.: The difficulty of sit-up tests: an empirical investigation. Research Quarterly for Exercise and Sport, 63:277, 1992.
29. Jorgensen, K, & Nicolaisen, T.: Two methods for determining trunk muscle endurance: a comparative study. European Journal of Applied Physiology, 55:639, 1986.
30. Johns, R.J., and Wright, V.: Relative importance of various tissues in joint stiffness. Journal of Applied Physiology, 17:824, 1962.
31. Jackson, A.W., and Baker, A.A.: The relationship of the sit and reach test to criterion measures of hamstring and back flexibility in young females. Research Quarterly for Exercise and Sport, 57:183, 1986.
32. Norkin, C.C., and White, D.J.: Measurement of Joint Motion: A Guide to Goniometry. Philadelphia, FA Davis, 1995.
33. Biering-Sorensen, F.: Physical measurements as risk indicators for low-back trouble over a one-year period. Spine, 9:106, 1984.
34. Hyytiainen, K., et al.: Reproducibility of nine tests to measure spinal mobility and trunk muscle strength. Scandinavian Journal of Rehabilitative Medicine, 23:3, 1991.
35. Gehlsen, B.M., and Whaley, M.H.: Falls in the elderly, part II. Balance, strength, and flexibility. Archives of Physical Medicine and Rehabilitation, 71:739, 1990.
36. Glencross, D.J.: The measurement of muscular power: a test of leg power and a modification for general use. Doctoral dissertation, University of Western Australia, Nedlands, 1960. Reported in B.L. Johnson and J.K. Nelson, Practical Measurement for Evaluation in Physical Education, 4th ed. Edina, MN, Burgess, 1986.
37. Eckert, H.M.: Practical Measurement of Physical Performance. Ann Arbor, MI, Books on Demand, 1974.

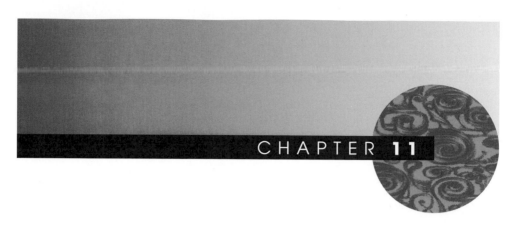

CHAPTER 11

Assessing Sport Skills

Motor skill competence is the unique contribution of physical education to the school curriculum and the primary goal of school and community athletic programs. The purpose of this chapter is to show the student and the practitioner who works in these settings how to employ sport skill tests to achieve motor skill learning and performance goals. This chapter presents a wide variety of specific sport skill tests. Each is described in enough detail to allow the practitioner to administer the test and interpret test scores without additional sources. Many of the tests in this chapter were reviewed and described by Dr. Andrea Farrow in the fourth edition of this textbook (1). I sincerely thank Dr. Farrow for her contributions to this chapter.

As you read this chapter, watch for the following keywords:

Closed skills	Open skills	Sport skill test
Multiple-repetition test	Psychomotor taxonomy	

Psychomotor Taxonomies

Classification schemes, commonly called taxonomies, have been developed for all three domains of learning. Cognitive-domain taxonomies (discussed in Chapter 17) classify intellectual processes; affective taxonomies classify interests, attitudes, beliefs, and appreciations. **Psychomotor taxonomies** classify motor abilities and skills. An understanding of taxonomic relationships is essential to the process of setting objectives, designing appropriate lessons, and assessing the extent to which stated objectives are attained. Good physical education teachers and athletic coaches are aware of the physical demands of the objectives they set for their students and players; they attempt to challenge their charges with tasks requiring motor responses that span the levels of the psychomotor taxonomy.

> Psychomotor taxonomy is a classification scheme for motor abilities and skills.

Over the past decades a number of psychomotor taxonomies have been developed (2–5). Only the Goldberger and Moyer taxonomy is presented here, because it specifically addresses the relationship between physical fitness (Chapters 8 to 10) and motor skills (Chapter 11). This is especially important for a psychomotor taxon-omy because, as Seefeldt and Vogel (6) posited in a 1987 article, "It is the mastery of motor skills and the ability of children [and adolescents and adults] to incorporate these skills into the games, dances, and sports of their culture that provides the stim-ulus for movement, and the stimulus for a series of mechanical, chemical, psycholog-ical and social events which in combination contribute to total fitness" (p. 332).

Goldberger and Moyer Taxonomy

The Goldberger and Moyer taxonomy (Fig. 11-1) provides a scheme for classifying all human movement, that is, reflexive movements, movements that reflect physical fitness, and movements that demonstrate purposeful motor skills (2). Their model suggests that every human movement can be classified according to three dimen-sions: its *psychomotor attributes*, which underlie the movement and allow the movement to occur, its *anatomical division* of body parts used and developed by the movement, and its *psychomotor form*. For example, a pull-up test demands mus-cular strength and endurance, develops the arms and shoulder girdle, and is a univer-sal movement form. A football punt demands coordination and power, employs the arms, legs, and trunk, and is a skilled movement form.

The taxonomy of psychomotor forms can also be studied in more detail. Gold-berger and Moyer use the term *psychomotor forms* to refer to various kinds of movements hierarchically ordered according to the developmental sequence that

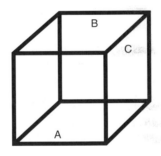

A—Psychomotor Attribute	B—Anatomical Division	C—Taxonomy of Psychomotor Forms
Reaction Time	Neck	1.0 Reflexive Movement Forms
Rhythm (timing	Shoulders	1.1 Inherited Reflexive Forms
Balance	Arms	1.2 Exploratory Forms
Coordination (accuracy)	Back	1.3 Conditioned Reflexive Forms
Power	etc.	2.0 Universal Forms
Agility		2.1 Basic Movement Forms
Flexibility		2.2 Conceptual Movement Forms
Muscular Endurance		3.0 Skilled Forms
Cardiorespiratory Endurance		3.1 Algorithmic Movement Forms
Speed		3.2 Low Organization Forms
Strength		3.3 Complex Organization Forms
Relation		4.0 Expansive Forms
etc.		4.1 Interpretive Movement Forms
		4.2 Creative Movement Forms

FIGURE 11-1

The Goldberger and Moyer three-dimensional model of developmental movement. (Adapted from Goldberger, M., and Moyer, S.: A schema for classifying educational objectives in the psychomotor domain. Quest, 342:136, 1982.)

humans follow in learning to move skillfully. Physical educators generally begin their work with elementary school children at the level of universal forms. Sublevel 2.11 identifies nonlocomotor forms that allow the creation of a variety of body shapes. Sublevel 2.12 specifies universal locomotor forms such as walking and running. Sublevel 2.13 identifies environment interaction forms, in which an obstacle is manipulated. Level 2.2 addresses conceptual movement forms. These are basic movement forms that have been refined into more general forms. Examples include the overarm throw, the vertical jump, striking, and static balances.

Middle- and secondary-school physical education teachers teach objectives that draw primarily from levels 3.0 and 4.0 of the taxonomy. Algorithmic movement forms, level 3.1, are short-sequenced, self-paced, **closed skills** such as shooting an arrow or putting a golf ball. Low-organization forms, level 3.2, include both continuous closed and discrete open skills such as are needed for most sport skill drills and lead-up activities. Level 3.3 identifies complex movement forms, also known as **open skills,** that require the performer to adjust to a continually changing environment. Tennis ground and net strokes, basketball dribbling and passing, and baseball fielding and throwing are all examples of movement forms at this level (Fig. 11-2). Highly skilled performers, especially in gymnastics and figure skating, often work at the 4.1 level of interpretive movement forms, in which an existing movement form is used to express feelings. In those same sports one may also see creative movement forms at the 4.2 level. At this level the performer expresses something both new and unique, such as a new dismount from the balance beam. Goldberger and Moyer suggested that a classic example of a creative movement form was Dick Fosbury's development of his flop in high jumping.

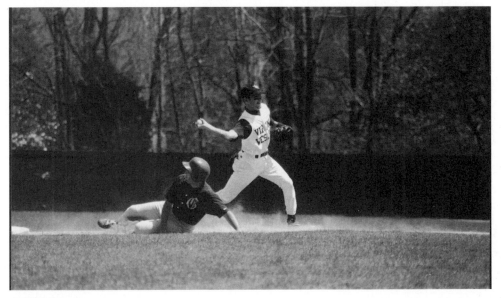

FIGURE 11-2

Baseball fielding and throwing skills are open skills because the performer must adjust the skills to a constantly changing environment. (Photo by John Bell, Touch a Life Photography, Greensboro, NC.)

> Closed skills are performed in a stable, unchanging environment; the practice goal of closed skills is consistency.

> Open skills are performed in an unstable, changing environment; the practice goal of open skills is successful adaptation to conditions.

This chapter presents tests and rating scales that can be used to assess a variety of sport motor skills. Most of these tests assess the qualities of movement forms at or higher than the 3.2 level on the Goldberger and Moyer taxonomy.

Ways to Assess Sport Skill Proficiency

There are at least three ways to assess proficiency in performance of a sport: by observation of performance, by use of a rating scale, and by use of a sport skill test. The most obvious way to assess skill proficiency is by observing an actual game or competition. Scouts do this all the time. While observing a game, they record subjective and objective information about the play. In some cases game statistics are used alone or in combination with other information to assess skill proficiency.

A rating scale may be used either in a controlled environment or while observing a game. In either case, rating scales help to objectify observation by providing specific performance criteria. The rating scale criteria focus either on the process or form or on a combination of process and product. The rating scale may be a checklist, a numerical scale, a descriptive scale, or graphic scale.

A **sport skill test** can also be used to assess proficiency. While they have been developed for nearly every imaginable skill used in nearly every imaginable sport, sport skill tests have the following characteristics:

They commonly modify the usual game environment by addition of targets, stationary obstacles, ropes, line, and so on for the purpose of standardizing the conditions under which each examinee performs the skill.

They usually focus on a single skill and sometimes on a single aspect of a skill, such as accuracy or power.

They usually focus on the product of performance, not the process. The product is typically scored by measuring time, distance, accuracy, or velocity.

They usually test one person at a time.

> A sport skill test is an instrument or procedure that elicits an observable response that provides information about a motor skill used in a sport.

Reasons for Use of Sport Skill Tests

There are many reasons to employ a sport skill test. Among them:

To Classify Performers for Instruction or Competition.   A common use of sport skill tests is to identify learners or performers who are at different levels of skill development. Once identified, they can be grouped homogeneously for instruction or competition.

To Assess Achievement or Improvement. Whether by a teacher to assign a grade (i.e., summative evaluation) or for one's own benefit, sport skill tests can be used to identify a learner's progress in development of a skill. Many athletes like to chart their personal bests in a log or journal. Because sport skill tests standardize the conditions for testing, the score gives a true indication of changes in performances over time. Performers can take and retake a test every few months to ascertain the effectiveness of their practice.

To Identify Skill Deficiencies. Sport skill tests can be formative evaluations to diagnose specific deficiencies. For example, analysis of the subscores on a tennis serve test might reveal problems in serving to the left-hand court, and instruction can be modified to focus on this deficiency. In team sports opportunities to observe a player performing a particular skill may be limited, but the skill may easily be evaluated by testing. When a weakness is noted, instruction can be provided to remedy the weakness.

For Motivational Purposes. Having access to objective information about one's level of skill is motivating to many people. If one has confidence in a particular sport skill test, a good score on the test may reinforce positive behaviors and increase the likelihood that these behaviors will be repeated. A low score may motivate greater effort and adoption of new behaviors.

To Provide Practice in Skills. One of the best uses of skill tests is for practice. Motor skill learning occurs best when a motivated learner engages in productive and accurate practice while receiving information about the results of his or her motor responses (7). Most sport skill tests modify the physical environment within which the skill is performed, for example by adding targets, ropes, cones, and so on. The modified environment augments the feedback available to the learner and contributes to productive and accurate practice.

To Help Select Team Members. Making cuts during tryouts for athletic teams is notoriously difficult, because the coaches must predict success on the basis of limited information about each player. The process is highly subjective and prone to errors. (You have probably heard that as a sophomore, Michael Jordan was cut from his high-school basketball team. OOPS!) Sport skill tests, especially norm-referenced tests, can play a part in the team selection process by providing objective data that can be used to compare players who may appear to be equally skilled.

To Improve Public Relations. Twentieth-century American culture has brought us popular national youth competitions such as the Punt, Pass, and Kick competition sponsored by Ford Motor Company and the Pepsi Hot Shot competition. While these competitions are clearly public relations campaigns with advertising motives, schools and other nonprofit organizations can also use sport skill competitions or reports of them to improve public relations. One such test that is a lot of fun is the Sports Skill Quotient Test (8). This is a comprehensive battery that requires examinees to perform a number of skills from various sports. Similarly, individual skill tests can be used to promote interest in specific sports.

Criteria for Selection of a Sport Skill Test

The practitioner who wishes to use an existing sport skill test can find many of them in the published literature. A particularly useful text by Strand and Wilson (9) reviews more than 300 sport skill tests in 29 sports and activities. Also useful is an earlier text by Collins and Hodges (10); published 20 years ago, it has much excellent information on a wide variety of sport skill tests. The high-school or college physical education teacher may want to invest in these two books.

Once a sport skill test is found, the practitioner must evaluate it. General procedures for evaluation of tests are described in Chapter 3, but the following criteria are especially applicable to the selection of sport skill tests.

Administrative Feasibility

Is the test practical and appropriate for your setting in terms of administration time, pretest setup time, need for special equipment, and so on? Can you set up and administer the test in the allotted class time? Some tests are amazingly simple, but others are amazingly complex. Some tests require special court markings and series of ropes strung at specific heights. Some require multiple trials per examinee. Some have complicated scoring systems or require subjective judgments on the part of the scorer.

Also important is whether the test is consistent with your objectives. The test is not an end in itself; it is a means to an end. It is intended to support and reinforce your teaching emphases. This means the test must be appropriate for the developmental levels of the students. Most skill tests are designed for high-school or college-age beginner or intermediate learners. This is not meant to imply that one cannot use a test developed for college men with junior-high girls, but the instructor must ascertain that this is appropriate. Norms developed for college men cannot be used for junior-high girls, but there may be other problems even if the test is used merely for practice. Because of differences in height and strength, the target areas and scoring schemes may encourage the younger girls to use poor form or technique to achieve higher scores. This is not what a teacher wants!

Instructors must also be wary of old tests. Some old tests are excellent, and there is no reason they should not be used. In some sports, however, new rules and technique changes have invalidated old tests. Similarly, the norms of old tests may not be appropriate for today's learners, who are on average physically larger and stronger at some ages than similar cohorts from 2 or 3 decades past.

Psychometric Concerns

Validity is, of course, the primary psychometric concern for any test. Sport skill tests are commonly criticized for questionable content validity. By modifying the environment in which the skill is performed, the test may lose some of the qualities associated with performance of the skill in the game. In other words, they lack authenticity. (This issue is discussed further in Chapter 18.) For example, a softball batting test that uses a batting tee to standardize conditions for batters may be questioned because the relationship between batting a stationary ball and batting a pitched ball in a softball game is not known. Similarly, it is not clear whether one's score on an unguarded basketball shooting skill test predicts one's shooting in an actual basketball game. So what is gained by standardization of conditions in a test may be offset by some loss of validity. This concern must be acknowledged by anyone who chooses to employ a sport skill test.

A **multiple-repetition test** requires examinees to manipulate balls or other objects rebounding from a wall. These tests, which are common to a number of sports, include such activities as volleyball passing, soccer passing, basketball passing, tennis rally, badminton underhand drive, and softball field and throw. All multiple-repetition tests, or repeated wall volley tests, are subject to criticism, because they also are perceived to be ungamelike. In no sport in actual play are players expected to repeat a single skill over and over, nor are they expected to respond to their own last attempt.

> Multiple-repetition tests are sport skill tests that require the examinee to perform a particular skill repeatedly: to manipulate a ball or other object that rebounds from a wall target. These tests are also sometimes called repeated wall volley tests.

Also potentially problematic are tests that make use of a partner. An example is the Kemp-Vincent Rally Test for tennis (11). This test specifies that two players "of similar ability" rally a ball back and forth across the net on a singles court for 3 minutes. Each player's score is determined by subtracting his or her errors from the total number of hits for both players combined. Clearly, a score can be hugely affected by the performance of the partner. How does one interpret such a score? This is, of course, why so many sport skill tests make use of rebound walls, that is, to eliminate the problems associated with partners' performances. Neither approach is completely satisfactory.

Although most tests focus on a single skill, some combine various skills into a single test. An example is the Kehtel Softball Fielding and Throwing Accuracy Test (12). Although fielding and throwing naturally occur in combination in softball, the issue for a sport skill test is how to interpret a low score for diagnostic purposes. Does a low score reflect poor fielding, poor throwing, or both? Which skill or skills should be worked on? The test score itself must be supplemented by the instructor's observation and analysis of skill deficiencies.

The final concern is scoring. Scoring problems can reduce both validity and reliability of sport skill tests. Scores whose range is too narrow (e.g., pass-fail or hit-miss scoring) do not provide good discrimination between skill levels and are not stable in a test-retest reliability check. To be valid, scoring must be consistent with effective use of the skill in the game. If a time or point penalty is imposed for a violation, the penalty must also reflect the actual game. Tests of accuracy must include sufficient trials to yield good reliability; most test experts recommend at least 10 trials. And finally, sport skill tests that employ trials must treat the final score in a realistic way. In most sports it is more realistic to sum or average trial scores than to record a single best score.

Recent Approaches to Sport Skill Testing

Two recent changes to sport skill testing were made in response to the concerns addressed in the previous section. One change is that tests and assessment procedures are being designed with greater attention to the need to preserve as much of the natural game environment as is reasonable. An example is the approach to measuring soccer-playing ability proposed by Ocansey and Kutame (13). Their Pioneer Instrument for Measuring Soccer Playing Ability in a Regular Setting (PIMSPARS) is used to assess the skills of an examinee during an actual soccer match. Increased gamelikeness improves test validity but may result in lower reliability because test conditions are more variable.

The other promising approach is the development of testing to criterion. An example is assessing basketball free-throw skills by having each examinee shoot until sinking 5 free throws. The number of trials to reach the criterion is recorded. A good free-throw shooter may sink 5 free throws in 6 attempts, while a poor one may take 11 or 12 attempts. This approach may increase test feasibility by reducing the total amount of time needed to assess skills during mass testing.

Tests of Specific Sport Skills

Presented here are a number of tests and rating scales for many specific sport skills for individual, dual, and team sports. Some are tests of single skills; others are batteries. Comments follow the presentation of each test or scale. In some cases alternative uses for the test or scale are suggested. Remember, any changes to the procedures or scoring affect the psychometric qualities of the test.

Aerobics

Jeffreys Rhythmic Aerobics Rating Scale

Purpose

The purpose of the Jeffreys Rhythmic Aerobics Rating Scale (Jeffreys, A.: A rating scale for rhythmic aerobics, unpublished paper, University of North Carolina at Greensboro, 1987) is to measure ability and knowledge in rhythmic aerobics, especially for grading large classes. The components to be measured are (*a*) quality of movement and body alignment area, (*b*) effectiveness of the warm-up and stretching exercises, (*c*) effectiveness of the cardiovascular conditioning phase, and (*d*) effectiveness of the cool-down phase. The scale may also be used as a content guide for a rhythmic aerobics routine.

Gender and Age

This test is appropriate for beginning rhythmic aerobics classes at the college level and for both genders.

Psychometric Information

No validity or reliability data are given. Interjudge agreement between the two judges performing the rating was reported to be high.

Personnel

This test requires two judges.

Facility Needs

This test requires a dance room or gymnasium.

Equipment

This test requires record, CD, or tape player; recorded music; scoring forms; and pencils.

Procedure

This scale is a group measure. Groups of three to five students design a routine that they feel will combine all the elements of the rating scale. They perform their routine for two evaluators.

Scoring

Group members receive one grade based on *the combined average ratings of the two judges*. The scale has 14 elements, each rated from 1 to 3.

There are 42 possible points (Fig. 11-3).

Comments

This scale can also be used with smaller groups. Although it was developed for college classes, it can be used for any age group for whom rhythmic aerobics is appropriate. If use of two judges is not practical, a single instructor may use this form to rate the groups. As this scale is set up, each element has equal value. The user may choose to adapt the elements or their weightings to fit the situation or the philosophy of the instructor. (Remember that any changes will affect the psychometric qualities.) In some situations it may be appropriate to use the results of this scale along with the results of a routine constructed by the instructor.

Archery

The rounds used in competitive archery are generally too difficult for beginners because the target distances are too great. Consequently, many beginner students fail to make even minimal scores. Thus target distance must be considered when constructing an archery skills test. Another factor that must be considered is the number of arrows; the number of arrows shot must be high enough to assure reliability. Ishee and Shannon (14) found that practice improves the reliability of scores. Thus it is wise to use a practice end of six arrows prior to administration of the following tests.

McKenzie-Shifflett Archery Test

Purpose

The purpose of the McKenzie-Shifflett Archery Test (McKenzie, R., and Shifflett, B.: Skill evaluation in a coeducational beginning archery class, unpublished paper, San Diego State University, 1986) is to measure the skill level of students enrolled in beginning classes on the same scale by adjusting the shooting distances.

Gender and Age

This test is appropriate for college students enrolled in beginning coeducational classes.

Psychometric Information

When 54 men and 54 women beginning archery students shot from 30 yards, there was a significant difference between the scores of men and women. When 35 men and 13 women beginning archery students shot from varying distances based on bow weight and draw length, there were no significant differences between the genders. The authors concluded that the score was a function of strength rather than gender. Reliability was calculated by using the best three scores of each student. The resulting reliability scores were respectively .90, .93, and .93 for women,

Jeffreys Rhythmic Aerobics Rating Scale
Scoring Form

Directions: Using the following as a guide, rate the group rhythmic aerobics routine on a 1 to 3 scale on each of the 14 elements.

1 (Poor)	Group shows lack of organizaiton and preference for this activity. Group is not at ease.
2 (Average)	Group is at ease, working together, and sharing the experience by contributing and communicating. All members contribute to the performance.
3 (Good)	Group is very enthusiastic. Bouts are unique, innovative, and creative.

I. Movement and Body Alignment Cues

____ 1. Move with the music, proper tempo and rhythm.

____ 2. Correct body positions to reduce compromising positions and injuries.

____ 3. Transitions and progressions noted by adding/combining several arm works to the same leg movement. Blending of movements smooth, permitting participants to follow with little difficulty.

____ 4. Eye contact along with verbal, body, and directional cues, singly or in combination.

II. Warm-up and/or Stretches

____ 5. Static stretches held 10 to 15 seconds. Stretching several muscle groups without compromising body alignment.

____ 6. Standing and floor stretches appropriate (correct sequencing).

____ 7. Duration adequate, includes most major muscle groups.

III. Cardiovascular Phase

____ 8. Interval training combining low, nonimpact aerobics with recovery periods.

____ 9. Duration and intensity sufficient to reach medium and submaximal rates, gradually increasing, intensifying and decreasing. Follows the aerobic curve.

____ 10. Heart rate monitored 2 to 3 times with the last count being after a recovery period of 3 minutes.

____ 11. Bout dense enough to allow most to reach and sustain their targeted heart rate for 15 to 20 minutes without overtaxing and causing strain.

IV. Cool Down Phase

____ 12. Static stretching of the legs and Achilles tendon sufficient.

____ 13. Relaxation, stretching, walking movements included. Supportive, encouraging and informative.

____ 14. Time for questions and answers, sharing before departure.

____ **TOTAL POINTS (42 Possible)**   **GROUP MEMBERS**   _____

_____

_____

_____

_____

FIGURE 11-3

Scoring form for Jeffreys Rhythmic Aerobics Rating Scale. (Used with permission from Jeffreys, A.: A rating scale for rhythmic aerobics, unpublished paper, University of North Carolina at Greensboro, 1987.)

men, and both genders combined. Archery experts attending the world archery center reviewed the test to establish logical validity.

Facility Needs
This test requires indoor or outdoor shooting area with targets at 25, 30, 35, and 40 yards.

Equipment
This test requires bows of varying weights, at least 10 arrows per examinee, several standard 80-cm F.I.C.A. targets on tripods, score sheets, and pencils.

Procedure
Each day during the last third of a course each examinee shoots one round of 10 arrows from his or her designated distance. The designated distance is based on the bow weight plus or minus 2 lb for every inch the draw deviates from the 28-inch standard. For example, an archer pulling a 25-pound bow 24 inches has a draw weight of 17 pounds (28-inch standard draw − 24-inch draw = 4; 4 × 2 [lb] = 8; 25 [pull of bow] − 8 = 17). Since it is impractical to have everyone at a different distance, the weights are divided into ranges as follows:

BOW WEIGHT (pounds)	DISTANCE (yards)
Under 20	25
20–23	30
24–29	35
30 or more	40

Scoring
The three best scores are averaged. All examinees are graded on the same scale.

Comments
Some caution must be exercised in interpreting the results of this study because there were only 13 women in the sample. This is, however, a better method than having all students shoot from the same distance. Additional work is probably needed to determine the best distance for shooting for each bow weight and draw length. Biomechanical analyses could aid in this determination. Also, the appropriateness of using this method with younger students should be investigated. The authors suggested that if space is limited, the instructor may experiment with varying the target sizes instead of the target distances.

Shifflett and Shuman Criterion-Referenced Archery Test (15)
Purpose
The purpose of this test is to use a criterion-referenced approach for assessment of archery skill.

Gender and Age
This test is appropriate for all levels, both genders.

Psychometric Information

Based on the instructed versus uninstructed approach to validation, scores from college men and women yielded a validity coefficient of .73. Reliability was estimated by calculating the proportion of agreement between two administrations of the test to college women; P was found to be .87.

Facility Needs

This test requires a shooting area of 20 yards.

Equipment

This test requires bows of appropriate weights, six arrows per examinee, 48-inch targets on tripods, score sheets, and pencils.

Procedure

All examinees shoot 2 ends, that is, 12 arrows, from 20 yards.

Scoring

Target scores of 9 and 7 are converted to 1 point; target scores of 5, 3, and 1 are converted to 0 points. *The total test score is the sum of the converted scores for 12 arrows*. An examinee whose test score is 5 or greater is classified as a master; examinees with scores less than 5 are classified as nonmasters.

Comments

The test authors suggested that this test can be used as a proficiency test to exempt students from a beginning archery class. It can also be used for pass-fail grading in a physical education class.

Badminton

Lockhart-McPherson Badminton Wall Volley Test (16)

Purpose

The purpose of this test is to assess general badminton playing by measuring skill in repeatedly volleying a shuttlecock against a wall.

Gender and Age

This test was originally developed for college women but later adapted for college men. It is also appropriate for use in junior and senior high school.

Psychometric Information

Concurrent validity coefficients ranged between .71 and .90, using criteria of judges' ratings of ability and tournament rankings. Test-retest reliability was .90.

Facility Needs

Each test station requires a 10- by 10-foot smooth wall surface and 10- by 10-foot floor space.

Equipment

This test requires rackets, shuttlecocks, stopwatch, score sheets, and pencils.

Court Markings

Each test station should be marked as illustrated in Figure 11-4. A 1-inch net line is marked on the wall 5 feet high. A starting line is marked on the floor 6 feet 6

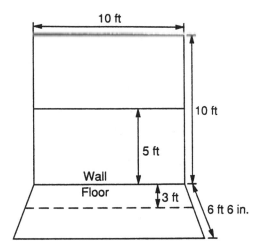

FIGURE 11-4

Wall and floor marking specifications for the Lockhart-McPherson Wall Volley Test for badminton. (Reprinted with permission from Lockhart, A., and McPherson, F.A.: The development of a test of badminton playing ability. Research Quarterly, 20:402, 1949.)

inches from the base of the wall; a restraining line is marked on the floor 3 feet from the base of the wall.

Procedure

The examinee starts behind the starting line with a racket and a shuttlecock. On a signal of "ready, go," the shuttlecock is to be legally served to the wall on or above the 5-foot net line. The served shuttlecock is volleyed back to the wall as many times as possible in 30 seconds. After the service, the examinee may move up to the restraining line and play the shuttlecock from there. If the restraining line is crossed, the shuttlecock may remain in play but the hits are not counted. If a shuttlecock is missed or goes out of control, the examinee is to retrieve the shuttlecock and put it back into play with a serve from behind the starting line. Double hits and carries are disregarded. The examinee gets three trials with rest periods between them. A 15-second practice is allowed prior to the first trial.

Scoring

The final score is the sum of all legal hits made from behind the restraining line that hit the wall on or above the 5-foot net line during the three 30-second trials. A timer is needed; the examinee may self-score or have a scorer count the legal hits.

Norms

Table 11-1 provides achievement scales for college women.

Comments

This test is subject to the criticisms of most multiple-repetition tests noted earlier in the chapter. It is, however, a commonly used test of general playing ability. It is perhaps most useful for classifying players for future instruction or competition or as a warm-up practice task. Some students have to be reminded to maintain a correct grip and use good striking form.

TABLE 11-1	Achievement Scales for the Lockhart-McPherson Badminton Wall Volley Test
RATING	**TEST SCORE (SUM OF THREE TRIALS)**
Superior	126 and up
Good	90–125
Average	62–89
Poor	40–61
Inferior	39 and below

Reprinted with permission from Lockhart, A., and McPherson, F.A.: The development of a test of badminton playing ability. Research Quarterly, 20:402, 1949.

French Short Serve Test (17)

Purpose

The purpose of this test is to assess ability to use the badminton short serve to serve low and accurately.

Gender and Age

This test is appropriate for intermediate and advanced players who have developed some skill in the short serve.

Psychometric Information

A concurrent validity coefficient of .66 was reported using a criterion of tournament rankings. Test-retest reliability was .96.

Facility Needs

This test requires a regulation badminton court.

Equipment

This test requires nets, rope, rackets, at least five shuttlecocks per examinee, score sheets, and pencils.

Court Marking

A rope is stretched taut 20 inches above the top of the net. Four concentric quarter-circles are drawn on the right service court (Fig. 11-5). Each curved line is 1.5 inches wide, and its width is included in the radius. The use of different colors for the lines makes scoring more objective.

Procedure

The examinee stands in the regulation right court for serving and serves 20 times into the opposite right service court for the doubles game. The serve must be legal, and the shuttlecock should go between the rope and the top of the net. Serves should be taken in groups of at least 5.

Scoring

For each serve, record the numerical value for the area in which it first lands. Shuttlecocks that land on a line receive the higher value. Serves that fail to go between the rope and the net, that are out of the bounds of the right service court for

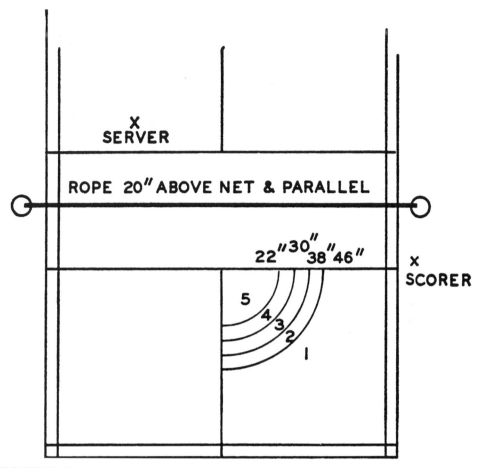

FIGURE 11-5

Specifications for the French Short Serve Test for badminton. (Reprinted with permission from Scott, M.G., Carpenter, A., French, E., and Kuhl, L.: Achievement examinations in badminton. Research Quarterly, 12:242, 1941.)

doubles, or that are otherwise illegal receive a score of 0. The final score is the total for 20 serves.

Comments

This test may be used to increase awareness that the short serve should be low, as a self-testing instrument for motivation, and to indicate touch. Reliability does not hold up for beginning badminton players; a rating of the short serve may be more appropriate for them.

GSC Badminton Clear Test (18)

Purpose

The purpose of this test is to assess skill in the clear stroke.

Gender and Age

This test is appropriate for beginning-level college students of both genders.

Psychometric Information

The test was administered to 61 men and 65 women students in seven beginning classes at Georgia Southern College. A badminton expert and each class instructor independently ranked each student on the ability to hit a deep clear. Using a combination of the expert's and teacher's ratings as the criterion, concurrent validity was reported as .85 for both genders. Intraclass reliability for 10 trials was .87 for men and .89 for women.

Facility Needs

This test requires regulation badminton courts, rope, and standards or wall mounts to stretch the rope across the court 8 feet high and 13.5 feet from the net.

Equipment

This test requires rackets, shuttlecocks, rope, score sheets, and pencils.

Court Markings

The badminton court is marked as shown in Figure 11-6, with the scoring area on the right and the receiving areas on the left. The receiving area for women is 2 feet closer to the net than the area for the men. A rope is stretched across the court 8 feet high and 13.5 feet back from the net.

Procedure

Examinees should warm up on a nearby court. The test administrator stands at point A on the court; the examinee is positioned in the appropriate receiving area. The administrator attempts to serve the shuttlecock to the midpoint of the receiving area. The examinee does not have to play any poorly placed serve, but any swing is considered a trial. The test consists of 10 trials.

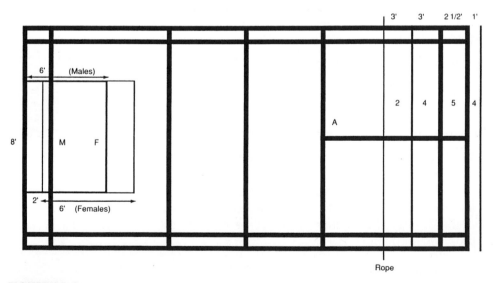

FIGURE 11-6

Court markings for the GSC Badminton Clear Test. (Reprinted with permission from Cotten, D.J., Cobb, P.R., and Fleming, J.: Development and validation of a badminton clear test. Research Abstracts. American Alliance of Health, Physical Education, Recreation, and Dance National Convention, Las Vegas, April 13–17, 1987, p. 168.)

Scoring

The zone in which the shuttlecock first lands is recorded as the score. The value of the zones from the net, respectively, are 2, 4, 5, and 4. No points are awarded for any shuttlecock failing to clear the rope or land in the scoring zones. A shuttlecock that lands on a line receives the higher point value. *The test score is the sum of the points for 10 trials.*

Norms

No norms are provided, but the test authors suggest that separate scoring scales be developed for men and women.

Comments

This test assesses ability to clear; it is not intended as a test of overall playing ability. A player or instructor who can consistently serve high and deep to the middle of the receiving area is essential for the administration of this test.

Bobrich Badminton Observational Rating Scale (19)

Purpose

The purpose of this test is to assess development of the basic skills of badminton as the examinee participates in a regulation doubles badminton game.

Gender and Age

This rating scale was developed for high-school girls, but it may be appropriate for boys and older persons of either gender.

Psychometric Information

This scale was adapted from the original Bobrich scale, which assessed strategies, knowledge, and several additional skills. The subscales presented here are for the skills that are most often taught in a beginning badminton class. The tool was developed with two classes of 67 girls enrolled in a high-school beginning badminton course. Logical validity is claimed. Reliability coefficients from .77 to .87 were calculated by test-retest using three qualified judges, Pearson r, and analysis of variance techniques.

Facility Needs

This test requires a regulation doubles badminton court.

Equipment

This test requires a racket for each examinee, one shuttlecock, a scoring form, and pencil.

Administrative Considerations

A trained student leader and a qualified physical education teacher can administer the rating scale. A 20-minute period is needed for one evaluator to rate four students in a doubles match.

Procedure

While examinees are participating in a doubles match, each examinee is rated on the criteria shown in Figure 11-7. The criteria are worded for a right-handed player. The score of 1 to 3 for each skill should be based on consistency in form and execution.

(text continues on page 336)

Bobrich Badminton Observational Rating Scale
Skill Criteria & Scoring Form

EXAMINEE _____   DATE _____

PARTNER _____

OPPONENTS _____

<u>Directions</u>: Using the criteria below, assign 0 to 3 points for each of the following skills. The rating should be based on consistency in form and execution. Circle the rating for each skill.

Short Serve

0   Skill not observed or not attempted.

1   If the shuttle is hit more than 3 feet over the top of the net, lands more than 4 feet beyond the front service line, or lands out of bounds.

2   If the shuttle is hit to cross the net within 1 to 3 feet over the top of the net and lands within 4 feet of the front service line.

3   If the shuttle is hit to skim the top of the net, loses height immediately, and lands along the front service line or near the corner of the opposite service court.

Short Serve Return

0   Skill not observed or not attempted.

1   If the shuttle is returned out of bounds, or in the attempt to return the shuttle the footwork is slow, causing the body to become off balance, resulting in a poor return.

2   If the receiver moves forward to meet the shuttle and successfully returns it into the opponent's court.

3   If the receiver moves forward to meet the shuttle and makes an effective return.

Long Serve

0   Skill not observed or not attempted.

1   If the shuttle height is medium or low; if there is not direction of the shuttle to the opposite court; or if the shuttle falls out of bounds or close to the short service line of the opposite court.

2   If the shuttle is hit to travel high and lands in the middle of the opposite service court.

3   If the shuttle is hit to travel high and deep to land on the back service line or is directed to land in either corner of the opposite service court.

FIGURE 11-7

Skill criteria and scoring form for the Bobrich Badminton Observational Rating Scale. (Reprinted with permission from Bobrich, M.N.: Reliability of an evaluative tool used to measure badminton skill. Master's thesis, George Williams College, 1972.)

Long Serve Return

0   Skill not observed or not attempted.
1   If the attempt made shows slow footwork in a backward direction causing the body to become off balance and results in a poor return or a failure of the shuttle to cross the net.
2   If quick footwork is used in moving backward; some body balance is observed as the shuttle is successfully returned over the net.
3   If the receiver uses quick footwork in moving backward to get behind the shuttle; body balance is in good control; and the shuttle is returned by any overhead stroke, preferably the smash.

Clear

0   Skill not observed or not attempted.
1   If the body is off balance or the shuttle is improperly contacted, causing a poor return or a fault.
2   If the body is aligned with the shuttle so contact is made overhead and shuttle flight is high so that it lands in the opponent's midcourt.
3   If the body is aligned so that contact with the shuttle is made overhead with a full swing, and the return is high into the opponent's backcourt landing just inside the baseline.

Smash

0   Skill not observed or not attempted.
1   If the body is off balance, no wrist snap is present, or the shuttle is hit over the net as in any return with no aim or direction present.
2   If the body is aligned with the oncoming shuttle; or contact is made but the wrist snap is weak and the shuttle is moved downward without the necessary speed for a successful stroke.
3   If the body is aligned with the oncoming shuttle so that contact is made high and on top of the shuttle; there is definite wrist snap at point of contact so that the shuttle is forced downward with great speed aimed at opponent's body, his left side, to baseline, or to sidelines.

Drop

0   Skill not observed or not attempted.
1   If the body is not aligned with the shuttle for proper execution of the stroke, a forward drive is used instead of an overhead stroke, or the shuttle does not fall in bounds.
2   If the body is aligned with the shuttle for contact overhead but is hit behind the short service line with either too much arc or too much speed.
3   If the body is aligned with the shuttle so contact is made in front of the body, the shuttle is "patted" down so it falls in a steep angle just over the net in front of the short service line, and the swing is overhead but slow so as to deceive the opponent.

_____ **TOTAL POINTS (21 Possible)   EXAMINER** _____

FIGURE 11-7

Continued

Scoring

Point values for each skill: 0 points for skill not observed or not attempted; 1 for fair ability; 2 for good ability; and 3 for excellent ability. Total scores can range from 0 to 21.

Comments

This rating scale can be used for grading, for classification for tournament groupings, and for assessing individual achievement. Parts of it can be used to focus on specific aspects of the game. It can be used by players to make peer evaluations. Because the ratings occur in the natural setting of a doubles game, it is a relatively authentic assessment (see Chapter 18).

Basketball

AAHPERD Basketball Test for Boys and Girls (20)

Purpose

The purpose of this test is to assess the four essential skills in basketball.

Gender and Age

This test is appropriate for male and female subjects aged 10 through college.

Psychometric Information

Six test items were administered in developing this battery. The four presented here are the items chosen for the final American Alliance of Health, Physical Education, Recreation, and Dance (AAHPERD) basketball battery because they cover the essential skills and can be administered to an average-sized class in two periods.

Validity and reliability coefficients for each test item for each gender and academic level were established by administering the battery of tests in school settings at the conclusion of a basketball unit of instruction. Multiple trials of the test items were administered to 50 students per gender per grade. Intraclass reliability estimates ranged from .82 to .98. Concurrent validity coefficients were determined by correlating subjective ratings for both the specific skill and game performance with each test. The concurrent validity coefficients ranged from .37 to .91. The lower values were for college-age men and women and for girls at the elementary and junior-high level. These low coefficients may have been affected by a lack of agreement among the raters, and the college age coefficients may also have been affected by the homogeneity of the sample due to the testing of elective physical education classes. Validity estimates for the entire test battery ranged from .65 to .95. The degree of agreement among raters was much greater for overall game performance than for specific skills. Construct validity estimates were determined by identifying test performance differences between groups of varsity and nonvarsity players.

Scoring

The manual provides complete percentile and T-score norms for male and female examinees separately for ages 10 through college. A total score for playing ability can be obtained by converting raw scores for each of the four tests to T-scores and then totaling or averaging the T-scores. Table 11-2 provides selected percentile rank values.

Comments

This battery can be used for assessing playing ability for grading, grouping, practice, diagnosis, and showing improvement. It can also aid in team selections. Individual items can be used for these same purposes. Norms can be used if deemed appropriate, or local norms may be developed.

ITEM 1: SPEED SPOT SHOOTING
Purpose

The purpose of this test is to assess skill in rapidly shooting from specified positions and indirectly to assess agility and ball handling.

Court Markings

As shown in Figure 11-8, five markers 2 feet long and 1 inch wide are placed on the floor. For grades 5 and 6 the markers are 9 feet from the backboard; for grades 7, 8, and 9, markers are 12 feet from the backboard; for grades 10 though college, the markers are 15 feet from the backboard. The distances for spots B, C, and D must be measured from the center of the backboard; those for spots A and E must be measured from the center of the basket.

| TABLE 11-2 | Selected Percentile Norms for the AAHPERD Basketball Skills Test Battery |

		BOYS AND MEN				
Test	Percentile	Age 10	Age 12	Age 14	Age 16–17	College
SPEED SPOT SHOOTING						
	99	31	32	48	30	61
	75	17	19	23	22	25
	50	13	15	18	16	22
	25	10	11	13	12	19
PASSING						
	99	43	52	60	65	78
	75	35	40	45	49	58
	50	31	35	40	41	53
	25	25	30	35	25	47
CONTROL DRIBBLE						
	99	6.4	7.4	5.8	6.8	4.9
	75	10.4	9.5	8.5	8.1	7.3
	50	11.7	10.5	9.3	9.0	7.8
	25	13.7	11.7	10.3	10.0	8.5
DEFENSIVE MOVEMENT						
	99	8.9	7.8	8.0	5.0	8.0
	75	11.5	10.7	10.1	9.6	9.4
	50	12.7	11.9	11.3	10.3	10.3
	25	13.9	13.0	12.4	11.5	11.2

(continued)

TABLE 11-2	Selected Percentile Norms for the AAHPERD Basketball Skills Test Battery *(Continued)*

| GIRLS AND WOMEN | | | | | |
Test	Percentile	Age 10	Age 12	Age 14	Age 16–17	College
SPEED SPOT SHOOTING						
	99	33	43	38	37	44
	75	11	13	15	14	21
	50	8	10	11	11	17
	25	5	7	9	7	13
PASSING						
	99	38	48	49	59	65
	75	30	35	39	39	47
	50	25	31	34	34	42
	25	21	26	29	24	37
CONTROL DRIBBLE						
	99	8.6	7.0	6.9	5.5	6.9
	75	12.3	10.6	9.6	9.8	8.5
	50	14.3	11.9	10.7	10.7	9.3
	25	16.6	13.3	12.0	12.2	10.4
DEFENSIVE MOVEMENT						
	99	8.8	7.4	6.1	8.6	7.3
	75	11.8	11.5	11.0	11.1	10.3
	50	13.2	12.8	12.0	12.0	11.0
	25	14.6	14.1	13.2	13.2	12.0

Adapted from Hopkins, D.R., Shick, J., and Plack, J.J.: Basketball Skills Test Manual for Boys and Girls. Reston, VA, AAHPERD, 1984.

Procedure

Examinees perform three trials of 60 seconds each. The first is a practice trial; the next two are recorded. The examinee stands behind any marker designated for his or her age level. On a "ready, go" signal, the examinee shoots, retrieves the ball, dribbles, and shoots from another designated spot. One foot must be behind the marker during each attempt. A maximum of four layups may be attempted during each trial, but no two may be in succession. Also, the examinee must attempt at least one shot from each designated spot. The examinee continues until a stop signal is given.

Scoring

Two points are awarded for each shot made. One point is awarded for an unsuccessful shot that hits the rim from above either initially or from a rebound off the backboard. If a ball-handling infraction (e.g., traveling, double dribbling) occurs, the shot following the infraction is scored as zero points. If two layups in succession are taken, the second layup is scored as zero points. If more than four layups are at-

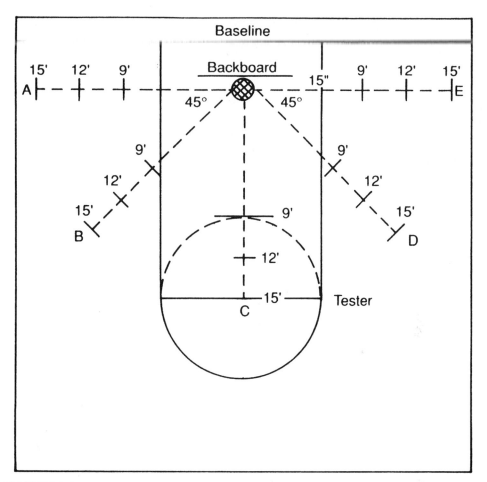

FIGURE 11-8

Court markings for the AAHPERD Basketball Speed Spot Shooting Test. (Reprinted with permission from Hopkins, D.R., Shick, J., and Plack, J.J.: Basketball Skills Test Manual for Boys and Girls. Reston, VA, AAHPERD, 1984.)

tempted, the extras are scored as zeros. If the examinee does not shoot from all designated spots, the trial must be repeated. *The final score is the total of two legal trials.*

ITEM 2: PASSING
Purpose
The purpose of this test is to assess skill in passing (chest pass) and recovering the ball accurately while moving.

Court Markings
As shown in Figure 11-9, six 2-foot squares are marked on a smooth wall so that the base of the square is either 3 or 5 feet from the floor. As shown in Figure 11-10, adjacent squares are 2 feet apart. A restraining line is marked on the floor 8 feet from the wall.

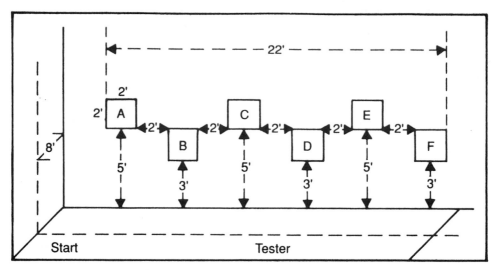

FIGURE 11-9

Court markings for the AAHPERD Basketball Passing Test. (Reprinted with permission from Hopkins, D.R., Shick, J., and Plack, J.J.: Basketball Skills Test Manual for Boys and Girls. Reston, VA, AAHPERD, 1984.)

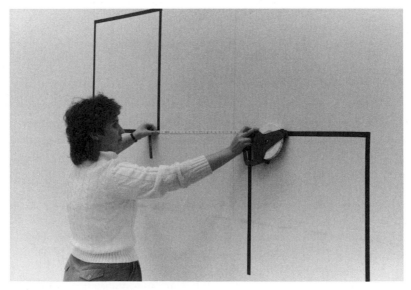

FIGURE 11-10

Adjacent targets for the AAHPERD Basketball Passing Test are 2 feet apart. (Photo by Dr. Karen Uhlendorf, University of Vermont, Burlington, VT.)

Procedure

Three trials of 30 seconds each are administered. The first is a practice trial; the last two are recorded. The examinee holds a ball and stands behind the restraining line, facing the target on the far left. On a "ready, go" signal, the examinee chest-passes to target A, recovers the rebound while moving to a location behind the second target and behind the restraining line, then chest-passes to target B. This pattern continues until target F is reached, where two chest passes are executed; then the examinee changes direction and passes to target E. The sequence continues until a "stop" signal is given.

Scoring

Each pass that hits the target or the target lines counts two points. Each pass hitting the intervening spaces on the wall counts one point. If a pass is made from a point in front of the restraining line, no points are awarded. If passes are made at target B, C, D or E twice in succession, no points are awarded for the second pass. If the pass is not a chest pass (Figure 11-11), no points are awarded for the pass. *The final score is the total of the two trials.*

ITEM 3: CONTROL DRIBBLE
Purpose

The purpose of this test is to assess skill in ball handling while the body is moving.

Court Setup

As shown in Figure 11-12, an obstacle course is marked by six cones set up in the free throw lane.

Procedure

Three timed trials are given. The first is a practice trial; the last two are recorded. The examinee, who has a ball, takes a position with cone A next to the nondominant hand. A. On a "ready, go" signal, the examinee dribbles with the nondominant hand to the nondominant side of cone B. The examinee then follows the course using the preferred hand, changing hands as deemed appropriate. If control is lost, the examinee retrieves the ball and continues from where control was lost. The trial is stopped and repeated if a ball-handling infraction occurs, if the examinee or the ball remains outside the cone, or if the examinee fails to begin at the point in the course where control was lost.

Scoring

The score for each trial is the elapsed time to complete the course legally. The clock is started on the go signal and stopped when both feet cross the finish line. Scores are recorded to the nearest 0.1 second for each trial. *The final score is the sum of two legal trials.*

ITEM 4: DEFENSIVE MOVEMENT
Purpose

The purpose of this test is to assess skill in defensive movement.

Court Markings

The test perimeters are marked by the free-throw line, the out-of-bounds line behind the basket, and the rebound lane markers, which are marked into sections by a square and two lines. Only the middle line (rebound lane marker) is a target point

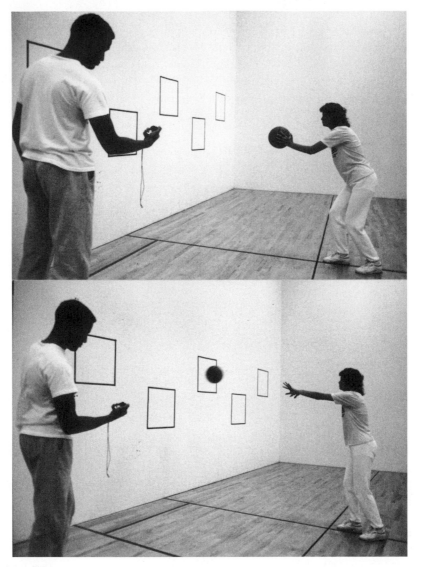

FIGURE 11-11

A chest pass is used for the AAHPERD Basketball Passing Test. (Photos by Dr. Karen Uh-lendorf, University of Vermont, Burlington, VT.)

for this test. Additional spots outside the four corners of the area should be marked with tape at points A, B, D, and E (Fig. 11-13).

Procedure

Three trials are given. The first is a practice trial; the other two are timed for the record. The examinee begins at point A, facing away from the basket. On a "ready, go" signal, he or she slides to the left without crossing feet and continues to point B, touches the floor outside the lane with the left hand, executes a drop step

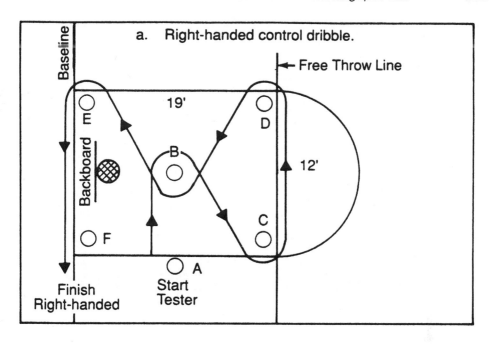

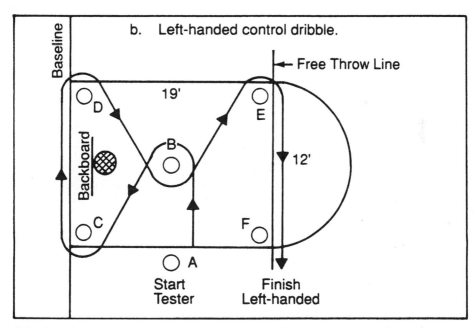

FIGURE 11-12

Court setup for AAHPERD Basketball Control Dribble Test. *a.* Right-handed control dribble. *b.* Left-handed control dribble. (Reprinted with permission from Hopkins, D.R., Shick, J., and Plack, J.J.: Basketball Skills Test Manual for Boys and Girls. Reston, VA, AAHPERD, 1984.)

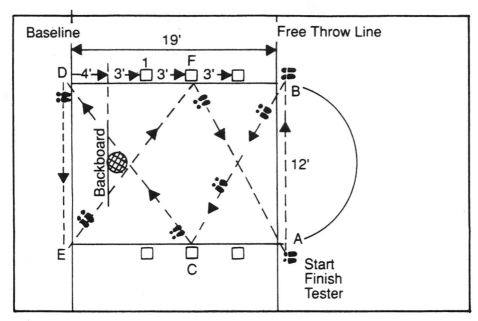

FIGURE 11-13

Court markings for the AAHPERD Basketball Defensive Movement Test. (Reprinted with permission from Hopkins, D.R., Shick, J., and Plack, J.J.: Basketball Skills Test Manual for Boys and Girls. Reston, VA, AAHPERD, 1984.)

(Figure 11-14), slides to point C, and touches the floor outside the lane with the right hand. The examinee continues the course as diagrammed. The trial is stopped and repeated if the examinee crosses his or her feet during the slide or turns and runs, if he or she fails to touch the floor outside the lane, or if he or she executes the drop step before the hand touches the floor.

Scoring

The score for each trial is the elapsed time required to complete the course legally. The clock is started on the go signal and stopped when both feet cross the finish line. Scores are recorded to the nearest 0.1 second for each trial. *The final score is the sum of two legal trials.*

Boetel Basketball Rating Scale (21)

Purpose

The purpose of this test is to evaluate the physical performance of basketball players in a game.

Gender and Age

This rating scale was developed for high school girls in competitive basketball.

Psychometric Information

A 96-item rating scale was designed to represent seven categories of basketball performance, including shooting and offensive moves, defensive moves and tactics, ball handling, rebounding, speed and quickness, body control and balance, and general floor play. These categories were derived from a review of the literature and in-

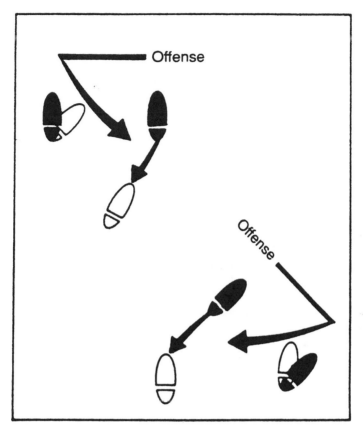

FIGURE 11-14

Footwork pattern for the drop step used in the AAHPERD Basketball Defensive Movement Test. (Reprinted with permission from Hopkins, D.R., Shick, J., and Plack, J.J.: Basketball Skills Test Manual for Boys and Girls. Reston, VA, AAHPERD, 1984.)

terviews with basketball coaches, players, and physical education teachers. The scale was used to evaluate 38 interscholastic and intercollegiate female basketball players. Means and standard deviations were calculated for each of the 96 items, and a correlation matrix for each category was created. From this matrix each of the seven categories was factor-analyzed independently of the other six categories. An abbreviated rating scale is based on the factor structure after rotation. The original seven categories were retained, and 17 items were developed or selected to represent the original 96 items. This scale was used to evaluate 34 high-school girls playing in a state B tournament. The interjudge reliability using Kendall's coefficient of concordance was .86, significant at the .01 level. The relationship between the total scores of players on the scale and a subjective ranking of the players was .65, significant at the .01 level.

Procedure

The rating scale (Fig. 11-15) is used by an observer during game play. Raters should judge each of the 17 items on a five-point scale. Figure 11-16 shows dribbling technique defined as desirable by the Boetel scale.

Boetel Basketball Rating Scale
Scoring Form

PLAYER _____   DATE _____

Directions: Check (✓) a rating for the player on each of the 17 scale items using the following key below. Judges should attempt to rate each item and choose only one response for each item. An N in front of an item indicates a negative statement.

    HA   *Highly Agree* the statement is descriptive of the player.
    A   *Slightly Agree* the statement is descriptive of the player.
    NN   *Neither Disagree Nor Agree* the statement is descriptive of the player.
    D   *Slightly Disagree* the statement is descriptive of the player.
    HD   *Highly Disagree* the statement is descriptive of the player.

Shooting Ability and Offensive Moves	HA	A	NN	D	HD
1. Player is accurate in shooting with the proper alignment of the body and shooting arm.					
2. When shooting, the player has a smooth, balanced hand release and follow-through.					
3. The player gains an offensive advantage by using evasive moves (fakes, cuts, pivots, and dribbles).					
N4. The shooter takes shots when he or she is off balance and has *not* squared his or her body toward the basket.					
5. Player uses a variety of shots.					
6. The shooter can go both left and right to successfully get the shot started from the dribble.					
Defensive Moves and Tactics	HA	A	NN	D	HD
7. The player uses the appropriate defense stance to counteract the opponents' movements on offense.					
8. The player works efficiently as part of the total defense team plan by being alert for possible interceptions and aiding teammates on defense.					
9. The player blocks attempted shots by his or her opponents.					

FIGURE 11-15

Scoring form for Boetel Basketball Rating Scale. (Reprinted with permission from Boetel, N.A.: Factorial approach in the development of a basketball rating scale to evaluate players in a game situation. Doctoral dissertation, University of North Carolina at Greensboro, 1976.)

Ball Handling	HA	A	NN	D	HD
10. The player executes the dribble with the head and shoulders up and keeps the ball from bouncing too high.					
11. When dribbling the ball the player uses either hand to change directions and pace efficiently.					
12. Passes are accurate and relative (lob, bounce, straight) to each situation.					
Rebounding (Offensive and Defensive)	HA	A	NN	D	HD
N13. When rebounding, the player consistently jumps over a positioned defender.					
14. The player is consistent in acquiring the rebound.					
Speed and Quickness	HA	A	NN	D	HD
15. The player maintains his or her weight on the balls of the feet, enabling quick movements.					
Body Control and Balance	HA	A	NN	D	HD
16. The player maintains body control and balance through the execution of proper footwork.					
General Floor Play	HA	A	NN	D	HD
17. The player is at the right place at the right time consistently.					

_____ **TOTAL POINT (85 Possible)**   **EXAMINER** _____

FIGURE 11-15

Continued

Scoring

Values for the scale ratings are highly agree (HA), 5; agree (A), 4; neither agree nor disagree (NN), 3; disagree (D), 2; and highly disagree (HD), 1. Negative items are scored by reversing the scale. The total number of points is the player's score. The maximum score is 85 points.

Comments

The Boetel scale can be used to evaluate players participating in competitive basketball and to aid in selecting players for competition. It may also be useful to diagnose weaknesses. Although the scale was developed for high-school girls, it can be used for boys and for members of other age groups who are at or near the beginning level of competitive play.

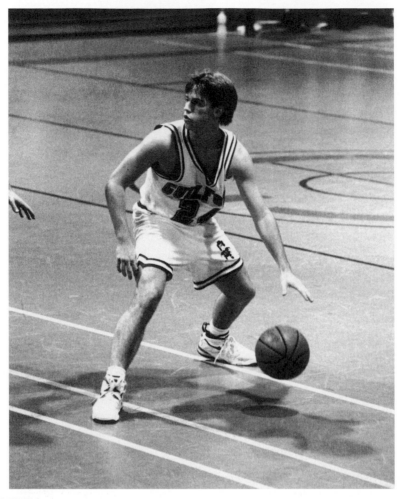

FIGURE 11-16

The rater would "highly agree" with Boetel's item 10 statement: the player executes the dribble with the head and shoulders up and keeps the ball from bouncing too high. (Photo by John Bell, Touch a Life Photography, Greensboro, NC.)

Each item on the Boetel scale is equal in value. Consequently, categories contribute different proportions to the total score. For example, shooting ability and offensive moves, with 6 items, contributes twice as heavily in the overall scoring as defensive moves and tactics, which has only 3 items. The scoring can be adjusted to match the philosophy and needs of the teacher or coach.

Field Hockey

Chapman Ball Control Test (22)

Purpose

The purpose of this test is to assess ball control skills in field hockey and more specifically, to assess the examinee's ability to combine quickness in wrist and hand movements needed to manipulate the stick with ability to control the force element when contacting the ball.

Gender and Age
The test was designed for high-school through adult women playing competitive field hockey.

Psychometric Information
This test was administered to 11 varsity and 12 junior-varsity intercollegiate women field hockey players at Illinois State University. Their years of experience ranged from 1 to 7. To estimate test reliability a one-way analysis of variance (ANOVA) was used on the scores of the three first-day trials, and from that an intraclass correlation was calculated to estimate reliability of the sum of the trials. Reliability was .89. Validity was established in two ways. First-day trial scores were subjected to a t-test and revealed a statistical difference between the means of scores of members on the two teams, significant at the .01 level. Before the test, players on each team were asked to rank the first three players on their team. The Pearson product-moment correlation between the varsity team and test scores and the junior varsity and test scores were both .63.

The test was given to 106 women and high-school girls who were trying out for the U.S. Olympic women's field hockey team. The players were rated subjectively by a panel of coaches appointed by the U.S. Field Hockey Association. Players were classified at level A, B, or C according to their potential for selection as participants on the U.S. team. The test accurately classified players 58.49% of the time. The weakest part of this evaluation was the differentiation between members of the A and B levels. This might have been affected by the fact that many B players were experienced but were not selected for the A level because of age.

Floor Markings
The target is placed on a gymnasium floor. The target pattern (Fig. 11-17) is made of self-adhesive plastic measuring 9.5 inches in diameter, with an inner circle of 4.5 inches. The larger circle is divided into three equal segments of 120°. Lines an eighth of an inch wide originating in the center of the circle and extending to its outer edge are marked on the target to define the boundaries of the segments. The color of the ringlike pattern should contrast with the color of the floor.

Personnel
The movement is so quick that a test administrator and a separate timekeeper are needed.

Procedure
This is a timed test in which the subject is required to send the ball into and out of the center circle by tapping it with the stick.

Scoring
A point is scored each time the ball is clearly tapped *into* or *through* the center circle and each time it is tapped from the center to beyond the larger circle, provided it is sent out through a segment other than the one through which it entered. Examples of basic scoring techniques are shown in Figure 11-18. No point is awarded for a ball that is tapped while it is in the area between the two circles or with the rounded side of the stick. *The final score is the sum of all points scored on*

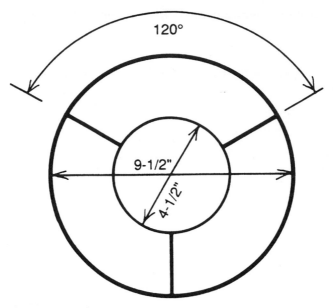

FIGURE 11-17

Floor target measurements for Chapman Ball Control Test. (Reprinted with permission from Chapman, N.L.: Chapman ball control test: field hockey. Research Quarterly for Exercise and Sport, 53(1):239, 1982.)

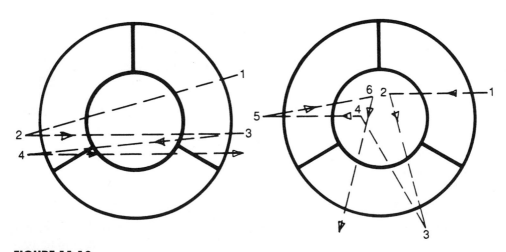

FIGURE 11-18

Basic scoring techniques for the Chapman Ball Control Test. (Reprinted with permission from Chapman, N.L.: Chapman ball control test: field hockey. Research Quarterly for Exercise and Sport, 53:239, 1982.)

three 15-second trials. A brief practice period and rest between each trial should be provided.

Comments

The Chapman Ball Control Test was designed to assess ball control skills of advanced players. In fact, it is one of relatively few sport skill tests in the published literature that is specifically for advanced players. It has not been tested on players with lesser skills. It can be used to aid in the selection of competitive teams or to help in classifying advanced players. It can also be used for practice by players who wish to improve their ball handling. The test assesses field hockey playing ability to some degree but should not be used as the sole criterion for ability. Although most field hockey players in the United States are women and girls, there appears to be no reason why this test could not be used with men and boys.

Football

Jacobson-Borleske Touch Football Test (23)

Purpose
The purpose of this test is to assess three essential skills used in football.

Gender and Age
This test was designed for boys in grades 7 to 9.

Psychometric Information
The Jacobson-Borleske Touch Football Test is a revision of an earlier battery by Borleske that was designed for college-age men (24). Using expert judges' ratings of overall playing ability as the criterion, a concurrent validity coefficient of .88 was reported for the three-item battery. Reliability was not reported for the individual items or the battery as a whole.

Facility Needs
This test requires a regulation football field.

Equipment
This test requires several footballs, markers, measuring tapes, stopwatch, scorecards, and pencils.

Scoring
Each item is scored as described later. The raw scores can be converted to T-scores using the chart in Table 11-3. *An overall score for the battery is obtained by averaging the T-scores for the three tests.*

Comments
This battery is appropriate for beginners, regardless of age or gender, in touch, flag, or regulation football. It may be used for a variety of purposes in school or youth sport settings. A junior-size football may be more appropriate for young players than a regulation football.

ITEM 1: FORWARD PASS FOR DISTANCE
Purpose
The purpose of this test is to assess skill in passing a football for distance.

TABLE 11-3   T-Scores for the Jacobson-Borleske Football Test

T SCORE	PASS FOR DISTANCE			PUNT FOR DISTANCE			RUN FOR TIME			T SCORE
	7th Grade	8th Grade	9th Grade	7th Grade	8th Grade	9th Grade	7th Grade	8th Grade	9th Grade	
85	41	48	53	38	43	47				85
80	39	45	50	36	40	44	6.3	5.8	5.7	80
75	36	41	46	33	37	41	6.7	6.2	6.0	75
70	34	38	43	31	34	38	7.0	6.6	6.3	70
65	31	35	39	28	31	34	7.3	7.0	6.7	65
60	28	32	36	26	28	32	7.7	7.4	7.0	60
55	25	29	33	23	25	28	8.0	7.7	7.3	55
50	23	26	29	20	22	25	8.3	8.1	7.6	50
45	20	23	26	18	19	22	8.6	8.5	7.9	45
40	18	20	23	16	16	19	9.0	8.9	8.3	40
35	15	17	19	13	13	16	9.3	9.2	8.6	35
30	13	14	16	11	10	13	9.6	9.6	8.9	30
25	10	10	13	8	7	10	10.0	10.0	9.2	25
20	8	8	10	6		7	10.3	10.4	9.5	20
15	5	6					10.6	10.7	9.9	15

Reprinted with permission from Jackson, T.V.: An evaluation of performance in certain physical ability tests administered to selected secondary school boys. Unpublished master's thesis, University of Washington, Seattle, 1960.

Procedure

The examinee stands, holding a football, behind a restraining line. When ready, the examinee passes the ball as far as possible down the field along a sideline. The examinee may take any number of preparation steps but may not step beyond the restraining line prior to release of the ball. A brief warm-up period precedes three measured trials.

Scoring

A marker is placed where the ball first lands for the first trial; the marker is moved to locate subsequent longer throws. Distance is measured along the sideline. A ball that deviates from the line is measured at right angles to the sideline. *The final score for this item is the distance of the best of three passes, measured to the nearest whole yard.*

ITEM 2: PUNT FOR DISTANCE
Purpose

The purpose of this test is to assess skill in punting a football for distance.

Procedure

The examinee stands in a ready position 7 yards behind a center at a restraining line. The center snaps the ball to the examinee, who punts the ball as far as possible down the field. The ball must be punted within 2 seconds of receiving the snap. Bad snaps are repeated. A brief warm-up period should precede the three measured trials.

Scoring

A marker is placed where the ball first lands for the first trial; the marker is moved to locate subsequent longer punts. Distance is measured along a straight line. A ball that deviates from a straight line is measured at right angles to the line. *The final score for this item is the distance of the best of three punts measured to the nearest whole yard.*

ITEM 3: RUN FOR TIME
Purpose

The purpose of this test is to assess skill in running for speed while carrying a football.

Procedure

The examinee begins in a 3-point backfield stance on the goal line. The center is on the 5-yard line. Upon receiving a snap from the center, the examinee immediately runs 50 yards as fast as possible while carrying the football. Bad snaps are repeated. One trial is given.

Scoring

The score is the elapsed time to the nearest 0.1 second from when the examinee receives the snap to when he crosses the 50-yard line.

Golf

Shick-Berg Indoor Golf Skill Test (25)

Purpose

The purpose of this test is to evaluate 5-iron driving skill indoors.

Gender and Age
This test is designed for junior-high boys.

Psychometric Information
This test was developed with 63 boys in junior high school who had just completed a golf unit. The scores from three rounds of nine holes each were used as the criterion measure for establishing validity. The reliability coefficient for the play of these rounds was .91. Validity coefficients were calculated for the best of the three rounds and the total of the three rounds for both 10 and 20 trials on the test. They ranged from −.79 to −.84. (The negative values of these coefficients resulted from the best score on the test being high and the best score on the rounds of golf being low.) The test-retest reliability coefficients for 10 and 20 trials, respectively, were .90 and .97.

Facility Needs
This test may be administered outdoors on a calm day or indoors. Each test station requires an area approximately 70 by 45 feet.

Equipment
Equipment for the actual test includes 5-irons; plastic golf balls; golf driving mats; cone; tape, chalk, or small flags; score sheets; and pencils.

Personnel
Two persons are needed at each test station; one spots and announces where balls land, and the other records scores.

Course Layout
The target area is shown in Figure 11-19. The target can be marked on a gymnasium floor with tape or outside with chalk. The test authors also found that the target could be designated simply by marking the intersections of the scoring areas with small colored flags.

Procedure
The examinee stands on a golf driving mat and uses a 5-iron to hit a plastic golf ball. The driving mat is positioned so that the front edge is 1 foot from the target line. The examinee is told to hit the ball as far and as straight as possible, aiming for the cone. The student takes 2 practice trials, then either 20 or 10 consecutive test trials. (If time, space, or equipment is limited, 10 trials are recommended.)

Scoring
The score for each trial is the point value of the area where the ball first lands. Balls landing on a line are given the higher value. Balls traveling beyond the target area but in line with it are awarded either 6 or 4 points as if those areas were extended. A topped ball that enters the scoring area is awarded 1 point. No points are recorded for a swing and a miss or for a ball landing outside the target area. *The final score is the sum of the trials.*

Comments
This test can be used for grading, pretesting and posttesting to show improvement, practice, and classification. It is very advantageous that it can be administered indoors or outdoors. Although designed and validated with junior-high boys, the Shick-Berg Golf Skill Test can be used with other beginning groups. The distance between the mat and the target area may have to be adjusted for some groups. Neal, as

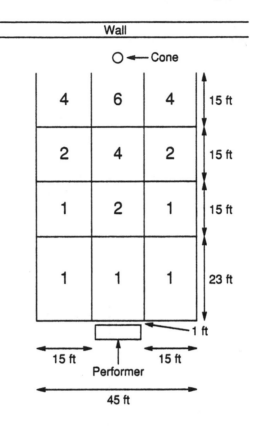

FIGURE 11-19

Gymnasium markings for Shick-Berg Indoor Golf Skill Test. (Reprinted with permission from Shick, J., and Berg, N.G.: Indoor golf skill test for junior high school boys. Research Quarterly for Exercise and Sport, 54:75, 1983.)

reported by Shick and Berg, found that golfers drive a plastic golf ball approximately 10% of the distance that they drive a regulation golf ball (26). This figure can be used to adjust target distance to fit the group being tested.

Gymnastics and Tumbling

Ellenbrand Gymnastics Skills Test (27)

Purpose

The purpose of this test is to assess gymnastics skills in four official women's gymnastics events: balance beam, floor exercise, uneven parallel bars, and vaulting.

Gender and Age

This test is appropriate for beginner to advanced college women. Because the examinee makes the choice of item within each event, difficulty can be matched to the examinee's abilities.

Psychometric Information

This test was developed on 56 college women. From a list of skills for each event, examinees were asked to select the one stunt of highest difficulty that they could perform with the best execution score. Using judges' ratings as the criterion, the validity coefficients ranged from .88 to .99 for the four items. Intraclass reliabilities ranged from .94 to .99. The agreement of judges and examiners ranged from .97 to .99. Correlations between events ranged from .44 to .70. On the basis of these low correlations, it was concluded that the events were assessing different aspects of skill in gymnastics.

Equipment

This test requires a regulation balance beam, Reuther board, and mats; mats for floor exercise; uneven parallel bars and mats; regulation vaulting horse, Reuther board, and landing mats. Also needed are score sheets, clipboards, and pencils.

Administrative Considerations

A copy of the test should be distributed to examinees before the test period. They should be allowed practice to select the skills to match their abilities and in some cases to combine the selected skills into a gymnastics routine.

Procedure

Each examinee performs each of the four events according to the directions given later. The events may be performed in any order.

Scoring

The score for each test item is the product of the difficulty value and the execution rating for the skill selected. If an examinee is incapable of performing any skill listed for a test item, a difficulty value of zero is recorded. The sum of all test items in each event is the score for that event. *The final test score is the sum of all events.* The score sheet is shown in Figure 11-20.

Execution ratings for the selected skills must be recorded on the score sheet during or immediately after the performance. The ratings are based upon the proper execution of each skill and the characteristics for each basic movement pattern. The general rating scale for all skills:

POINTS	CRITERIA
3	Correct performance; proper mechanics; executed in good form; performer shows balance, control, amplitude
2	Average performance; errors evident in either mechanics or form; may show some lack of balance, control, or amplitude
1	Poor performance; errors in both mechanics and form; performer shows little balance, control, or amplitude
0	Improper or no performance; incorrect mechanics or complete lack of form; no display of balance, control, or amplitude

There are no deductions for falls or repeated skills. However, a stunt performed with assistance from a spotter earns a zero.

EVENT 1: BALANCE BEAM

A Reuther board may be used to mount, and the beam may be approached from any direction. Positioning of the arms is optional, but since arm movements are considered part of the form, they may add or detract from the execution rating. One skill from each test item should be selected and performed.

Ellenbrand Gymnastics Skills Test
SCORESHEET

Name _____ Class Period _____ Date _____

Balance Beam Event

Item	Difficulty	Execution		
1.	_____	X _____	=	_____
2.	_____	X _____	=	_____
3.	_____	X _____	=	_____
4.	_____	X _____	=	_____
5.	_____	X _____	=	_____
		Balance Beam	=	_____

Floor Exercise Event

Item	Difficulty	Execution		
6.	_____	X _____	=	_____
7.	_____	X _____	=	_____
8.	_____	X _____	=	_____
9.	_____	X _____	=	_____
		Floor Exercise Total	=	_____

Uneven Parallel Bars Event

Item	Difficulty	Execution		
10.	_____	X _____	=	_____
11.	_____	X _____	=	_____
12.	_____	X _____	=	_____
13.	_____	X _____	=	_____
14.	_____	X _____	=	_____
		Bars Total	=	_____

Vaulting Event

Item	Difficulty	Execution		
15.	_____	X _____	=	_____
16.	_____	X _____	=	_____
		Vault Total	=	_____

EVENT TOTALS

Balance Beam _____
Floor Exercise _____
Bars _____
Vault _____
Final Test Score _____

FIGURE 11-20

Score sheet for Ellenbrand Gymnastics Skills Test. (Reprinted with permission from Ellenbrand, D.A.: Gymnastics skills test for college women. Master's thesis, Indiana University, 1973.)

Test Item 1:	Mounts

DIFFICULTY	SKILLS
1.0	a. Front support mount
2.0	b. Single-knee mount
3.0	c. Single-leg squat on
3.0	d. Straddle on
4.0	e. Forward roll mount
5.0	f. Single leg step on (to stand)
6.0	g. Handstand mount

Test Item 2:	Locomotor Skills

DIFFICULTY	SKILLS
0.5	a. Slide forward or sideways
1.0	b. Walk forward
2.0	c. Plié walk (dip step) forward
3.0	d. Step-hop forward (skip step)
4.0	e. Walk backward
5.0	f. Run forward
6.0	g. Cross-step sideways

Test Item 3:	Heights

DIFFICULTY	SKILLS
0.5	a. Hop on 1 foot
1.0	b. Two-foot jump
2.0	c. Jump with change of legs
3.0	d. Hitch kick forward
3.0	e. Cat leap
4.0	f. Stride leap
4.0	g. Tuck or arch jump
5.0	h. Stag or split leap
6.0	i. Series of leaps or jumps

Test Item 4:	Turns

DIFFICULTY	SKILLS
0.5	a. Half turn standing (2 feet)
1.0	b. Half turn squat
2.0	c. Half turn on 1 foot
3.0	d. Full turn on 2 feet (walking turn)
4.0	e. Full turn on 1 foot
5.0	f. Jump with half turn
5.0	g. 1.5 turn on 1 foot
6.0	h. Leap with half turn

Test Item 5:	Tumbling Skills On Beam

DIFFICULTY	SKILLS
0.5	a. Supine position
1.0	b. Roll backward to touch toes over head and return
2.0	c. Back shoulder roll
2.0	d. Forward shoulder roll
3.0	e. Forward head roll to back lying
4.0	f. Shoulder stand
4.0	g. Forward head roll to feet
4.0	h. Bridge position (push to a back-arch position)
4.0	i. Cartwheel off or walkover off
4.5	j. Handstand quarter-turn dismount
5.0	k. Cartwheel on
5.0	l. Back walkover on
5.5	m. Handstand forward roll
5.5	n. Front walkover on
5.5	o. Free forward roll
6.0	p. Series of cartwheels or walkovers
6.0	q. One-handed cartwheel or walkover
6.0	r. Handspring on forward or backward
7.0	s. Aerials on

EVENT 2: FLOOR EXERCISE

Perform skills on the length of mats provided. A return trip may be used if necessary. Connecting skills may be added if needed for preparation of a selected skill (e.g., round off to prepare for a back handspring). However, extra steps and runs should be avoided, as they detract from the execution rating.

Test Item 6:	Tumbling Skills—Rolls

DIFFICULTY	SKILLS
0.5	a. Forward roll to stand
0.5	b. Backward roll to knees
1.0	c. Back roll to stand
2.0	d. Pike forward or backward roll
2.0	e. Straddle roll forward or backward
3.0	f. Dive forward roll pike
4.0	g. Handstand forward roll
4.0	h. Back roll to headstand
4.5	i. Back extension
5.0	j. Dive forward roll layout
6.0	k. Back tuck somersault aerial
6.5	l. Back pike somersault
6.5	m. Forward tuck somersault
7.0	n. Back layout somersault
8.0	o. Somersault with a twist

Test Item 7:	Tumbling Skills—Springs

DIFFICULTY	SKILLS
1.0	a. Handstand snap-down
2.0	b. Round off
2.5	c. Neck spring (kip)
3.0	d. Headspring
3.5	e. Front handspring to squat
4.0	f. Front handspring arch to stand
4.5	g. Front handspring walk-out
5.0	h. Back handspring
5.0	i. Front handspring on 1 hand or with change of legs
5.5	j. Series of front handsprings
6.0	k. Series of back handsprings
6.5	l. Back handspring to kip (cradle)
6.5	m. Back handspring with twist

Test Item 8:	Acrobatic Skills

DIFFICULTY	SKILLS
1.0	a. Mule kick (three-quarter handstand)
1.0	b. Bridge (back-arch position)
2.0	c. Handstand
2.0	d. Cartwheel
2.5	e. ackbend from standing
3.0	f. Front limber
3.0	g. One-handed cartwheel
4.0	h. Walkover forward and backward
4.0	i. Dive cartwheel
4.0	j. Tinsica
4.5	k. Dive walkover
5.0	l. Handstand with half turn or straddle-down to a sit
5.0	m. One-handed walkover
6.0	n. Butterfly (side aerial)
7.0	o. Aerial cartwheel or walkover

Test Item 9:	Dance Skills

DIFFICULTY	SKILLS
1.0	a. Half turn (1 foot), run, leap
2.0	b. Half turn, step, hitch kick forward, step, leap
3.0	c. Half turn, slide, tour jeté, hitch kick
4.0	d. Full turn (1 foot), step, leap, step, leap
5.0	e. Full turn, tour jeté, cabriole (beat kick forward)
6.0	f. 1.5 turn, step, leap, step, leap with a change of legs

EVENT 3: UNEVEN PARALLEL BARS

Connecting stunts may be added as preparation for selected skills (e.g., back hip circle as preparation for eagle catch). Dismounting between items is allowed but not necessary.

Test Item 10:	Kips

DIFFICULTY	SKILLS
1.0	a. Single knee swing-up
2.0	b. Two-leg stem rise to high bar
3.0	c. Single-leg stem rise to high bar
4.0	d. Kip between bars from sit on low bar
4.5	e. Glide kip with single-leg shoot-through
5.0	f. Glide kip
5.5	g. Glide, kip, regrasp high bar
5.5	h. Drop, glide kip
6.0	i. Kip from long hang
6.5	j. Rear or reverse kip

Test Item 11:	Casts

DIFFICULTY	SKILLS
0.5	a. Cast rearward off low bar to stand
1.0	b. Cast and return to bar
2.0	c. Cast to squat (1 hand on low bar, 1 hand on high bar)
3.0	d. Cast, single-leg shoot-through
4.0	e. Cast to long hand from high bar
4.5	f. Cast to squat, stoop, or straddle stand on either bar
5.0	g. Cast, half turn to catch high bar
5.0	h. Eagle catch
5.5	i. From front support on high bar facing low bar, cast to low bar, cast to handstand on
6.0	j. Cast, full turn to regrasp either bar

Test Item 12: Hip Circles

DIFFICULTY	SKILLS
1.0	a. Forward somersault over high bar to a hang
2.0	b. Back pullover high bar or low bar
3.0	c. Back hip circle
4.0	d. Forward hip circle
5.0	e. Forward hip circle, regrasp high bar
5.0	f. Flying back hip circle (hands on high bar, circle low bar)
6.0	g. Free back hip circle to hang
6.0	h. Forward hip circle directly to a handstand

Test Item 13: Seat Circles

DIFFICULTY	SKILLS
1.0	a. Half seat circle backward (skin-the-cat)
2.0	b. Single knee circle backward
3.0	c. Single-knee circle forward (modified split-leg circle)
4.0	d. Split-leg circle forward (straight legs)
4.0	e. From straddle or rear sit, circle backward and release to rear stand
5.0	f. Seat circle forward or backward
6.0	g. Seat circle forward to straddle cut-and-catch
6.0	h. From a seat circle backward on high bar, release to a front support on low bar

Test Item 14: Underswings

DIFFICULTY	SKILLS
1.0	a. From sit on low bar, facing high bar, underswing dismount
2.0	b. From front support, half hip circle backward (underswing)
3.0	c. Half sole circle backward to dismount
3.5	d. Underswing on high bar to dismount over low bar
4.0	e. Sole circle backward or forward to regrasp high bar
4.5	f. Underswing on high bar to dismount over low bar with half twist
5.0	g. Straddle or sole circle backward, half turn to regrasp high bar in a hang
5.5	h. Straddle or flank cut on return swing of half seat circle backward
6.0	i. Straddle cut-and-catch

EVENT 4: VAULTING

Two vaults with different degrees of difficulty must be performed. The Reuther board should be used for takeoff and may be adjusted to any distance from the horse.

Test Items 15 and 16:	Two Vaults

DIFFICULTY	SKILLS
1.0	a. Knee mount
2.0	b. Squat mount
2.5	c. Straddle mount
3.0	d. Squat vault
3.5	e. Flank vault
4.0	f. Straddle vault
4.0	g. Wolf vault
4.5	h. Rear vault
5.0	i. Front vault
6.0	j. Thief vault
6.5	k. Headspring vault
7.0	l. Straddle half twist
9.0	m. Horizontal squat
9.5	n. Horizontal straddle
10.0	o. Horizontal stoop
11.0	p. Layout squat
11.5	q. Layout straddle
12.0	r. Layout stoop
13.0	s. Handspring vault
13.0	t. Giant cartwheel
14.0	u. Hecht vault
15.0	v. Yamashita
15.0	w. Handspring with half twist (on or off)

Lacrosse

Ennis Multi-Skill Test in Lacrosse (28)

Purpose

The purpose of this test is to assess skill and knowledge of lacrosse technique and the flexibility to adapt skills to new situations.

Gender and Age

This test is appropriate for women lacrosse players beyond the beginning level of skill development.

Psychomotor Information

Ennis developed a one-item multiskill test to resemble the game. Development of the test was based on performance scores from 95 players from five Virginia colleges. Varsity lacrosse coaches from each college rated their players into five categories using a revision of the Hodges Rating Scale (29). A validity coefficient using Kendall's rank correlation coefficient, tau, between the coaches' ratings and mean time scores on the multiskill test was .66. Construct validity was demonstrated by the ability to discriminate between players at different levels. Coefficients of reliability between levels and between trials were respectively R = .89 and R = .78.

Facility Needs
This test requires a grassy field at least 180 feet long.

Equipment
This test requires lacrosse sticks and balls, eight cones, score sheets, and pencils.

Field Markings
Cone placements and field markings are shown in Figure 11-21. The lines are not drawn on the field; only the circles are drawn on the field.

Instructions for Examinees
The following explanation occurs simultaneously with walk-through:

Begin in the area of cone 3.
Run forward to pick up a stationary ball next to cone 1. Time begins as you touch the ball.
Turn to your left and go around cone 1. Run to the right of cone 2, to the left of cone 3, and to the right of cone 4.
Once past cone 4, continue running and toss and catch the ball twice above your head. The examiner must be able to see the ball above your head for each toss. If the ball is not above your head, the examiner will call, "Repeat."
After tossing and catching the ball twice, shoot for the goal. There is no penalty if you miss, but if you are successful, 1 second will be deducted from your time. You may shoot from anywhere; there is no restraining line.
Without the ball, run goal side of cone 5. Turn and run backward to cone 6 and then forward to pick up a ball beside cone 7.
Run around cone 7 and throw the ball beyond cone 8. You may throw from anywhere; there is no restraining line. The ball may bounce. If the ball stops before passing cone 8, you must use your stick to propel it again. Time will be recorded as the ball passes cone 8.

Instructions for Examiner
The examiner leads the examinees through the test, repeating key words for each task. There is no demonstration, and no reference is made to specific ways to perform the various tasks.

A group of about eight examinees follows the examiner through the complete test, while the examiner repeats word cues for each task and explains that many movement and skill shortcuts can be used to cut seconds from the time. The examinees should practice to discover ways to move as quickly and efficiently as possible. The examinees should take a second practice trial as the examiner repeats word cues when necessary. After the second practice trial, three actual trials are timed and recorded.

Allow examinees to begin when ready.
Begin time when examinee touches stationary ball, even if pickup is unsuccessful.

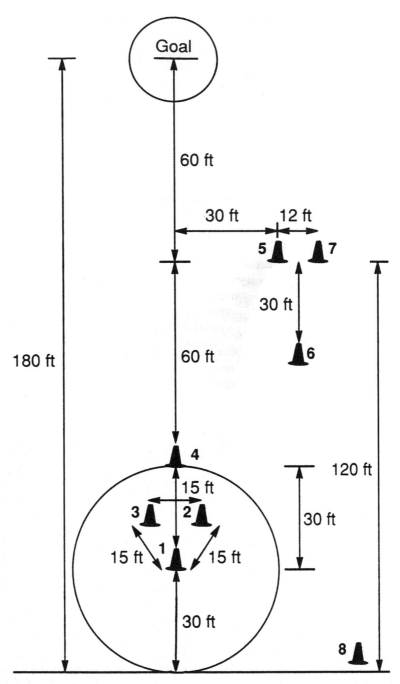

FIGURE 11-21

Field layout for Ennis Multi-Skill Test in Lacrosse. (Reprinted with permission from Ennis, C.D.: The development of a multi-skill test in lacrosse for college women. Master's thesis, University of North Carolina at Greensboro, 1977.)

Observe that tosses are above examinee's head. If not, call, "Repeat." Examinee should repeat only unsuccessful tosses.

Record success of shot on goal.

Backward running: observe whether player's back is square with cone 8. If not, call, "Backward." No penalty.

Move opposite cone 8. If throw is unsuccessful, encourage player to propel ball again. Record time as the ball passes cone 8.

Scoring

Time is recorded to the nearest 0.1 second. Score is time for trials minus 1-second deduction for successful goal. *Final score is the sum of three trials.*

Comments

The directions for this test are complex. It is important to make sure that examinees understand what they are supposed to do and can go smoothly from one part of the test to the next. Although this test is gamelike, the final score yields little diagnostic information. It may, however, be useful for summative grading, classification, practice, and team selection.

Racquetball

Valcourt Racquetball Skills Test Battery (30)

Purpose

The purpose of this test is to assess overall racquetball ability.

Gender and Age

This test is appropriate for adult racquetball players of both genders at the beginner or intermediate level.

Psychometric Information

Subjects for the development study were beginner and intermediate adult racquetball players. All subjects were volunteers from either college beginning racquetball classes or a racquetball club. Beginners were tested after 4 or 5 weeks of instruction; intermediates were tested in the same time frame. All subjects played two singles games with at least five opponents of the same gender and skill level. Scores from these matches were the criteria for validation of the skills tests. The total number of wins and losses (winning percentage) and the total number of points scored and lost by a player (point differential) were computed for each subject.

The recommended final test battery included two tests, Buschner's Ceiling Shot Placement Test and a variation of Hensley, East, and Stillwell's Wall Volley Test (31, 32). For beginner men, the Ceiling Shot Placement Test had a .82 correlation with the criteria of winning percentage and a .75 correlation with point differential. For beginner women, the Long Wall Volley Test had a .75 correlation with winning percentage. For intermediate men players, the Wall Volley test had a .83 correlation with winning percentage and a .78 correlation with point differential. For intermediate women players, the Long Wall Volley Test had a correlation of .77 with winning percentage and .60 with point differential. Reliability coefficients were not reported.

Battery Scoring

Multiple correlations and stepwise regression analyses were computed. Seven prediction equations were based on these results. (None of the variables was able to predict point differentials for intermediate women.) The equations for winning percentage and point differential for each group can be used separately or together for grading or other purposes. The prediction equations:

Winning percentage for male beginners: 0.014 (Ceiling Shot Placement Test score) + 0.011 (Long Wall Volley Test score) + 0.092

Point differential for male beginners: 0.023 (Ceiling Shot Placement Test score) + 0.794

Winning percentage for female beginners: 0.028 (Long Wall Volley Test score) + 0.019 (Ceiling Shot Placement Test score) − 0.260

Point differential for female beginners: 0.068 (Ceiling Shot Placement Test score) + 0.648

Winning percentage for male intermediates: 0.569 (Long Wall Volley Test score) − 1.0172

Point differential for male intermediates: 0.156 (Long Wall Volley Test score) − 3.202

Winning percentage for female intermediates: 0.031 (Long Wall Volley Test score) + 0.013 (Ceiling Shot Placement Test score) − 0.549

Comments

The individual test items can be used for practice. The test battery with the appropriate equations can be used for grading both beginner and intermediate adult players. It can also be used to classify players for different levels of instruction or to rank players for a ladder tournament.

The tests and the battery may also be found to be appropriate for younger players, but such testing has not yet been done. Some beginners may have trouble doing the lob serve that is needed to set up the ceiling shot for the Ceiling Shot Placement Test.

ITEM 1: CEILING SHOT PLACEMENT TEST

Purpose

The purpose of this test is to assess the defensive abilities of a player by assessing skill in placement of the ceiling shot.

Facility Needs

This test requires a regulation racquetball court marked with scoring lines.

Equipment

This test requires a racquet and several balls, goggles, score sheets, and pencils.

Court Markings

As shown in Figure 11-22, two lines are marked on the back wall at 2.5 and 5 feet. Three more lines are marked on the floor at 2, 4, and 6 feet from the back wall.

Procedure

The examinee stands behind the short line and strokes the ball using a lob serve to the front wall. When the ball rebounds, the examinee moves into position and performs a ceiling shot; 10 trials are taken.

Scoring

The ceiling shot must hit the ceiling first, then the front wall, then rebound near midcourt, and then rebound again in the backcourt. When the ball hits the floor the second time in the backcourt, it is scored according to the point values shown in Figure 11-22. A ball hitting a line receives the higher value. If the ball does not strike

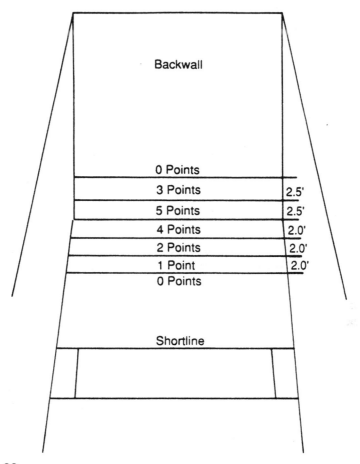

FIGURE 11-22

Court markings for Valcourt's Ceiling Shot Placement Test for racquetball. (Reprinted with permission from Valcourt, D.F.: Development of a racquetball skills test battery for male and female beginner and intermediate players. Master's thesis, Springfield College, Springfield, MA, 1982.)

any of the score zones, a zero is recorded for that trial. The examinee must attempt a ceiling shot for each of the setups. No extra trials are permitted. *The total of the 10 trials is the score for the test;* 50 points are possible.

ITEM 2: LONG WALL VOLLEY TEST
Purpose
The purpose of this test is to assess the speed and power components of the racquetball drive strokes.

Court Markings
A restraining line is marked across the width of the court 12 feet behind the short line.

Facility Needs
This test requires a regulation racquetball court with markings.

Equipment

This test requires a racquet, two balls, stopwatch, score sheet, and pencil.

Procedure

The test item is explained and demonstrated. The examinee is permitted a 5-minute warm-up on an adjacent court and a 1-minute warm-up on the test court. The test consists of two 30-second trials that are taken in succession with no rest between the trials. The examinee begins the test positioned behind the restraining line and holding two racquetballs. He or she drops a ball and volleys it against the front wall for 30 seconds. The time begins when the examinee first drops the ball. The examinee should hit the ball from behind the restraining line. Any stroke may be used to keep the ball in play. The ball may be stroked in the air or after bouncing; there is no restriction on the number of bounces the ball may take before being hit. In case the ball fails to return past the restraining line, the examinee may step into the front-court to retrieve the ball but must return behind the restraining line for the succeeding stroke. If the examinee should miss the ball, a second ball may be put into play in the same manner as the first, or the examinee may retrieve the first ball and continue to volley it. If both balls are missed, the player may retrieve either ball and put it in play in the same manner.

Scoring

One point is scored each time the ball legally hits the front wall. A legal hit requires that the ball travel from the face of the racquet and hit the front wall before hitting the floor during the 30-second trial. *The total score is the sum of all legal hits for the two trials.* No points are scored when the examinee steps over the restraining line to volley the ball or when the ball hits the floor on the way to the front wall.

Soccer

Mor-Christian General Soccer Ability Skill Test Battery (33)

Purpose

The purpose of this test battery is to assess overall soccer playing ability.

Gender and Age

This battery was developed for college men of varying skill levels.

Psychometric Information

This battery was developed with 45 male college students of varying skill levels, including varsity team players, intramural champion players, and physical education soccer class players. Five skill tests were initially studied. The three presented here make up a battery with acceptable validity and reliability that can be administered without the need for any special equipment.

The criterion for the estimation of validity was a rating by three soccer experts who observed players during actual matches. A multiple correlation analysis was used to select the items for the test battery. Coefficients for various test battery components were passing, .776; passing plus dribbling, .790; and passing plus dribbling plus shooting, .913. Other findings are as shown in the table. The three-item test battery is recommended.

	DRIBBLING	PASSING	SHOOTING
Concurrent validity coefficient	.731	.776	.912
Test-retest reliability coefficient	.795	.961	.984
Interjudge objectivity coefficient	.998	1.000	.999

Battery Scoring

Scores from any of the tests can be used separately. To obtain an overall test battery score, individual test scores should be converted to T-scores based on local group data. The T-scores can then be averaged.

Comments

The Mor-Christian battery can be used for grading, classification, practice, and to aid in team selection. Since the battery was designed for a wide skill level, it may be appropriate for use with other age groups and women and girls (Figure 11-23). The passing and shooting tests may be quite difficult for some less-skilled groups. The passing test may be modified by moving the line closer to the target or increasing the size of the target. The shooting test may be modified by giving some credit to shots that go into the middle of the goal area between the circular targets. However, modifications affect the validity and reliability estimates.

Motor learning theorists recommend randomized practice for better learning of open skills (7). This suggests that if practice for learning is the goal, the four trials

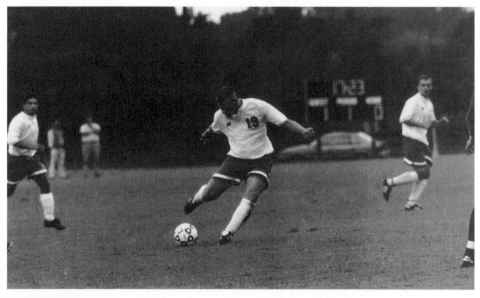

FIGURE 11-23

The Mor-Christian soccer battery was designed for a wide range of skill levels for college men, but it may also be used with other groups. (Photo by John Bell, Touch a Life Photography, Greensboro, NC.)

from the three angles on the passing test should be randomly ordered rather than consecutive. Similarly, the four trials to each of the four target areas on the shooting test should also be randomly ordered rather than consecutive. Again, however, such modifications would affect validity and reliability estimates.

ITEM 1: DRIBBLING
Field Markings

As shown in Figure 11-24, a circular course with a diameter of 20 yards is marked on a soccer field. The starting line is a 3-foot line drawn perpendicular to the circle. Cones 18 inches tall are placed at 5-yard intervals around the circle.

Facility Needs

This test requires a grassy field.

Equipment

This test requires a soccer ball, a dozen 18-inch cones, stopwatch, score sheets, and pencil.

Procedure

A soccer ball is placed on the starting line. On a "ready, go" signal, the examinee dribbles the ball around the course by weaving through the cones back to the starting line, attempting to traverse the course as quickly as possible. Three trials are

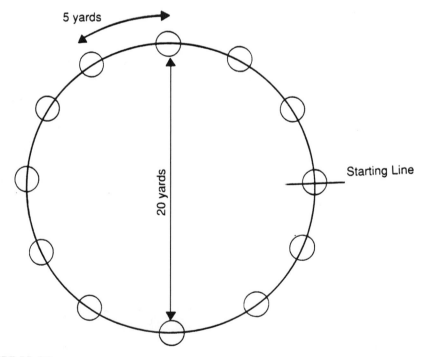

FIGURE 11-24

Field layout for Mor-Christian Dribbling Test. (Reprinted with permission from Mor, D., and Christian, V.: The development of a skill test battery to measure general soccer ability. North Carolina Journal of Health and Physical Education, 15(1):30, Spring 1979.)

taken, recorded to the nearest 0.1 second. The first trial is performed clockwise, the second counterclockwise, and the third in the direction of the examinee's choice.

Scoring
The test score is the combined best two of the three timed trials.

ITEM 2: PASSING
Field Markings
As shown in Figure 11-25, a goal 1 yard wide and 18 inches high is marked with two cones and a rope. Three other cones are placed 15 yards from the center of the goal at 90° and 45°.

Facility Needs
This test requires a grassy field.

Equipment
This test requires several soccer balls, five 18-inch cones, 4-foot rope, score sheet, and pencil.

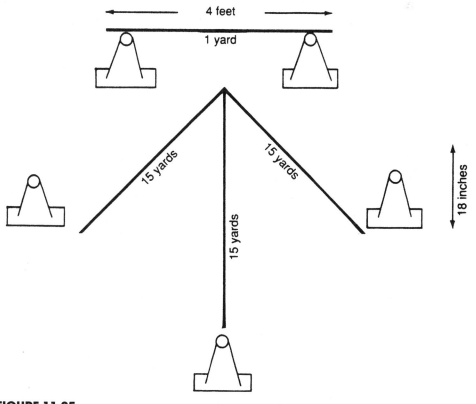

FIGURE 11-25

Field layout and target for Mor-Christian Passing Test. (Reprinted with permission from Mor, D., and Christian, V.: The development of a skill test battery to measure general soccer ability. North Carolina Journal of Health and Physical Education, 15(1):30, Spring 1979.)

Procedure

Examinees pass a stationary ball with their preferred foot into the small goal from the three angles marked by the cones. Four consecutive trials are taken from each angle for a total of 12 trials. Two practice trials at each angle are allowed.

Scoring

One point is awarded for passes that go between the cones or rebound off one of the cones. *The test score is the total of the 12 trials.*

ITEM 3: SHOOTING
Field Markings

A regulation soccer goal is divided into scoring areas by two ropes suspended from the crossbar 4 feet from each goal post. In addition, each scoring area is divided into an upper and lower target area by hanging two hula hoops. A shooting line is marked 16 yards from the goal (Fig. 11-26).

Facility Needs

This test requires a grassy field with regulation soccer goal.

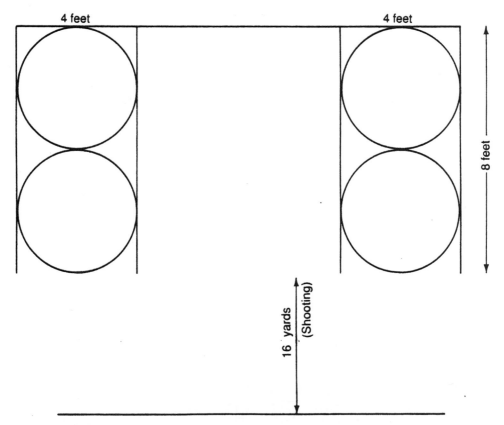

FIGURE 11-26

Field layout and target for Mor-Christian Shooting Test. (Reprinted with permission from Mor, D., and Christian, V.: The development of a skill test battery to measure general soccer ability. North Carolina Journal of Health and Physical Education, 15(1):30, Spring 1979.)

Equipment
This test requires several soccer balls, four hula hoops, score sheets, and pencil.

Procedure
The examinee shoots a stationary ball with the preferred foot from any point along the 16-yard shooting line. Four practice trials are given, then four consecutive shots are attempted at each of the four hula hoops. There is a total of 16 trials.

Scoring
If the ball is shot through or rebounds from the intended target, 10 points are awarded; 4 points are scored if the ball is shot through or rebounds from the target adjacent to the intended target. No points are given for shots that go between the target areas or that roll or bounce through the target areas. The maximum score is 160 points.

McDonald Volleying Soccer Test (34)

Purpose
The purpose of this test is to assess general soccer ability.

Gender and Age
This test was designed for collegiate men varsity soccer players of varying skill levels.

Psychometric Information
The criterion for estimates of concurrent validity was coaches' ratings of playing ability. Coefficients were .94 for varsity players, .63 for junior varsity players, and .76 for freshman varsity players. The concurrent validity coefficient for all groups combined was .85. No reliability estimates were reported.

Facility Needs
This test requires an indoor gymnasium with a large smooth wall surface.

Equipment
This test requires three soccer balls, stopwatch, score sheets, and pencil.

Court Markings
The wall target area is 30 feet wide and 11.5 feet high; a restraining line is marked 9 feet from the wall.

Procedure
One ball is placed on the restraining line; two spare balls are placed 9 feet back from the restraining line. The examinee begins on a "ready, go" signal, then repeatedly kicks the ball against the wall from or behind the restraining line as many times as possible during a 30-second trial. Any type of kick may be used. Any body part, including the hands, may be used for retrieving an out-of-control ball. If needed, a player may put one of the spare balls into play from behind the restraining line. Four trials are taken.

Scoring
The score for each trial is the number of legal kicks in a 30-second period. *The overall test score is the best of the four trials.*

Comments

The McDonald test can be given indoors and is quick and easy to administer. This test does, however, have the concerns of other repeated wall volley tests because in an actual game the soccer player does not respond repeatedly to his or her own kicks. While the test can be used for many reasons, perhaps its best use is for classification for future instruction or for competition. It may be used as is or modified to accommodate other age groups or women and girls.

The Pioneer Instrument for Measuring Soccer Playing Ability in a Regular Setting (13)

Purpose

The purpose of the Pioneer Instrument for Measuring Soccer Playing Ability in a Regular Setting (PIMSPARS) is to assess soccer ability in a natural game setting.

Psychometric Information

Using expert ratings on a 5-point Likert scale, mean ratings of importance of the 10 ability attributes included in the PIMSPARS ranged from 4.5 to 5.0. Interobserver agreement ratings ranged from .80 to 1.00, with an average interobserver agreement rating of .83. The authors concluded, "The PIMSPARS appears to be scientifically purposeful for accurate evaluation of playing ability in natural settings" (13, p. 57).

Facility Needs

This test requires a marked soccer field with goals.

Equipment

This test requires observation sheet, pencil, and clipboard but no special equipment besides standard game equipment.

Personnel

The recorder must be knowledgeable about soccer and a skilled observer.

Procedure

While the examinee engages in game play, the recorder observes for 10 key behaviors and records observations on the PIMSPARS observation form. The key behaviors are defined in Table 11-4; the PIMSPARS observation form is shown in Figure 11-27. For each condition that presents itself, the following five steps are followed. The conditions are numbered chronologically.

Step 1. The recorder identifies a condition in the game that has the potential to elicit a key behavior from the examinee.

Step 2. The recorder determines whether the examinee responded to the condition. If the condition was ignored, the recorder marks an X in the I (ignored) column corresponding to the condition. The recorder writes in the symbol for the key behavior that was ignored under the BS (behavioral symbol) column.

Step 3. If the examinee recognizes and responds to the condition, the I column is left blank and the symbol for the key behavior that was attempted is recorded in the BS column.

Step 4. The recorder determines the appropriateness or accuracy of the examinee's response to the condition. The recorder makes an X under the A (appropriate) column to designate an appropriate response. If the response is inappropriate

TABLE 11-4	Operational Definitions of Key Behaviors for the PIMSPARS
KEY BEHAVIOR	**DEFINITION**
Relocating for a pass	Deliberate movement into open space to receive a pass from a teammate. Give-and-go passes are included in this category.
Defensive relocation	Deliberate movement toward player's own goal area to help on defense; does not include hustles to regain possession of a ball immediately after the ball has been lost to an opponent.
Maneuvering and faking	Attempt to create illusion with body movements that causes an opponent to hesitate, take eyes off the ball, or lose balance; places opponent at a momentary disadvantage.
Jockeying	Movement into space or away from ball in attempt to create opportunity for response by teammate in possession of ball or to increase attacking potential of team; does not include relocating for a pass or defensive relocation. Jockeying movements occur in the opposite direction of the teammate with the ball to draw defender away from ball and to create space for teammate with ball.
Hustling	Attempt to gain or regain possession of the ball from an opponent; includes tackling to gain possession of ball or gaining possession of space to contain opponent or halt opponent's offensive maneuver; also includes regaining possession of ball immediately after losing it to an opponent.
Passing	Attempt to send ball to teammate by kicking with either foot or other part of the body except hands. Use of head, chest, thigh, knee, or shin is included; does not include pass that results in successful shot at goal by another teammate.
Assisting	Pass to teammate preceding successful shot at goal. Ball may be passed by kicking with either foot or other part of body except hands. Use of head, chest, thigh, knee, or shin is included.
Shooting	Attempt to send ball through goal by kicking with leg, head, or any part of body except hands to score a goal.
Trapping	Attempt to receive a ball from a throw-in or kick with any part of body except hands so that ball remains under player's control or within player's reach. Trap is unsuccessful if player takes more than a step to recover ball.
Defensive save	Any attempt by a player to stop a shot at goal with any part of the body except the hands. All goalie actions intended to prevent the ball from scoring are included in this category. It includes clearances around the goal area that are intended to break offensive actions.

Reprinted with permission from Ocansey, R.T.A., and Kutame, M.A.: Measuring soccer playing ability in natural settings. Journal of Physical Education, Recreation, and Dance, 62(7):54, September 1991.

Student _____ Recorder _____ Date _____
Time _____ to _____ Game Type _____

Key Behaviors

RP:	Relocating for a pass	H:	Hustling	S:	Shooting
DR:	Defensive Relocation	P:	Passing	T:	Trapping
M:	Maneuvering and Faking	A:	Assisting	DS:	Defensive Save
J:	Jockeying				

Assessment Keys

OTR:	Opportunity to Respond	BS:	Behavioral Symbol	I:	Ignore
A:	Appropriate	S:	Successful	US:	Unsuccessful
IA:	Not Appropriate				

OTR	I	BS	A	IA	S	US		OTR	I	BS	A	IA	S	US
1								16						
2								17						
3								18						
4								19						
5								20						
6								21						
7								22						
8								23						
9								24						
10								25						
11								26						
12								27						
13								28						
14								29						
15								30						

Summary Report

OTRs: _____ Actual Responses: _____ I = _____

Ratio of OTR/Actual response: _____ / _____

A: _____ IA: _____ Ratio of A/IA: _____ / _____ Percent of A: _____ %
S: _____ US: _____ Ratio of S/US: _____ / _____ Percent of S: _____ %

Key behaviors

RP: _____ DR: _____ M: _____ H: _____ S: _____
T: _____ A: _____ DS: _____ P: _____ J: _____

FIGURE 11-27

Observation recording form for the Pioneer Instrument for Measuring Soccer Playing Ability in a Regular Setting. (Reprinted with permission from Ocansey, R.T.A., and Kutame, M.A.: Measuring soccer playing ability in natural settings. Journal of Physical Education, Recreation, and Dance, 62(7):54, September 1991.)

or incongruous with the condition presented, the recorder makes an X under the IA (inappropriate) column.

Step 5. The recorder determines the result or product of the examinee's response. If the result is successful, the recorder makes an X under the S (successful) column. If the result is not successful, the recorder makes an X under the US (unsuccessful) column.

For example, if a *defensive save* opportunity arose and the examinee *appropriately* responded but was *unsuccessful* in the attempt, the recorder would mark a DS in the BS column, an X in the A column, and an X in the US column.

Scoring

After completing the observational data, the recorder completes the summary report for all opportunities to respond collectively and/or individual key behaviors. The data are analyzed to reveal patterns of behaviors.

Comments

Both physical education teachers and soccer coaches find the PIMSPARS useful for evaluation of the abilities of their charges. It may be used for grading, classification, and diagnostic purposes. The authors did not report the age, gender, or skill level of the subjects for whom they developed the PIMSPARS, but it is probably appropriate for many types of examinees. Clearly, the major appeal of this instrument is its authenticity. It does, however, require that the recorder be both knowledgeable about soccer and a keen observer.

Softball

AAHPERD Softball Skills Test (35)

Purpose

The purpose of this test is to assess skills that are essential to softball, that is, batting, fielding, throwing, and base running.

Gender and Age

The tests were designed for both genders from grade 5 to college.

Norms

Selected percentile norms for all four individual tests are given in Table 11-5.

Comments

Individual tests and/or the full battery can be used for a variety of purposes, including assessing achievement, classification, and diagnosis. They may also be used to aid in team selection.

TEST 1: BATTING

Purpose

The purpose of this test is to assess power and placement in softball batting.

Psychometric Information

Validity and reliability data and norms were calculated from a national sample of data for both genders from grades 5 through college. Using judges' ratings of skill as the criterion, concurrent validity coefficients ranged from .54 to .85. Logical validity was also claimed. Intraclass test-retest reliability coefficients ranged from .69 to .91.

Field Markings

As shown in Figure 11-28, nine scoring areas are created by dividing the outfield of a regulation softball field into three power zones and three placement areas. Different power zone distances are used for grades 5 to 8 and for grades 9 through college. Cones may be used to mark the division lines between zones.

Equipment

This test requires a batting tee, bats, softballs, eight cones; score sheet, and pencil.

| TABLE 11-5 | Selected Percentile Norms for the AAHPERD Softball Skills Test Battery (continues on page 381) | | | | |

		BOYS AND MEN				
Test	Percentile	Grade 5	Grade 7	Grade 9	Grade 11	College
BATTING						
	99	36	36	36	36	36
	75	21	29	26	24	32
	50	14	23	20	20	26
	25	9	16	14	16	20
FIELDING						
	99	24	24	24	24	24
	75	23	23	23	24	24
	50	20	20	20	20	21
	25	16	17	16	18	18
THROWING						
	99	129	195	218	238	268
	75	99	136	166	182	200
	50	85	118	141	160	180
	25	68	98	120	140	159
BASE RUNNING						
	99	6.5	6.1	5.9	5.6	5.7
	75	7.3	6.8	6.5	6.1	6.0
	50	7.8	7.3	6.9	6.4	6.3
	25	8.4	7.8	7.2	6.9	6.7

Procedure

With the ball on a batting tee adjusted to a proper height, the examinee hits the ball as long and as straight as possible. Two warm-ups are allowed, and then six test trials are taken.

Scoring

Each trial is scored according to the value for the zone in which the hit ball comes to rest. A ball landing on a line receives the higher zone value. Zero points are awarded for a swing and a miss, a topped ball, a pop-up, and a foul ball. *The total test score is the sum of the six test trials.*

Comments

The validity of this test is limited by the use of a batting tee. Some players perform well on this test but hit poorly from a pitched ball, and vice versa.

TEST 2: FIELDING GROUND BALLS
Purpose
The purpose of this test is to assess skill in fielding ground balls.

GIRLS AND WOMEN					
Test	Percentile	Grade 5	Grade 7	Grade 9	Grade 11	College
BATTING						
	99	26	32	28	32	34
	75	13	15	16	18	24
	50	8	9	10	11	19
	25	5	6	7	7	12
FIELDING						
	99	24	24	24	24	24
	75	21	20	22	22	22
	50	18	17	18	18	18
	25	12	14	14	16	14
THROWING						
	99	111	112	132	161	180
	75	59	75	82	108	125
	50	46	62	67	86	104
	25	38	50	54	66	86
BASE RUNNING						
	99	7.0	6.6	6.8	6.3	6.5
	75	7.8	7.3	7.4	7.0	7.0
	50	8.2	7.8	7.9	7.5	7.3
	25	8.8	8.4	8.4	8.0	7.7

Adapted from Rikli, R.E. (ed.): Softball Skills Test Manual. Reston, VA, AAHPERD, 1991.

Psychometric Information
Using judges' ratings of skill as the criterion measure, concurrent validity coefficients ranged from .60 to .85 for both genders in grade 5 through college. Logical validity was also claimed. Test-retest intraclass reliability coefficients ranged from .75 to .89.

Field Markings
A large, smooth, grassy field is marked as shown in Figure 11-29. Distance for the velocity indicator is 65 feet for grades 5 and 6, 75 feet for grades 7 and 8, 90 feet for grades 9 to 12, and 100 feet for college students.

Equipment
This test requires gloves, softballs, three cones, score sheet, and pencil.

Personnel
A minimum of two trained testers are necessary for this test.

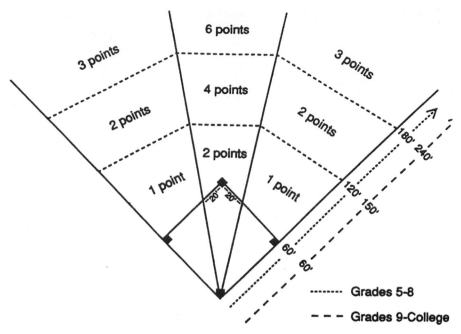

FIGURE 11-28

Field markings for the AAHPERD Softball Batting Test. (Reprinted with permission from Rikli, R.E. (ed.): Softball Skills Test Manual. Reston, VA, AAHPERD, 1991.)

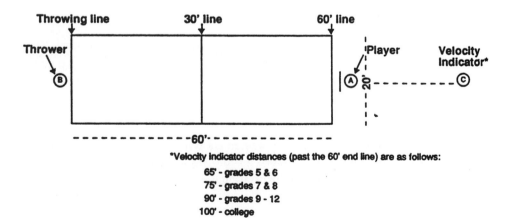

Velocity indicator distances (past the 60' end line) are as follows:

65' - grades 5 & 6
75' - grades 7 & 8
90' - grades 9 - 12
100' - college

FIGURE 11-29

Field markings for the AAHPERD Softball Fielding Test. (Reprinted with permission from Rikli, R.E. (ed.): Softball Skills Test Manual. Reston, VA, AAHPERD, 1991.)

Procedure

A thrower, positioned at cone B, throws to the examinee, positioned at cone A. Each thrown ball must hit the ground in front of the 30-foot line with sufficient velocity to roll to the velocity indicator at cone C if not intercepted. A total of two practice trials and six test trials are taken. Balls are to be thrown in a random order, with two balls thrown directly to the examinee, two thrown to the examinee's left, and two thrown to the examinee's right.

Scoring

Points are based on how cleanly the examinee fields the ball and where the ball is fielded. Four points are given for balls cleanly fielded in front of the 60-foot line. Two points are given for bobbled balls taken in front of the 60-foot line. The score is halved if the ball is fielded behind the 60-foot line; that is, two points are given for a ball cleanly fielded behind the 60-foot line and 1 point is given for a bobbled ball taken behind the 60-foot line. *The test score is the sum of the six test trials.*

TEST 3: OVERHAND THROWING
Purpose

The purpose of this test is to assess skill in the overhand throw by measuring distance and placement.

Psychometric Information

Using judges' ratings as the criterion, concurrent validity coefficients ranged from .64 to .94; logical validity was also claimed. Test-retest intraclass reliability coefficients ranged from .90 to .97.

Field Markings

As shown in Figure 11-30, a throwing line lies perpendicular to a restraining line. A back boundary line is also marked.

Equipment

This test requires several softballs, cones, measuring tape, score sheet, and pencil.

Procedure

After warming up with short throws for several minutes, the examinee begins just in front of the back boundary line. When ready, he or she takes a few steps and throws the ball as far and as straight along the throwing line as possible. The ball must be released before the restraining line. Two trials are taken.

Scoring

The throw is scored by subtracting the deviation score (i.e., the perpendicular distance from the throwing line) from the distance score. Scores are rounded to the nearest whole foot. *The test score is the net throwing score for the longer of the two throws.*

TEST 4: BASE RUNNING
Purpose

The purpose of this test is to assess skill in base running by measuring speed in running two bases.

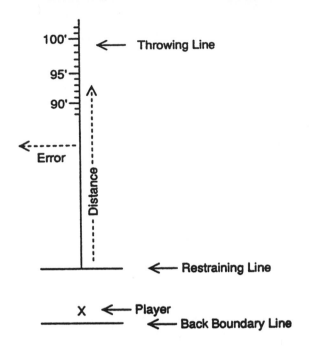

FIGURE 11-30

Field markings for the AAHPERD Softball Throwing Test. (Reprinted with permission from Rikli, R.E. (ed.): Softball Skills Test Manual. Reston, VA, AAHPERD, 1991.)

Psychometric Information

Using judges' ratings as the criterion, concurrent validity coefficients ranged from .79 to .92; logical validity was also claimed. Test-retest intraclass reliability coefficients ranged from .89 to .95.

Facility Needs

This test requires a regulation softball diamond with regulation bases and 60-foot base paths.

Equipment

This test requires a stopwatch,; score sheet, and pencil.

Procedure

The examinee begins at home plate, indicated by position A on Figure 11-31. He or she runs as fast as possible from point A around first base to second base. (For safety the examinee should run through second base.) One warm-up run is allowed; two test trials are timed by a timer who begins at B1 and moves to B2 (Fig. 11-31).

Scoring

The trial is timed to the nearest 0.1 second. *The test score is the faster of the two trials.*

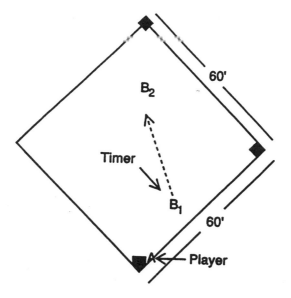

FIGURE 11-31

Field markings for the AAHPERD Softball Base Running Test. (Reprinted with permission from Rikli, R.E. (ed.): Softball Skills Test Manual. Reston, VA, AAHPERD, 1991.)

Batting Test From the Maver Softball Skills Test Battery

Purpose

The purpose of this test (Maver, D.J.: Maver softball skills test battery, unpublished paper, University of North Carolina at Greensboro, 1986) is to assess the skill with which an examinee can hit a pitched ball.

Gender and Age

This test is appropriate for high-school girls and college women of varying abilities.

Psychometric Information

This test is one of four that Maver recommends for a softball skills battery. The tests were administered to 15 female intercollegiate softball players, 15 female college students, 15 female high-school varsity softball players, and 15 female high-school students. An additional 10 female college students were administered the test while two persons scored and recorded to assess interscorer agreement.

A comparison of the means of the four test groups revealed that athletes performed better than students on the batting test. Intercorrelations between the batting test and the other three tests were low, suggesting that the tests assessed different skills. The batting test also had a high predictive value. Somewhat problematic is that the test-retest reliability for the batting test, at .42, was very low. The problem with the results of the batting test may have been that the subjects were tested in terms of slow or fast pitch according to the type of game they were playing. Three of the groups were playing slow pitch; only the college athletes were playing fast pitch. In essence, the subjects took two different tests that may not have combined well statistically.

Facility Needs

This test requires a regulation softball diamond, with personnel stationed as shown in Figure 11-32.

Equipment

This test requires bats, batting helmets, softballs, score sheet, and pencil.

Personnel

This test uses a pitcher who must be skilled at delivering a pitch consistent in speed and placement for fast pitch or consistent in arc and placement for slow pitch. Also needed are a trained observer who judges the type of hit made by the batter and an umpire who calls balls and strikes. For consistency, the same administrative personnel should be used for all examinees.

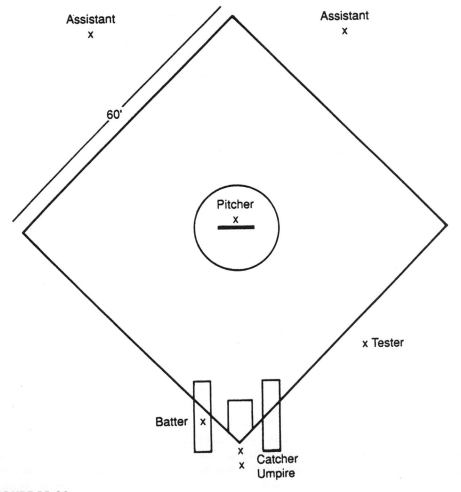

FIGURE 11-32

Field markings and personnel placement for the Maver Softball Batting Test. (Used with permission from Maver, D.J.: Maver softball skills test battery, unpublished paper, University of North Carolina at Greensboro, 1986.)

Procedure

The examinee, wearing a batting helmet, is positioned in the batter's box and receives nine opportunities to hit a pitched ball. The pitcher throws a fast ball or arc depending on whether the test is fast pitch or slow pitch. To achieve the highest possible score, the examinee should attempt to hit a line drive on each pitch. The test administrator says "pitch" prior to each pitch. If the examinee does not swing and the umpire calls it a ball, it does not count as one of the nine attempts; if a strike is called, it counts as an attempt. If the examinee swings, it counts as an attempt regardless of the umpire's call. Two practice swings are allowed.

Scoring

Zero points are given for a swing and miss, for a called strike when the examinee does not swing, and if the examinee steps out of the batter's box or onto home plate while swinging. One point is given for a foul or fly ball. A grounder receives two points. A line drive, defined as a ball hit in virtually a straight line from the point of contact with the bat, receives three points. *The test score is the sum of the points for the nine attempts.* The maximum score is 27.

Comments

Despite the low reliability coefficient that was reported for this test, it is included here as an alternative to the AAHPERD batting test that uses a tee. The Maver batting test is more gamelike. However, the test consumer should be aware of the reliability concerns. The Maver batting test is appropriate for practice and may also be useful for assessing improvement, for classification, and even as one factor in team selection.

Swimming

Rosentswieg Revision of the Fox Swimming Power Test (36)

Purpose

The purpose of this test is to assess power and form for the five basic swimming strokes: the front crawl, back crawl, side crawl, breaststroke, and elementary backstroke.

Gender and Age

This test is designed for college women.

Psychometric Information

Rosentswieg revised the Fox test by changing the starting procedures, by adding a rating form, and by testing five strokes (37). Test subjects included 184 college women. The form rating was correlated with the better of the power scores to show the relationship between the two components. These coefficients were .72 for the front crawl, .63 for the back crawl, .81 for the side crawl, .74 for the breaststroke, and .83 for the elementary backstroke. Test-retest reliability coefficients ranged from .89 to .96.

Pool Markings

The pool deck is marked off in 1-foot intervals beginning 8 feet from the shallow end to designate the starting line.

Equipment
This test requires a stopwatch, recording sheet, and pencil.

Procedure
The test is started by having an assistant stand to the side of the examinee, cradling the examinee's legs with the forearms so that the examinee's feet are at the surface of the water. The examinee sculls or floats horizontally with shoulders in line with the starting line. When ready, the examinee swims away from the assistant, using an arm stroke first. If a kick is made prior to the arm stroke, the trial is immediately halted. Trials include 12 arm strokes or six cycles, depending on the stroke. Two trials are taken.

Scoring
At the end of the allotted arm strokes, the distance at the shoulders is measured to the nearest whole foot. At the same time, a form is subjectively rated on a 5-point scale. The distance score is the better of the two trials. Both distance and the form rating are considered in the final assessment.

Comments
Although designed for college women, there is no apparent reason this test may not be used with other groups. These tests can be used for grading, assessment of improvement, and practice. Because no push-off from the side of the pool is permitted, this is a good assessment of stroke and kick efficiency.

Team Handball

Zinn Team Handball Skills Battery

Purpose
The purpose of this battery (Zinn, J.L.: Construction of a battery of team handball skills tests, unpublished master's thesis, University of Iowa, Iowa City, 1981) is to assess passing and throwing skills for team handball.

Gender and Age
This battery is designed for male and female high-school team handball players.

Psychometric Information
Using judge's ratings as the criterion, concurrent validity coefficients were .76 for the 9-m front throw, .71 for the dominant-hand speed pass, and .77 for the overhead pass. Test-retest reliability coefficients ranged from .82 to .89.

Comments
Team handball is gaining popularity in the United States. These three tests assess essential skills for this sport. The tests are appropriate for a variety of examinees and a variety of uses.

TEST 1: NINE-METER FRONT THROW
Purpose
The purpose of this test is to assess skill in the front throw for scoring.

Court Markings
A team handball goal is divided into scoring areas with ropes placed as shown in Figure 11-33. The free throw line at 9 m (29 feet 6 inches) should be clearly marked.

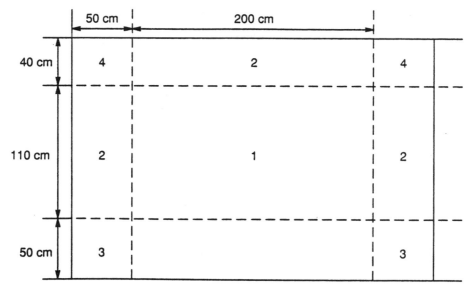

FIGURE 11-33

Target markings for the Zinn Team Handball Nine-Meter Throw Test. (Used with permission from Zinn, J.L.: Construction of a battery of team handball skills tests, unpublished master's thesis, University of Iowa, Iowa City, 1981.)

Equipment
This test requires team handballs, marked goal, ropes, score sheet, and pencil.

Procedure
The examinee takes 5 jump throws and 5 set throws at the marked goal. Up to three preparatory steps may be taken, but the examinee must not step on or over the free-throw line.

Scoring
Points based on difficulty are awarded for each throw. Zero points are given for throws that hit the court surface before entering the goal. *The test score is the sum of points awarded for 10 throws.* A maximum of 40 points is possible.

TEST 2: DOMINANT-HAND SPEED PASS
Purpose
The purpose of this test is to assess skill in the speed pass with the dominant hand.

Court Markings
A restraining line is marked 2.5 meters from and parallel to a smooth wall surface.

Equipment
This test requires team handball, stopwatch, score sheet, and pencil.

Procedure
The examinee is positioned behind the restraining line with a team handball. On a "begin" signal the examinee throws the ball to the wall with the dominant hand.

He or she catches the rebound with both hands. These actions are repeated as quickly as possible until 10 bounces have hit the wall. All throws must be from behind the restraining line. A stopwatch is started when the ball first contacts the wall and is stopped when the ball hits the wall on the 10th bounce. Two trials are given.

Scoring
Time is recorded to the nearest 0.1 second. *The test score is the better of the two timed trials.*

TEST 3: OVERHEAD PASS
Purpose
The purpose of this test is to assess skill in the overhead pass.

Court Markings
A target is marked on a wall (Fig. 11-34). The concentric circles have diameters of 45, 95, and 150 cm. The bottom edge of the outer circle is 100 cm high. A restraining line is marked 15 m from the wall target.

Equipment
This test requires team handballs, score sheet, and pencil.

Procedure
From behind the restraining line, the examinee does a total of 10 one-armed overhead passes at the target.

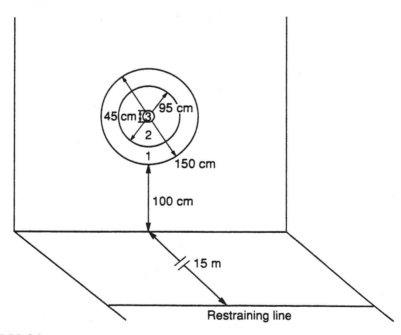

FIGURE 11-34

Target markings for the Zinn Team Handball Overhead Pass Test. (Used with permission from Zinn, J.L.: Construction of a battery of team handball skills tests, unpublished master's thesis, University of Iowa, Iowa City, 1981.)

Scoring

A pass that hits on or within the inner circle earns three points; a pass that hits on or within the middle circle earns two points; a pass that hits on or within the outer concentric circle earns 1 point. *The test score is the sum of the points for 10 passes.* A maximum of 30 points is possible.

Tennis

AAHPERD Tennis Skills Test (38)

Purpose

The purpose of this battery is to assess skill in the essential skills of tennis.

Gender and Age

This battery is designed for both genders, grade 9 through college.

Psychometric Information

Using judges' ratings as the criterion, concurrent validity coefficients for both genders of high school and college age ranged from .78 to .91 for the serve test and from .76 to .86 for the groundstroke test. Intraclass test-retest reliability coefficients ranged from .79 to .95 for the serve test and from .80 to .88 for the groundstroke test.

Comments

The AAHPERD tennis skills test battery consists of a serve test, a groundstroke test, and an optional volley test. Only the serve and groundstroke tests are presented here. Both tests employ an interesting and effective approach to the assessment of placement and power. Selected percentile norms are presented in Table 11-6. The interested test consumer should see the test manual for further information.

TEST 1: SERVE

Purpose

The purpose of this test is to assess placement and power in the tennis serve.

Court Markings

A regulation tennis court is marked as shown in Figure 11-35.

Equipment

This test requires tennis rackets and balls, score sheet, and pencil.

Procedure

The examinee serves eight balls from each of the two serving positions labeled with an S in Figure 11-35. Four balls are to be served to the outside target area and four are to be served to the inside target area.

Scoring

Each serve attempt is scored for both placement and power (Fig. 11-36). Placement is scored according to the target area where the ball lands. Two points are given for a ball landing in the intended target area; one point is given for an otherwise legal serve that lands outside the intended target. Power is scored according to the power zone where the ball lands on its *second* bounce. *The test score is the sum of the placement and power points for the 16 serves.* The maximum test score is 64. A balls that lands on a line is scored at the higher value.

TABLE 11-6	Selected Percentile Norms for the AAHPERD Tennis Skills Test Battery

BOYS AND MEN					
Test	Percentile	Grade 9	Grade 10	Grade 11	Grade 12	College
SERVE						
	99	44	50	54	52	64
	75	21	26	31	33	37
	50	15	19	25	27	29
	25	8	12	18	21	21
GROUNDSTROKE						
	99	97	108	107	109	124
	75	57	65	63	66	77
	50	45	53	51	54	63
	25	33	41	38	42	49

GIRLS AND WOMEN					
Test	Percentile	Grade 9	Grade 10	Grade 11	Grade 12	College
SERVE						
	99	34	50	49	52	50
	75	16	26	26	31	28
	50	11	19	19	25	22
	25	6	12	13	19	16
GROUNDSTROKE						
	99	94	92	108	104	105
	75	46	49	56	62	63
	50	32	37	41	50	50
	25	18	25	27	38	38

Adapted from Hensley, L.D. (ed.): Tennis Skills Test Manual. Reston, VA, American Alliance for Health, Physical Education, Recreation and Dance, 1989.

Comments

If this test is used for diagnosis, the placement and power scores should be recorded separately.

TEST 2: GROUNDSTROKE TEST

Purpose

The purpose of this test is to assess power and placement of the forehand and backhand groundstrokes.

Court Markings

A regulation tennis court is marked as shown in Figure 11-37.

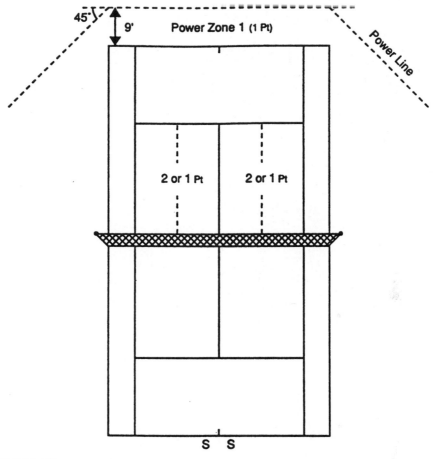

FIGURE 11-35

Court markings for the AAHPERD Tennis Serve Test. (Reprinted with permission from Hensley, L.D. (ed.): Tennis Skills Test Manual. Reston, VA, AAHPERD, 1989.)

Equipment
This test requires tennis rackets and balls, score sheet, and pencil.

Procedure
The examinee is positioned just behind the baseline at the center of court at point S, and the test administrator is positioned close to the net at point T. The tester tosses 12 balls to the examinee's forehand side and 12 balls to the examinee's backhand side. The first two balls on each side are practice trials; the other 10 are scored. For each trial the examinee attempts to drive the ball deep into the opposite court.

Scoring
Each groundstroke is scored for both placement and power (Fig. 11-38). Placement is scored according to the target area in which the ball first bounces. The max-

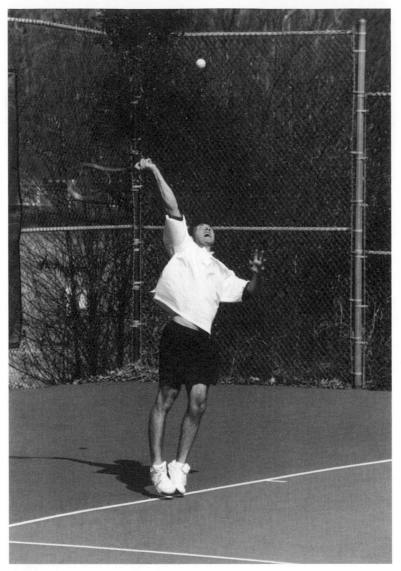

FIGURE 11-36

A serve that bounces first in the intended serve target area and then bounces to the deep power zone receives 4 points. (Photo by John Bell, Touch a Life Photography, Greensboro, NC.)

imum placement score for the 20 groundstrokes is 80. Power is scored according to the power zone where the ball lands on its *second* bounce. The maximum power score for the 20 groundstroke is 60. *The test score is the sum of the placement and power points for the 20 groundstrokes.* The maximum test score is 140. A ball that lands on a line is scored at the higher value.

Comments

If this test is used for diagnosis, the placement and power scores should be recorded separately for the forehand and backhand strokes.

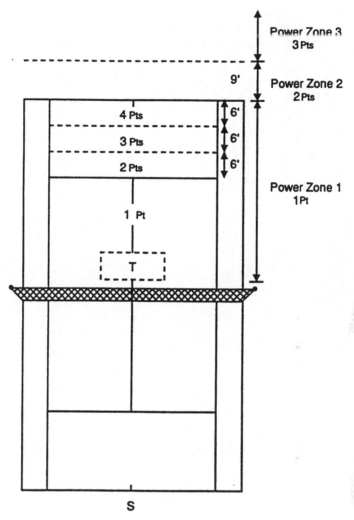

FIGURE 11-37

Court markings for the AAHPERD Tennis Groundstroke Test. (Reprinted with permission from Hensley, L.D. (ed.): Tennis Skills Test Manual. Reston, VA, AAHPERD, 1989.)

Hamer Mini-Match of Tennis Ability (39)

Purpose

The purpose of this test is to assess overall playing ability using a test that simulates actual play.

Gender and Age

This test is designed for college women at the beginning level.

Psychometric Information

Hamer used four beginning college tennis classes to investigate the appropriateness of a minimatch tournament to assess overall tennis playing ability. The official rules of the United States Lawn Tennis Association (USLTA) 7-out-of-12 tie break

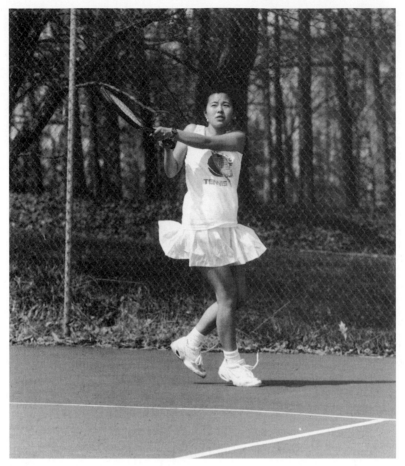

FIGURE 11-38

A groundstroke that bounces first in the deepest placement zone and then bounces to the deepest power zone receives 7 points. (Photo by John Bell, Touch a Life Photography, Greensboro, NC.)

were used for the minimatch round robin tournament in each class. The minimatch tournament was conducted during the fifth and sixth weeks of instruction. Each student was ranked within her class according to the number of wins and losses recorded. At the same time two judges rated each student once per week. Each student was ranked on the basis of the average of the four subjective ratings by the two judges.

Validity and reliability coefficients were calculated for each of the four classes. Validity coefficients ranged from .72 to .81, using Spearman rho for the correlation between the two rankings. Test-retest reliability coefficients, using chi square, ranged from .43 to .75. The reliability of the judges' ratings were calculated using ANOVA; estimates ranged from .87 to .93.

Procedures and Scoring

A group of players plays a round robin tournament in the minimatch format. Player A serves points 1 and 2, from the right, then left, courts. Player B serves points 3 and 4. Player A serves points 5 and 6. The players change sides. Player B serves points 7 and 8. Player A serves points 9 and 10. Player B serves points 11 and 12.

An examinee wins the match by winning 7 points or more and being at least 2 points ahead of the opponent. If the score reaches 6 points each, the players change sides and play continues with the serve alternating on every point until one player establishes a margin of 2 points, as follows: player A serves point 13 from the right court. Player B serves point 14 from the right court. Player A serves point 15 from the left court. Player B serves point 16 from the left court. If the score is still tied, the players change sides every 4 points and repeat this procedure.

Comments

This test can be used as a motivational technique, as an assessment of playing improvement during a teaching unit, and as a partial measure of overall tennis playing ability. One advantage of the test is that it is very gamelike and has high validity. Ideally the reliability coefficients should be higher. This might be achieved with a double round robin tournament conducted later in a unit, when skill performance is more stable.

Volleyball

North Carolina State University Volleyball Skills Test Battery (40)

Purpose
The purpose of this battery is to assess skill in the volleyball serve, forearm pass, and set in gamelike situations.

Gender and Age
This battery is designed for college-age volleyball players of both genders at the beginning level.

Psychometric Information
The authors claimed logical validity. Reliability data were collected on 313 male and female college students enrolled in beginning volleyball classes. Intraclass test-retest reliability coefficients with 2 days between administrations of each test were .65 for the serve test, .73 for the forearm pass test, and .88 for the set test.

Comments
The gamelike qualities of these tests are very appealing. The individual tests and the entire battery may serve many purposes. Net height, string height, and court positions can be modified if needed for use with different groups.

TEST 1: SERVE
Purpose
The purpose of this test is to assess consistency and accuracy of the overhand or underhand serve.

Court Markings
The court is marked as shown in Figure 11-39.

Facility Needs
This test requires a regulation volleyball court with net at 7 feet 11⅝ inches and antennae mounted on net.

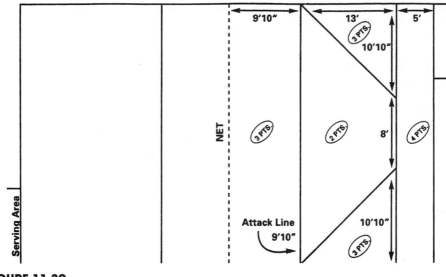

FIGURE 11-39

Court setup for the North Carolina State University Volleyball Serve Test. (Reprinted with permission from Bartlett, J., Smith, L., Davis, K., and Peel, J.: Development of a valid volleyball skills test battery. Journal of Physical Education, Recreation, and Dance, 62(2):19, 1991.)

Equipment

This test requires volleyballs, score sheet, and pencil.

Procedure

From the service area the examinee attempts either 10 overhand or 10 underhand serves.

Scoring

Points are awarded for each of the 10 serve attempts. Balls landing on a line receive the higher point value. Zero points are given for serves that go out of bounds or that hit the net or antennae. *The test score is the sum of all 10 serve attempts.* The maximum score possible is 40.

TEST 2: FOREARM PASS TEST

Purpose

The purpose of this test is to assess accuracy, height, and consistency in the forearm pass.

Court Markings

The court is marked as shown in Figure 11-40. In addition to the markings, an 8-foot-high string is extended over the court in line with the attack line.

Equipment

This test requires volleyballs, 30-foot-long string, two 8-foot vertical poles, score sheet, and pencil.

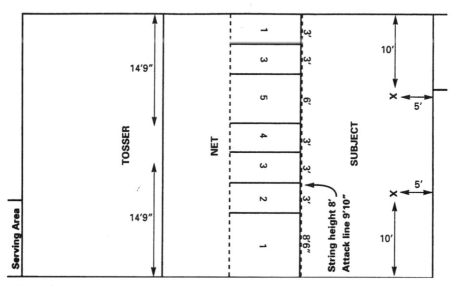

FIGURE 11-40

Court setup for the North Carolina State University Volleyball Forearm Pass Test. (Reprinted with permission from Bartlett, J., Smith, L., Davis, K., and Peel, J.: Development of a valid volleyball skills test battery. Journal of Physical Education, Recreation, and Dance, 62(2):19, 1991.)

Procedure

Examinees receive a total of 10 pass attempts; five are taken from the right back position and five from the left back position. For each attempt a tosser tosses a ball over the net to the intended receiving area using a two-handed overhead toss. Poor tosses should be repeated. The examinee uses a forearm pass to send the ball over the 8-foot string and into a target area.

Scoring

Points are awarded according to the target values. Balls that land on a line receive the higher point value. Zero points are given for passes made with illegal contact, for passes that hit or go under the string, and for passes that go over or hit the net. *The test score is the sum of the points for the 10 attempts.* The maximum possible score is 50 points.

TEST 3: SET
Purpose

The purpose of this test is to assess consistency, height, and accuracy of the high set.

Court Markings

The court is marked as shown in Figure 11-41. In addition to the court markings, a 10-foot-high string is extended over the court perpendicular to the net.

Equipment

This test requires volleyballs, 11-foot string, two 10-foot vertical poles, score sheet, and pencil.

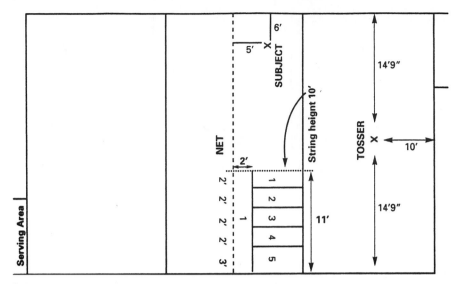

FIGURE 11-41

Court set-up for the North Carolina State University Volleyball Set Test. (Reprinted with permission from Bartlett, J., Smith, L., Davis, K., and Peel, J.: Development of a valid volleyball skills test battery. Journal of Physical Education, Recreation, and Dance, 62(2):19, 1991.)

Procedure

The examinee begins at a point 6 feet from the right sideline and 5 feet back from the net. A tosser is positioned near the center of the court 10 feet from the back line. The tosser tosses a ball underhand to the examinee. Poor tosses should be repeated. The examinee attempts to set the tossed ball over the 10-foot string and into the target area. The examinee performs 10 set attempts.

Scoring

Points are awarded according to the target values. Balls that land on a line receive the higher point value. Zero points are given for illegal contact, sets that hit or go under the string, and for sets that go over or hit the net. *The test score is the sum of the points for the 10 attempts.* The maximum possible score is 50 points.

Chapter Summary

Motor skill competence is the unique contribution of physical education to the school curriculum and the primary goal of school and community athletic programs. It is important, therefore, that practitioners who work in these settings be prepared to assess sport skill proficiency. This chapter begins with a presentation and explanation of a psychomotor taxonomy by Goldberger and Moyer. The Goldberger and Moyer taxonomy can be used to classify all human movements on the basis of their psychomotor attributes, anatomical division of body parts used, and psychomotor form. The psychomotor taxonomy provides practitioners with a context for the motor skill learning and performance goals that they set for their clients.

The many reasons to use a sport skill test are reviewed. Much of the rest of the chapter is devoted to the presentation of 41 sport skill tests or rating scales in 16 sports. Each test is presented in detail so the practitioner can administer the test and interpret test scores.

SELF-TEST QUESTIONS

1. What is the Goldberger and Moyer taxonomic classification of the skills that are assessed by most traditional sport skill tests?
   A. Algorithmic movement forms
   B. Complex movement forms
   C. Interpretive movement forms
   D. Universal movement forms

2. Which of the following is used to assess sport skill during play?
   A. Bobrich Badminton Rating Scale
   B. Hamer Mini-Match of Tennis Ability
   C. The PIMSPARS
   D. All of the above

3. Which of the following is a common characteristic of traditional sport skill tests?
   A. They assess the form used by the examinee.
   B. They assess combinations of skills.
   C. They are used to assess the skill levels of several examinees simultaneously.
   D. The performance conditions are standardized.

4. According to motor learning specialists, why are sport skill tests especially effective for practice?
   A. The performer may be motivated by the test conditions.
   B. The performer receives objective feedback about his or her performance.
   C. The performer may perceive the practice as meaningful.
   D. All of the above.

5. What psychometric characteristic is most threatened by a softball skills test battery that does *not* include a batting test?
   A. Concurrent validity
   B. Content validity
   C. Test-retest reliability
   D. All of the above

6. What is the minimum number of trials needed to ensure good reliability for a sport skill test that assesses accuracy (e.g., an archery or golf putting test)?
   A. 2 trials
   B. 3 trials
   C. 10 trials
   D. 20 trials

7. An archer shoots two ends of arrows from 20 yards. He misses the target on two arrows and scores the following on the other arrows:

POINT VALUE (TARGET AREA)	NUMBER OF ARROWS
9 (gold; bull's-eye)	1
7 (red)	2
5 (blue)	2
3 (black)	2
1 (white)	3

According to the Shifflett & Shuman Criterion-Referenced Archery Test, is this archer a master? _____

8. Which test is most appropriate for use with advanced players?
   A. Boetell Basketball Rating Scale
   B. Chapman Ball Control Test for field hockey
   C. French Short Serve Test for badminton
   D. Jacobson-Borleske Touch Football Test Battery

9. What is the mean T-score for an 8th-grade boy who receives the following scores on the Jacobson-Borleske Touch Football Test?

   _____

TEST	RAW SCORE
Forward pass for distance	20 yards
Punt for distance	25 yards
Run for time	10.0 seconds

10. A gymnast performs a tinsica (a floor exercise move) with good form and good balance and control, but the tinsica lacks amplitude because of a mechanical flaw. How many points would she receive for this move on the Ellenbrand Gymnastics Skills Test?
    A. 2 points
    B. 3 points
    C. 6 points
    D. 8 points

11. Calculate the winning percentage value for a female beginning racquetball player who scores 20 points on the Valcourt Ceiling Shot Placement Test and 30 points on the Valcourt Long Wall Volleying Test. _____

12. Which PIMSPARS key behavior is defined as "movement into space or away from the ball in an attempt to create opportunity for a response by a teammate in possession of the ball or to increase the attacking potential of the team"?
    A. Assisting
    B. Hustling
    C. Jockeying
    D. Maneuvering and Faking

ANSWERS

1. B	2. D	3. D	4. D	5. B	6. C
7. No	8. B	9. 40	10. D	11. 96%	12. C

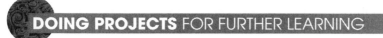

DOING PROJECTS FOR FURTHER LEARNING

1. Nothing beats hands-on experience. Select a sport skill test or rating scale that you may one day want to use and administer it to an appropriate group. This may be some of your classmates, some of your intramural teammates, students at a local school, or youth involved in a local community sport program. Before administering the test, plan for efficient and effective administration using some of the ideas you learned in Chapter 3. After the test, analyze the test scores using some of the techniques learned in Chapters 4 to 6. Finally, sit down with the examinees and explain their test results to them.

2. Construct your own sport skill test. This is easier said than done, but there are some excellent references to help you. In particular, we recommend Chapter 15, "Constructing Sports Skills Tests," in *Introduction to Measurement in Physical Education and Exercise Science* by Safrit and Wood (41). Another excellent reference is Chapter 2, "Selecting and Constructing Tests," in *Assessing Sport Skills* by Strand and Wilson (9).

REFERENCES

1. Barrow, H.M., McGee, R., and Tritschler, K.A.: Practical Measurement in Physical Education and Sport. 4th ed. Baltimore, Williams & Wilkins, 1989.
2. Goldberger, M., and Moyer, S.: A schema for classifying educational objectives in the psychomotor domain. Quest, 34(2):134, 1982.
3. Harrow, A.J.: A Taxonomy of the Psychomotor Domain: A Guide for Developing Behavioral Objectives. 2nd ed. White Plains, NY, Longman, 1979.
4. Jewett, A., Jones, L.S., Luneke, S., and Robinson, S.: Educational change through a taxonomy for writing physical education objectives. Quest, 15(1):32, 1971.
5. Simpson, E.J.: The classification of educational objectives, psychomotor domain. Illinois Teacher of Home Economics, 3(1):110, 1966.
6. Seefeldt, V., and Vogel, P.: Children and fitness: a public health perspective. Research Quarterly for Exercise and Sport, 58:331, 1987.
7. Schmidt, R.A.: Motor Learning and Performance. 2nd ed. Champaign, IL, Human Kinetics, 1999.
8. Achtzehn, R.H.: Sports skill quotient test. Journal of Physical Education and Recreation, 50(3):72, March 1979.
9. Strand, B.N., and Wilson, R.: Assessing Sport Skills. Champaign, IL, Human Kinetics, 1993.
10. Collins, D.R., and Hodges, P.B.: A Comprehensive Guide to Sports Skills Tests and Measurement. Springfield, IL, Thomas, 1978.
11. Kemp, J., and Vincent, M.F.: Kemp-Vincent rally test of tennis skill. Research Quarterly, 39:1000, 1968.
12. Kehtel, E.H.: The development of a test to measure the ability of a softball player to field a ground ball and successfully throw it at a target. Master's thesis, University of Colorado, Boulder, 1958.

13. Ocansey, R.T.A., and Kutame, M.A.: Measuring soccer playing ability in natural settings. Journal of Physical Education, Recreation, and Dance, 62(7): 54, 1991.

14. Ishee, J.H., and Shannon, J.L.: Scoring collegiate archery. Perceptual and Motor Skills, 57:525, 1983.

15. Shifflett, B., and Shuman, B.J.: A criterion-referenced test for archery. Research Quarterly for Exercise and Sport, 53:330, 1982.

16. Lockhart, A., and McPherson, F.A.: The development of a test of badminton playing ability. Research Quarterly, 20:402, 1949.

17. Scott, M.G., Carpenter, A., French, E., and Kuhl, L.: Achievement examinations in badminton. Research Quarterly, 12:242, May 1941.

18. Cotten, D.J., Cobb, P.R., and Fleming, J.: Development and validation of a badminton clear test. Research Abstracts. American Alliance of Health, Physical Education, Recreation, and Dance National Convention, Las Vegas, April 13–17, 1987, p. 168.

19. Bobrich, M.N.: Reliability of an evaluative tool used to measure badminton skill. Master's thesis, George Williams College, 1972.

20. Hopkins, D.R., Shick, J., and Plack, J.J.: Basketball Skills Test Manual for Boys and Girls. Reston, VA, American Alliance of Health, Physical Education, Recreation, and Dance, 1984.

21. Boetel, N.A.: Factorial approach in the development of a basketball rating scale to evaluate players in a game situation. Doctoral dissertation, University of North Carolina at Greensboro, 1976.

22. Chapman, N.L.: Chapman ball control test: field hockey. Research Quarterly for Exercise and Sport, 53:239, 1982.

23. Jacobson, T.V.: An evaluation of performance in certain physical ability tests administered to selected secondary school boys. Master's thesis, University of Washington, Seattle, 1960.

24. Borleske, S.E.: A study of achievement of college men in touch football. Master's thesis, University of California, Berkeley, 1936.

25. Shick, J., and Berg, N.G.: Indoor golf skill test for junior high school boys. Research Quarterly for Exercise and Sport, 54:75, 1983.

26. Neal, C.: The value of variation in grip in selected sports for women in compensating factors for sex difference in strength. Master's thesis, University of Iowa, Iowa City, 1951.

27. Ellenbrand, D.A.: Gymnastics skills test for college women. Master's thesis, Indiana University, 1973.

28. Ennis, C.D.: The development of a multi-skill test in lacrosse for college women. Master's thesis, The University of North Carolina at Greensboro, 1977.

29. Hodges, D.R.: Construction of an objective knowledge test and skills tests in lacrosse for college women. Master's thesis, University of North Carolina at Greensboro, 1967.

30. Valcourt, D.F.: Development of a racquetball skills test battery for male and female beginner and intermediate players. Master's thesis, Springfield College, 1982.

31. Buschner, C.A.: The validation of a racquetball skills tests for college men. Doctoral dissertation, Oklahoma State University, Stillwater, 1976.

32. Hensley, L.D., East, W.B., and Stillwell, J.L.: A racquetball skills test. Research Quarterly, 50:114, March 1979.

33. Mor, D., and Christian, V.: The development of a skill test battery to measure general soccer ability. North Carolina Journal of Health and Physical Education, 15(1):30, Spring 1979.

34. McDonald, L.G.: The construction of a kicking skill test as an index of general soccer ability. Master's thesis, Springfield College, 1951.

35. Rikli, R.E. (ed.): Softball Skills Test Manual. Reston, VA, American Alliance for Health, Physical Education, Recreation and Dance, 1991.

36. Rosentswieg, J.: A revision of the power swimming test. Research Quarterly, 39:818, 1968.

37. Fox, M.G.: Swimming power test. Research Quarterly, 28(10):233, October 1957.

38. Hensley, L.D. (ed.): Tennis skills test manual. Reston, VA, American Alliance for Health, Physical Education, Recreation and Dance, 1989.

39. Hamer, D.R.: The "mini-match" as a measurement of the ability of beginning tennis players. Doctoral dissertation, Indiana University, 1974.

40. Bartlett, J., Smith, L., Davis, K., and Peel, J.: Development of a valid volleyball skills test battery. Journal of Physical Education, Recreation, and Dance, 62(2):19, 1991.

41. Safrit, M.J., and Wood, T.M.: Introduction to Measurement in Physical Education and Exercise Science. 3rd Ed. St. Louis, Mosby–Year Book, 1995.

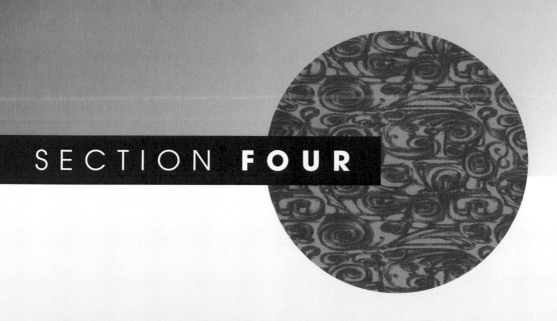

SECTION **FOUR**

Special Assessment Concerns

CHAPTER **12**

Assessing Body Image

Elizabeth A. Hart

Body image (Fig. 12-1) has been the subject of study during much of this century. Traditional approaches to body image assessment by psychologists, sociologists, and cultural anthropologists were instrumental in stimulating advances in the understanding of this interesting construct. More recently, researchers in exercise and sport science (ESS) have entered into the examination of body image. ESS researchers have been particularly concerned with the relationship between body image and physical activity because body image is thought to play an important part in our selection of physical activities and in our continued adherence to exercise programs. Measurement techniques developed by exercise and sport scientists have been used to compare different groups of individuals (e.g., athletic, sedentary, old, young, physically challenged), and to track changes in body image resulting from various interventions. Whether we are trying to lose a few pounds at the fitness club, rehabilitate from an injury, or prepare for an athletic event, our perceptions of our bodies can either motivate or deter us. Body image measurement and assessment are therefore important tools for the ESS practitioner.

This chapter presents and discusses a number of body image measures. It begins with a review of some of the traditional body image measurement techniques and tools, then focuses on several tools developed by ESS researchers. This chapter also addresses relationships of body image to eating and exercise behaviors. As you read this chapter, think creatively about what exercise and sport practitioners may learn from body image assessment of their clients.

As you read this chapter, watch for the following keywords:

Body image	Distorting image technique	Social physique anxiety
Discrepancy score	Physical self-worth	

What Is Body Image?

Despite extensive research by scientists from many disciplines, no commonly accepted definition of body image has emerged. This is because body image has been interpreted in many ways. Some researchers define it as the concept of one's body

409

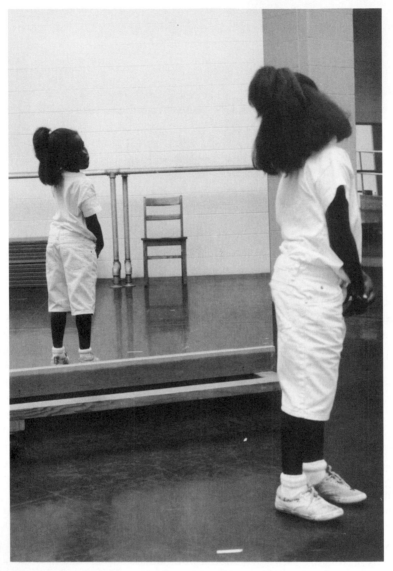

FIGURE 12-1

Body image concerns begin at an early age. (Photo by Marvin Arrington, Heritage Photography, Greensboro, NC.)

that grows out of the personality and affects the way one relates to others (1). Others suggest that body image is simply the mental representation of the body or the perceptual experience of one's body size (2). Still others consider it to be the subjective feelings associated with one's body (3). Rita Freedman, researcher and author of the popular nonfiction text *Bodylove*, offered the following definition of body image:

> 66 Each of us carries around an inner view of our outer self. This is your body image: a picture of the body as seen through the mind's eye. While this image is built on physical characteristics, it's also separate and distinct from them. . . .

Although it's imaginary, body image can feel as real as the body itself. It can be a constant source of strength or a chronic cause of pain. . . . Body image is a complex combination of attitudes, feelings and values. . . . In some ways it's a bit like intelligence (4)."

Also at issue among researchers is whether body image is exclusively a function of the overall appearance of one's body or is influenced by the appearance and functioning of selected body parts. In this chapter the term **body image** includes people's thoughts, feelings, and perceptions about their general appearance, body parts, and the physiological structures and functions of the body. These thoughts, feelings, and perceptions may or may not be consistent with reality.

> Body image is a psychological construct that develops from thoughts, feelings, and perceptions about one's own general appearance, body parts, and physiological structures and functions.

Traditional Body Image Assessment

Reflecting the many definitions of body image, traditional body image assessment tools are remarkably varied. They range from the clinical projective tests used by psychologists to the simple self-report questionnaires found in popular mainstream magazines. Most measures can be classified as either perceptual or attitudinal. Perceptual tools attempt to measure the degree to which one accurately assesses one's own body size. They require subjects to estimate the size of various body regions; their estimates are usually compared with actual measurements. Attitudinal measures explore the thoughts and feelings one has about one's body; they commonly take the form of self-report inventories.

Perceptual Measures of Body Image

Perceptual measures of body image include *body size estimation, distorting image techniques,* and *silhouette* techniques. These methods include body region or whole-body size estimation. Perceived dimensions are usually compared with true dimensions as measured by standard anthropometric tools or as assessed by an objective observer. Discrepancies between the perceived and actual measurements are interpreted as evidence of body image distortion.

Body Size Estimation

Body size estimation techniques include visual size estimation (VSE), the image marking procedure (IMP), and the body image detection device (BIDD). These techniques require calculation of a *body perception index* (BPI) for specified body regions such as the waist, hips, or thighs. BPI is calculated by Formula 12-1:

$$\text{BPI} = \frac{\text{Perceived size}}{\text{True size}} \times 100 \qquad \text{Formula 12-1}$$

where perceived size is a person's estimate of a specific body region and true size is the actual measured size of that body region.

VSE uses adjustable beams of light to simulate a person's perception of the sizes of various body regions. The IMP is a similar but simpler procedure. The subject of an IMP stands before a large piece of paper mounted on a wall. Imagining that he or she is standing in front of a mirror, the subject holds a pencil in each hand and marks the points where specific body regions would be seen in the reflection. Figure 12-2 shows a variation of the IMP. Use of the BIDD entails manipulation of templates on a standard overhead projector to adjust bands of light projected onto the wall to represent perceived body part size.

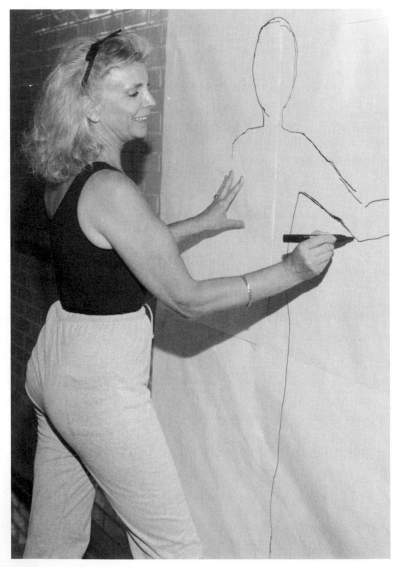

FIGURE 12-2

A variation of the Image Marking Procedure. (Photo by Marvin Arrington, Heritage Photography, Greensboro, NC.)

The BIDD, a relatively new perceptual technique, also has an attitudinal dimension. After estimating body part sizes, subjects are asked to provide a subjective appraisal of each body width on a scale of 0 to 100. An appraisal of 0 refers to physical dimensions grossly below the norm for the individual's age, gender and height, an appraisal of 50 represents normative physical dimensions, and an appraisal of 100 refers to physical dimensions grossly above the norm for the individual's age, gender and height. Higher scores occur when clients perceive their own body parts as larger than those of other persons similar to them in age, gender, and so on.

Distorting Image Techniques

Use of **distorting image techniques** entails estimation of overall body size rather than regions of the body. An early distorting image technique used an adjustable body-distorting mirror. This mirror could be bent to provide distorted images of the body. Subjects could adjust the mirror such that the resultant reflection represented how they "saw" their body. Similarly, the distorting photograph technique uses a variable camera lens that can distort a slide photograph by as much as 20% in directions of appearing fat and thin. More recent technology has created the video distortion technique, which electronically distorts the body image via a modified television camera.

> Distorting image techniques allow a person to alter an image of himself or herself so that it reflects that person's body image.

Silhouette Rating Scales

The use of silhouettes, or body size drawings, is a simple, time-efficient, and highly affordable way to assess perceptions of overall body size. A series of silhouettes representing various body sizes is presented to the subject, who is asked to select the silhouette that most closely resembles him or her. Both male and female silhouette series are available, with body sizes ranging from extremely thin to very obese. An example of male and female silhouette series is shown in Figure 12-3.

In addition to estimating current body image, individuals are sometimes asked to identify their "ideal" size using these techniques. Body size dissatisfaction is assessed by comparing the perceived current body size and shape (CBS) with the perceived ideal body size and shape (IBS). The IBS silhouette rating is subtracted from the CBS rating, and the resulting difference is the **discrepancy score.** The discrepancy score reveals the degree of body size dissatisfaction. Researchers hypothesize that discrepancy scores may offer evidence of unrealistic body image expectations.

> The body image discrepancy score is the difference between the perceived body size and shape and the ideal body size and shape.

The degree to which the CBS is elevated from norms assesses body image distortion, whereas the degree to which the IBS is depressed from norms indicates preference for a thin body size. Although the discrepancy score derived from CBS and IBS is regarded as body size dissatisfaction, it does not include attitudinal components. Therefore, it cannot be considered a comprehensive measure of body image disturbance.

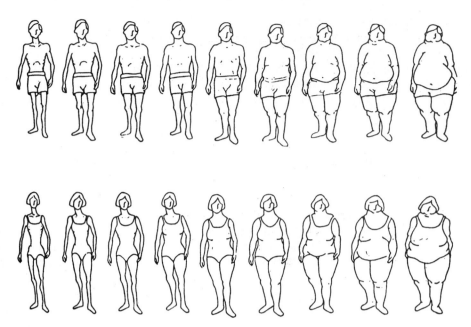

FIGURE 12-3

Full body silhouettes represent a continuum of various full body sizes. (Reprinted with permission from Stunkard, A., Sorensen, T., and Schulsinger, F.: Use of the Danish Adoption Register for the study of obesity and thinness. In Kety, S. (ed.): The Genetics of Neurological and Psychiatric Disorders. Philadelphia, Lippincott-Raven, 1980, pp. 115–120.)

In an effort to tap a wide range of physical self-perceptions, a variety of instructional protocols and related rating procedures have been developed for use with silhouettes. In addition to the standard instructions, which include "choose your ideal figure" and "choose the figure that reflects how you think you look," clients may be asked to "choose the figure that reflects how you feel most of the time." Alternative directions may also be given, such as "choose the figure that you think is most preferred by men," "choose the figure that you think is most preferred by women," or "pick the opposite-sex figure that you find most attractive."

Silhouette ratings can be transformed into three discrepancy measures that reflect various aspects of subjective body dissatisfaction. These include feel-ideal, think-ideal, and feel-think discrepancies. The use of these discrepancy scores allows

What Do YOU Think?

Subjects for a recent study were 35 male-and-female couples. Each of the 35 partnered women was asked to look at a series of photographs and identify the figure that she thought her partner would ideally want her to have. Results revealed that the women chose significantly thinner figures than their partners (5). What do YOU think about this research finding? Why do you suppose these women misjudged their partners' feelings?

for a finer evaluation of the affective aspects of body image. For example, the distance between affective and cognitive size ratings (indicating that a subject feels larger than he or she thinks he or she looks) has been positively associated with greater eating disturbance and lower self-esteem (6). In fact, investigations that rely solely on current size ratings may not capture the subtle affective aspects of body image disturbance. It is important to distinguish between the cognitive and affective aspects of body image, as these may suggest different treatments.

Other advances in silhouette techniques have resulted in greater specificity of body size estimation. For example, to accommodate variations in body regions, recent silhouette techniques include separate upper-body and lower-body series (Fig. 12-4).

The use of silhouettes for assessment of body image is conceptually straightforward and practically feasible. You may wonder, however, whether silhouette scales are also valid and reliable. Few psychometric investigations have been conducted on silhouette scales, yet the standard nine-silhouette rating scale has been widely used in several seminal studies on body image and eating disorders. Most studies demonstrate that silhouette scales have at least adequate validity and good test-retest reliability (7).

Analog Scales

Perceptions of body weight also constitute a major approach to body image assessment. Some researchers have constructed analog scales on which subjects are asked to indicate a point representing their body weight. One such analog scale, the Body

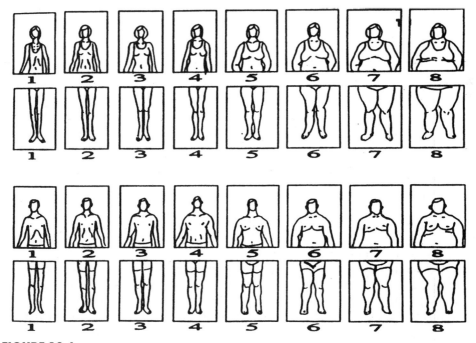

FIGURE 12-4

Split-body silhouettes offer dual continuums representing upper and lower body choices. (Reprinted with permission from Rodin, J.: Body Traps: Breaking the Binds that Keep You From Feeling Good About Your Body. New York, William Morrow, 1992.)

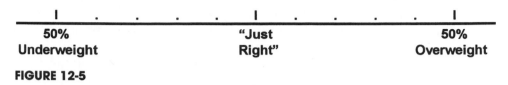

FIGURE 12-5

The Body Image Distortion Questionnaire. (Adapted from Mable, H.M., Balance, W.D.G., and Galgan, R.J.: Body-image distortion and dissatisfaction of university students. Perceptual and Motor Skills, 63:907, 1986.)

Image Distortion Questionnaire, shown in Figure 12-5, consists of a line with end points of 50% underweight and 50% overweight and a midpoint designated as just right (8). Use Formula 12-2 to quantify body image distortion:

$$\% \text{ Distortion} = \frac{\text{Perceived weight deviation}}{\substack{\text{Deviation of reported weight} \\ \text{from standard height-weight norms}}} - 1 \, (\times 100) \qquad \text{Formula 12-2}$$

 Body Build Computer Program

In addition to the perceptual measures already discussed, a computer program assesses body image perceptions (9). The program, Body Build, runs on a personal computer using a graphics adapter and color display. The subject interactively manipulates a body image until he or she is satisfied with the figure's appearance. The subject is asked to create three figures, the ideal body for the opposite sex (to familiarize them with the program), his or her ideal body, and his or her current body. Instructions are given by the computer before the participant draws each figure. For each drawing, the participant is presented with same-gender front and side images on which he or she can selectively manipulate the size of nine body parts by entering a value from 1 to 9. The introduction of computer technology offers exciting possibilities for future developments in body image assessment.

Attitudinal Measures

As stated earlier, attitudinal measures assess thoughts and feelings associated with body image perceptions. These assessments may focus on satisfaction with the gestalt (i.e., the whole body) or with specific body parts. Thoughts and feelings about one's body are related to perceived images, not actual images. For example, by objective standards of body fat and lean muscle mass, a ballet dancer may seem to have a "perfect body." If, however, the dancer perceives himself or herself as large and overweight, his or her body image will reflect these negative feelings. Perhaps you have witnessed this body image distortion in others who claim they are so fat, yet to you they look great.

Most body attitude measures are self-report inventories that are highly practical and efficient. Interview techniques requiring one-on-one attention are most often reserved for professional clinical assessments. Numerous self-report body attitude measures are available; they are often identified by such descriptors as body esteem, body dissatisfaction, body cathexis, or body self-relationships. Because of a relationship between eating disorders and body image, body image subscales are also included in some eating disorder inventories.

Body Cathexis Scale

Early attitudinal measures were characterized by the evaluation of individual body parts. The Body Cathexis Scale by Secord and Jourard (10) was one of the first instruments developed to assess feelings about the body. Respondents are asked to rate their feelings about 46 body parts and functions (e.g., "thighs," "appetite") using the following scale: 1, wish strongly a change could somehow be made; 2, don't like, but can put up with; 3, have no particular feelings one way or the other; 4, am satisfied; and 5, consider myself fortunate. The Body Cathexis Scale considers body image to be unidimensional, so it is scored by summing responses across all 46 items. Thus, a positive body image is represented by a high score, whereas a negative body image is represented by a low score.

Body Attitude Scale

Developers of the Body Attitude Scale (BAS) introduced body image as a multidimensional construct. The BAS assesses 30 body aspects along the three dimensions of evaluation, potency, and activity (11). Subjects are asked to rate each body aspect (e.g., width of shoulders, size of waist) on nine bipolar seven-point adjective scales. The evaluative dimension scales consist of good to bad, awkward to graceful, and beautiful to ugly. The potency dimension scales consist of weak to strong, hard to soft, and thin to thick. The activity dimension scales consist of active to passive, cold to hot, and fast to slow.

Initial research employing the BAS explored gender differences in body attitudes; women and girls were found to have more clearly differentiated ideas of what they liked and disliked about their bodies than men and boys (11). Male subjects, however, viewed their bodies as more potent and active. It was hypothesized that these differences were the result of gender role socialization. A related study found that there are many more advertisements for diet foods and "figure-enhancing" products in women's magazines than in men's magazines (12).

Body Consciousness Questionnaire

In addition to perceptions of shape and size or degrees of satisfaction and dissatisfaction with body parts, body feelings can be assessed in terms of general awareness. Applying the concept of self-consciousness to the body, the Body Consciousness Questionnaire (BCQ) was developed to measure the extent to which people distinguish private aspects of the body (internal sensations and feelings observed only by the person experiencing them) from the public aspects of the body (appearances and behaviors observable by others) (13). The BCQ is a 15-item self-report instrument with subscales for private body consciousness (PRBC), public body consciousness (PBBC), and body competence (BC). Respondents answer each item on a scale ranging from 0 (extremely uncharacteristic of me) to 4 (extremely characteristic of me). The PRBC subscale includes items such as "I know immediately when my mouth or throat gets dry" and "I'm very aware of changes in my body temperature." The PBBC subscale includes items such as "I think a lot about my body build" and "I'm concerned about my posture." The BC subscale includes items such as "For my size I'm pretty strong" and "I'm capable of moving quickly." Adequate test-retest reliability has been demonstrated for all three subscales (PRBC, r = .69; PBCS, r = .73; BC, r = .83) using a sample of 130 undergraduates who completed the BCQ over a 2-month period.

The BCQ offers a unique twist to the area of body perception and may be one of the more useful tools in physical activity settings. Rather than focusing on specific body parts or global attitudes about physical appearance, this inventory allows for assessment of internal body awareness and concern with social presentation of the body. Participation in exercise and sport involves both an awareness of body competence and private and public body consciousness. For example, some individuals may be more privately body conscious than others. A highly trained runner may notice even the slightest changes in body temperature and adjust his or her pace to accommodate this sensation. A novice tennis player, on the other hand, may be forced to forfeit because of heat exhaustion before recognizing the physiological sensations of overexertion. Similar differences can be demonstrated in public self-consciousness; for example, a professional body builder may be more closely aware of how his or her body is observed by others than is a recreational golfer.

Body Esteem Scale

Expanding on the original Body Cathexis Scale, the Body Esteem Scale (BES) was developed to explore the multidimensionality of body esteem (14). To develop the BES, the Body Cathexis Scale was administered to 366 women and 257 men undergraduate students. Students rated each item on a 5-point Likert scale. Factor analysis revealed three distinct body esteem factors for each gender: upper-body strength, attractiveness, and physical condition for men; attractiveness, weight concern, and physical condition for women. Items with low factor loadings were dropped. Several items deemed relevant to the newly defined factors were added, and a second principal component factor analysis was conducted with another sample of undergraduate students (301 men and 182 women). The result was the final 35-item Body Esteem Scale (Fig. 12-6).

Summing across all items of the BES produces an overall body esteem score, with high scores indicating body image satisfaction and low scores, dissatisfaction. For men and women separately, the three subscale scores are obtained by summing responses to items in each scale. Reliability coefficients of .81 for attractiveness, .85 for upper body strength, and .86 for physical condition were reported for 331 male undergraduates. Coefficients of .78 for attractiveness, .87 for weight concern, and .82 physical condition were reported for 633 female undergraduates.

Researchers using the BES have reported some notable trends that vary by gender (14). Body parts loading on the attractiveness factor for women tend to be those that cannot be changed through exercise and/or dietary restraint (e.g., nose, lips, breasts, eyes, cheekbones); change in these body parts would require cosmetic intervention (i.e., surgery, not just make-up). Body parts and processes that can be altered through exercise or diet tended to load on the weight concern factor (e.g., waist, hips, thighs, appetite, stomach). Not surprisingly, many of these body charac-

Instructions: On this page are listed a number of body parts and functions. Please read each item and indicate how you feel about this part or function of *your own body* using the following scale:

1. Have strong negative feelings
2. Have moderate negative feelings
3. Have no feelings one way or the other
4. Have moderate positive feelings
5. Have strong positive feelings

_____ 1. Body scent	_____ 19. Arms
_____ 2. Appetite	_____ 20. Chest or breasts
_____ 3. Nose	_____ 21. Appearance of eyes
_____ 4. Physical stamina	_____ 22. Cheeks and cheekbones
_____ 5. Reflexes	_____ 23. Hips
_____ 6. Lips	_____ 24. Legs
_____ 7. Muscular strength	_____ 25. Figure and physique
_____ 8. Waist	_____ 26. Sex drive
_____ 9. Energy level	_____ 27. Feet
_____ 10. Thighs	_____ 28. Sex organs
_____ 11. Ears	_____ 29. Appearance of stomach
_____ 12. Biceps	_____ 30. Health
_____ 13. Chin	_____ 31. Sex activities
_____ 14. Body build	_____ 32. Body hair
_____ 15. Physical coordination	_____ 33. Physical condition
_____ 16. Buttocks	_____ 34. Face
_____ 17. Agility	_____ 35. Weight
_____ 18. Width of shoulders	

Scoring Keys

Females

Sexual attractiveness: body scent, nose, lips, ears, chin, chest or breasts, appearance of eyes, cheeks and cheekbones, sex drive, sex organs, sex activities, body hair, face.

Weight concern: appetite, waist, thighs, body build, buttocks, hips, legs, figure or physique, appearance of stomach, weight.

Physical condition: physical stamina, reflexes, muscular strength, energy level, biceps, physical coordination, agility, health, physical condition.

Males

Physical attractiveness: nose, lips, ears, chin, buttocks, appearance of eyes, cheeks/cheekbones, hips, feet, sex organs, face.

Upper body strength: muscular strength, biceps, body build, physical coordination, width of shoulders, arms, chest or breasts, figure or physique, sex drive.

Physical condition: appetite, physical stamina, reflexes, waist, energy level, thighs, physical coordination, agility, figure or physique, appearance of stomach, health, physical condition, weight.

To determine an individual's score for a particular subscale of the BES, simply add up the individual scores given items on the subscale. For example, for female physical condition you would add up the individual's ratings of the items comprising the physical condition subscale (9 items).

FIGURE 12-6

Body Esteem Scale. (Reprinted with permission from Franzoi, S.L., and Shields, S.A.: The Body Esteem Scale: multidimensional structure and sex differences in a college population. Journal of Personality Assessment, 48:173, 1984.)

teristics are closely scrutinized by women in our society, as the media often portray unrealistic ideals. Unfortunately, some women may develop eating and/or exercise disorders as a result of pursuing mediated ideals of "the perfect body."

Men revealed a different trend. The attractiveness subscale included body parts associated with being handsome (e.g., chin, eyes, and body hair), as well as physique items (e.g., buttocks, hips). Unlike women, men did not demonstrate a clear distinction between factors influenced by diet and/or exercise and less easily modifiable physical characteristics. Upper body strength, however, appeared to have similarly unrealistic social ideals for men as weight concern did for women. For example, body characteristics associated with masculinity, (e.g., strength, biceps, chest, shoulders, and stomach) loaded on this factor (Fig. 12-7). As was found among

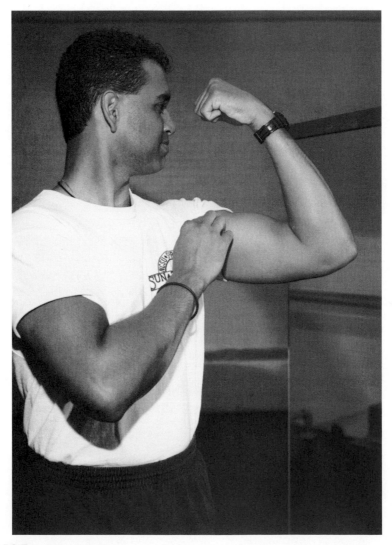

FIGURE 12-7

Men may associate biceps size with masculinity. (Photo by Marvin Arrington, Heritage Photography, Greensboro, NC.)

women, men may also be influenced by cultural ideals of the "perfect body." Mediated images of muscle-bound superheroes and the broad-shouldered, V-torsoed, tall, dark, and handsome man contribute to unrealistic body image aspirations for some men. This mediated male ideal may contribute to the observed increase in steroid use for cosmetic reasons among adolescent boys and young adult men.

The physical conditioning factor for both men and women included the obvious items of stamina, strength, and agility. Interestingly, the majority of the women's items on this factor typically do not come under public scrutiny unless physical activity is demonstrated (e.g., energy level, physical coordination, and condition). Men included items such as waist, stomach, and appetite not as appearance-related or weight concern items, but rather as physical condition items. It appears that men interpret these body parts and processes as interfering with or enhancing their physical condition. For example, the thirty-something recreational basketball player may be more concerned with how his "spare tire" affects his performance than with how it affects his appearance. ESS practitioners may use the BES to assess physical conditioning concerns.

Body Esteem Scale for Children

Because of assumptions of physical maturity and difficulty in use of Likert scales, use of the BES is limited to adult populations, which led to development of the Body Esteem Scale for Children (BES-C) (15). This 24-item self-report instrument is appropriate for second-grade readers. Similar to the adult BES, the BES-C assesses how a child values his or her appearance and body, using yes and no answers to 24 items such as "I like what I look like in pictures," "I wish I were thinner," and "I often wish I looked like someone else." The BES-C also assesses public self-consciousness by items such as "Kids my own age like my looks" and "Other people make fun of the way I look." The BES-C has demonstrated acceptable concurrent validity as indicated by a +.67 ($p < .002$) correlation with the Physical Appearance and Attributes subscale of the Piers-Harris Children's Self-Concept Scale. Body esteem scores calculated separately for odd and even items are significantly correlated ($r = .85, p < .002$), indicating that the BES-C yields good internal reliability.

Body Self-Relations Questionnaire

The Body Self-Relations Questionnaire (BSRQ) describes body image as a multidimensional self-attitude consisting of three psychological dimensions or dispositions: affective, cognitive, and behavioral. Unlike the BES, the BSRQ allows for direct gender comparisons because it has identical factors and items for both genders. Particularly interesting to ESS professionals, the BSRQ clearly distinguishes among the affective somatic (i.e., body) domains of appearance, fitness, and health. The BSRQ consists of a 140-item inventory with the three domains: appearance, fitness, and health, each having three conceptual subscales (evaluation, attention or importance, and activity), resulting in nine subscales. The affective component of body image is assessed by the evaluation subscale (i.e., liking, attainment, satisfaction). The cognitive component is assessed by the attention or importance subscale, and the behavioral component is indicated by the activity subscale (i.e., grooming, clothing, activity).

The Body-Self Relations Questionnaire: Short Form is a 54-item inventory developed from the original BSRQ (16). Each of the three domains has two attitudinal subscales for evaluation and orientation, resulting in six factors: appearance evaluation, appearance orientation, fitness evaluation, fitness orientation, health evaluation, and health orientation. The evaluation subscale assesses satisfaction, whereas the orientation subscale addresses the degree of importance and the behaviors related to maintaining or improving the domain. The integration of the importance and behavior items into a single orientation subscale was based on the high probability that people who value and attend to events in a given somatic domain are also likely to maintain and enhance activities in that domain.

The revised BSRQ: Short Form also includes illness orientation. The emergence of the illness orientation factor revealed that both genders regard motivation to maintain and enhance bodily wellness as relatively distinct from alertness to symptoms of physical illness. This distinction may be particularly useful for professionals interested in assessing health promotion, disease prevention, and illness profiles in selected populations. Selected items drawn from the revised BSRQ: Short Form are shown in Figure 12-8.

The revised BSRQ: Short Form along with a 9-item body areas satisfaction scale and six weight-related items received widespread exposure in 1985 when presented in a nationwide readership survey in *Psychology Today* (17). The authors were interested in changes in body image in the decade following a previous *Psychology Today* body image survey (18). A 2,000-person sample was selected from nearly 30,000 people who responded to the 1985 survey. As in the earlier survey, results with the revised multidimensional format revealed that women were more critical of and dissatisfied with their bodies than were men. And in the decade between the

Appearance

Evaluation: *I like the way I look without my clothes.*
Orientation: *It is important that I always look good.* (Importance)
              I check my appearance in a mirror whenever I can. (Behavior)

Physical Fitness

Evaluation: *I dislike my physique.*
Orientation: *It is unimportant that I have superior physical strength.* (Importance)
              I work to improve my physical stamina. (Behavior)

Health

Evaluation: *From day to day I never know how my body will feel.*
Orientation: *Good health is one of the most important things in my life.*
                                                              (Importance)
              I often read books and magazines that pertain to my health.
                                                              (Behavior)

Illness

Orientation: *I pay close attention to my body for any signs of illness.*

FIGURE 12-8

Sample items from the Revised BSRQ: Short Form. (Adapted from Cash, T.F.: The Multidimensional Body-Self Relations Questionnaire User's Manual. Norfolk, VA, Old Dominion University, 1994.)

surveys, the pressure to look good had intensified, particularly for men. Interestingly, women evaluated their fitness more harshly than men yet placed less importance and did fewer things, such as regular exercise, to improve it. In addition, men reported that exercise made them feel better about their bodies, while women reported exercise simply as a means of improving appearance, specifically by reducing body weight. A finding of particular relevance to ESS practitioners is that those who cared about fitness and health had more positive feelings about their appearance than did those who were primarily concerned with their appearance.

It was suggested that the findings reflect differences in the way the genders in our culture learn to regard their bodies. Even today there is evidence that boys are taught to be proud of themselves because they are strong and athletic, whereas girls are taught to value beauty. But among both genders, increasing numbers of children report a desire to lose weight primarily to improve their appearance. To contribute to a healthy body image, it is important that coaches and teachers emphasize the aspects of physical activity, such as the fitness and health benefits, that are not matters of appearance.

The 1997 version of the *Psychology Today* body image survey revealed that *both* genders are even more preoccupied with how they look than they were a decade ago (19). The results also indicated that our body shape preferences are growing thinner. The good news was that those who exercised regularly had more positive body feelings; this finding was true for both genders but very strong among the men. The relationship between body image and physical activity is not quite as simple as it might first seem. This is discussed in the next section.

Body Image and Physical Activity

There seems to be an obvious relationship between body image and physical activity. It is quite complicated, however, as illustrated by the following examples of body image experiences encountered in physical activity settings:

A college athlete takes pride in her athleticism and feels satisfied with the way her body moves on the basketball court yet perceives herself as fat.

A middle-aged man likes his facial features yet longs for greater muscularity when comparing himself with others in the weight room.

A woman is pleasantly surprised because she thought she had a 32-inch waist, but the tape measure reports it as only 29 inches.

A 70-year old woman perceives herself as weak, although she frequently picks up her 30-pound grandson with ease.

Although weighing exactly the same as when he walked his personal best, a recreational race walker feels fat one day and consequently does not give his total effort.

A professional bodybuilder perceives her biceps as small and does not feel confident about an upcoming competition.

There are obvious questions regarding the relationship between body image and physical activity. One is whether body image affects whether an individual exercises or not. If one does exercise, does body image affect the choice of activities? Related questions include whether body image influences who we exercise with, what we wear, and why we participate in the first place. Another interesting question is the reverse of the first question, that is, whether participation in physical activity affects one's body image. If so, are the changes positive or negative? What types of physical activity affect body image? Such questions are beginning to be investigated. For example, participation in Outward Bound programs has been found to improve self-scores on both physical ability and appearance (20). Involvement in exercise programs, such as aerobic dance and weight training, has resulted in positive body and self image scores (21–24).

ESS researchers and practitioners have traditionally focused their attention on objective body measurements, largely ignoring assessment of the attitudes and perceptions of the very foundation that creates movement, the human body. This is unfortunate because our attitudes and perceptions about our bodies can motivate or deter us from physical activity. For example, consider the case of two people who have recently put on some extra weight and are feeling dissatisfied with their bodies. One may be motivated to begin an exercise program; the other may be too embarrassed to be seen exercising. In support of this, exercise scientists have demonstrated that feelings about one's body determine whether one is likely to initiate and adhere to a physical activity program (25, 26). For example, overweight persons may not feel comfortable exercising in the presence of others whom they perceive as fit and lean.

The exercise and sport arena can be a significant environment for shaping one's body image. Consistently being picked last for kickball may contribute to a child's feeling of physical inadequacy and may discourage future participation in physical activity. Public weigh-ins and strict weight limits can be humiliating to athletes and may encourage unhealthy eating and exercise practices. It is important for ESS professionals to recognize the influence of experiences of physical activity on body attitudes and perceptions and the influence of body attitudes and perceptions on experiences of physical activity.

The interplay between physical activity and body image may have implications more far reaching than originally thought. According to recent research, improvement in specific physical subdomains (e.g., strength, body attractiveness) positively influences general physical self-perception, which in turn affects global self-esteem (26). Increased self-esteem is a common objective of exercise and sport programs. Traditionally, self-esteem has been viewed as unidimensional; more recent research suggests that it is multidimensional, involving a variety of domains including physical self-worth (27). For example, one may feel confident about his or her athletic skills but not academic skills. As depicted in Figure 12-9, self-perception is hierarchical, with global self-esteem representing the apex and physical self-worth representing a general domain. **Physical self-worth** is regarded as the general feeling of pride, self-respect, satisfaction, and confidence in the physical self. Physical self-worth contains specific physical self-perception subdomains, including sports competence, body attractiveness, physical strength, and physical condition. Therefore, one may feel that one's body is attractive yet may not feel confident about one's physical condition.

> Physical self-worth is the general feeling of pride, self-respect, satisfaction, and confidence in one's physical self.

According to this hierarchical model, physical self-worth mediates the relationship between global self-esteem and the four subdomains of physical self-perception. Thus, an individual's global self-esteem could be greatly affected by the

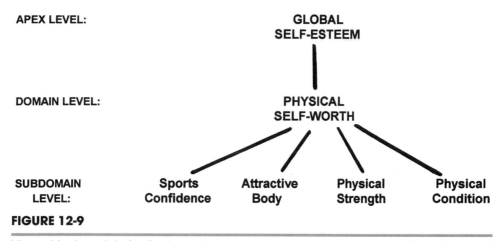

FIGURE 12-9

Hierarchical model of self-esteem includes a domain level of physical self-worth, as well as specific physical subdomains. (Reprinted with permission from Fox, K.R., and Corbin, C.B.: The Physical Self-Perception Profile: development and preliminary validation. Journal of Sport and Exercise Psychology, 11:408, 1989.)

perception of his or her physical appearance, but only if this subdomain significantly affects his or her physical self-worth.

Body Image Assessment and ESS

This section of text includes a number of body image assessment tools developed by ESS researchers. These tools are especially applicable for use in physical activity settings.

Physical Self-Perception Profile

The Physical Self-Perception Profile (PSPP) consists of five six-item subscales, each with a four-choice alternative format (28). Four of the subscales address four subdomains: sports competence, perceived body attractiveness, physical strength, and physical condition. A series of factor analyses refined the subscales and indicated that subjects' responses to the PSPP were adequately described by the four factors. The fifth subscale consists of items designed to measure the more general domain of physical self-worth.

The Perceived Importance Scale (PIP) was developed in conjunction with the PSPP to measure the subjective importance of each subscale (28). The combination of the PSPP and the PIP allows for greater specificity in physical self-perception analysis. For example, if a woman perceives physical strength as very important and general physical condition as relatively unimportant, her self-assessment on strength has greater influence on her physical self-worth than her assessment of her physical condition.

Physical Self-Efficacy Scale

The Physical Self-Efficacy Scale (PSES) was developed to address the limitations of global measures of self-concept for prediction of specific behaviors (26, 29). The PSES includes items relating to individuals' perceived physical competence, that is, assessing their beliefs in their physical abilities. Rather than specific body part perceptions such as "I like my legs," the 10-item perceived physical ability (PPA) subscale focuses on perceptions of bodily skills, such as "I am not agile and graceful" and "I can't run fast." In addition, PSES includes a unique 12-item physical self-presentation confidence (PSPC) subscale addressing confidence in displaying bodily skills to others, such as "People think negative things about me because of my posture" and "Because of my agility, I have been able to do things which many others could not do." Subjects are asked to respond to all items using a 6-point Likert scale. Overall physical self-efficacy (PSE) is calculated by summing PPA and PSPC.

Alpha-coefficients of .81 for the PSE subscale, .84 for the PPA subscale, and .74 for the PSPC subscale indicate that the PSES is internally stable. Test-retest reliability coefficients across a 6-week interval for PSE, PPA, and PSPC were .80, .85, and .69, respectively. Convergent, discriminant, and predictive validity have also been demonstrated.

Social Physique Anxiety Scale

A construct identified as social physique anxiety expanded the construct of physical self-presentation confidence by noting the effects of perceived social evaluation of one's body. As mentioned at the beginning of this chapter, unfavorable perceptions of one's body can either motivate or deter people from exercising. Intentions to engage in physical activity can be sabotaged by social factors. For example, the perception that others are evaluating one's body may lead to uncomfortable feelings in settings such as health clubs. A person may feel as if everyone is staring when no one is. Obviously, in some situations one's body is the subject of evaluation, such as during a body fat measurement. Regardless of whether the body is indeed being evaluated, the individual's perception that he or she is being scrutinized results in **social physique anxiety** (30). Most of us have been subjected to this phenomenon from time to time. Imagine the feelings you might have walking down a crowded beach in a bikini (Fig. 12-10). Imagine how you might feel entering a fitness facility filled with bodies notably leaner and better toned than your own.

> Social physique anxiety is a psychological construct resulting from uncomfortable feelings associated with the perception that one's body is being scrutinized by others.

The Social Physique Anxiety Scale (SPAS) (Fig. 12-11) was developed to assess anxiety in response to the prospect of or actual evaluation of one's body by others. The SPAS has demonstrated criterion-related validity, indicating that scores on the SPAS are related to anxiety during an actual evaluation of the physique. In a study designed to evaluate one's body shape and size, including body fat and muscle tone, highly socially physique-anxious (SPA) women reported more stress during the physique evaluation performed by a fitness professional than did low-SPA women. In addition, high-SPA women indicated that they felt less comfortable having their body evaluated by the fitness professional and had more frequent negative thoughts about their body's appearance during the evaluation than did the low-SPA women. Social physique anxiety may influence the degree to which people participate in social

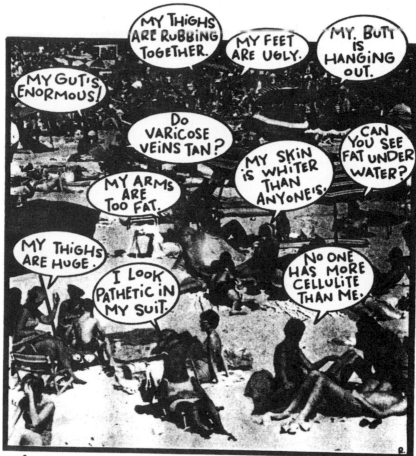

ANOTHER FUN DAY AT THE BEACH.

FIGURE 12-10

Certain environments may lead us to feel particularly self-conscious about our bodies. (Reprinted with permission from Hallmark Cards.)

exercise experiences. Related effects may include position selection and clothing preferences in social exercise settings (Hart, E., and Gill, D.L.: Protective self-presentation and exercise behavior. Unpublished paper, 1993). Have you met members of group exercise programs, such as aerobic dance, who prefer to exercise in the back of the room because they feel uncomfortable in the front? High-SPA individuals may feel uncomfortable in form-fitting exercise clothes and may cover up even when inappropriate (e.g., exercising outside in the summer heat in a long-sleeved sweatshirt and sweat pants versus shorts and a T-shirt).

Awareness of the influence of real or imagined body evaluation on physical activity participation can enable the ESS practitioner to make affected persons more comfortable. A negative body image may decrease one's motivation to participate in physical activity. Ironically, this very same body image may be a significant reason for engaging in sport and exercise.

Instructions: The following questionnaire contains statements concerning your body physique or figure. Physique or figure refers to body form and structure; specifically, body fat, muscular tone, and general proportions.

Read each item carefully and indicate how characteristic it is of you according to the following scale:

1. Not at all characteristic
2. Slightly characteristic of me
3. Moderately characteristic of me
4. Very characteristic of me
5. Extremely characteristic of me

_____   1. I am comfortable with the appearance of my physique/figure.
_____   2. I would never worry about wearing clothes that might make me look too thin or overweight.
_____   3. I wish I wasn't so uptight about my physique/figure.
_____   4. There are times when I am bothered by thoughts that other people are evaluating my weight or muscular development negatively.
_____   5. When I look in the mirror I feel good about my physique/figure.
_____   6. Unattractive features of my physique/figure make me nervous in certain social settings.
_____   7. In the presence of others, I feel apprehensive about my physique/figure.
_____   8. I am comfortable with how fit my body appears to others.
_____   9. It would make me uncomfortable to know others were evaluating my physique/figure.
_____ 10. When it comes to displaying my physique/figure to others, I am a shy person.
_____ 11. I usually feel relaxed when it's obvious that others are looking at my physique/figure.
_____ 12. When in a bathing suit, I often feel nervous about how well proportioned my body is.

Scoring

To determine an individual's score:
First, reverse scoring on items 1, 2, 5, 8, and 11. (If scored 1, change to 5; if scored 2, change to 4, and so on; a score of 3 is 3). Second, add up total score.

Norms
Original Means and Standard Deviations

Sample 1
Males (n = 98)	30.2	(7.50)
Females (n = 97)	37.9	(9.78)

Sample 2
Males (n = 115)	30.1	(8.49)
Females (n = 114)	37.0	(10.01)

FIGURE 12-11

Social Physique Anxiety Scale. (Reprinted with permission from Hart E.A., Leary M.R., and Rejeski, W.J.: The measurement of social physique anxiety. Journal of Sport and Exercise Psychology, 11(1):98, 1989.)

Reasons for Exercise Inventory

The Reasons for Exercise Inventory (REI) (Fig. 12-12) was constructed in an effort to assess why people engage in physical activity (31). This 24-item inventory includes seven general reasons for exercise: weight control, fitness, health, improving body tone, improving overall physical attractiveness, improving one's mood, and enjoyment. The seven subscales have adequate internal consistency. As we have discussed, weight control, body tone and physical attractiveness are related to body image, especially for women. Women, significantly more than men, report that they exercise for weight control (32, 33). Similarly, we noted earlier how men interpret fitness and health as significantly influencing body image.

Other Measures of Body Image

Often body image items or themes are included in broad sport science measurement instruments that assess global feelings of sport confidence or motivations for physical activity (34, 35). In addition, measures of perceived physical competence and physical estimation and attraction have been studied (36, 37). Many of these measures have been developed from more global psychological constructs such as general self-esteem and self-efficacy (38, 39). Although many sport-related affective measures include body image items, they usually focus more on sport skills than on body experiences.

Additional Reasons to Assess Body Image

During the 1990s body image gained increased attention as a result of its clinical role in disorders such as anorexia and bulimia, steroid use, *exercise dependence*, and obesity. ESS practitioners must be aware of the relationship between body image and these factors, as we may have to deal with these concerns.

Body Image and Eating Disorders

Body image distortion is common among those who have anorexia nervosa or bulimia nervosa. Literature consistently documents greater incidence of body image dysfunction and eating disturbance in women and girls than in men and boys. The extreme motivation to attain a low body weight and a very thin body is called drive for thinness, a characteristic of some eating disorders (Fig. 12-13). Many of the measures designed to assess eating disorders include a body image subscale. A few of these inventories are briefly discussed next. For a more comprehensive discussion of these eating disorder inventories, please refer to the referenced sources. The following tools should be used by a trained clinician only; they are included here for informational purposes only. If you suspect an eating disorder, you must refer the person to a trained clinician.

Eating Attitudes Test

The Eating Attitudes Test (EAT) is a 26-item self-report measure of attitudinal and behavioral characteristics commonly found in persons with anorexia nervosa or bulimia nervosa (40). Individual items are rated on a 6-point scale from never to always, and an overall score is obtained by summing all 26 items. The higher the scores, the more strongly it suggests disturbed attitudes toward food, weight, and eating. The EAT has

People exercise for a variety of reasons. When people are asked why they exercise, their answers are sometimes based on the reasons they believe they *should* have for exercising. What we want to know are the reasons people *actually* have for exercising. Please respond to the items below as honestly as possible. To what extent is each of the following an important reason you have for exercising? Use the scale below, ranging form 1 to 7, in giving your answers.

          1   2   3   4   5   6   7

    not at all   moderately   extremely

    important   important   important

Weight Control

_____   To be slim

_____   To lose weight

_____   To maintain my current weight

Fitness

_____   To improve my muscle tone

_____   To improve my strength

_____   To improve my endurance, stamina

_____   To improve my flexibility, coordination

Mood

_____   To cope with sadness, depression

_____   To cope with stress, anxiety

_____   To increase my energy level

_____   To improve my mood

Health

_____   To improve my cardiovascular fitness

_____   To improve my overall health

_____   To increase my resistance to illness and disease

_____   To maintain my physical well-being

Attractiveness

_____   To improve my appearance

_____   To be sexually desirable

_____   To be attractive to members of the opposite sex

Enjoyment

_____   To meet new people

_____   To socialize with friends

_____   To have fun

Tone

_____   To redistribute my weight

_____   To improve my overall body shape

_____   To alter a specific area of my body

Scoring

Note: In the questionnaire items are presented in random order without category headings. Headings are included here for appropriate categorization of questions for scoring. Add scores given to each item within each category to determine specific category scores.

FIGURE 12-12

Reasons for Exercise Inventory. (Reprinted with permission from Silberstein, L.R., Striegel-Moore, R.H., Timko, C., and Rodin, J.: Behavioral and psychological implications of body dissatisfaction: do men and women differ? Sex Roles, 19:219, 1988.)

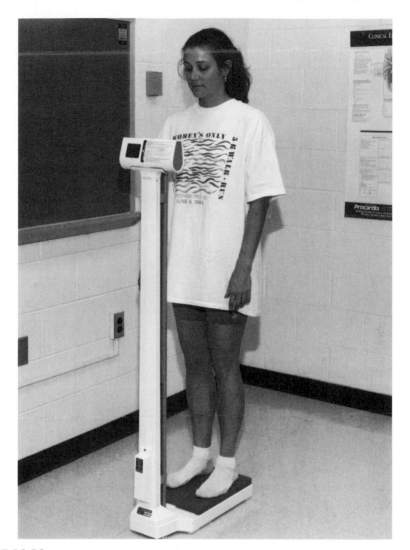

FIGURE 12-13

Excessive concern with body weight may be associated with an eating disorder. (Photo by Marvin Arrington, Heritage Photography, Greensboro, NC.)

satisfactory test-retest reliability (r = .88), and has been found to differentiate among various populations (i.e., those with anorexia, those with bulimia, and normals).

Bulimia Test

The Bulimia Test is a self-report inventory that identifies those with bulimia nervosa (41). This self-report inventory, which is scored to yield a total, demonstrates adequate test-retest reliability (r = .87).

Eating Disorders Inventory

The Eating Disorders Inventory (EDI) is a comprehensive, widely used self-report measure for the assessment of many aspects of eating disorders (42). The EDI has subscales for bulimia, drive for thinness, and body dissatisfaction. The bulimia subscale measures the tendency to binge, purge, and engage in other bulimia-associated behaviors. Cronbach alphas of .90 and .83 have been reported for persons with anorexia and female controls, respectively, indicating internal consistency. The drive for thinness subscale assesses the intensity of one's desire to lose weight and fear of weight gain. Cronbach alphas of .85 for independent samples of persons with anorexia and female controls have been reported. The body dissatisfaction subscale measures the extent to which individuals are satisfied with specific parts of the body (e.g., waist, hips, thighs). Cronbach alphas of .90 for persons with anorexia and .91 for female controls have been reported.

Steroids

Body image concerns affect both genders. In an effort to achieve the male muscular ideal, some males resort to steroid use. Recent research suggests that while 58% of high-school boys take steroids in the hope of improving sport performance or to prevent or treat a sport-related injury, 34% stated appearance and social reasons for their steroid use (43). Unfortunately, whether taken for performance or appearance, steroids pose major risks to physical health.

Exercise Dependence

Exercise dependence, defined as feeling compelled to exercise daily and feeling unable to live without it, is a relatively new area of study. Dependence exists in various degrees, and therefore it is often difficult to determine the point at which exercise behaviors become "unhealthy." Body image may play an important role in exercise dependence, particularly if the obsessive activity is motivated by unrealistic body image goals. Figure 12-14 presents interview questions that may help assess whether a per-

1. Are there times during the day when you feel unable to stop thinking about exercise, even if you want to?
2. Do you feel anxious, irritable, or uncomfortable when you miss an exercise session?
3. If you miss an exercise session, do you feel that you need to make up for it (e.g., by staying later or getting up earlier to do it, by increasing the amount of exercise you do the next day)?
4. Have you sometimes exercised despite being advised against it (i.e., by a doctor, friend, family member)? What advice was given? Why did you exercise?
5. Do you try to increase your exercise session (or add additional exercise) when you feel you have overeaten or when you eat junk foods?
6. Do you worry about putting on weight or becoming fat if you miss an exercise session?
7. When you exercise, do you think about the calories or the amount of fat you are burning off?

FIGURE 12-14

Interview Questions to Assess the Potential of Exercise Dependency. (Reprinted with permission from Grilo, C.M., and Wilfley, D.E.: Weight control: exercise adherence and abuse. Weight Control Digest, 2(3):161, 1992.)

son is exercise dependent (44). As with eating disorders, you must refer to a trained clinician anyone who exhibits possible patterns of unhealthy exercise behavior.

Obesity

Actual body composition can influence body image. Obese persons have been found to have negative body images. This is most likely due to the high value our culture places on being lean. Overweight persons are keenly aware of this and therefore may feel self-conscious about their body. Although you should support a proper body weight for overall health, not everyone is so fortunate. It is important, therefore, to do what you can to deemphasize cultural demands for thinness and encourage all persons to appreciate their own body and the bodies of others for what they can do rather than focusing solely on physical appearances.

Chapter Summary

This chapter defines body image as thoughts, feelings, and perceptions about one's own general appearance, body parts, and physiological structures and functions. Traditional body image assessment tools designed by psychologists, sociologists, and cultural anthropologists are either perceptual or attitudinal. Perceptual measures include techniques to determine body size estimation, distorting image, and silhouette ratings. Attitudinal measures are largely self-report inventories that assess satisfaction with body image perceptions. Several of these inventories have been used to identify gender differences in body image. Researchers in ESS have also studied body image and have developed instruments for use in the study of the relationship between body image and physical activity. Body image may play a part in disorders such as anorexia and bulimia, steroid use, *exercise dependence*, and obesity. The ESS practitioner should be familiar with the concept of body image and know how this factor can be assessed.

SELF-TEST QUESTIONS

1. Which of the following professionals is most likely to use a clinical projective test to identify a body image disturbance in a client?
   A. An athletic trainer
   B. A physical education teacher
   C. A psychologist
   D. A sociologist

2. Which of the following is *not* classified as a perceptual measure of body image?
   A. Image marking procedure
   B. Body silhouette ratings
   C. Body Esteem Scale
   D. Body Image Detection Device

3. Using Formula 12-1, calculate the BPI for a man who perceives his waist as 36 inches but whose actual waist measurement is only 30 inches.
   A. 60
   B. 90
   C. 120
   D. 150

4. Using Formula 12-1, calculate the BPI for a woman who perceives her bust measurement as 36 inches but whose actual measurement is 40 inches.
   A. 60
   B. 90
   C. 120
   D. 150

5. On a standard 9-point silhouette rating, a client answered 6 to the statement, "Choose the figure that reflects how you think you look." She answered 8 to the statement, "Choose the figure that reflects how you feel most of the time." She answered 3 to the statement, "Choose your ideal figure." What is her feel-think discrepancy score?
   A. −2
   B. +2
   C. −3
   D. +5

6. Which of these attitudinal measures treats body image as a unidimensional construct?
   A. Body Attitude Scale
   B. Body Cathexis Scale
   C. Body Consciousness Questionnaire
   D. Body Esteem Scale

7. According to research using various attitudinal measures, which of the following is *not* generally true?
   A. Males have less definite ideas of what they like and dislike about their own bodies than do females.
   B. Males view their bodies as more active than do females.
   C. Males believe more strongly that the buttocks ("buns of steel") contributes to male attractiveness than do females.
   D. Males are more concerned with the attractiveness of body parts such as lips and cheekbones than are females.

8. According to Fox (Fig. 12-6), improvement in which of the following is likely to cause an increase in physical self-worth?
   A. Improved aerobic fitness
   B. Improved body fat percentage
   C. Learning a new sport
   D. All of the above

ANSWERS

1. C	2. C	3. C	4. B
5. B	6. B	7. D	8. D

DOING PROJECTS FOR FURTHER LEARNING

1. Explore your own body image in the following ways:
   A. Focus on your body-specific thoughts and feelings in various environments. For example, visit a beach, a weight training gym, a weight loss center, a running

club. Pay attention to your thoughts and feelings about your body that emerge in these environments. Were you proud? embarrassed? motivated to exercise? Explain.

   B. Experiment by wearing or imagining yourself wearing various types of clothing, such as a bathing suit or a sweat suit, in these places. Are you self-conscious in certain clothing? More comfortable in others?

   C. Surround yourself with persons of various body shapes and sizes. Do you consciously compare your body with others'? How do you feel about the comparisons?

2. Use the IMP to estimate the size of your neck, shoulders, waist, hips, thighs, calves, and ankles. Use a ruler or yardstick to measure the actual width of each of these body parts. Compare the measurements and calculate BPIs using Formula 12-1 for any body parts for which there is a discrepancy between your drawing and the actual measurement.

3. Using the body silhouettes in Figures 12-3 and 12-4, ask several friends of both genders to identify the figures that they think represent the ideal for females and the ideal for males. Analyze the data. (You may want to calculate means and standard deviations for your analysis.) Do the genders agree about the ideal female and male figure?

REFERENCES

1. Gottesman, E.G., and Caldwell, W.E.: The Body Image Identification Test: a quantitative projective technique to study an aspect of body image. Journal of Genetic Psychology, 108:19, 1966.

2. Hutchinson, M.G.: Transforming body image: your body, friend or foe? Women and Therapy, 1:59, 1982.

3. Whitbourne, S.K.: The Aging Individual: Physical and Psychological Perspectives. New York, Springer, 1996.

4. Freedman, R.: Bodylove: Learning to Like Our Looks and Ourselves. New York, Harper Collins, 1990.

5. Cooke, K.: Real Gorgeous: The Truth About Body and Beauty. New York, Norton, 1996.

6. Thompson, J.K., and Thompson, C.M.: Body size distortion and self-esteem in asymptomatic, normal weight males and females. International Journal of Eating Disorders, 5:1061, 1986.

7. Thompson, J.K., and Altabe, M.N.: Psychometric qualities of the Figure Rating Scale. International Journal of Eating Disorders, 10:615, 1991.

8. Mable, H.M., Balance, W.D.G., and Galgan, R.J.: Body-image distortion and dissatisfaction in university students. Perceptual and Motor Skills, 63:907, 1986.

9. Dickson-Parnell, B., Jones, M., and Braddy, D.: Assessment of body image perceptions using a computer program. Behavior Research Methods, Instruments, and Computers, 19:353, 1987.

10. Secord, P.F., and Jourard, S.M.: The appraisal of body-cathexis: body-cathexis and the self. Journal of Consulting Psychology, 17:343, 1953.

11. Kurtz, R.M.: Sex differences and variations in body attitudes. Journal of Consulting and Clinical Psychology, 33:625, 1969.

12. Silverstein, B., Perdue, L., and Peterson, B.: The role of the mass media in promoting a thin standard of bodily attractiveness for women. Sex Roles, 14:519, 1986.

13. Miller, L.C., Murphy, R., and Buss, A.H.: Consciousness of body: private and public. Journal of Personality and Social Psychology, 41:397, 1981.

14. Franzoi, S.L., and Shields, S.A.: The Body-Esteem Scale: multidimensional structure and sex differences in a college population. Journal of Personality Assessment, 48:173, 1984.

15. Mendelson, B.K., and White, D.R.: Relation between body-esteem and self-esteem of obese and normal children. Perceptual and Motor Skills, 54:899, 1982.
16. Cash, T.F.: The Multidimensional Body-Self Relations Questionnaire Users' Manual. Norfolk, VA, Old Dominion University, 1994 (available from the author).
17. Cash, T.F., Winstead, B.A., and Janda, L.H.: Your body, yourself: a Psychology Today reader survey. Psychology Today, 19(7):22, 1985.
18. Berscheid, E., Walster, E., and Bohrnstedt, G.: The happy American body: a survey report. Psychology Today, 7(11):119, 1973.
19. Garner, D.M.: The 1997 body image survey results. Psychology Today, 30(1):30, 1997.
20. Marsh, H.W., Richards, G.E., and Barnes, J.: Multidimensional self-concepts: the effect of participation in an Outward Bound program. Journal of Personality and Social Psychology, 50:195, 1986.
21. Davis, T.: Effect of cardiovascular fitness on the body concept of women. Dissertation Abstracts International, 41(8-B):3173, 1981.
22. Tucker, L.A., and Maxwell, K.: Effects of weight-training on the emotional well-being and body image of females: predictors of greatest benefit. American Journal of Health Promotion, 6:338, 1992.
23. Hawkins, D.L.: The effect of exercise on self-esteem and body image. Dissertation Abstracts International, 42(5-A):2031, 1981.
24. Seggar, J.F., McCammon, D.L., and Cannon, L.D.: Relations between physical activity, weight discrepancies, body-cathexis, and psychological well-being in college women. Perceptual and Motor Skills, 67(2):659, 1988.
25. Dishman, R.K.: Advances in Exercise Adherence. Champaign, Illinois, Human Kinetics, 1994.
26. Fox, K.R., and Corbin, C.B.: The Physical Self-Perception Profile: development and preliminary validation. Journal of Sport and Exercise Psychology, 11:408, 1989.
27. Harter, S.: Competence as a dimension of self-evaluation: toward a comprehensive model of self-worth. In Leahy, R. (ed.): The Development of the Self. New York, Academic Press, 1985.
28. Fox, K.R., and Corbin, C.B: The Physical Self-Perception Profile Manual. Champaign, IL, Human Kinetics, 1990.
29. Ryckman, R.M., Robbins, M.A., Thornton, B., and Cantrell, P.: Development and validation of a physical self-efficacy scale. Journal of Personality and Social Psychology, 42:891, 1982.
30. Hart, E.A., Leary, M.R., and Rejeski, W.J: The measurement of social physique anxiety. Journal of Sport and Exercise Psychology, 11:94, 1989.
31. Silberstein, L.R., Striegel-Moore, R.H., Timko, C., and Rodin, J.: Behavioral and psychological implications of body dissatisfaction: do men and women differ? Sex Roles, 19:219, 1988.
32. Cash, T.F., Novy, P.L., and Grant, J.R.: Why do women exercise? Factor analysis and further validation of the Reasons for Exercise Inventory. Perceptual and Motor Skills, 78:539, 1994.
33. Yates, A.: Compulsive Exercise and the Eating Disorders: Toward an Integrated Theory of Activity. New York, Brunner-Mazel, 1991.
34. Kenyon, G.S.: Six scales for assessing attitude toward physical activity. Research Quarterly, 39:566, 1968.
35. Schultz, R.W., Smoll, F.L., Carre, F.A., and Mosher, R.E.: Inventories and norms for children's attitudes toward physical activity. Research Quarterly for Exercise and Sport, 56:256, 1985.
36. Harter, S.: The Perceived Competence Scale for Children. Child Development, 53:87, 1982.
37. Sonstroem, R.J.: Physical estimation and attraction scales: rationale and research. Medicine and Science in Sports, 10:97, 1978.

38. Rosenberg, M.: Society and the Adolescent Self-Image. Hanover, NH, University Press of New England, 1989.

39. Bandura, A.: Self-efficacy: toward a unifying theory of behavioral change. Psychological Review, 84(2):91, 1977.

40. Garner, D.M., Olmsted, M., Bohr, V., and Garfinkel, P.E.: The Eating Attitudes Test: psychometric features and clinical correlates. Psychological Medicine, 12:871, 1982.

41. Smith, M.C., and Thelen, M.H.: Development and validation of a test for bulimia. Journal of Consulting and Clinical Psychology, 52:863, 1984.

42. Garner, D.M., Olmsted, M., and Polivy, J.: Development and validation of a multidimensional eating disorder inventory for anorexia nervosa and bulimia. International Journal of Eating Disorders, 2:15, 1983.

43. Dukes, W.: Is body image related to exercise? New Zealand Journal of Sports Medicine, 18(2):34, 1990.

44. Grilo, C.M., and Wilfley, D.E.: Weight control: exercise adherence and abuse. Weight Control Digest, 2(3):161, 1992.

CHAPTER 13

Nutritional Assessment

Carolyn Dunn

Good nutrition is essential for good health. Both the quality and quantity of foods eaten affect a person's total well-being. Nutritional assessment, the focus of this chapter, is the evaluation of nutritional status of an individual or group. In the early part of this century nutritional assessment was focused mainly on deficiency diseases, such as scurvy and beriberi. Diets poor in vitamins and/or minerals were common both in the United States and in other countries, and the deficiencies were a major threat to health. Although deficiency diseases are for the most part a thing of the past, nutritional assessment is more important than ever. Chronic diseases such as obesity, heart disease, and certain forms of cancer have been linked to diet. Nutritional assessment can help health professionals identify those who would benefit from changes in their diet and determine the appropriate dietary changes (Fig. 13-1).

Many techniques can be used to assess nutritional status. These methods fall into four categories. Anthropometric assessment of nutritional status is discussed in Chapter 8. This chapter discusses the three remaining categories of nutritional assessment: dietary analysis, biochemical analysis, and methods based on clinical signs and symptoms. Measurement of nutrition knowledge and its relationship to dietary habits will also be discussed.

As you read this chapter, watch for the following keywords:

Flat-slope syndrome	Nutrient dense
Inadequate intake	RDA

Dietary Analysis Methods

This section discusses four dietary analysis methods. The following section is a discussion of ways to evaluate the data collected by these methods.

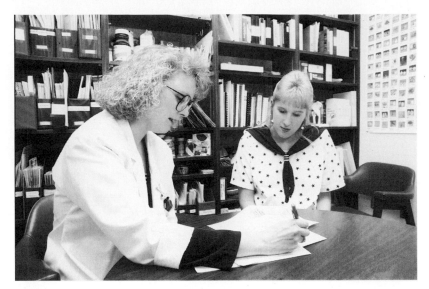

FIGURE 13-1

Nutritional assessment interview.

24-Hour Recall

The *24-hour recall* is one of the most common methods of collecting dietary data. Subjects or caregivers of the subject are asked to recall what they consumed over the past 24 hours. The recall is collected by a trained interviewer who obtains as much detail as possible about the foods and beverages consumed. The interviewer is interested not only in what foods and beverages were consumed but also in the amounts, methods of preparation, sauces added, and brand names or restaurant names when appropriate. Responses are usually recorded on a data sheet for consistency and ease (Fig. 13-2).

The interviewer is the key in obtaining a valid and reliable 24-hour recall. He or she should be trained in use of a standard procedure. It is essential to avoid asking judgmental or leading questions. For example, the interviewer should not ask, "What did you have for breakfast?" This simple question may lead a subject to fabricate a breakfast. A better approach, therefore, is to ask subjects what time they got up and what they did first. Step them through the day in that manner, giving them opportunities to recall foods and beverages consumed without specifically asking, "What did you have for lunch?" Similarly, don't ask leading questions about serving sizes or method of preparation. If a subject indicates that he or she ate white bread, do not respond, "Just one piece?" Instead ask about serving sizes without giving an answer; let the subject tell you how much was eaten. The same holds true when inquiring about method of preparation. If the subject mentions having chicken for dinner, do not assume the chicken was fried. Let the subject tell you how it was prepared and whether it was served with a sauce or condiment.

The following is an example of an exchange between a trained interviewer and a subject:

Interviewer: "What did you do after practice was over?"

Name_____   **Date**_____

Interviewer_____   **Day of the Week**_____

Place	Time	Food/Beverage Consumed	Amount	Comments/Code

Was your food/beverage intake on this day usual?   Yes   No
  If yes, why?

Do you take any vitamins, minerals, or protein supplements?   Yes   No
  If yes, what are they?
  How often do you take them?

FIGURE 13-2

Data collection form for a 24-hour dietary recall.

Subject: "I went to the student union to study."

Interviewer: "Did you start studying right away or talk with friends, watch TV, or anything?"

Subject: "I talked with friends at the snack bar."

Interviewer: "Did you have anything to eat or drink while you were with your friends?"

Subject: "I had a cola."

Interviewer: "Was that a fountain or can cola?"

Subject: "It was a can cola."

Interviewer: "Was it regular or diet?"

Subject: "It was diet."

Interviewer: "Did you have anything to eat with it?"

Subject: "Oh yeah, a friend gave me some cookies."

Interviewer: "What kind of cookies?"

Subject: "Chocolate chip."

Interviewer: "Show me how big they were and how many you ate."

By asking good questions the interviewer helped the subject recall what and how much was drunk and eaten. The interviewer must also collect information about any nutritional supplements the subject is taking. The interviewer should inquire about vitamin, mineral, and protein supplements and collect details about the type, amount, and frequency of consumption.

Several tools can be very helpful in collecting accurate 24-hour recalls. Food models (Fig. 13-3) are commonly used to spark a subject's memory and help with estimating serving sizes. In addition to food models, household measuring cups, measuring spoons, bowls, and plates can help a subject estimate how much of a given food was eaten. A deck of cards or pieces of cardboard can help estimate the size of a piece of meat.

There are several advantages to using 24-hour recall for collecting dietary data. It is relatively easy and inexpensive. It is quick and requires little effort on the part of the subject. And if the subject does not know that a recall will be taken, it does not affect normal eating patterns.

The 24-hour recall does, however, have several limitations. Because we all eat differently from day to day, the 24-hour recall is not meant to be used to estimate the dietary intake of an individual (1–5). Recalls of 24-hour eating patterns can be used

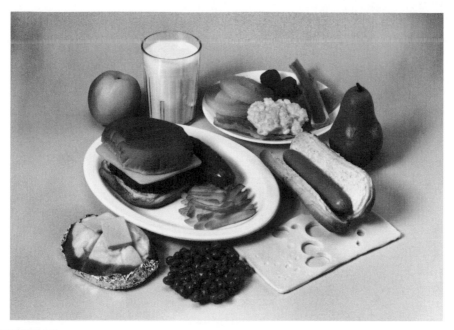

FIGURE 13-3

Use of food models can help in collecting dietary intake data. (Food models by Nasco, Inc., Fort Atkinson, WI.)

to estimate the dietary intake of large groups of people. If no great deal of accuracy is required, multiple 24-hour recalls spaced over several months may provide a reasonable estimate of an individual's intake (6–8). There is also the problem of overestimation or underestimation of intake, commonly called the **flat-slope syndrome** (9, 10). People tend to overestimate underconsumption and underestimate overconsumption. In other words, they tell you what they think you want to hear.

> Flat-slope syndrome is the tendency of subjects to overestimate actual underconsumption and to underestimate actual overconsumption of food and beverages.

The 24-hour recall also has the disadvantage of relying on memory. This may be more of a problem in the elderly and in children than in others. Young children may not remember what they ate yesterday and may confuse yesterday with last week. The child's caregiver may be able to help. However, many children attend day care and have several caregivers throughout the day. Another limitation of the 24-hour recall is that it may overestimate or underestimate certain nutrients, depending on the season the recall is collected (11, 12). People tend to vary their diet according to the season. For example, subjects may have beef stew only in the winter and strawberries only in the spring, when they are plentiful and inexpensive.

For all of its limitations, the 24-hour recall remains one of the most common methods of estimating food intake. When using it, remember its limitations and be persistent to collect complete and accurate data.

Food Record

Estimating dietary intake by using a *food record* requires the subject to keep a record of all food and beverages consumed for a specified number of days. The subject is given instructions and a special form to record food and beverages consumed (Figs. 13-4 and 13-5). The subjects are instructed to keep the record immediately after eating.

The number of days collected depends on the accuracy needed. Food records, sometimes called food diaries, are usually collected for 3, 5, or 7 days (13). Generally speaking, the more days collected, the more accurate the picture of the normal eating pattern of the subject. Collecting 5-day or 7-day records is not always possible, however, and a 3-day record must be used. If a 3-day food record is used, only one of the days should be a weekend or non–working day. Try not to collect food records during holidays or other times (such as final examination week) when the intake is likely to be unusual.

There are two types of food records, estimated and weighed. The weighed food record is considered the more accurate of the two. This method requires that the subject weigh all foods on a small kitchen scale. Weighing food and beverages provides an accurate picture of an individual's intake, but the limited use of kitchen scales in this country may make this method difficult for many subjects. If using this method, you may have to provide a scale. The weighed food record is also problematic if food must be weighed in a restaurant or cafeteria. For these reasons, an estimated food record is often used. The estimated food record uses common household measures such as ounces, cups, and tablespoons to estimate serving sizes. A ruler may be used to measure pieces of meat or baked goods.

There are several advantages to both weighed and estimated food records. Unlike the 24-hour recall, the food record can provide good insight regarding a person's diet. If multiple days are collected (especially for as many as 7 days), the food record can provide a reasonable estimate of dietary intake. If information such as time and place eaten are recorded, the food record can also reveal eating habits. The food record does not require that the subject remember what was eaten but provides detailed information about foods and beverages consumed.

Collecting dietary intake data by food record also has some limitations. The major one is that the act of recording what one eats may alter intake. Subjects may not eat foods they perceive as bad for them if they know they are going to have to write it down. They also may choose basic foods to simplify the recording process. For example, it is a lot easier to record "hamburger on a bun" than the multiple ingredients in a casserole. The food record requires cooperation on the part of the subject and his or her commitment to recording intake for the specified period. The subject must also be literate and have a certain degree of education. The food record provides more information than the 24-hour recall, but analysis of it is more expensive and time consuming. If a weighed record is used, there is also the added expense of providing subjects with scales.

Considering the advantages and limitations, the food record is a very useful tool for assessing dietary intakes. Give subjects accurate instructions, and go over their records with them when they return them. Clarification at this time gives a fairly reasonable picture of what and how that subject eats.

1. Record all foods and beverages consumed on the form provided immediately after eating.
2. Include time eaten, place eaten, preparation method and amount in appropriate column.
3. Using household measurements, estimate the serving size of each food and beverage. Record only portion eaten, for example 1 cup of milk, 3 ounces of turkey, 1 small apple, 1 tablespoon butter, 1 slice of bread.
4. Include all sauces and condiments, including but not limited to catsup, mustard, mayonnaise, hollandaise sauce, and so on.
5. Be as specific as possible about method of preparation, including fats used in cooking. For example, 1 egg scrambled in 1 teaspoon of margarine.
6. Include brand names when appropriate and whenever possible attach food labels or packages from foods consumed. If this isn't possible, write down pertinent information from the label, such as tuna packed in oil or pineapple in its own juice.
7. For combination foods such as casseroles or stews, include as much information about the contents as possible. For example, if you had tuna casserole, indicate each ingredient and the amount consumed.
8. If you eat at a restaurant, include the name of the restaurant and as much information about the food as possible. Use the description on the menu or ask the server for further clarification on cooking method when needed.
9. Try to consume your normal diet while keeping this record. Keep the record for the number of days requested.

Example

TIME	PLACE	FOOD OR BEVERAGE CONSUMED	PREPARATION	AMOUNT
6:30 AM	Kitchen	Coffee	Brewed	1 cup
		Sugar		1 tsp
		Nondairy creamer		2 tsp
8:00 AM	Car	Bread, whole wheat	Toasted	2 slices
		Margarine		2 tsp
12:00	Office	Turkey sandwich		
		Turkey	Smoked	3 ounces
		Lettuce		1 leaf
		American cheese		1 ounce
		Bread, whole wheat		2 slices
		Mayonnaise		1 tsp
		Mustard		1 tsp

FIGURE 13-4

Instructions for keeping a food record.

Name_____ **Date**_____

Interviewer_____ **Day of the Week**_____

Place	Time	Food/Beverage Consumed	Amount	Comments/Code

FIGURE 13-5

Data collection form for a food record.

Dietary History

Burke (14) developed the dietary history in the 1940s to assess usual intake. Unlike the 24-hour recall and the food record, which assess recent intake for a short period, the diet history assesses usual intake for an extended period, usually a month to a year.

Burke's procedure has four steps. The first is to collect general information about the subject's health habits, including such things as tobacco use, exercise patterns, stress, and work habits. The second step is to collect information on usual eating habits, such as number of meals eaten per day, snacking patterns, likes and dislikes, and seasonal variances in eating patterns. At this step a 24-hour recall is also collected. The third step is to collect information about frequency of consumption of specific foods. For example, how often do you drink milk? This step also serves as a check on the information given in step two. If the subject indicates that he or she drinks cola every day as a snack but answers never when asked how often soft drinks are consumed, the interviewer must clarify the responses. The fourth and final step is to have the subject collect a 3-day food record. This step is sometimes omitted, since it is only another measure of recent intake and it adds to the cost and time needed to complete the analysis.

The diet history has several advantages over other methods of dietary assessment. It gives an overall picture of eating habits and patterns, not just an estimate of recent intake. Information such as whether or not the subject's job or school interferes with eating habits or whether the subject usually eats breakfast can be obtained. Foods that are consumed only seasonally can be assessed, especially if the history is collected for a full year's intake.

The diet history also has some limitations. Because of the large amount of information collected, the history is very difficult to analyze. It also takes as much as 2 hours to collect it, and it requires a skilled interviewer. The subject must have a relatively good memory, especially if data are collected on usual intake for a full year. Despite these limitations plus limitations of cost and time, the diet history can provide valuable information about eating habits.

Food Frequency Questionnaire

The *food frequency questionnaire* (Fig. 13-6) is a checklist of foods and frequencies of consumption. The subject is asked to indicate how often he or she consumes a given food or foods within a food group. The list of foods may focus on particular foods, food groups, preparation methods, or nutrients, or it may be a general list to assess overall consumption. The frequency of consumption can range from never to more than once a day. Categories such as once a month or once every 3 months can be included if seasonal differences in consumption are an issue.

Depending on the type of dietary information needed, the food frequency questionnaire can include questions about serving size. If only a general sense of serving sizes is needed, the subject may be asked to indicate whether the servings were small, medium, or large, with a standard given for the medium serving. For example, "if medium is half a cup, were your servings of juice small, medium, or large?" Some questionnaires may ask subjects to estimate serving sizes; these are called semiquantitative (15–17).

The food frequency questionnaire has several advantages. It is relatively inexpensive and easy to administer. Although better data are obtained if an interviewer collects

FOODS	DAILY				WEEKLY		NEVER
	1	2	3	MORE	1-2	3-4	
Milk, yogurt, cheese, or cottage cheese							
Carrots, broccoli, tomatoes, green beans, collards, potatoes, or other vegetable							
Banana, apple, grapes, orange, or other fruit							
Beef, chicken, pork, fish, turkey, or eggs							
Nuts, dried peas, lentils, or dried beans							
Rice, pasta, noodles, bread, crackers, cereal, oatmeal, or other food from grains							

FIGURE 13-6

Food frequency questionnaire.

the data, the food frequency questionnaire can be self-administered. It asks about intake over time and is therefore more representative of usual intake than a 24-hour recall or food record. It gives a good overall picture of a person's intake and is valuable in estimating the intake of large groups. The questionnaire can be specific about foods or groups of foods to investigate the relationship between diet and disease. For example, if you are interested in the relationship between calcium intake and osteoporosis, you can assess calcium intake by use of a food frequency questionnaire that asks only about foods high in calcium. (This is, of course, just the first of many steps to assess the relationship between calcium intake and osteoporosis.) Or if you are interested in the fruit and vegetable consumption of college students, you can structure a questionnaire that addresses those foods only. The instrument may also contain questions about preparation techniques, such as fried or baked, if these data are a point of interest.

Several versions of the food frequency questionnaire to collect information on one specific nutrient have been developed. An example of this is the calcium wheel shown in Figure 13-7. This is an excellent tool to assess calcium intake from all food sources, with the pictures on the wheel serving to spark the respondent's memory. It also teaches respondents about calcium content of various foods.

The food frequency questionnaire also has some limitations. The most serious one is that it requires the subject to have a good memory of intake over weeks, months, or sometimes years. The limited number of foods listed may cause the subject to underestimate consumption, or the subject may eat things that are not listed on the questionnaire and not remember to list them. The food frequency questionnaire may not estimate serving sizes, hence not provide a quantitative estimate of intake. This limitation can be partially overcome by using a semiquantitative questionnaire.

A comparison of all of the dietary intake collection methods discussed and their advantages and limitations can be found in Table 13-1. Under what conditions would each of the methods be best?

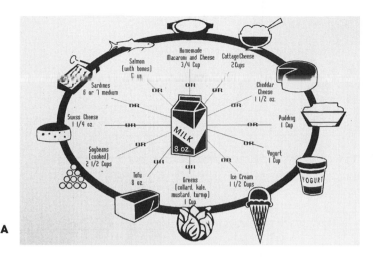

A

AM I GETTING ENOUGH CALCIUM?

To compare the amount of calcium you're *now* getting from food, with calcium you *need,* fill in the six boxes on this page.

- First, look at the RDA Table (Table 13–2). Write the number of mg/day you need in Blank (2). Divide that number by 300 and put in Blank (1).

- Next, try to remember what you ate yesterday. Look at the diagram provided. Mark an "X" in the boxes next to every food you ate yesterday. If you ate more than one serving of that food, write "X" for each serving.

- Count each "X" as one, and enter that total in Blank (3). This is the amount of calcium you're now getting from food, *in terms of equivalent glasses of milk.*

- Next, multiply the number in Blank (3) by 300. Put that number into Blank (4). That is the amount of calcium you're getting from food *in milligrams a day.*

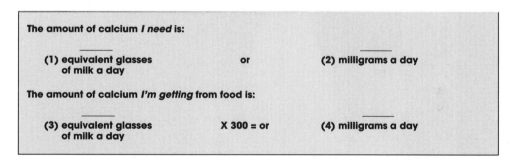

- Compare what you're *getting* from food, Blanks (3) and (4), with the amount of calcium you *need,* in Blanks (1) and (2). Next, consider what you have eaten over the past few days. If your calcium need *is* being met from the foods you eat, keep it up! Remember, your calcium needs change, so become familiar with the calcium turning points.

- If your calcium need is *not* being met from your diet, write the amount of calcium you must add to your diet to meet your needs in Blanks (5) and (6).

FIGURE 13-7

A. The calcium wheel. **B.** Calculations to determine whether calcium intake is adequate. (Reprinted courtesy of the Nutrition Information Center of the New York Hospital Cornell University Medical Center, Memorial Sloan-Kettering Cancer Center.)

TABLE 13-1	Advantages and Limitations of Various Methods of Assessing Dietary Intake	
DATA COLLECTION METHOD	**ADVANTAGES**	**LIMITATIONS**
24-hour recall	Quick to collect Relatively inexpensive Requires only short-term memory Does not alter eating patterns Good estimate of intake of groups or communities Does not require much effort from subject	Not representative of individual intake Subject to underreporting or overreporting of serving size May omit foods Relies on memory May vary with season
Food record	May provide information about eating habits Can get estimate of an individual's intake Multiple days are more representative Doesn't rely on memory Provides detail about intake	Takes cooperative subject May alter diet Requires subject to be literate Expensive and time consuming
Dietary history	Assesses usual eating habits, not just recent intake Can detect seasonal differences	Requires highly skilled interviewer Difficult to analyze Requires good memory of subject Can take 1 to 2 hours to collect
Food frequency	May better represent usual intake than several days of food record or 24-hour recall Good choice to identify diet and disease relationships Relatively easy to administer and inexpensive Can identify specific foods or groups of foods that are overconsumed or underconsumed	May not give good estimate of quantity consumed Requires subject to have good memory of diet over weeks or months

What Do YOU Think?

"According to diet lore, 'indulging,' or 'giving in to temptation' is a 'sin' " (18). A sin? Like murder and adultery? Come on now! How can eating possibly be a sin? Will a client who believes that eating is naughty be honest in reporting food consumption? Will a client who believes that eating is sinful actually consume a healthy diet? What do YOU think?

Evaluation of Dietary Data

Now that you have taken great care to choose the right method of collecting dietary data and taken every precaution to get the most accurate record of intake possible, what do you do with it? This section outlines several ways to evaluate dietary data. There are two general approaches. You can either analyze individual foods for nutrients and get an average for each day's intake, or you can use a more general food grouping plan. Intakes may also be evaluated by comparisons with intake recommendations, such as the dietary guidelines from the U.S. government.

There are two ways to evaluate dietary data if you are interested in specific amounts of nutrients. The more common method is to look up each item in a reference that contains the nutrient breakdown of foods. *Handbook 8*, from the U.S. Department of Agriculture is the mother of all food composition books and tables (19). *Handbook 8* consists of several volumes of material containing information about foods that you may not even know exist. If you need to know the calorie content of ostrich eggs or the vitamin A content of polar bear meat, this is the place to look. If you are analyzing a diet made up of common foods, however, an abridged version of *Handbook 8* will do just fine. The famous *Bowes and Church's* (now edited by Pennington) (20) is another reference for food composition; you will find it on all nutritionists' desks. *Bowes and Church's* contains every food you will probably ever need for dietary analysis.

To use one of these food composition books, you simply look up the food or foods at issue and record their nutrient content. To produce an accurate analysis you have to keep several things in mind. First, pay close attention to serving size. If the subject had half a cup of cornflakes and the analysis in the food composition table is for a whole cup, be sure to make the adjustment. Second, be conscious of preparation method and cooked versus raw foods. Choose the entry in the table that is closest to what was taken. This brings up another point. What if you are using one of the abridged versions of *Handbook 8* and the food is not listed? You must choose the closest approximation. If you are not sure what is closest, seek the advice of a person trained in nutrition.

An easier and sometimes more accurate method of analyzing dietary data is to use a computer program. Several good programs have a wide selection of foods. One that I like is *Food Processor* from ESHA research (21). *Food Processor* lists more than 5,000 foods, including name-brand and fast-food restaurant foods; the price is about $500. Figure 13-8 is a printout from a *Food Processor* analysis of a 24-hour recall from Jane Doe.

A computer program yields a great deal of information in a relatively short period, including a comparison of the intake with the recommended dietary al-

```
--------------------------------------------------------------------------
| Analysis: Jane Doe
| % RDA: Jane Doe                      Wgt: 1832 g (64.6 oz.)
| Cost:                                Water:  75%
--------------------------------------------------------------------------

        Amount     Item                                          Code
--------------------------------------------------------------------------
        1 cup      Cheerios Cereal                               1166
        .5 cup     Nonfat Skim Milk                                73
        1 each     Banana                                         190
        1 cup      Fresh Orange Juice                             270
        2 piece    Whole Wheat Bread                             1014
        3 piece    Ham Lunchmeat-Extra Lean-Slice                 940
        1.5 oz-wt  American Processed Cheese                         1
        2 tsp      Prepared Mustard                              1666
        1 each     Medium Apple w/Peel                            154
        3 each     Soft Chocolate Chip Cookie                    1052
        1.5 cup    Diet Cola/Coke w/Aspartame-Bottle/Can         1407
        2 oz-wt    Potato Chips                                   593
        5 oz-wt    Swordfish-Baked/Broiled                        776
        1 each     Baked Potato w/Skin-Long                       563
        1 tbs      Butter                                        1462
        1 tbs      Cultured Sour Cream                             57
        .5 cup     Green Peas-Canned-Drained                      527
        1 each     Chocolate LoFat Frozen Yogurt Cone-Small      1257

NUTRIENT          VALUES   Goal% |---------25--------50--------75-------100----->
--------------------------------------------------------------------------
Calories          2082      96% ###################################
Protein           97.8 g   207% ##################################### |#####>>
Carbohydrates      259 g    82% #############################
Fat - Total       78.5 g   108% #################################### |##
Saturated Fat     33.3 g   138% ##################################### |#####>>
Mono Fat          26.6 g   110% ##################################### |###
Poly Fat          13.1 g    54% ###################
Omega 3 FA        2.27 g    --
Omega 6 FA        10.4 g    --        |         |        |
Cholesterol        196 mg   65% ########################
Dietary Fiber     24.9 g   114% ##################################### |#####
Total Vit A        839 RE  105% ##################################### |#
A - Retinol        674 RE   --
A - Carotenoid     165 RE   --
Thiamin-B1        2.26 mg  208% ##################################### |#####>>
Riboflavin-B2     1.91 mg  146% ##################################### |#####>>
Niacin-B3           36 mg  251% ##################################### |#####>>
Niacin Equiv.       36 mg  251% ##################################### |#####>>
Vitamin B6        3.61 mg  226% ##################################### |#####>>
Vitamin B12       5.79 mcg 290% ##################################### |#####>>
Folate             254 mcg 141% ##################################### |#####>>
Pantothenic       4.81 mg   69% ######################### |
Vitamin C          232 mg  386% ##################################### |#####>>
Vitamin D         4.64 mcg  46% ################# |
Vit E-Alpha E     5.39 mg   67% ######################### |
Calcium            762 mg   63% #######################
Copper            2.02 mg   81% ############################
Iron              15.4 mg  103% ###################################
Magnesium          401 mg  143% #####################################|#####>>
```

FIGURE 13-8

Computer analysis of Jane Doe's dietary intake.

lowances (RDAs), discussed in the next section. Information that is pertinent to the analysis, such as age, gender, and physical activity can be entered, giving a more personal analysis. Computer analysis does have several limitations. It is not available to all people, and the lack of equipment and/or the cost may be prohibitive. Computer programs typically have a limited number of foods in the database, which may cause a problem when a certain degree of accuracy is needed. This may be overcome by choosing a good program and having a good knowledge of foods, so that appropriate substitutions can be made.

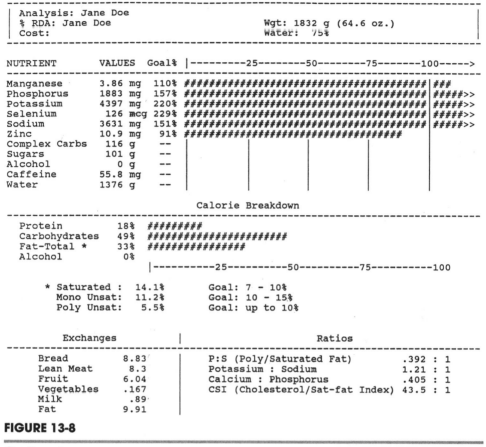

```
-------------------------------------------------------------------------
| Analysis: Jane Doe
| % RDA: Jane Doe                         Wgt: 1832 g (64.6 oz.)
| Cost:                                   Water:  75%
-------------------------------------------------------------------------

NUTRIENT         VALUES  Goal% |---------25--------50--------75-------100---->
-------------------------------------------------------------------------
Manganese         3.86 mg  110% ##################################### |###
Phosphorus        1883 mg  157% #####################################|####>>
Potassium         4397 mg  220% #####################################|####>>
Selenium           126 mcg 229% #####################################|####>>
Sodium            3631 mg  151% #####################################|####>>
Zinc              10.9 mg   91% ##################################
Complex Carbs      116 g    --    |         |         |         |
Sugars             101 g    --    |         |         |         |
Alcohol              0 g    --    |         |         |         |
Caffeine          55.8 mg   --    |         |         |         |
Water             1376 g    --    |         |         |         |

                         Calorie Breakdown
-------------------------------------------------------------------------
   Protein          18%  ########
   Carbohydrates    49%  #####################
   Fat-Total *      33%  ###############
   Alcohol           0%
                       |----------25----------50----------75----------100

     * Saturated :   14.1%      Goal: 7 - 10%
       Mono Unsat:   11.2%      Goal: 10 - 15%
       Poly Unsat:    5.5%      Goal: up to 10%


       Exchanges           |              Ratios
-------------------------------------------------------------------------
    Bread        8.83    | P:S (Poly/Saturated Fat)             .392 : 1
    Lean Meat    8.3     | Potassium : Sodium                  1.21 : 1
    Fruit        6.04    | Calcium : Phosphorus                 .405 : 1
    Vegetables    .167   | CSI (Cholesterol/Sat-fat Index)     43.5 : 1
    Milk          .89    |
    Fat          9.91    |
```

FIGURE 13-8

Continued

Recommended Dietary Allowances

Once you have your dietary data summarized, you need guidelines for comparisons. Knowing that the subject consumed 85 mg of vitamin C on Monday does not tell you much on its own. Is that too much, too little, or just right? The RDAs provide a useful standard for evaluating dietary data.

RDAs are the "levels of intake of essential nutrients that, on the basis of scientific knowledge, are judged by the Food and Nutrition Board to be adequate to meet the known nutrient needs of practically all healthy persons" (22). The RDAs are set by a group of scientists, using the latest information on nutrient requirements. It is their intent to set RDAs that are safe and adequate for most of the population of the United States. The RDAs are not applicable to people with special dietary needs.

> RDAs are the levels of essential nutrients deemed to be adequate to meet the nutrient needs of most healthy persons.

Using research data, the Food and Nutrition Board estimates a population's average need for a nutrient. The RDA for a given nutrient is then set 2.0 standard deviations above the mean level of need. Setting the RDAs higher than the mean theoretically covers the needs of 97.5% of the population. The only RDA that is not set in this manner is the one for energy or caloric intake. Because it does not want to encourage overconsumption, the Food and Nutrition Board has set the RDA for energy at the mean need for a given group. Figure 13-9 illustrates RDAs in relation to population percentages.

Because age, gender, and reproductive status can greatly affect need for nutrients, separate recommendations are made for various groups, such as pregnant or lactating women and adolescent boys. RDAs by gender and age are listed in Table 13-2. There is not an RDA for every nutrient known to be essential for humans. The Food and Nutrition Board sets an RDA only when there is sufficient research to support a recommendation. Data for some nutrients are sufficient to estimate a range of requirements but not sufficient to set RDAs. Ranges of intake recommended for these nutrients are called *estimated safe and adequate daily dietary intake* (ESADDI). ESADDIs are provided in Table 13-3.

RDAs are used for many purposes, such as food labeling, setting standards for school lunches, and nutrition counseling. They are also commonly used to evaluate nutrient intake for an individual or group. Because RDAs were not meant to be used in this manner, however, the following should be considered: *RDAs are* not *amounts of nutrients that are absolutely required by individuals.* They are merely estimates of need that include safety margins to allow for nutrient loss during digestion and absorption and for individual variations in requirements. For many people this means that the RDA is much higher than the actual need. For this reason nutrition professionals often set cutoff points to define **inadequate intake.** A cutoff commonly used is two-thirds, or 60 to 70%, of the RDA.

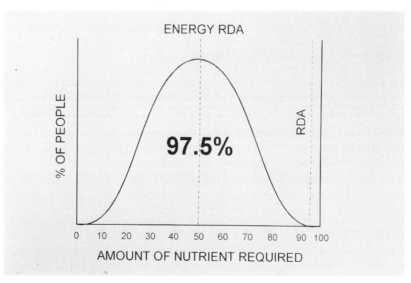

FIGURE 13-9.

The RDA for a nutrient covers the needs of most persons.

Inadequate intake is consumption of a nutrient at or below a level that is approximately two-thirds of the RDA for that nutrient.

Look at Figure 13-8 again. Jane consumed at least 60% of each RDA. These data suggest that for that day, Jane was doing okay with respect to her nutrient intake. Let's discuss another scenario. Assume you analyzed your diet for 7 days and found that your vitamin A intake was 50% of the RDA. What does that mean? If the 7 days were typical of your normal eating habits, it means that your consumption is somewhat lower than the RDA set for the nation. It does *not* necessarily mean you are deficient in that nutrient or even that you have a poor diet. You may just happen to need substantially less vitamin A than the RDA. Of course, it could mean that you need more vitamin A–rich foods. Keep in mind how RDAs are set. Remember that they are *not* absolute levels that must be met by all persons to have a good diet. They are estimates of adequate intake for most healthy Americans. They are best used as guides to healthy eating.

U.S. Dietary Goals and U.S. Dietary Guidelines

The U.S. Dietary Goals (Fig. 13-10) were set in 1977 by the U.S. Senate Select Committee on Nutrition and Human Needs (23). They are a series of goals and recommendations for all Americans, offered in an attempt to decrease risks of chronic diseases such as obesity and heart disease. The crux of the dietary goals report was that (*a*) Americans should get no more than 30% of their calories from fat, with only 10% coming from saturated sources (e.g., predominantly animal products); (*b*) 12% of calories should come from protein; (*c*) 58% of calories should come from carbohydrate sources; and (*d*) only 10% of calories should come from refined

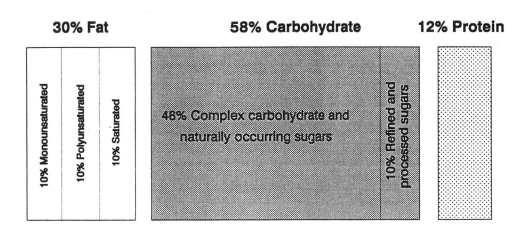

Dietary Goals

FIGURE 13-10.

U.S. Dietary Goals for a healthy diet.

TABLE 13-2	Food and Nutrition Board, National Academy of Sciences, National Research Council Recommended Dietary Allowances,[a] Revised 1989, *Designed for the Maintenance of Good Nutrition of Practically All Healthy People in the United States* (continues on page 457)

| | | | | | | | FAT-SOLUBLE VITAMINS | | | |
CATEGORY	AGE (YEARS) OR CONDITION	WEIGHT[b] (kg)	(lb)	HEIGHT[b] (cm)	(in)	PROTEIN (g)	VITA-MIN A (μg RE)[c]	VITA-MIN D (μg)[d]	VITA-MIN E (mg α-TE)[e]	VITA-MIN K (μg)
Infants	0.0–0.5	6	13	60	24	13	375	7.5	3	5
	0.5–1.0	9	20	71	28	14	375	10	4	10
Children	1–3	13	29	90	35	16	400	10	6	15
	4–6	20	44	112	44	24	500	10	7	20
	7–10	28	62	132	52	28	700	10	7	30
Males	11–14	45	99	157	62	45	1,000	10	10	45
	15–18	66	145	176	69	59	1,000	10	10	65
	19–24	72	160	177	70	58	1,000	10	10	70
	25–50	79	174	176	70	63	1,000	5	10	80
	51+	77	170	173	68	63	1,000	5	10	80
Females	11–14	46	101	157	62	46	800	10	8	45
	15–18	55	120	163	64	44	800	10	8	55
	19–24	58	128	164	65	46	800	10	8	60
	25–50	63	138	163	64	50	800	5	8	65
	51+	65	143	160	63	50	800	5	8	65
Pregnant						60	800	10	10	65
Lactating	1st 6 months					65	1,300	10	12	65
	2nd 6 months					62	1,200	10	11	65

[a]The allowances, expressed as average daily intakes over time, are intended to provide for individual variations among most normal persons as they live in the United States under usual environmental stresses. Diets should be based on a variety of common foods in order to provide other nutrients for which human requirements have been less well defined.

[b]Weights and heights of reference adults are actual medians for the U.S. population of the designated age, as reported by NHANES II. The median weights and heights of those under 19 years of age were taken from Hamill, P. V., et al.: Physical growth: National Center for Health Statistics percentiles. Journal of Clinical Nutrition, 32(3):607–629, 1979. The use of these figures does not imply that the height-to-weight ratios are ideal.

and processed sugars (e.g., colas and candy bars). The goals can be used for evaluations of dietary intake. They provide an excellent guide for how much fat, protein, and carbohydrate we should get. It is simple to figure the percentages of calories from fat, protein, and carbohydrate. These calculations are given in Formulas 13-1 to 13-3.

$$\% \text{ calories from carbohydrates} = \frac{\text{grams of carbohydrates in diet} \times 4}{\text{total calories consumed}} \times 100 \qquad \text{Formula 13-1}$$

$$\% \text{ calories from proteins} = \frac{\text{grams of proteins in diet} \times 4}{\text{total calories consumed}} \times 100 \qquad \text{Formula 13-2}$$

WATER-SOLUBLE VITAMINS							MINERALS						
VITA-MIN C (mg)	THIA-MIN (mg)	RIBO-FLAVIN (mg)	NIACIN (mg NE)[f]	VITA-MIN B$_6$ (mg)	FO-LATE (µg)	VITA-MIN B$_{12}$ (µg)	CAL-CIUM (mg)	PHOS-PHORUS (mg)	MAG-NESIUM (mg)	IRON (mg)	ZINC (mg)	IODINE (µg)	SELE-NIUM (µg)
30	0.3	0.4	5	0.3	25	0.3	400	300	40	6	5	40	10
35	0.4	0.5	6	0.6	35	0.5	600	500	60	10	5	50	15
40	0.7	0.8	9	1.0	50	0.7	800	800	80	10	10	70	20
45	0.9	1.1	12	1.1	75	1.0	800	800	120	10	10	90	20
45	1.0	1.2	13	1.4	100	1.4	800	800	170	10	10	120	30
50	1.3	1.5	17	1.7	150	2.0	1,200	1,200	270	12	15	150	40
60	1.5	1.8	20	2.0	200	2.0	1,200	1,200	400	12	15	150	50
60	1.5	1.7	19	2.0	200	2.0	1,200	1,200	350	10	15	150	70
60	1.5	1.7	19	2.0	200	2.0	800	800	350	10	15	150	70
60	1.2	1.4	15	2.0	200	2.0	800	800	350	10	15	150	70
50	1.1	1.3	15	1.4	150	2.0	1,200	1,200	280	15	12	150	45
60	1.1	1.3	15	1.5	180	2.0	1,200	1,200	300	15	12	150	50
60	1.1	1.3	15	1.6	180	2.0	1,200	1,200	280	15	12	150	55
60	1.1	1.3	15	1.6	180	2.0	800	800	280	15	12	150	55
60	1.0	1.2	13	1.6	180	2.0	800	800	280	10	12	150	55
70	1.5	1.6	17	2.2	400	2.2	1,200	1,200	320	30	15	175	65
95	1.6	1.8	20	2.1	280	2.6	1,200	1,200	355	15	19	200	75
90	1.6	1.7	20	2.1	260	2.6	1,200	1,200	340	15	16	200	75

[c]Retinol equivalents, 1 retinol equivalent = 1 µg retinol or 6 µg β-carotene.
[d]As cholecaliferol. 10 µg cholecaliferol = 400 IU of vitamin D.
[e]α-Tocopherol equivalents. 1 mg d-α-tocopherol = 1 α-TE.
[f]1 NE (niacin equivalent) is equal to 1 mg of niacin or 60 mg of dietary tryptophan.
Reprinted with permission from Recommended Dietary Allowances: 10th ed. Courtesy of the National Academy Press, Washington, 1989.

$$\% \text{ calories from fats} = \frac{\text{grams of fats in diet} \times 9}{\text{total calories consumed}} \times 100 \qquad \text{Formula 13-3}$$

The 4, 4, and 9 in these formulas refer respectively to the calories per gram of carbohydrate, protein, and fat.

The U.S. Dietary Guidelines (Figure 13-11), which were developed cooperatively in 1990 by the U.S. Department of Agriculture and the U.S. Department of Health and Human Services (24), were written for all healthy Americans over age 2 years. They are general and nonquantitative, but they can be a good tool in evaluating the quality of a diet. The guidelines were written to show what Americans

TABLE 13-3A	Estimated Safe and Adequate Daily Dietary Intakes of Selected Vitamins and Minerals[a]

		VITAMINS	
CATEGORY	AGE (years)	BIOTIN (μg)	PANTOTHENIC ACID (mg)
Infants	0–0.5	10	2
	0.5–1	15	3
Children and adolescents	1–3	20	3
	4–6	25	3–4
	7–10	30	4–5
	11+	30–100	4–7
Adults		30–100	4–7

		TRACE ELEMENTS[b]				
CATEGORY	AGE (years)	COPPER (mg)	MANGANESE (mg)	FLUORIDE (mg)	CHROMIUM (μg)	MOLYBDENUM (μg)
Infants	0–0.5	0.4–0.6	0.3–0.6	0.1–0.5	10–40	15–30
	0.5–1	0.6–0.7	0.6–1.0	0.2–1.0	20–60	20–40
Children and adolescents	1–3	0.7–1.0	1.0–1.5	0.5–1.5	20–80	25–50
	4–6	1.0–1.5	1.5–2.0	1.0–2.5	30–120	30–75
	7–10	1.0–2.0	2.0–3.0	1.5–2.5	50–200	50–150
	11+	1.5–2.5	2.0–5.0	1.5–2.5	50–200	75–250
Adults		1.5–3.0	2.0–5.0	1.5–4.0	50–200	75–250

[a]Because there is less information on which to base allowances, these figures are not given in the main table of RDA and are provided here in the form of ranges of recommended intakes.
[b]Since the toxic levels for many trace elements may be only several times usual intakes, the upper levels for the trace elements given in this table should not be habitually exceeded.

(continues on page 459)

should eat to stay healthy. The emphasis was on reduction of risks of contracting chronic disease and a call for moderation.

Food Group Plans

Food group plans pay less attention to the specific foods eaten and more attention to the type of foods eaten. Food group plans categorize foods according to nutrient content. I'm sure you remember the Basic 4 from your early years in school. The Basic 4 plan has been replaced by the Food Guide Pyramid plan (Fig. 13-12). The Food Guide Pyramid was developed by the U.S. Department of Agriculture's Human Nutrition Information Service in 1992 (25). It builds on the idea of the Basic 4 by grouping foods into categories; however, there are five categories in the Food Guide Pyramid because fruits and vegetables are treated separately. Each food category has

TABLE 13-3B	Estimated Sodium, Chloride, and Potassium Minimum Requirements of Healthy Persons[a] *(Continued)*			
AGE	WEIGHT (kg)[a]	SODIUM (mg)[a,b]	CHLORIDE (mg)[a,b]	POTASSIUM (mg)[c]
Months				
0–5	4.5	120	180	500
6–11	8.9	200	300	700
Years				
1	11.0	225	350	1,000
2–5	16.0	300	500	1,400
6–9	25.0	400	600	1,600
10–18	50.0	500	750	2,000
>18[d]	70.0	500	750	2,000

[a]No allowance has been included for large, prolonged losses from the skin through sweat.
[b]There is no evidence that higher intakes confer any health benefit.
[c]Desirable intakes of potassium may considerably exceed these values (~3,500 mg for adults—see text).
[d]No allowance included for growth. Values for those below 18 years assume a growth rate at the 50th percentile reported by the National Center for Health Statistics (Hamill et al., 1979) and averaged for males and females. See text for information on pregnancy and lactation.
Reprinted with permission from Recommended Dietary Allowances: 10th ed. Courtesy of the National Academy Press, Washington, 1989.

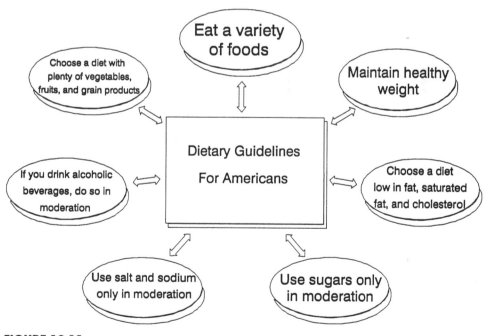

FIGURE 13-11

U.S. Dietary Guidelines for Americans, U.S. Department of Agriculture, U.S. Department of Health and Human Services, 1990.

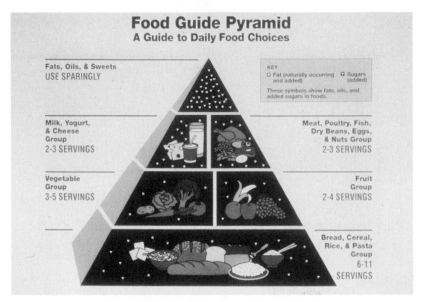

FIGURE 13-12

The Food Guide Pyramid. (From The Food Guide Pyramid, Home and Garden Bulletin Number 252, U.S. Department of Agriculture.)

recommendations for numbers of servings a person should consume daily. The pyramid shape graphically depicts what our diet should look like. Grains, the bulk of our diet, form the large base of the pyramid, while the small tip of the pyramid represents fats, oils, and sweets. Fat, both naturally occurring and added, is represented by small circles; added sugar is represented by small triangles. You will notice these symbols in the tip of the pyramid as well as sprinkled elsewhere. For example, the meat group has some naturally occurring fat, so there are several circles in that part of the pyramid.

The food guide pyramid indicates a range of servings for each category. The number of servings that is right for you depends on how many calories you consume, your age, gender, and activity level. Most people should consume at least the minimum number of servings indicated. Serving sizes, which vary with the category, are given in Table 13-4. Some foods appear in more than one category. For example, a piece of pizza counts as a serving of bread from the crust, milk group from the cheese, and vegetable from the tomato sauce. It also has some fat from the cheese and any added oil.

A drawback to the Food Guide Pyramid and to food group plans in general is that there is no true qualitative measure. A serving of food in a given group counts as one serving whether or not it is **nutrient dense,** that is, has high levels of nutrients relative to the number of calories. To help address this problem, you can use the Food Guide Pyramid in combination with the U.S. Dietary Goals or the U.S. Dietary Guidelines. Despite its shortcomings, the Food Guide Pyramid is an excellent tool for teaching nutrition and for evaluating the adequacy of dietary intake.

A nutrient-dense food has high levels of nutrients relative to its number of calories.

TABLE 13-4	Serving Sizes for the Food Guide Pyramid

FOOD GROUP	SERVING SIZE
Bread, cereal, rice, pasta	1 slice bread 1 oz ready-to-eat cereal 1/2 cup cooked cereal, rice, or pasta
Vegetable group	1 cup raw leafy vegetables 3/4 cup vegetable juice 1/2 cup other vegetables, cooked, chopped, or raw
Fruit group	1 medium apple, banana, orange 3/4 cup fruit juice 1/2 cup chopped, cooked, or canned fruit
Milk, yogurt, cheese	1 cup milk or yogurt 1/2 oz natural cheese 2 oz processed cheese
Meat, poultry, fish, dry beans, eggs, nuts	2–3 oz cooked lean meat, poultry, or fish 1/2 cup cooked dried beans, 1 egg, or 2 Tb peanut butter count as 1 serving of meat

Biochemical Methods

There are several different types of biochemical tests used to assess nutritional status. They can be broken down into two very broad categories, functional and static. Functional tests assess the task a given nutrient is supposed to perform in the body. For example, since vitamin A is involved in the eye's ability to adapt to dim light, a functional test for vitamin A is to assess a person's ability to see in dim light. Static tests are more commonly used; they measure a nutrient in a body fluid or tissue. You probably had a static test for part of your medical examination to enter college. (Remember when the nurse pricked your finger?) Among common blood analyses is the one for hemoglobin, an indicator of iron status.

Static tests can be performed on any body fluid or tissue. While blood, components of blood, and urine tests are most common, tests can also be performed on saliva, amniotic fluid, skin, fingernails, and so on. Blood tests that measure whether a certain nutrient is within normal range can be used both to assess the status of a given nutrient and to screen for risk factors (e.g., plasma cholesterol). The major limitation of a blood test for nutrition assessment is that it measures only what is circulating in the blood; it may not be a good indicator of what is stored elsewhere in the body. A hemoglobin test can be normal despite low levels of storage forms of iron. Similarly, abnormal blood levels of a given nutrient may not mean there is a problem with the person's diet. The abnormal reading may be a result of stress, illness, infection, or inappropriate testing methods. For example, high blood glucose can signal a problem metabolizing glucose (a symptom of diabetes) or recent consumption of a candy bar. Furthermore, normal amounts of glucose may appear in the blood even if dietary intake of carbohydrate is low. Because of hormonal controls, calcium in the blood remains constant regardless of the amount in the diet. If the diet is low in cal-

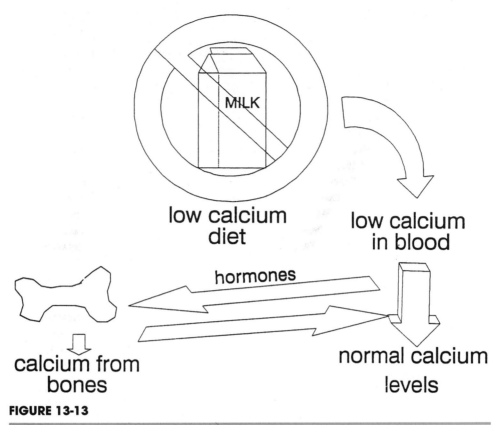

low calcium
diet

low calcium
in blood

hormones

calcium from
bones

normal calcium
levels

FIGURE 13-13

The amount of a nutrient in the blood does not always reflect dietary intake. Even when calcium in the diet is low, the calcium in the blood remains relatively constant because of the mobilization of calcium from the bones. Thus there is little if any relation between dietary calcium and blood calcium levels.

cium, calcium will be drawn from the bones so that blood levels remain within a narrow range (Fig. 13-13).

Urine tests are used to measure excretion rates of a given nutrient or its metabolites. Urine tests can offer valuable information as to general nutritional status and the presence of disease.

Both urine and blood tests are commonly used biochemical measures, and they are very useful in assessing nutritional status. For further information on specific tests for urine, blood, or blood components, or for ranges of normal values, consult *Common Diagnostic Tests: Use and Interpretation* (26). This reference is used by many hospital dietitians.

Another biochemical measure of nutritional assessment is hair analysis. However, I mention it only because you should be aware of its low validity and reliability. Hair analysis is unlikely to be trustworthy for nutritional assessment unless it is being used in large population studies for comparing mineral contents. For use with individuals, there are several problems associated with it. Foremost, there are no standards for nutrients in hair. Even if a laboratory report indicates that your hair has *X* amount of a nutrient, without standards you do not know whether that is good or bad. Another problem with hair analysis is that use of products such as shampoo and dyes can affect the results of an analysis (27). Also, many laboratories that advertise hair analysis are not dependable, and they send back faulty results (28). So save your money and avoid using hair analysis as a means of nutritional assessment.

Clinical Signs and Symptoms

A person's physical appearance can sometimes be used as a very rough estimate of nutritional status. Many types of malnutrition, including some vitamin and mineral deficiencies, have outward signs, sometimes called clinical signs and symptoms. A deficiency of vitamin A, for example, may cause dry, scaling skin. A protein deficiency may change the texture or color of a person's hair and allow it to be easily plucked.

The problems with using this method of assessing nutritional analysis are twofold. First, few people in the United States have malnutrition severe enough to produce obvious external changes. Possible exceptions are the elderly and someone with a prolonged illness. Second, using outward appearance to assess nutritional status is inexact at best, and even trained professionals cannot always correctly identify malnutrition. (Was that a vitamin A deficiency or just chapped skin?)

Although use of clinical signs has its weaknesses, it can be useful as a screening device to alert a health care provider that there may be a nutritional problem and bring about detailed nutrition analysis. Clinical signs and symptoms may also be useful when working in developing countries, where nutritional deficiencies are more common.

Assessing Nutrition Knowledge

Nutrition knowledge is a nebulous term for a person's knowledge and understanding of food and nutrition (29). We are interested in this attribute because of the assumption that what people know may affect what they do. In other words, if they know what to eat or what not to eat, they are more likely to do so. Research indicates that this may be true (29). Although the correlation between nutrition knowledge and eating behaviors is weak, what people know about nutrition can affect their dietary behavior. For this reason, nutrition educators are constantly looking for methods to assess nutrition knowledge.

Most nutrition knowledge instruments are composed of true-false and/or multiple choice questions and are developed to assess the effectiveness of specific nutrition education programs. An instrument developed by researchers at North Carolina State University and East Carolina State University can be used to assess general nutrition knowledge (Figs. 13-14 and 13-15). The Nutrition Knowledge Test (NKT) can be used to compare nutrition knowledge of different groups or to rank the knowledge of individuals within a group. Their nutrition knowledge could then be correlated to their eating habits.

NUTRITION KNOWLEDGE TEST

Directions

This Booklet consists of True-False and Multiple Choice items. With a No. 2 pencil, blacken the circle immediately to the left of the response you choose. DO NOT USE ink, ballpoint or felt tip pens.

Items 1–14 are either true or false. If a statement is true, fill in the circle immediately to the left of "TRUE." If the statement is false, fill in the circle immediately to the left of "FALSE."

Items 15–40 are multiple choice. Choose the best answer from the alternatives provided. Fill in the circle immediately to the left of the answer you have selected.

IT IS IMPORTANT THAT YOU ANSWER ALL QUESTIONS EVEN IF YOU ARE NOT SURE OF YOUR ANSWERS.

Fill in circle completely and erase totally any answer you wish to change.

AGAIN, USE A NO. 2 LEAD PENCIL TO BLACKEN THE CIRCLE IMMEDIATELY TO THE LEFT OF THE RESPONSE YOU CHOOSE. DO NOT USE INK, BALLPOINT OR FELT TIP PENS.

FIGURE 13-14

The Nutrition Knowledge Test. (Reprinted with permission from Carolyn Lackey, East Carolina University, Greenville, NC.)

True-False

Answer the following questions by filling in the circle to the **left** of either "true" or "false."

1. All nutrients are chemicals.
   ○ True   ○ False

2. Vitamin E eaten or taken as a supplement beyond the body's requirements is stored in the body.
   ○ True   ○ False

3. An ounce of carbohydrate has more calories than an ounce of protein.
   ○ True   ○ False

4. Minerals provide the body with small amounts of calories.
   ○ True   ○ False

5. Some foods by themselves have all the nutrients in the amounts needed for adequate growth and health.
   ○ True   ○ False

6. The teenage habit of snacking can provide valuable nutrients.
   ○ True   ○ False

7. Pesticides and other pollutants are incidental food additives.
   ○ True   ○ False

8. Vitamin A is toxic when consumed in large quantities.
   ○ True   ○ False

9. As a person ages, generally, energy needs are reduced while nutrient needs remain the same.
   ○ True   ○ False

10. If a child refuses milk, an acceptable food to provide similar nutrients would be eggs.
    ○ True   ○ False

11. Nutrition labels are required on all canned goods.
    ○ True   ○ False

12. There are no known dietary cures for diseases such as diabetes and heart disease.
    ○ True   ○ False

13. If a food is high in fat it is also high in cholesterol.
    ○ True   ○ False

14. To be healthy, you have to eat meat.
    ○ True   ○ False

FIGURE 13-14

Continued

Multiple Choice

15. Decreasing calorie intake by 500 calories per day would mean a loss of about one pound of body fat in
    ○ 2 days   ○ 10 days
    ○ 7 days   ○ 14 days

16. Which of the following is a vitamin?
    ○ fluoride   ○ fructose
    ○ folacin   ○ iron

17. The RDAs (Recommended Dietary Allowances) are nutrient levels
    ○ used as guidelines for diet planning
    ○ which ensure good health for all indviduals
    ○ which represent minimum daily needs
    ○ all of the above

18. Weight gain results, if at all, when calorie intake
    ○ is from high-fat foods
    ○ is from high-sugar-content foods
    ○ is more than calorie expenditure
    ○ all of the above

19. Of the following, the best source of both vitamin A and vitamin C is
    ○ apple   ○ broccoli
    ○ apricot   ○ carrot

20. Which of the following is the best source of calcium?
    ○ butter   ○ tomato juice
    ○ kelp   ○ yogurt

21. The most concentrated source of calories is
    ○ fat   ○ starch
    ○ protein   ○ sugar

22. One of the first symptoms of vitamin A deficiency is
    ○ anemia   ○ night blindness
    ○ jaundice   ○ scurvy

23. The fat soluble vitamins include
    ○ A B_1 B_{12} and D
    ○ A   C   D and E
    ○ A   D   E and K
    ○ B_1 B_6 B_{12} and C

24. Vitamins are
    ○ a source of energy
    ○ indestructible
    ○ inorganic compounds
    ○ organic compounds

FIGURE 13-14

The Nutrition Knowledge Test. (Reprinted with permission from Carolyn Lackey, East Carolina University, Greenville, NC.) Continued

25. Which vitamin can be made in the body when sun rays contact the skin?
    ○ A   ○ C
    ○ B$_{12}$ ○ D

26. The chief function of carbohydrate we eat is to
    ○ maintain body fat
    ○ provide energy
    ○ provide essential amino acids
    ○ transport vitamin A

27. Sodium, found in table salt and in food,
    ○ can be deactivated by chloride
    ○ helps maintain water balance
    ○ helps prevent scurvy
    ○ is a nonessential nutrient

28. Enriched foods have nutrients
    ○ added that were not originally present or not present in the quantity
       needed
    ○ replaced that were removed during processing
    ○ that are chemically inferior to the natural ones present in food
    ○ that are chemically superior to the natural ones present in the food

29. If the cream is skimmed from milk, which nutrient will be reduced unless it is
    added back after processing?
    ○ calcium   ○ vitamin B$_{12}$
    ○ vitamin A   ○ vitamin C

30. According to the *Food Guide Pyramid,* it is recommended that children and
    adults have how many servings of vegetables per day?
    ○ 1–2   ○ 3–5
    ○ 2–4   ○ 4–8

31. People with hypertension may need to reduce their intake of
    ○ alcohol   ○ sodium
    ○ potassium   ○ sugar

32. Peanut butter belongs to which of the *Food Guide Pyramid* groups?
    ○ breads and cereals   ○ meat
    ○ fruits   ○ milk and dairy products
    ○ vegetables

33. Eggs belong to which of the *Food Guide Pyramid* groups?
    ○ breads and cereals   ○ meat
    ○ fruits   ○ milk and dairy products
    ○ vegetables

FIGURE 13-14

Continued

34. A child's lunch should supply how much of his nutritional needs for a day?
    - ○ 25%
    - ○ 33%
    - ○ 45%
    - ○ 50%

35. How many servings per day of milk are recommended in the *Food Guide Pyramid* for teenagers?
    - ○ 2–3
    - ○ 3–4
    - ○ 4–5
    - ○ 5–6

36. How many servings per day of meat are recommended in the *Food Guide Pyramid* for adults?
    - ○ 2–3
    - ○ 3–4
    - ○ 4–5
    - ○ 5–6

37. During pregnancy, most women (age 23 and above) should
    - ○ increase their food intake by 300 calories per day
    - ○ limit their weight gain to 15–20 pounds
    - ○ restrict their sodium intake
    - ○ take mega vitamin supplements

38. Labeling laws require that food product ingredients be listed on the container in descending order of their
    - ○ calories
    - ○ magnesium
    - ○ nutrients
    - ○ weight

39. Vitamin C found in an orange is chemically
    - ○ identical but more nutritious than vitamin C made in a lab
    - ○ identical to vitamin C made in a lab
    - ○ inferior to vitamin C made in a lab
    - ○ superior to vitamin C made in a lab

40. If a food additive is found to cause cancer in a laboratory rat, the FDA must, under the Delaney Clause of The Additive Amendment of 1958
    - ○ ban the use of that additive
    - ○ establish an allowable level for food additives
    - ○ order investigative hearings
    - ○ order lab testing in humans

THANK YOU FOR COMPLETING THE NUTRITION KNOWLEDGE TEST

FIGURE 13-14

The Nutrition Knowledge Test. (Reprinted with permission from Carolyn Lackey, East Carolina University, Greenville, NC.) Continued

Nutrition Knowledge Test
Answer Key

1. True
2. True
3. False
4. False
5. False
6. True
7. True
8. True
9. True
10. False
11. True
12. True
13. False
14. False
15. 7 days
16. folacin
17. used as guidelines for diet planning
18. is more than calorie expenditure
19. broccoli
20. yogurt
21. fat
22. night blindness
23. A, D, E, and K
24. organic compounds
25. D
26. provide energy
27. helps maintain water balance
28. replaced that were removed during processing
29. vitamin A
30. 3–5
31. sodium
32. meat
33. meat
34. 33%
35. 2–3
36. 2–3
37. increase food intake by 300 calories per day
38. weight
39. identical to vitamin C made in a lab
40. ban the use of that additive

FIGURE 13-15

Answer key for the Nutrition Knowledge Test. (Reprinted with permission from Carolyn Lackey, East Carolina University, Greenville, NC.)

Chapter Summary

This chapter reviews the major methods of nutritional assessment. Each method is described and its advantages and limitations discussed. Dietary analysis methods include 24-hour recalls, food records, food histories, and food frequency questionnaires. Data collected by these methods can be evaluated by comparing food nutrient values with RDAs, U.S. Dietary Goals, U.S. Dietary Guidelines, or the Food Guide Pyramid. Biochemical analyses and clinical signs and symptoms may also be used to assess nutritional status. What a person knows and understands about food and nutrition can be assessed by a paper-and-pencil tool such as the NKT.

SELF-TEST QUESTIONS

1. Which of the following nutritional assessment methods is *least* susceptible to the flat-slope syndrome?
   A. 24-hour recall
   B. 3-day food record
   C. Food history
   D. Food frequency questionnaire

2. Which of the following nutritional assessment methods is *least* affected by a subject's poor memory of what he or she has consumed?
   A. 24-hour recall
   B. 3-day food record
   C. Food history
   D. Food frequency questionnaire

3. Using Table 13-2, find the RDA for protein for a 16-year old boy.
   A. 45 g
   B. 58 g
   C. 59 g
   D. 63 g

4. Which of the following is inadequate intake for a pregnant woman?
   A. 50 g protein
   B. 20 mg iron
   C. 700 mg calcium
   D. 1 g phosphorus

5. Refer to Figure 13-8. Which of the following recommendations for Jane Doe is *not* consistent with the U.S. Dietary Goals?
   A. She should reduce consumption of saturated fats.
   B. She should increase consumption of polyunsaturated fats.
   C. She should reduce consumption of proteins.
   D. She should reduce consumption of carbohydrates.

6. A young woman consumes 2000 total calories, which includes 40 g fat. Approximately what percent of her total caloric intake is from fat sources?
   A. 8%
   B. 12%
   C. 18%
   D. 22%

7. Using Table 13-4, analyze the following breakfast: 2 oz Cheerios with half a cup of skim milk, half a cup of sliced strawberries, 1 tablespoon of sugar, a slice of whole wheat toast with 2 tablespoons of peanut butter, and a cup of black coffee. Which of the following is *not* a correct serving size for this breakfast?
   A. 3 servings from the bread group
   B. Half a serving from the fruit group
   C. 1 serving from the meat group
   D. Some fats, oils, and sweets

8. For the breakfast consumed in the previous question, how many additional servings from the bread group should be eaten during the rest of the day?
   A. 1 or 2 more servings
   B. 2 or 3 more servings
   C. 3 to 8 more servings
   D. No more bread group foods should be eaten

ANSWERS

1. B	2. B	3. C	4. C
5. D	6. C	7. B	8. C

DOING PROJECTS FOR FURTHER LEARNING

1. Using the 24-hour recall method, collect data about a friend's diet. If possible, arrange to have the recall interview videotaped. Evaluate your interviewing skills. Did you inadvertently ask any leading questions? Did your questions successfully elicit valid and reliable information about your friend's diet? Explain.

2. Using a 3, 5, or 7-day food record, collect information about your own diet. Evaluate your diet using each of the following standards: RDAs, U.S. Dietary Goals, U.S. Dietary Guidelines, and the Food Guide Pyramid. What recommendations might you make to improve your diet? Write a summary report.

3. Schedule an appointment with a nutrition specialist. Take along a copy of your food record and dietary analyses, and discuss your diet with the specialist.

4. Conduct a miniresearch study to determine the relation between nutrition knowledge and eating behaviors for some particular group. Administer the NKT to members of an intact group, such as members of an athletic team or residents in an elderly care center. (If you are working by yourself on this project, select a fairly small group or randomly select a sample from a larger group.) Rank the group members from high to low on the basis of their NKT score. Then, using one of the methods described in this chapter, collect information about each group member's diet. Figure out an analysis method that will allow you to rank the subjects according to the quality of their diets. Calculate the Spearman rank order correlation between rank on nutrition knowledge and rank on quality of diet. Interpret your findings. Are you surprised at the results? Explain.

REFERENCES

1. Freudenheim, J.L.: A review of study designs and methods of dietary assessment in nutritional epidemiology of chronic disease. Journal of Nutrition, 123:401, 1993.
2. Peddarinen, M.: Methodology in the collection of food consumption data. World Review of Nutrition and Dieting, 12:145, 1970.
3. Todd, K.S., Hudes, M., and Calloway, D.H.: Food intake measurement: problems and approaches. American Journal of Clinical Nutrition, 37:139, 1983.
4. Beaton, G.H., et al.: Source of variance in 24-hour dietary recall data: implications for nutrition study design and interpretation. Carbohydrate sources, vitamins, and minerals. American Journal of Clinical Nutrition, 37:986, 1983.
5. Block, G., et al.: A data-based approach to diet questionnaire design and testing. American Journal of Epidemiology, 124:453, 1986.
6. United States Department of Health and Human Services: Nutrition monitoring in the United States: an update report on nutrition monitoring. Washington, U.S. Government Printing Office, 1989.
7. Block, G.: Human dietary assessment: methods and issues. Preventive Medicine, 18:653, 1989.
8. Balogh, M., Kanh, H.A., and Medalie, J.H.: Random repeat 24-hour dietary recalls. American Journal of Clinical Nutrition, 24:304, 1971.
9. Karvetti, R.L., and Knuts, L.R.: Validity of the 24-hour dietary recall. Journal of the American Dietetic Association, 85:1437, 1985.
10. Gersovitz, M., Madden, J.P., and Smiciklas-Wright, H.: Validity of the 24-hour dietary recall and seven-day record for group comparisons. Journal of the American Dietetic Association, 73:48, 1978.
11. Rasanen, L.: Nutrition survey of Finnish rural children. VI. Methodological study comparing the 24-hour recall and the dietary history interview. American Journal of Clinical Nutrition, 32:2560, 1979.
12. van Stauersen, W.A., et al.: Seasonal variation in food intake, pattern of physical activity and change in body weight in a group of young adult Dutch women consuming self-selected diets. International Journal of Obesity, 10:133, 1986.
13. Block, G., et al.: A data-based approach to diet questionnaire design and testing. American Journal of Epidemiology, 124:453, 1986.
14. Burke, B.S.: The dietary history as a tool in research. Journal of the American Dietetic Association, 23:1041, 1947.
15. Willett, W.C., et al.: Reproducibility and validity of a semiquantitative food frequency questionnaire. American Journal of Epidemiology, 122:51, 1985.
16. Munger, R.G., et al.: Dietary assessment of older Iowa women with a food frequency questionnaire: Nutrient intake, reproducibility, and comparison with 24-hour dietary recall interviews. American Journal of Epidemiology, 136:192, 1992.
17. Hankin, J.H.: Development of a diet history questionnaire for studies of older persons. American Journal of Clinical Nutrition, 50:1121, 1989.
18. Cooke, K.: Real Gorgeous: The Truth About Body and Beauty. New York, Norton, 1996.
19. United States Department of Agriculture / Human Nutrition Information Service: Composition of Food: Agriculture Handbook Number 8 Series. Washington, United States Government Printing Office.
20. Pennington, J.A.T.: Bowes and Church's Food Values of Portions Commonly Used. 17th ed. Philadelphia, Lippincott-Raven, 1997.
21. ESHA Research: Food Processor Plus: Nutrition and Fitness Software, version 5.0. Salem, Oregon, 1992.
22. Institute of Medicine Staff: Recommended Dietary Allowances. 10th ed. Washington, National Academy Press, 1998.

23. Select Committee on Nutrition and Human Needs, United States Senate: Dietary Goals for the United States. Washington, United States Government Printing Office, 1977.

24. United States Department of Agriculture / United States Department of Health and Human Services: Nutrition and Your Health: Dietary Guidelines for Americans. 3rd ed. Washington, United States Government Printing Office, 1990.

25. United States Department of Agriculture / Human Nutrition Information Services: The Food Guide Pyramid. Washington, United States Government Printing Office, 1992.

26. Sox, H.C. (ed): Common Diagnostic Tests: Use and Interpretation. 2nd ed. Philadelphia, American College of Physicians, 1990.

27. Fosmire, G.L.: Hair analysis to assess nutritional status. Nutrition Today, Sept/Oct, 1986.

28. Barrett, S.: Commercial hair analysis: science or scam? Journal of the American Medical Association, 254:1041, 1985.

29. Axelson, M.L., and Brinberg, D.: The measurement and conceptualization of nutrition knowledge. Journal of Nutrition Education, 24:239, 1992.

CHAPTER **14**

Practical Assessment of Physical Activity

Barbara E. Ainsworth

Regular physical activity affords many health benefits, including reduced risks of coronary heart disease, diabetes mellitus, osteoporosis, and some types of cancer (1). People who engage in regular physical activity also report better health practices: they regularly wear seat belts and smoke less, eat a better-balanced diet, and maintain lower weight for height and body fat levels than do those who do not exercise (1). For these reasons physical educators and public health professionals are interested in promoting regular physical activity in populations.

Identifying the most accurate methods to measure physical activity habits is a challenge. Investigators may measure physical activity in many ways, ranging from simple one-item surveys to detailed measurements of physiological and metabolic body processes. No one method is accurate enough to be considered a gold standard. However, some methods are better than others. This chapter discusses and evaluates the types of tools available for measurement of physical activity in the laboratory and the field. It begins with definitions of common terms used in assessing physical activity habits.

As you read this chapter, watch for the following keywords:

Compendium of Physical Activities	Moderate intensity
Energy expenditure	Physical activity
MET	Vigorous intensity

Definitions

Common terms used in the measurement of human movement include physical activity, leisure activity, recreational activity, exercise, physical fitness, and energy expenditure. People often define these terms according to their experiences and familiarity with various types of activities, yet they differ markedly in terms of frequency, intensity, and duration. This may create wide variation in how investigators

475

record and interpret physical activity participation rates. Therefore, investigators must use common definitions for these terms to reduce measurement errors and to increase the accuracy of physical activity measurement data.

Before 1985 few people agreed about definitions of the terms used in measuring physical activity. Carl Caspersen, an epidemiologist with the U.S. Centers for Disease Control and Prevention (CDC), and colleagues (2) clarified much of the confusion by defining physical activity, exercise, and fitness. Professionals in leisure studies have contributed to the terminology of leisure activity, recreational activity, and free time. Exercise physiologists have defined frequency, intensity, and duration of activities. These definitions form the foundation for classifying types of physical activity assessment tools. The definitions follow:

- *Physical activity* is "any bodily movement produced by skeletal muscles that results in energy expenditure" (2). This definition includes all activities of daily living, home and child care, occupation, transportation, leisure, and various types of inactivity.
- *Exercise* is "planned, structured, repetitive, and purposive in the sense that improvement or maintenance of physical fitness is an objective" (2). Most people refer to organized sports and conditioning activities when defining an activity as exercise.
- *Physical fitness* has many definitions. This chapter recognizes the following two definitions: (*a*) "the ability to carry out daily tasks with vigor and alertness, without undue fatigue and with ample energy to enjoy leisure-time pursuits and to meet unforeseen emergencies" (3); and (*b*) "the ability to do moderate to vigorous levels of physical activity without undue fatigue and the capability of maintaining such ability throughout life" (4). Improved fitness is an outcome of regular exercise and some types of physical activity.
- *Leisure activity* is "physical activity that a person or a group chooses to undertake during their discretionary time" (1). Leisure professionals characterize leisure activities as enjoyable, relaxing, intrinsically self-rewarding, and free from constraints (5).
- *Free time* is "unobligated time, when activities are freely chosen" (5). Leisure activities, exercise, and other recreational activities are usually done in one's free time (5).
- *Recreational activity* is an activity "one does in his or her free time" (5). The context of recreational activities is wider than that of sport and exercise activities. Recreational activities may include but are not limited to cultural, outdoor, and home-based activities (5).
- *Occupational activity* results from "time spent at work for pay or in volunteer activities" (5). This may include, for example, the time spent in transportation to work.

Figure 14-1 shows the relations among these terms. In this framework **physical activity** includes all types of sedentary and active pursuits. Exercise, free-time, recreational, leisure, and occupational activities are subsets of physical activity. The subsets of physical activity have a common outcome of increased physical fitness. The resulting level of physical fitness depends on the intensity, frequency, and duration of physical activities. Because the subsets of physical activity intersect, the subsets are difficult to measure as independent categories.

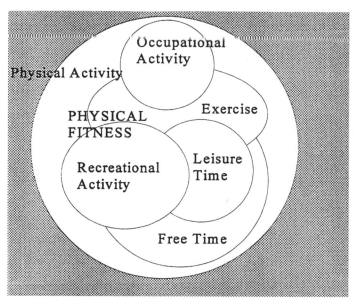

FIGURE 14-1

Relations among the various types of physical activity.

Physical activity is "any bodily movement produced by skeletal muscles that results in energy expenditure" (2). This includes all active pursuits and many sedentary pursuits.

Exercise specialists use the terms *frequency*, *intensity*, and *duration* to prescribe exercise programs and to define the types of activity necessary to improve cardiorespiratory fitness (6). The American College of Sports Medicine (ACSM) (6) defines these terms:

- *Frequency* is "the number of events of physical activity during a specific period (e.g., day, week, or month)."
- *Duration* is the "time, in minutes or hours, of participation in a single bout of physical activity."
- *Intensity* is the "physiological effort associated with participating in a specific activity."

Exercise physiologists distinguish between absolute and relative intensity. Absolute intensity is the actual rate of energy expenditure. It is expressed as the oxygen uptake (VO_2), heart rate, or **METs** (metabolic equivalents). Absolute intensity levels do not account for individual differences in age, gender, body mass, or body fatness. Absolute measures of physical activity intensity are useful when using surveys or other indirect methods to characterize activity habits. Relative intensity refers to the energy cost of an activity, expressed as a percentage of one's maximal oxygen uptake (VO_2max) or maximal heart rate. Relative intensities also account for age, gender, and maximal fitness levels. Exercise specialists use relative intensity levels to prescribe exercise to individuals and to describe exercise intensity in physiological studies.

A MET is the ratio of the metabolic rate for an activity divided by the resting metabolic rate; 1 MET is equivalent to 1 kcal per kg body weight per hour, or about 3.5 $mL \cdot kg^{-1} \cdot min^{-1}$.

Physiologists agree about definitions of intensity levels in laboratory and exercise settings. The ACSM defines activities of **moderate intensity** as requiring 40 to 60% VO_2max (or a maximum MET level) and as 50 to 75% of a maximum heart rate reserve. They define **vigorous intensity** activities as those requiring more than 60% of VO_2max or 75 to 85% of one's maximum heart rate reserve (6).

The heart rate reserve is the difference between the maximum and resting heart rates. The target heart rate reserve is computed as [(220 − age in years) − resting heart rate] × percent effort) + resting heart rate. There follows an example target heart rate reserve for a 20-year-old with a resting heart rate of 70 bpm and an exercise intensity of 75%:

$$
\begin{aligned}
\text{Target exercise heart rate} &= [(220 \text{ bpm} - 20) - 70 \text{ bpm}) \times 0.75] + 70 \text{ bpm} \\
&= [(130 \text{ bpm}) \times 0.75] + 70 \text{ bpm} \\
&= [97.5 \text{ bpm} + 70 \text{ bpm}] \\
&= 167.5 \text{ bpm}
\end{aligned}
$$

Unifying the definitions of physical activity intensities in public health is more difficult. Until recently most physical activity assessment studies used various definitions for light, moderate, and vigorous intensity physical activity levels (7–9). This has created considerable confusion when attempting to define public health guidelines for physical activity.

In 1995 the CDC and ACSM published recommendations on the levels of physical activity needed to promote good health (10). The levels defined for the recommendations were as follows: light, less than 3 METs; moderate, 3 to 6 METs; and vigorous, more than 6 METs. These intensity ratings are absolute levels; they do not account for the age, gender, or cardiorespiratory fitness levels of participants. To promote consistency among research findings, the CDC and ACSM recommended the use of these intensity levels in research and public health settings.

Moderate intensity is performance of a physical activity at 40 to 60% of VO_2max or at 50 to 75% of maximum heart rate reserve.

Vigorous intensity is performance of a physical activity at more than 60% of VO_2max or at 75 to 85% of maximum heart rate reserve. In absolute terms it is more than 6 METs.

Methods of Assessing Physical Activity

Methods for the assessment of physical activity may be categorized as either direct or indirect. Several options exist for both assessment methods (Table 14-1).

Direct Measures

Direct measures of physical activity reflect actual movement and/or energy expended during a period of physical activity. These methods include direct calorimetry, doubly labeled water, motion detectors, physiological monitors, physical activity

TABLE 14-1	Methods Used to Assess Physical Activity

DIRECT MEASURES	INDIRECT MEASURES
Direct calorimetry	Body composition
Doubly labeled water	Cardiorespiratory fitness
Motion detectors	Surveys
Physiological monitors	
Physical activity records	
Physical activity logs	
Direct observation	

records and logs, and direct observation. While none of these methods is adequate alone to characterize total physical activity, they are considered objective, quantitative measures of activity exposure. Therefore, direct measures of physical activity are often used to validate physical activity surveys and other subjective measures of physical activity.

Direct Calorimetry

Direct calorimetry assesses total body **energy expenditure** by measuring one's heat produced at rest or during exercise. This system is based on the principle of conservation of energy. From the food ingested (chemical energy), about 80% is transferred to heat and about 20% is transferred to muscular activity (11). Physiologists measure the kilocalories (kcal) of heat produced in a calorimetry chamber. By subtracting the heat produced from the kilocalories of food ingested, physiologists can compute muscular energy expenditure.

> Energy expenditure is the transfer of chemical energy to work and heat energy. Daily energy expenditure depends on the resting metabolic rate, the thermogenic effect of food consumed, and one's level of physical activity.

An adaptation of the calorimetry chamber is the respiratory chamber. This system is based on measuring the proportion of oxygen and carbon dioxide entering and leaving a closed chamber. The proportion of oxygen and carbon dioxide entering the chamber is constant ($O_2 = 20.09\%$; $CO_2 = 0.03\%$) (11). The proportion of oxygen and carbon dioxide leaving the chamber varies with the work done in the respiratory chamber. Physiologists assume that the difference between inspired and expired gases is the oxygen used and carbon dioxide produced by the person in the respiratory chamber. Caloric energy expenditure is calculated from respiratory chamber data using the following equation:

$$1 \text{ L } O_2 = 4.68 \text{ kcal for fat food sources} = 4.48 \text{ kcal for protein food sources}$$
$$= 5.06 \text{ kcal for carbohydrate food sources}$$

The major advantage of direct calorimetry is in the precision of measurement of the energy expenditure. However, the method is very costly and requires an elaborate metabolic chamber. It also puts the participant in an artificial setting (a small room), which does not reflect the variety of freely chosen physical activity usually done in a given period.

Doubly Labeled Water

Doubly labeled water measures total body energy expenditure using biochemical analysis of hydrogen and oxygen molecules used in cellular respiration. Ingesting a quantity of water with labeled hydrogen (deuterium, or ^2H) and oxygen (^{18}O) isotopes into the body initiates the process, called dosing. Within several hours the body completely mixes the labeled isotopes with body water. As part of the body's metabolic process, the labeled hydrogen molecules gradually leave the body as water, mainly in the forms of urine, sweat, and insensible water vapor loss. The labeled oxygen leaves the body as water and carbon dioxide . The isotopes are measured by collecting urine or saliva samples before dosing, 5 hours after dosing, and 7 to 14 days after dosing. Fast elimination of the isotopes indicates high energy expenditure over time. Energy expenditure is computed using the disappearance rate of ^2H and ^{18}O to compute the rate of production of carbon dioxide (12). Then, by knowing or estimating the respiratory quotient (CO_2 production $\div$ O_2 uptake), one may calculate the caloric energy expenditure during the sampling time.

Estimates of energy expenditure using doubly labeled water are very accurate and are often used as the gold standard to compare indirect methods of physical activity assessment (13). Physiologists have validated use of doubly labeled water with respiratory chambers and caloric balance studies with good results (14). However, while simple in theory, doubly labeled water is very difficult and expensive to carry out. The cost of obtaining and analyzing the isotopes is considerable. In addition, the types, frequencies, intensities, and durations of specific activities during the measurement period are unknown.

Motion Detectors

Motion detectors reflect physical activity by measuring the distance traveled in steps, deflections of body parts, or acceleration of the body (Fig. 14.2). Three types of motion detectors are pedometers, motion counters, and accelerometers.

Pedometers.   Pedometers count the number of steps taken to estimate distance walked. A lever arm does this by moving vertically to rotate a counting device when a participant takes each step. Advantages of pedometers are that they provide an objective measure of body movement, are easy to use, and are inexpensive. They also do not require the user to be literate. However, the accuracy of pedometers varies within and among the various brands. Bassett et al. compared the accuracy of five pedometers over a walking course (15). The pedometers studied were Eddie Bauer Compustep II (Redmond, Washington), Freestyle Pacer 798 (Camarillo, California), L. L. Bean (Freeport, Maine), Yamax Digiwalker DW-500 (Tokyo), and Accusplit Fitness Walker (San Jose, California). The Yamax was the best at tracking distance and the number of steps taken. The other models varied considerably when tested over different times and terrains.

Motion Counters.   Motion counters extend the information obtained from pedometers by detecting movements of other body parts, such as the trunk or limbs. Manufacturers design these instruments to detect deflections of body parts during movement. The monitors store the data for later interpretation. One type is the

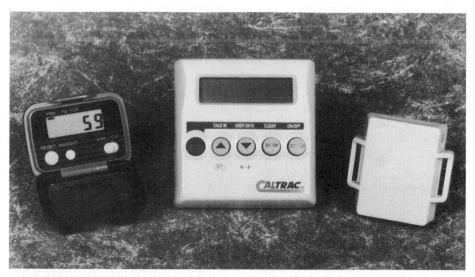

FIGURE 14-2

Motion detectors include pedometers, motion counters, and accelerometers. Accelerometers are usually more valid and reliable than pedometers and motion counters.

Large-Scale Integrated Motor Activity Monitor (L.S.I.) (GMM Electronics, Verona, Pennsylvania). The L.S.I. is the size of a wristwatch and can be worn at any of several places on the body. The L.S.I. contains a ball of mercury that triggers a mercury switch when the wearer moves. Investigators compute a movement score from the total number of deflections recorded during a period. Validation studies show inconsistent results when compared with laboratory measures of human movement and other measures of good health (16–19).

Advantages of motion counters are that they are inexpensive, easy to use, and do not require much effort by the respondent. However, motion counters are less valid and reliable than newer devices (e.g., accelerometers, multiple recorders), so use of motion counters to assess physical activity is relatively rare.

Accelerometers. Accelerometers detect motion produced by a change in the speed or pattern of bodily movements. Engineers have designed two types of accelerometers: vertical plane and multiple plane. Vertical plane accelerometers detect movement in a single plane. The Caltrac Accelerometer (Muscle Dynamics, Torrence, California) and Computer Science and Applications (C.S.A.) (Shalimar, Florida) are vertical-plane accelerometers. Multiple-plane accelerometers measure movement in horizontal and vertical planes. The Tri-Trac-R3D Activity Monitor (Hemokinetics, Madison, Wisconsin) is a multiple-plane accelerometer. Various studies of accelerometers show that they are accurate measures of body movement and energy expenditure (20–23). Multiple-plane accelerometers are considered more precise than single-plane accelerometers, as they capture more types of bodily movement.

Using accelerometers to record human movement has many advantages. They are easy to wear and do not interfere with movement patterns. Accelerometers also can record data in movement counts or as kilocalories. Both Tri-Trac and C.S.A. accelerometers can store minute-by-minute data that investigators download to a computer for analysis. However, these instruments are more expensive than the Caltrac accelerometer, which stores movement data but does not permit downloading to a computer. A general limitation of accelerometers is that they do not record the types of physical activity done. This may be a disadvantage if one is interested in knowing types of movement as well as energy expended in movement.

Physiological Monitors

Physiological monitors record the body's responses to physical activity. Measures of physiological responses associated with movement are the following: increases in heart rate, breathing depth and rate, body temperature, skeletal muscle activity, and heat production (11). Monitoring of physiologic data in the laboratory is easy and reliable. However, similar measurements are difficult to obtain in the field.

Heart Rate Monitors. Heart rate monitors record the heart's response to movement patterns. The basic assumption behind use of heart rate monitors to assess physical activity is that the heart rate increases linearly with the intensity of movement. A high heart rate implies a concomitantly high intensity of physical activity. In laboratory settings, where investigators control the environment, the heart rate response to an activity is considered very accurate. In field conditions many factors can affect the heart rate disproportionately to actual energy expenditure. Fatigue, state of hydration, air and body temperatures, and emotions can significantly increase the heart rate regardless of activity level. These conditions can invalidate data obtained from heart rate monitors. To standardize heart rate monitors, investigators develop heart rate–oxygen uptake curves for each person. This procedure creates a calibration curve that accounts for individual differences in the heart rate response to physical activity. However, the calibration curves do not account for all environmental conditions that may affect heart rates. Therefore, participants should keep a brief log of the activities engaged in while recording the heart rate. This may identify increases in the heart rate that are not associated with physical movement (14).

An advantage to using a heart rate monitor is the possibility of an objective physiological measure of physical activity. In addition, wearing a heart rate monitor is noninvasive and does not interfere with activities. However, the limitations of heart rate monitors are substantial. The heart rate response to movement varies considerably from person to person. Moreover, it is impossible to control environmental conditions that affect the heart rate independent of movement.

Multiple Recorders. Multiple recorders simultaneously record movement patterns and physiological responses to movement. The Vitalog PMS-8 (Redwood City, California) simultaneously records movement patterns and the heart rate response to movement (24). Multiple recorders help to explain the environmental factors that may increase the heart rate disproportionately to movement patterns. They also allow an investigator to identify the amount of time during which a person is engaged in moderate or vigorous activities.

Advantages of multiple recorder systems are that they provide more information about human movement than do single recorders. They also do not interfere with movement patterns. However, the recorders are expensive and are difficult to validate. Multiple recorders are also difficult to use in community settings with many people.

Physical Activity Records

Physical activity records provide a detailed account of activities done within a given time. They are useful for identifying the type, duration, and frequency of activities. Physical activity records may take the form of a written diary or record book or may be dictated to a tape recorder.

Details of the information in a physical activity record vary. One may describe activities precisely (e.g., reasons, types, subjective intensities, exact time records). Alternatively, one may simply write down the names and durations of the activities. The advantage of recording more detailed information is that laboratory staff can be more precise in assigning intensity scores to the activities.

Figure 14-3 is a detailed physical activity record. The respondent identifies the following items: (*a*) purpose (e.g., occupation, inactivity, household), (*b*) type (e.g., writing, sleeping, cooking), (*c*) body position (sitting, reclining, standing), (*d*) effort (e.g., light, moderate, hard) or speed (e.g., slow, moderate, fast) and, (*e*) time spent on the activity. Investigators can use this information to select appropriate intensities of the activities from available charts and to compute a physical activity score.

The **Compendium of Physical Activities** (25) provides standardized MET intensity levels for more than 500 activities (see Appendix D, Parts 1 to 3). The first activity in the Compendium is listed below:

CODE	MET	CATEGORY	ACTIVITY
01009	8.5	Bicycling	Bicycling, BMX or mountain

Column 1 shows a five-digit code that describes the class and type of activity. In this case 01 refers to bicycling in general and 009 refers specifically to BMX or mountain cycling. Column 2 shows the MET level. Columns 3 and 4 describe the category and activity. The activity in Figure 14-4 is coded 02050, and the activity in Figure 14-5 is coded 02100. A competitive sport such as is shown in Figure 14-6 is coded 15210. The Compendium of Physical Activities (25) contains a detailed description of the coding scheme and scoring format.

> The Compendium of Physical Activities is a comprehensive alphabetized listing of physical activities and their standard MET levels.

The advantage of using physical activity records is that they allow for the most detailed description of activities. Obtaining detailed information about activity habits is important when validating indirect methods, such as surveys, used to measure physical activity habits. They are also useful for determining daily physical activity patterns to compute caloric energy expenditure. However, physical activity records have many drawbacks. Keeping an ongoing record of all activities during the designated period is a tremendous burden on the respondent. Physical activity records are also expensive to code and impractical for people with poor reading and writing

PHYSICAL ACTIVITY RECORD

Day _____   Date _____   Time Period _____

Code (1–19)	Body Position (Sit, Std, Rec)	Activity	Effort (L, M, V)	Time (in min.)

Codes
1 = bicycling   6 = home repair   11 = occupation   16 = transportation
2 = calisthenics   7 = inactivity   12 = running   17 = walking
3 = dancing   8 = lawn/garden   13 = self care   18 = water activities
4 = fishing/hunting   9 = miscellaneous   14 = sexual activity   19 = winter activities
5 = home   10 = music playing   15 = sports

Body Position
Sit = Sitting   Std = Standing   Rec = Reclining

Effort
L = Light   M = Moderate   V = Vigorous

FIGURE 14-3

A physical activity record.

skills. For these reasons, physical activity records are used mainly in research settings.

Physical Activity Logs

A modified form of the physical activity record is the physical activity log book (26). Participants using a log book check items they did from a list of possible choices. Participants may check items as they are done or at the end of the day. The advantages of using log books over physical activity records are that they are easy to use, allow recording only data of interest, and simplify data processing. However, because investigators obtain less detailed information, it may not be possible to compute energy expenditure or other summary scores from log book data.

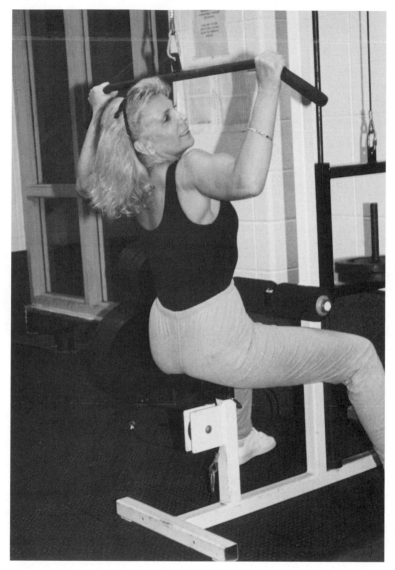

FIGURE 14-4

Weight lifting with vigorous effort is coded 02050. (Photo by Marvin Arrington, Heritage Photography, Greensboro, NC.)

Direct Observation

In direct observation investigators assess the physical activity of others by live observation or by reviewing films or videotapes. Direct observation is frequently used with children and other persons who are unable to complete written materials, recall, or judge the passage of time well. Common to all direct observation systems is the use of time intervals and coded scores to identify movement patterns (27–29). For example, in the Children's Activity Rating Scale (CARS), movement is coded on a five-point scale representing the quality of movement from low to high intensity. A

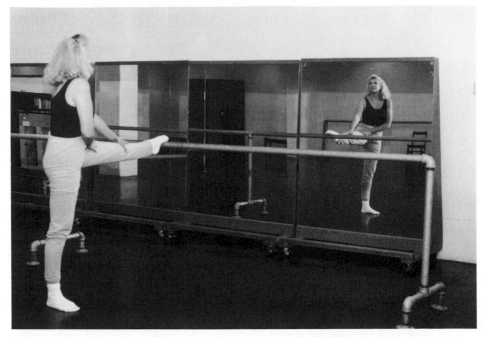

FIGURE 14-5

Stretching activities are coded 02100. (Photo by Marvin Arrington, Heritage Photography, Greensboro, NC.)

score of 1 indicates inactivity; a score of 5 indicates fast and strenuous movement. Detailed rules for coding ensure good objectivity among observers. Coders later transcribe the information to calculate physical activity scores.

A benefit of direct observation is that recall and self-reporting biases do not skew the score. However, direct observations are not practical for measuring physical activity in large groups or in distant locations. Direct observation is also costly and may modify the observed person's behavior.

Indirect Measures

Investigators use indirect measures of physical activity as surrogate markers. These methods include measures of body composition, cardiorespiratory fitness, and physical activity surveys (see Table 14-1).

Body Composition

Measures of body composition include percent body fat, lean body mass, bone mineral density, patterns of fat deposits, circumferences, and bone diameters. Correlations between physical activity levels and measures of body composition are as one would expect: high levels of physical activity are associated with low levels of total body fatness and abdominal adiposity and high levels of lean body mass and bone mineral density (30–32). Validation studies show the strongest correlations between

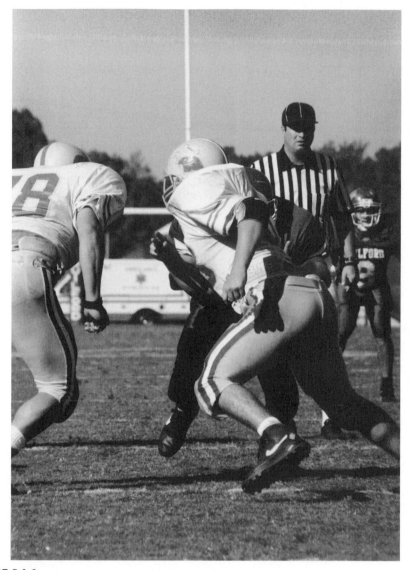

FIGURE 14-6

The code for participation in competitive football is 15210. (Photo by John Bell, Touch a Life Photography, Greensboro, NC.)

body composition measurements and measures of vigorous physical activity (30). Correlations between body composition and physical activity of light and moderate intensity are low and nonsignificant (30). These findings should be considered when using body composition as a surrogate measure of physical activity.

The advantage of using body composition as an indirect measure of physical activity is that it provides an objective measure of rates of participation in vigorous physical activity. However, as noted earlier, it correlates poorly with light and moderate physical activity. Neither do body composition measures provide information about the types and levels of activity done by the participant.

Cardiorespiratory Fitness

Cardiorespiratory fitness has become synonymous with physical fitness. High levels of cardiorespiratory fitness are positively associated with participation in vigorous physical activities; associations are weaker for measures of light and moderate physical activity.

Physiologists regard VO_2max as the best objective measure of cardiorespiratory fitness. One can compute VO_2max with either field or laboratory methods. Physiologists obtain the most precise measures in the laboratory with indirect calorimetry. Indirect calorimetry uses the same principle to compute caloric energy expenditure as does direct calorimetry. However, instead of using a respiratory chamber, physiologists conduct the procedure in an open laboratory. Participants inhale room air and exhale into a tube connected to a gas collection chamber. The volume of air inspired and the differences between the inspired and expired concentrations of oxygen and carbon dioxide are used to compute the VO_2 and the caloric equivalent of the work.

As one would expect, correlations between VO_2max and measures of vigorous physical activity are high (30). However, investigators observe lower correlations between VO_2max and measures of physical activity of light and moderate intensity (30). Therefore, the advantages of using cardiorespiratory fitness to measure physical activity are limited to vigorous activities. One who wants also to measure light and moderate levels of physical activity should include additional assessment tools in the test battery.

Surveys

Survey instruments measure physical activity behaviors from self-reported responses or interviews (Fig 14.7). Surveys vary in detail. They may be single-page instruments that give a global impression of one's activity status. They may also be long, detailed quantitative histories of an individual's physical activity habits over the past year or a even a lifetime.

The benefits of using surveys to measure physical activity status are that they are simple, inexpensive, unobtrusive, and generally do not require much effort on the

What Do YOU Think?

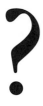

Physical activity surveys commonly show that women are typically less physically active than men (33). Is this really so? Or is this conclusion a result of asking women the wrong types of questions about their activities? Do women engage in different types of activities than their male counterparts? If physical activity is defined to include all bodily movements produced by skeletal muscles that result in energy expenditure, accurate surveys must ask respondents both about leisure activities such as traditional sports and exercise *and* about household activities such as meal preparation, child care, elderly care, laundry, shopping, and so on. In fact, if all of these types of activities were considered, might women actually be found to be *more* active than men? Must the cultural context of women's lives be taken into consideration to discover the truth about their activity patterns? What do YOU think?

LIPID RESEARCH CLINIC PHYSICAL ACTIVITY QUESTIONNAIRE

1. Thinking about the things you do <u>at work</u>, how would you rate yourself as to the <u>amount of physical activity</u> you get compared with others of your age and sex?

   1☐ Much more active
   2☐ Somewhat more active
   3☐ About the same
   4☐ Somewhat less active
   5☐ Much less active
   6☐ Not applicable

College Alumnus Health Questionnaire

1. How many flights of stairs do you climb <u>up</u> each <u>day</u>? _____flights per day
   (Let 1 flight=10 steps)

2. How many city blocks or their equivalent do you walk each <u>day</u>? _____
   (Let 12 blocks=1 mile)

3. List any sports or recreation you have participated in during the past <u>week</u>. Please include only the time you were physically active (i.e., actual playing time in jogging, bicycling, swimming, brisk walking, gardening, carpentry, calisthenics, etc.)

Sport, Recreation or Other Physical Activity	Number of Times per Week	Average Time per Episode		Number of Weeks per Year
		Hours	Minutes	

LEISURE TIME PHYSICAL ACTIVITIES

Listed below are a series of Leisure Time Activities. Related activities are grouped under general headings. Please read the list and check "YES" in column 3 for those activities which you have performed in the last 12 months, and "NO" in column 2 for those you have not. Do not complete any of the other columns.

For Clinic Personnel Use Only

To be completed by participant ACTIVITY (1)	Did you perform this activity? NO YES	DO NOT WRITE IN THIS SPACE	Month of Activity Jan Feb Mar Apr May Jun July Aug Sep Oct Nov Dec	Average number of times per month	Time per occasion Hrs. Min.
SECTION A: Walking and Miscellaneous					
010 Walking for Pleasure					
020 Walking to Work					
030 Using Stairs When Elevator is Available					
040 Cross Country Hiking					
050 Back Packing					
060 Mountain Climbing					
115 Bicycling to Work and/or for Pleasure					
125 Dancing-Ballroom, Square and/or Disco					
135 Dancing, Aerobic, Ballet					
140 Horseback Riding					

FIGURE 14-7

Sample physical activity questionnaire.

part of the respondent. The major drawback is their dependence on recall and lack of precision. Misclassification errors may occur if people exaggerate or underestimate their frequency, duration, intensity, or type of activity. They also occur if the survey omits some types of activities. Inaccuracies and inconsistencies in scoring systems used to estimate energy expenditure can also lead to false generalizations about activity levels and associated behaviors and/or health risks.

Global, recall, and quantitative history surveys are used to assess physical activity. Each type has benefits and limitations. Overall, validation studies show moderately high correlations with measures of vigorous activities; however, correlations for activities of light and moderate intensity are low (30). Table 14-2 lists the types of surveys used in research studies.

Global Surveys. Global surveys are limited to three or four questions about respondents' general physical activity or exercise habits. Epidemiologists use global surveys because they are easy to administer, take less than a minute to complete and have good repeatability. Global surveys have good validity when compared with indirect measures of vigorous activity (30, 34, 38). However, they do not give information about daily energy expenditure or physical activity during specific times.

Recall Surveys. Recall surveys ask about physical activity during the past 1 to 4 weeks. Depending on the questions, recall surveys can provide information about energy expended in various activities of differing types and intensities. Recall surveys usually have 10 to 30 questions. Summary scores may be presented as kilocalories per day or as other units. Validation studies of recall surveys show moderate correlations with objective measures of physical activities done at similar times (30, 39, 55).

Advantages of recall surveys are that they are easy to complete, provide information about specific activities, and allow quantification of physical activity exposure. However, recall surveys may not reflect the respondents' annual physical activity patterns, since the period is usually limited to the past 1 to 4 weeks.

TABLE 14-2	Surveys Used in Physical Activity Research[a]	
GLOBAL SURVEYS	**RECALL SURVEYS**	**QUANTITATIVE HISTORY SURVEYS**
Lipid Research Clinics (34)	7-Day Recall (7)	ACLS 3-Month Recall (35)
Minnesota Heart Health Plan (30)	CARDIA 7-Day Recall (36)	Minnesota LTPA (9, 30, 37)
Godin Leisure Time (38)	College Alumnus (39)	Tecumseh Occupation (37)
Stanford Usual (40)	Baecke (41)	4-Week History (30)
HIP-Job (42)	ARIC/Baecke (30)	3-Month Habitual (43)
St. Louis Heart Health (44)	ACLS 7-Day Recall (45)	CARDIA (30)
Finnish (46)	British Civil Servants (35)	Yale Elderly PA (47)
Parental Report (48)	Behavioral Risk Factor (49)	Diabetes PA (50)
Adventist Mortality (51)	PA Scale for Elderly[b]	Historical PA (52)

[a]For detailed information about each survey, see Ainsworth, Leon, and Montoye (53). Also see Kriska and Caspersen (54).
[b]Washburn, R.: PASE—Physical Activity Scale for the Elderly. Unpublished monograph, New England Research Institute, 1991.

Quantitative History Surveys. Quantitative history surveys are detailed records of the frequency, intensity, and duration of physical activities people did in the past year to a lifetime. These surveys may be self-administered. However, interviewers usually administer the survey so they may probe the respondent for accurate and complete answers. Investigators have validated quantitative history surveys against direct measures of physical activity (37, 56). Quantitative history surveys have also been validated against correlates of good health (52, 57, 58).

The primary advantage of using quantitative history surveys is that they provide a comprehensive accounting of physical activities. They also account for seasonal or lifetime variations in physical activity. However, the burden on the respondent and amount of time it takes to complete the survey sometimes offset these advantages.

Selecting A Suitable Physical Activity Assessment Tool

What is the best type of assessment tool to measure physical activity? The answer depends on the research question, setting, resources, and participants in the study.

Research Question. Investigators should select methods of assessing physical activity that answer the research questions. An investigator may want to use a quantitative history survey to relate an outcome variable (e.g., hypertension, diabetes, obesity) to the frequency, intensity, and duration of physical activities. However, if an investigator is interested in only a general impression of someone's physical activity status, a global survey may be used. An investigator who is attempting to validate a new physical activity assessment tool should use multiple direct-assessment tools to complete the project.

Another factor to consider in the use of a tool is the level of measurement needed to answer the research questions. Sometimes a simple categorical rating of one's physical activity status (e.g., active or inactive) is adequate. Other studies require a continuous interval or ratio variable (such as kilocalories per day) to describe the physical activity levels.

Setting. Laboratory settings permit complexity in measuring physical activity. However, they limit the types of measurement that the participants may take. Most physical activity assessment studies are done in the field using surveys and physical activity monitors. It is important to decide how feasible use of an assessment tool is before one begins the study. Detailed assessment tools are not practical for use with large groups. Thus, in studies with many participants, investigators are generally limited to survey methods to assess physical activity.

Resources. Resources include money, space, and personnel. A laboratory study requires considerable space and equipment. It also requires many personnel to collect the measurements. Lack of money often limits the types of assessment investigators can do. The most expensive methods of assessing physical activity are direct measures. The least expensive types are pencil-and-paper self-surveys.

Participants. Characteristics of the participants guide the type of measurement used in a research study. Important aspects are participants' level of education, age, physical abilities, and willingness to provide detailed information. Highly motivated participants complete nearly any assessment in exchange for information about the findings. On the other hand, one may have to pay less strongly motivated participants to complete a simple one-page survey.

Chapter Summary

Investigators can use direct or indirect methods to measure physical activity. The most precise but least practical are the direct methods. These include direct calorimetry, doubly labeled water, physiological measures, motion detectors, and behavioral observation. Indirect methods are easier to use but less precise. These include surveys and measures of cardiorespiratory fitness and body composition. It is important that investigators use common terminology to define physical activity. In addition, when measuring physical activity of groups, investigators should express the exercise intensities in absolute terms. Investigators should also be aware of practical matters when selecting physical activity assessment tools. Assessment tools should reflect the research questions and should be appropriate for the setting, affordable, and understood by the participants.

SELF-TEST QUESTIONS

1. According to the ACSM definition, which of the following is *not* a physical activity?
   A. Practicing a tennis serve.
   B. Practicing the piano.
   C. Practicing an oral presentation.
   D. All are examples of physical activity.

2. Driving oneself to and from work is _____.
   A. A free-time activity
   B. A leisure-time activity
   C. An occupational activity
   D. A physical activity

3. Which of the following defines an activity of vigorous intensity?
   A. An activity performed at greater than 60% of VO_2max
   B. An activity performed at 75 to 85% of maximum heart rate reserve
   C. An activity requiring more than 6 METs
   D. All of the above

4. Which one of the following provides an *indirect* measure of physical activity?
   A. Body composition
   B. Doubly labeled water
   C. Motion detector
   D. Physical activity log

5. Which one of the following measurement tools is *not* based on detection and measurement of bodily movement?
   A. Accelerometer
   B. Motion counter
   C. Pedometer
   D. Quantitative history

6. Which one of the following motion detectors is *least* valid and reliable?
   A. Vertical-plane accelerometer (Caltrac Accelerometer)
   B. Motion counter (Large-Scale Integrated Motor Activity Monitor)
   C. Multiple-plane accelerometer (Tri-Trac-R3D Activity Monitor)
   D. Multiple recorder (Vitalog PMS-8)

7. Using the Compendium of Physical Activities (see Appendix D), calculate the *total* number of MET-hours (hours × METs) for the following activities: 8 hours of chemical lab work, 1 hour of competitive racquetball, and 1 hour of sitting in a comfortable chair and reading. _____

8. According to figures given in the Compendium of Physical Activities (see Appendix D), what is the difference in MET-hours between playing golf while carrying your own clubs and riding in an electric cart? (Assume the average golf game takes 3 hours.) _____

9. Which of the following is *true* about the relationship between cardiorespiratory endurance (measured by VO_2max) and vigorous physical activity?
   A. There is a strong positive correlation.
   B. There is a weak positive correlation.
   C. There is a strong negative correlation.
   D. There is a weak negative correlation.

10. Which type of survey would best reveal the general exercise habits of the members of a large professional organization, such as the American Medical Association?
    A. A global survey.
    B. A recall survey.
    C. A quantitative history.
    D. All could be used equally well.

ANSWERS

1. D	2. C	3. D	4. A	5. D
6. B	7. 23.3	8. 6.0	9. A	10. A

DOING PROJECTS FOR FURTHER LEARNING

1. Use a 7-day recall survey to measure the physical activities of a group of people. What proportion of the group is vigorously active? What proportion is sedentary? Identify the strengths and weaknesses of the survey instrument in classifying the group members as vigorously active or sedentary.

2. Use 3-, 5-, or 7-day records to record information about your own daily physical activity habits. Use the MET levels from the Compendium of Physical Activities (see Appendix D) to decide the intensity level of the activities. Compute the daily kilocalorie score as follows: Duration (minutes ÷ 60) × intensity in METs × frequency in events per day × (body weight in kilograms ÷ 60). Use this information to answer the following questions:
   A. What proportion of the day did you spend doing the 19 categories of activities based on the first two digits of the five-digit codes listed in the Compendium of Physical Activities?
   B. What proportion of the day was spent doing activities of light (less than 3 METs), moderate (3 to 6 METs), and vigorous intensity (more than 6 METs)?
   C. The CDC and ACSM recommend that every adult do at least 30 minutes of moderate-intensity activities on most days of the week. Did you meet this requirement?

3. Complete project 2 in this chapter and project 2 in Chapter 13. Compare your energy balance in kilocalories by subtracting ingested kilocalories from kilocalories expended in physical activities. Are you in positive or negative energy balance? If needed, what type of changes can you make to modify either your caloric intake or energy expenditure?

4. Conduct a mini–research study to identify the relationship between physical activity status (exposure variable) and some outcome measure. Examples of outcome measures include physical fitness status (maximal oxygen uptake, muscular strength and endurance, or speed), body composition (percent body fat or regional fat deposits), and health status (blood pressure, smoking, mental health, other diseases). Use descriptive statistics to classify the distribution of the group's physical activity levels. Use other appropriate statistics (e.g., correlation, chi square, t-test, ANOVA) to test the hypothesis that physical activity is positively associated with measures of good health.

REFERENCES

1. Bouchard, C., Shephard, R.J., and Stephens, T. (eds.): Physical Activity, Fitness, and Health: International Proceedings and Consensus Statement. Champaign IL, Human Kinetics, 1994.
2. Caspersen, C.J., Powell, K.E., and Christenson, G.M.: Physical activity, exercise, and physical fitness: definitions and distinctions for health-related research. Public Health Reports, 100:126, 1985.
3. President's Council on Physical Fitness and Sports. Physical Fitness Research Digest. Series 1, No. 1. Washington, 1971.
4. American College of Sports Medicine.: ACSM position stand on the recommended quantity and quality of exercise for developing and maintaining cardiorespiratory and muscular fitness in healthy adults. Medicine and Science in Sports and Exercise, 30:975. 1998.
5. Henderson, K.A., Bialeschki, M.D., Shaw, S.M., and Freysinger, V.J.: A Leisure of One's Own: A Feminist Perspective on Women's Leisure. State College, PA, Venture, 1989.
6. American College of Sports Medicine: ACSM's Guidelines for Exercise Testing and Prescription. 5th ed. Baltimore, Williams & Wilkins, 1995.
7. Blair, S.N., et al.: Assessment of habitual physical activity by a seven-day recall in a community survey and controlled experiments. American Journal of Epidemiology, 122:794, 1985.
8. Caspersen, C.J., and Merritt, R.K.: Physical activity trends among 26 states, 1986–1990. Medicine and Science in Sports and Exercise, 27:713, 1995.
9. Taylor, H.L., et al.: A questionnaire for the assessment of leisure time physical activities. Journal of Chronic Disease, 31:741, 1978.
10. Pate, R.R., et al.: Physical activity and public health. A recommendation from the Centers for Disease Control and Prevention and the American College of Sports Medicine. Journal of the American Medical Association, 273:402, 1995.
11. Brooks, G.A., and Fahey, T.D.: Fundamentals of Human Performance. Paramus, NJ, Prentice Hall, 1987.
12. Schoeller, D.A., et al.: Energy expenditure by doubly labeled water: validation in humans and proposed calculation. American Journal of Physiology, 250:R823, 1986.
13. Stager, J.M., Lindeman, A., and Edwards, J.: The use of doubly labeled water in quantifying energy expenditure during prolonged activity. Sports Medicine, 19(3):166, 1995.
14. Montoye, H.J., Kemper, H.C.G., Saris, W.H.M., and Washburn, R.A.: Measuring Physical and Energy Expenditure. Champaign IL, Human Kinetics, 1996.
15. Bassett, D.R., et al.: Accuracy of five electronic pedometers for measuring distance walked. Medicine and Science in Sports and Exercise, 28:1071, 1996.

16. Montoye, H.J., et al.: Estimation of energy expenditure by a portable accelerometer. Medicine and Science in Sports and Exercise, 15:403, 1983.

17. Foster, F.G., McPartland, R.J., and Kupfer, D.J.: Motion sensors in medicine. Part 1: A report on reliability and validity. Journal of Inter-American Medicine, 3:4, 1978.

18. Cauley, J.A., et al.: Comparison of methods to measure physical activity in postmenopausal women. American Journal of Clinical Nutrition, 45:14, 1987.

19. Cook, T.C., Washburn, R.A., LaPorte, R.E., and Traven, N.D.: Chronic low level physical activity as a determinant of high density lipoprotein cholesterol and subfractions. Medicine and Science in Sports and Exercise, 18:653, 1986.

20. Richardson, M.T., et al.: Ability of the Caltrac accelerometer to assess daily physical activity levels. Journal of Cardiovascular-Pulmonary Rehabilitation, 15:107, 1995.

21. Welk, G.J., and Corbin, C.B.: The validity of the Tritrac-R3D monitor for the assessment of physical activity in children. Research Quarterly for Exercise and Sport, 66:202, 1995.

22. Janz, K.F.: Validation of the C.S.A. accelerometer for assessing children's physical activity. Medicine and Science in Sports and Exercise, 26:369, 1994.

23. Melanson, E.L., and Freedson, P.S.: Validity of the Computer Science and Applications, Inc. (C.S.A.) activity monitor. Medicine and Science in Sports and Exercise, 27:934, 1995.

24. Haskell, W.L., Yee, M.C., Evans, A., and Irby, P.J.: Simultaneous measurement of heart rate and body motion to quantitate physical activity. Medicine and Science in Sports and Exercise, 25:109, 1993.

25. Ainsworth, B.E., et al.: Compendium of physical activities: classification of energy costs of human physical activities. Medicine and Science in Sports and Exercise, 25:71, 1993.

26. Bouchard, C., et al.: A method to assess energy expenditure in children and adults. American Journal of Clinical Nutrition, 37:461, 1983.

27. Puhl, J., Greaves, K., Hoyt, M., and Baranowski, T.: Children's activity rating scale (CARS): description and calibration. Research Quarterly for Exercise and Sport, 61:26, 1990.

28. Baranowski, T., et al.: Reliability and validity of self-report of aerobic activity: family health project. Research Quarterly for Exercise and Sport, 55:309, 1984.

29. Wallace, J.P., McKenzie, T.L., and Nader, P.R.: Observed versus recalled exercise behavior: a validation of a seven-day exercise recall for boys 11 to 13 years old. Research Quarterly for Exercise and Sport, 56:161, 1985.

30. Jacobs, D.R., Ainsworth, B.E., Hartman T.J., and Leon, A.S.: A simultaneous evaluation of ten commonly used physical activity questionnaires. Medicine and Science in Sports and Exercise, 25:81, 1993.

31. Slattery, M.L., and Jacobs, D.R.: The inter-relationships of physical activity, physical fitness, and body measurements. Medicine and Science in Sports and Exercise, 19(6):564, 1987.

32. Forwood, M.R., and Burr, D.B.: Physical activity and bone mass: exercises in futility? Bone and Mineral, 21:89, 1993.

33. Ainsworth, B.E.: Women and physical activity. Lecture. St. Louis, American Alliance of Health, Physical Education, Recreation, and Dance, March 21, 1997.

34. Ainsworth, B.E., Jacobs, D.R., McNally, M.C., and Leon, A.S.: Validity and reliability of self-reported physical activity status: the Lipid Research Clinics Questionnaire. Medicine and Science in Sports and Exercise, 25:92, 1993.

35. Morris, J.N., Chave, S.P.W., Adam, C., and Sirey, C.: Vigorous exercise in leisure time and incidence of coronary heart disease. Lancet, 1:333, 1973.

36. Sidney, S., et al.: Comparison of two methods of assessing physical activity in the coronary artery risk development in adolescents (CARDIA) study. American Journal of Epidemiology, 133:1231, 1991.

37. Richardson, M.T., Ainsworth, B.E., Leon, A.S., and Jacobs, D.R.: Evaluation of the Minnesota LTPA Physical Activity Questionnaire. Journal of Clinical Epidemiology, 47:271, 1994.

38. Godin, G., and Shephard, R.J.: A simple method to assess exercise behavior in the community. Canadian Journal of Applied Sport Science, 10:141, 1985.

39. Ainsworth, B.E., Leon, A.S., Jacobs D.R., and Paffenbarger, R.S.: Accuracy of the College Alumnus Physical Activity Questionnaire. Journal of Clinical Epidemiology, 46:1403, 1993.

40. Sallis, J.F., et al.: Physical activity assessment methodology in the five-city project. American Journal of Epidemiology, 121:91, 1985.

41. Baecke, H.A.H., Burema, J., and Frijters, J.E.R.: A short questionnaire for the measurement of habitual physical activity in epidemiological studies. American Journal of Clinical Nutrition, 36:932, 1982.

42. Shapiro, S., Weinblatt, E., Frank, C.W., and Sager, R.V.: The HIP study of incidence and prognosis of coronary heart disease. Journal of Chronic Disease, 18:527, 1965.

43. Verschuur, R., and Kemper, H.: Habitual physical activity. Medicine and Sport Science, 20:56, 1985.

44. Schectman, K.B., Barzilai, B., Rost, K., and Fisher, E.B.: Measuring physical activity with a single question. American Journal of Public Health, 81:771, 1991.

45. Kohl, H.W., et al.: A mail survey of physical activity habits as related to measured physical fitness. American Journal of Epidemiology, 127:1228, 1988.

46. Salonen, J.T., Puska, P., and Tuomilheto, J.: Physical activity and risk of myocardial impaired cerebral stroke, and death. American Journal of Epidemiology, 115:526, 1987.

47. DiPietro, L., Caspersen, C., Ostfeld, A., and Nadel, E.: A survey for assessing physical activity among older adults. Medicine and Science in Sports and Exercise, 25:628, 1993.

48. Murphy, J.K., Alpert, B.S., Christman, J.V., and Willey, E.S.: Physical fitness in children: a survey method based on parental report. American Journal of Public Health, 78:708, 1988.

49. White, C.C., et al.: The behavioral risk factors survey: 4. The descriptive epidemiology of exercise. American Journal of Preventive Medicine, 3:304, 1987.

50. Kriska, A.M., et al.: Development of a questionnaire to examine relationship of physical activity and diabetes in Pima Indians. Diabetes Care, 13:401, 1990.

51. Lindsted, K.D., Tonstad, S., and Kuzma, J.W.: Self-report of physical activity and patterns of mortality in Seventh-Day Adventist men. Journal of Clinical Epidemiology, 44:355, 1991.

52. Kriska, A.M., et al.: The assessment of historical physical activity and its relation to adult bone parameters. American Journal of Epidemiology, 127:1053, 1988.

53. Ainsworth, B.E., Montoye, H.L., and Leon, A.S.: Methods of assessing physical activity during leisure and at work. In C. Bouchard, R.J. Shephard, & T. Stephens (eds.): Physical Activity, Fitness, and Health: International Proceedings and Consensus Statement. Champaign, IL, Human Kinetics, 1994.

54. Kriska, A.M., and Caspersen, C.J. (eds.): A collection of physical activity questionnaires for health-related research. Medicine and Science in Sports and Exercise, 29:S1, 1997.

55. Richardson, M.T., et al.: Ability of the Aric-Baecke to assess physical activity. International Journal of Epidemiology, 24:685, 1995.

56. Ainsworth, B.E., Jacobs, D.R., Leon, A.S., and Richardson, M.T.: Evaluation of Occupational Physical Activity Questionnaire data. Journal of Occupational Medicine, 35:1017, 1993.

57. Folsom, A.R., et al.: Leisure time physical activity and its relationship to coronary risk factors in a population-based sample: the Minnesota heart survey. American Journal of Epidemiology, 121:570, 1985.

58. Leon, A.S., Jacobs, D.R., DeBacker, G., and Taylor, H.L.: Relationship of physical characteristics and life habits to treadmill exercise capacity. American Journal of Epidemiology, 113:653, 1985.

CHAPTER 15

Assessing Physical Activity Injuries

Jerald D. Hawkins

As important as measurement and evaluation are in physical education and sport-related professions, nowhere are they more important than in the assessment of physical activity injuries. In fact, timely and accurate injury assessment, both on the playing field or court and in the clinical setting, may be the single most difficult and challenging responsibility confronting athletic trainers and other sport professionals. It is, after all, the data collected during assessment that form the basis for determining the appropriate disposition of an injury.

The answers to such critical questions as the precise nature and severity of an injury, whether it may be safely cared for by an athletic trainer or should be referred to a physician, when and whether the injured player may safely return to participation, and the appropriate care of the injury all depend upon the results of the assessment. For this reason, it is imperative that the athletic trainer (*a*) master the various techniques required for effective, comprehensive injury assessment, and (*b*) develop a systematic injury evaluation plan that will maximize the quantity and quality of pertinent data obtained while minimizing the likelihood of errors that may compromise the well-being of the injured athlete.

For a more detailed presentation of the concepts in this chapter, refer to *The Practical Delivery of Sports Services: A Conceptual Approach*, by Jerald D. Hawkins. Canton, OH, PRC Publishing, 1993. All rights reserved.

As you read this chapter, watch for the following keywords:

Crepitation	Injury assessment	Palpation
Edema	Medical diagnosis	Sign
Functional testing	Orthopaedic	Symptom

Criteria for Selecting an Assessment

When properly designed and performed, **injury assessment** procedures should have the same psychometric characteristics as cognitive, fitness, skill, and other types of physical activity tests: validity, reliability, objectivity, and freedom from assessment bias. There follows a brief overview of these four criteria and their relation to assessment of physical activity injury.

> Injury assessment is the evaluation of a possible injury by nonmedical personnel, such as athletic trainers.

Validity

Validity is simply the extent to which a given test does the job for which it is used. A volleyball skill test used to evaluate the serving ability of players may be considered to have validity if the results of the test accurately reflect (i.e., are consistent with) the serving performances of the players in games. A test that purports to identify a specific injury may be deemed valid if more direct and invasive diagnostic procedures (e.g., surgical examination) verify that the test, when properly performed, accurately and consistently identifies the injury. A good example is the Lachman test (Fig. 15-1) for evaluating anterior cruciate ligament sprains and tears. Most athletic

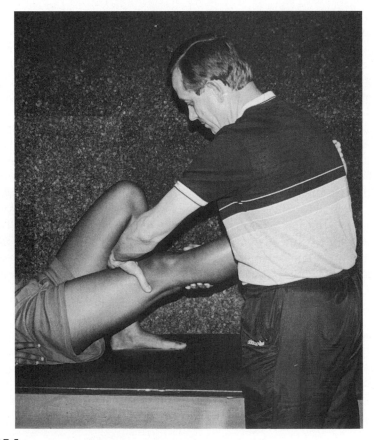

FIGURE 15-1

The Lachman Test is deemed valid because follow-up surgical evaluation verifies anterior cruciate ligament sprains or tears. (Photo by Joel Nichols, Greenwood, SC.)

injury assessments are criterion-referenced tests. They are used to establish the presence or absence of a particular injury; that is, the subject's injury passes or fails the test. Therefore, the first criterion for selecting a particular procedure is its validity, or the extent to which it does the job. Use of an injury assessment procedure of unknown or questionable validity increases rather than minimizes the risk of error.

Reliability

The second essential criterion, reliability, is the extent to which a test produces consistent results. In the case of criterion-referenced tests, reliability is consistency of classification. A volleyball serving test that yields significantly different results on several consecutive examinations lacks acceptable reliability. When assessing the nature and severity of a possibly serious injury, a high degree of reliability (consistency of classification) is essential, since the failure of a specific diagnostic procedure to yield consistent results reduces the assessment process to little more than a game of chance. Strict adherence to a specific assessment protocol when using a valid assessment procedure (e.g., careful and systematic evaluation of the ABCs—airway, breathing, and circulation—in an unconscious athlete) is necessary for establishing and maintaining reliability.

Objectivity

Objectivity is the extent to which a test or procedure is free from examiner bias, or the uniformity with which various persons with equivalent training, expertise, and experience can successfully employ it. In the absence of objective criteria, 10 volleyball coaches, asked to evaluate the serving skills of a group of players, might produce significantly different evaluations based upon their personal criteria. An excellent example of poor objectivity (even though objective criteria are supposedly employed) are the scores awarded to figure skaters, gymnasts, and boxers by judges who view the same activity yet perceive significantly different performances. When assessing a possibly serious injury, such a lack of objectivity can threaten not only the health and well-being of the injured athlete but possibly even his or her life. Therefore, to the extent possible, injury evaluation should include objective criteria that may be employed by the athletic trainer, maximizing the objectivity of the procedure. The Glasgow Coma Scale for evaluating the severity of head injuries (Fig. 15-2) is a good example of an objective assessment tool for injury.

Freedom From Assessment Bias

Injury assessment procedures are generally believed to be free of the influence of gender, race, and age biases. For example, it is unlikely that an assessment instrument such as the Glasgow Coma Scale would yield different results because the athlete was male as opposed to female, black as opposed to white, or young as opposed to old. Orthopaedic injury assessment procedures are designed to be socially neutral. The scales and tests are administered and interpreted the same for persons of both genders, any race, and any age.

However, because injury assessment requires subjective judgment on the part of the examiner, the issue of bias is not entirely irrelevant. Bias can subtly affect how the examiner interprets signs and symptoms. For example, if an athletic trainer

Best eye-opening response	Purposeful and spontaneous	4
	To verbal command	3
	To painful stimuli	2
	No response	1
Best motor response	Obeys verbal commands	6
	Localizes pain (painful stimuli)	5
	Withdraws from pain	4
	Flexion abnormal (decorticate rigidity)	3
	Extension abnormal (decerebrate rigidity)	2
	No response	1
Best verbal response	Oriented and converses	5
	Disoriented and converses	4
	Inappropriate words	3
	Incomplete sounds	2
	No response	1

FIGURE 15-2

The Glasgow Coma Scale is a subjective assessment with good objectivity.

holds the erroneous belief that women athletes have lower pain thresholds than their male counterparts, the trainer may unwittingly practice gender bias when assessing severity of an injury according to pain self-reports, facial grimaces, and such. Any source of bias poses a threat to valid, reliable, and objective assessment!

Principles of Injury Assessment

The initial step in maximizing the validity, reliability, and objectivity of the injury assessment process is by establishing and adhering to sound principles of assessment. The following seven principles are suggested as the basis for effective injury assessment.

1. "First, Do No Harm." One of the unique characteristics of injury assessment as compared with other forms of testing is that the physical health and well-being of the client are the focus of concern. Although there may be several valid tests for the assessment of a specific suspected injury, the relative safety of each test must be considered before the assessment is begun. As with any injury, the assessment itself may, if performed inappropriately, worsen the injury. Therefore, it is important to evaluate the injury in such a way as to avoid exacerbating it. For example, if there is any reason to suspect a head or neck injury, the initial evaluation should be performed without moving the injured person.

2. Have a Thorough Working Knowledge of Anatomy and Physiology. To select the proper sequence of evaluative procedures, an athletic trainer must develop the ability to look at an area of the body or specific body structure and visualize the anatomical makeup and physiological processes that lie beneath the skin. Often the absence of definitive signs of a specific injury makes accurate assessment extremely difficult or impossible for the trainer. However, even in the absence of such key information, knowledge of underlying anatomy enables the trainer to consider what specific structures may be injured, and knowledge of regional physiology may provide a basis for understanding such general signs as impairment of normal function.

3. Have a Thorough Knowledge of the Signs and Symptoms of Injuries. Objectivity of the assessment process may be enhanced through the systematic identification of specific **signs** and **symptoms**. Each individual item of data provides the athletic trainer with a valuable piece of the puzzle. Common symptoms such as generalized pain and **edema** may indicate the general area and possibly the severity of an injury, and specific signs, such as Babinski's sign in neurologic trauma and Kehr's sign in acute spleen injury, often provide critical definitive information. Although the learning of signs and symptoms is never ending and often tedious, there is no substitute for such knowledge when the health and safety of an injured person are at stake.

> A sign is a single specific condition that indicates a single specific injury or illness, e.g., Battle's sign.

> A symptom is a condition or behavior associated with a number of injuries or illnesses, e.g., swelling.

> Edema is an excessive accumulation of serous fluid in the tissues, that is, swelling.

4. Examine All Injuries as Soon as Possible. For a variety of reasons, the evaluation of an athletic injury is sometimes postponed until after a practice or game or even until the next day. Whether due to a coach's or player's insistence on waiting until later, an injured player's reluctance to acknowledge the injury, or any other reason, delaying the examination often makes the assessment more difficult, increases the severity of the injury, and/or increases the injured athlete's vulnerability to further injury. Common injury-related symptoms such as swelling, pain, and muscle spasticity generally become more pronounced with time. When the evaluation of an injury is delayed, such conditions may make accurate assessment by an athletic trainer virtually impossible and may necessitate referral to a physician for an otherwise needless extensive medical evaluation. In essence, failure to examine an injury in a timely manner may render assessment by the athletic trainer impossible. Therefore, it is wise to evaluate all injuries as soon as possible.

5. Use an Appropriate Place to Conduct the Assessment. The environment where an assessment is done may either contribute to or undermine the validity, reliability, and objectivity of the assessment process. Injury assessment on the field or court is difficult enough without having to contend with the confusion, distractions, and pressure from interested teammates, coaches, officials, parents, and fans. Therefore, once the initial evaluation indicates that it is safe to move the injured athlete, he or she should be taken to an appropriate place for further assessment. While it is not always practical, when possible injury assessment should be performed away from the playing area, preferably in a nearby training room or locker room. This not only affords privacy, it provides relief from the distractions and pressures of a crowded public place.

6. Avoid Haste.   Injury assessment, as with any other form of testing, should not be rushed. The scene is often charged with emotion. Officials may be anxious for play to resume, and coaches hope the player can continue, especially when the injury does not appear to them to be serious. When an injury occurs, however, the trainer must take the position that until a thorough evaluation is complete and it is deemed safe to remove the athlete from the field, the trainer and/or medical personnel—rather than officials, coaches, administrators, or fans—are in charge of the area. If it is considered unsafe to move the injured athlete, play must remain suspended until appropriate medical assistance is obtained and the athlete has been safely transported from the playing area. Acting hastily for any reason jeopardizes the effectiveness of the assessment and threatens the health and safety of the injured athlete.

7. Develop a System for Assessing All Injuries.   As stated previously, the assessment of injuries should be systematic. The reliability of otherwise valid assessment procedures may be jeopardized if assessment is haphazard. One of the most effective ways to enhance the reliability of the assessment process is through the development and use of a strategic plan for assessment. Just as the correct performance of cardiopulmonary resuscitation (CPR) and the proper taping of an ankle require a logical, step-by-step sequence of events, the assessment of sport injuries should be well organized. A suggested plan is described in the next section.

Systematic Injury Assessment: The Process

Injury assessment plans, like well-constructed cognitive and skill tests, should not be copied but should reflect the specific needs and resources of the program in which they are used. However, it is imperative that a logical, systematic plan for injury assessment be developed and used. Doing so maximizes both the reliability and objectivity of the assessment process. Although an experienced athletic trainer moves smoothly through the process step by step in much the same way that a skilled gymnast or figure skater negotiates a series of difficult maneuvers, the beginning athletic trainer may find it helpful to follow a written checklist until the steps of the plan are second nature. The following nine steps provide a system of injury assessment.

Step 1: See.   The initial step in the assessment of acute injuries is seeing:

1. What happened? How did the injury occur? What was the position of the athlete at the time of injury? What was he or she doing? How did the athlete move or fall following the injury?
2. What was the likely mechanism of injury? Was the athlete hit by another player or an object? Did he or she move in an awkward manner that might indicate a joint stress injury?
3. What obvious signs or symptoms of injury do you see upon reaching the scene? The primary concern is to establish whether the athlete is conscious. If so, attention should be turned to obvious concerns such as bleeding and bone deformity. If the athlete is unconscious, immediate attention should be focused on vital processes (the ABCs of basic life support: airway, breathing, and circulation). It is beyond the scope of this text to discuss the care of an unconscious athlete, so the remaining steps in the assessment plan are presented with the assumption that the injured athlete is conscious.

Step 2: Ask. Following the initial visual check, the injured athlete should be queried:

1. What happened? When questioning the injured athlete, resist the temptation to put words into his or her mouth with leading questions. Such actions may threaten the validity of the assessment, since suggestions made by the examining trainer may be verified by the injured athlete even if they don't exist on the assumption that the trainer knows what happened, so his or her suggestion must be accurate.
2. Where is the pain? Ask the injured athlete to point at or touch the specific pain site, if possible, since verbal descriptions are often vague and may be misleading. Also, actively involving the athlete in the assessment may alleviate the fear and apprehension often associated with injury.
3. Did the injured athlete hear or feel anything unusual? The athlete may report hearing or feeling a pop or snap that may indicate fracture or ligament rupture or feeling the subluxation (partial dislocation) or dislocation of a joint.

Step 3: Listen. During this initial communication with the injured athlete, listen carefully to the athlete's answers and statements or questions of concern. Also, other players who witnessed the injury may provide additional information.

Step 4: Observe. The first hands-on assessment of the specific injury site should include a careful, thorough observation of the injury to seek out such key symptoms as swelling, deformity, and bleeding. Throughout this process and during the remainder of the evaluation, watch the athlete's face closely, since nonverbal expressions of pain and apprehension are often more accurate than verbal responses.

Step 5: Feel. If there is doubt concerning whether the player may be safely moved, gentle **palpation** of the injured body part may be advisable. This initial palpation allows the evaluating trainer to feel for signs:

1. Pain or deformity of the head or neck may indicate serious head or neck injury. In such circumstances the athlete should not be moved until after further medical examination.
2. Bone or joint deformity may indicate fracture or dislocation, in which case the athlete should not be moved until the injury site is properly stabilized or splinted.
3. Significant bleeding in an area not readily visible to the athletic trainer should be controlled before any attempt is made to remove the athlete from the field or court.

Palpation is the examination or exploration of an area of the body by touching.

Step 6: Decide. At this point it may be appropriate to make a decision regarding the advisability of moving the injured athlete. If there is doubt concerning the safety of moving the athlete, steps should be taken to stabilize the injury and medical assistance should be obtained. Care of the injured athlete must always take precedence over the resumption of play regardless of the time involved.

Step 7: Examine.   Assuming that the injured athlete has been safely moved from the field or court, a more thorough examination of the injury may be warranted.

1. Visual comparison of an injured limb or joint with the contralateral limb or joint provides a frame of reference for further evaluation. Often what appears to be swelling or deformity upon initial examination is discovered to be a quite normal structural characteristic when the same appearance is noted in the uninjured body part.
2. Careful palpation may reveal important information about the precise nature and extent of the injury. In the case of limb or joint injury, palpation of the uninjured contralateral structure may serve two valuable functions: provide a point of reference for evaluation of the injured structure and alleviate the athlete's fear and apprehension concerning the examination. Information gained through palpation may include differentiation of general tenderness from point tenderness, edema from deformity, and any **crepitation**.
3. Results of this examination may suggest that the athlete should be referred to a physician.

Crepitation is a palpable or audible sound, such as crunching, grating, creaking, rattling, or crackling.

Step 8: Test.   If deemed safe and appropriate, a series of tests may be used to gain additional information about the injury.

1. Manipulation of the injured body part may be used to assess passive range of motion (athletic trainer moves the joint without assistance from the athlete), joint laxity, and so on.
2. Specific tests may be used to determine the specific nature and severity of the injury. Examples of such tests are presented later in this chapter.
3. **Functional testing** may be used to assess the extent to which normal function of the injured body part is possible. Such testing may include assistive range of motion (athletic trainer moves the joint with the athlete's assistance), active range of motion (athlete moves the joint without assistance), resistive range of motion (athlete moves the joint against controlled manual resistance from the athletic trainer), functional strength, functional weight bearing, the ability to walk, jog, or run without limping, and so on.
4. Successful completion of manipulative, joint-specific, and functional testing may indicate that the athlete may safely return to participation with few or no restrictions. However, failure to complete one or more of these tests successfully may indicate the need for specific injury care and/or referral to a physician.

Functional testing consists of performance-based assessment procedures.

Step 9: Monitor.   An injured athlete, whether returned to play or not, should be carefully monitored until fully recovered, since subtle symptoms such as recurrent swelling and/or pain, diminished functional capacity, and/or failure of the injury to respond to conventional therapy may indicate the need for medical consultation.

Specific Procedures for Injury Assessment

Assessment of injuries requires the gathering and interpretation of valid, reliable, and objective data. Unlike cognitive assessment, which may use a simple question-and-answer answer format, or skill testing, which may include the observation of highly objective behaviors and results, accurate assessment of a single injury may entail the use of a variety of assessment procedures. This often includes (*a*) the identification and interpretation of key symptoms and signs, (*b*) the performance of specific functional tests, and (*c*) the use of medical diagnostic procedures ordered by a physician.

Evaluation of Symptoms

The most fundamental form of injury assessment data is identification of symptoms. As noted earlier in this chapter, symptoms are conditions or behaviors that may be associated with one or more particular injuries or illnesses. There are two major characteristics of symptoms: (*a*) A single symptom by itself is rarely sufficient to identify the specific injury or illness. (*b*) Although often easily identified, many symptoms defy objective quantification, while others may be quantified with a high degree of reliability and objectivity.

When performing an injury assessment, the athletic trainer should identify and record as many symptoms as possible. For example, swelling around a joint may be the result of any one of a host of acute conditions (e.g., fracture, sprain, strain) or chronic conditions (e.g., bursitis, tendinitis). Therefore, swelling by itself provides only a small piece of the puzzle. However, several other symptoms in combination with swelling may enable the athletic trainer to identify the probable injury or illness more precisely.

An excellent example of the value of multiple-symptom evaluation can be seen when an eating disorder, such as anorexia nervosa or bulimia, is suspected. Figure 15-3 illustrates several symptoms and/or behaviors, any one of which by itself reveals little about a dangerous eating disorder. However, several of these symptoms in combination offer legitimate evidence of a health-threatening and possibly life-threatening condition.

As desirable as it is to base assessment only on objective data, some symptoms are not easily quantified. Point tenderness (the pain elicited when a specific structure is palpated) may appear severe in one athlete when in fact it is no greater than the apparently moderate pain in another athlete. Where possible, attempts are made to establish objective rating systems by which difficult-to-quantify symptoms (e.g., pain, soreness, skin coloration) may be objectively measured. The Glasgow Coma Scale (Fig. 15-2) is just such an instrument. A standard instrument for the assessment of an injured athlete's level of consciousness, the scale permits numeric description of activity in three critical areas: eye opening, motor responses, and verbal responses.

Evaluation of Signs

Unlike symptoms, which may be somewhat generic and are most useful when found in combination, signs are often so specifically related to a particular injury or illness that they are given unique names that reflect the specific nature of the sign or credit

ANOREXIA NERVOSA

- Exaggerated fear of being overweight or getting fat even though underweight
- Preoccupation with body image and diet
- Distorted perception of body image; seeing oneself as fat even while becoming thinner
- Preoccupation with increasing exercise
- Skipping meals and/or avoiding eating with others
- Wearing bulky clothing in an obvious attempt to hide the contours of the body
- Light-headedness and/or fainting without apparent cause
- Weight loss during normal growth periods
- Mood changes (e.g., irritability, depression)

BULIMIA

- Symptoms of anorexia nervosa
- Recurrent binge eating without weight gain
- Reliance on vomiting, laxatives, and/or diuretics for weight loss
- Frequent weight fluctuations of more than 10 lb
- Frequently excusing oneself immediately after meals to "go to the bathroom," "catch a quick shower," and so on, often returning with bloodshot eyes

FIGURE 15-3

Symptoms of eating disorders. These indications in combination may be a better indicator of disordered eating than any single symptom by itself. Also, they do not necessarily indicate an eating disorder but may nevertheless be cause for concern.

the person who identified the significance of its use. Such diagnostic signs are generally recognized for the validity, reliability, and objectivity with which they enable trained examiners to identify one specific injury or illness. The following are several of the common injury signs used in sport- and exercise-related injury assessment.

Battle's Sign: Fracture of the Temporal Bone or Basilar Skull

Following a blow to the head and up to 24 hours later, discoloration over the mastoid area may indicate a fracture of the temporal bone or basilar skull fracture. This is Battle's sign.

Cullen's Sign: Internal Hemorrhage

Following a blow to the abdominal area, discoloration (bruise type of bleeding) around the umbilicus may indicate peritoneal bleeding. This is Cullen's sign.

Kehr's Sign: Spleen Rupture

Following a blow to the abdominal area, pain that radiates to the left shoulder and upper arm may indicate a ruptured spleen. This is Kehr's sign.

Romberg's Sign: Intracranial Trauma

Following a blow to the head, the inability to maintain balance while standing with feet together, arms to the side, and eyes closed may indicate intracranial injury. This is Romberg's sign.

Piano Key Sign: Third-Degree Acromioclavicular Sprain

Following an injury to the shoulder girdle area, the distal end of the clavicle protrudes upward. When pressed downward, it springs back to its elevated position. This sign, which may indicate a third-degree acromioclavicular sprain, is the piano key sign.

Tapping Sign: Carpal Tunnel Syndrome

When tapping repetitively with the finger over the transverse carpal ligament produces pain or tingling, it may indicate carpal tunnel syndrome. This is the tapping, or Tinel's, sign.

Selected Orthopaedic Tests

Most physical activity injuries involve **orthopaedic** structures (bones, joints, muscles, tendons, ligaments, and related soft tissues). Therefore, a wide variety of specific tests for the assessment of orthopaedic injuries have been developed. It is not the purpose of this text to present a complete list and description of all such tests. However, the following section contains some of the more common tests used in the assessment of orthopaedic injuries resulting from participation in sports and exercise.

> Orthopaedic refers to the bones, joints, muscles, tendons, ligaments, and related soft tissues of the body.

Drawer Test: Ligament Rupture Associated With Ankle Sprain

In the drawer test, with the injured ankle in a neutral position at 90°, the examiner grasps the lower leg firmly just above the malleolus and the foot firmly at the calcaneus (Fig. 15-4). The examiner applies manual traction to the ankle in an attempt to pull the talus forward from its normal articulation with the distal tibia or fibula. If the ankle opens up (i.e., the talus glides forward with traction), it may indicate that the anterior talofibular ligament has been ruptured.

Manual Compression Test: Tibial or Fibular Fracture Associated With Sprain

An acute ankle sprain may result in fracture of the tibial or fibular malleolus. Therefore, in such cases the manual compression test is in order. The examiner manually compresses the proximal tibia and fibula (Fig. 15-5). Such compression producing pain on or above one of the malleoli suggests a fracture.

Thompson Test: Achilles Tendon Rupture

In the Thompson test, with the injured athlete prone with both knees fully extended the examiner firmly grasps the calf muscles on the injured side and applies manual compression (Fig. 15-6). Failure of the ankle to plantar-flex when the calf muscle is compressed indicates Achilles tendon rupture.

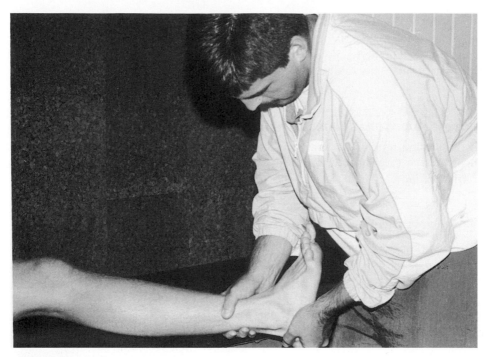

FIGURE 15-4

Drawer test to evaluate ligament rupture associated with ankle sprain. (Photo by Joel Nichols, Greenwood, SC.)

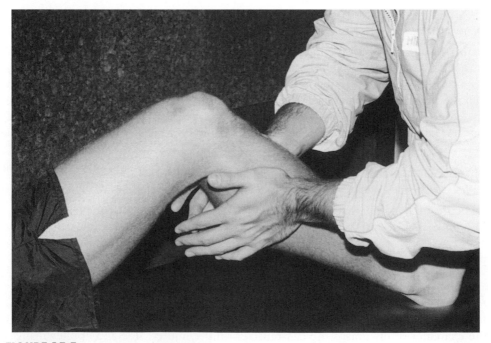

FIGURE 15-5

Manual compression test to evaluate tibial or fibular fracture associated with sprain. (Photo by Joel Nichols, Greenwood, SC.)

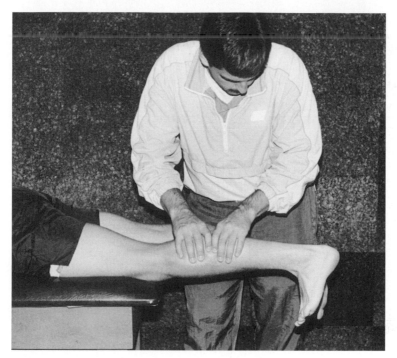

FIGURE 15-6

Thompson test to evaluate Achilles tendon rupture. (Photo by Joel Nichols, Green-wood, SC.)

Valgus and Varus Test of the Knee: Collateral Ligament Strain or Tear

In the valgus and varus test, with the athlete lying supine and the injured knee in full extension the examiner places one hand firmly against the lateral joint line and with the other grasps the lower leg just above the ankle. Use of opposing force (upper hand applying force medially, lower hand applying lateral force) allows evaluation of the medial stability of the joint. The test is repeated with one hand applying lateral force at the medial joint line while the other hand applies medial force just above the ankle (Fig. 15-7).

Abnormal instability may indicate collateral ligament sprain or tear and possible structural damage to the posterior capsule (posterior supporting structures). If no instability is detected, the knee should be passively flexed approximately 20° and the test repeated. This position eliminates the influence of posterior capsule support. Therefore, instability may indicate collateral ligament damage without posterior capsule disruption.

Apley Distraction Test of the Knee: Collateral Ligament Sprain or Tear and/or Capsular Damage

In the Apley distraction test (Fig. 15-8), with the athlete lying prone, the examiner flexes the knee 90°. The examiner stabilizes the thigh by placing his or her knee on the back of the thigh just above the knee or by having an assistant hold the thigh down during testing. The examiner firmly grasps the ankle and exerts upward pres-

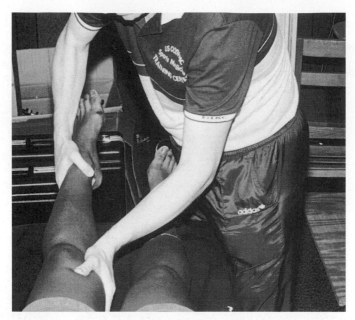

FIGURE 15-7

Valgus and varus test to evaluate collateral ligament strain or tear. (Photo by Joel Nichols, Greenwood, SC.)

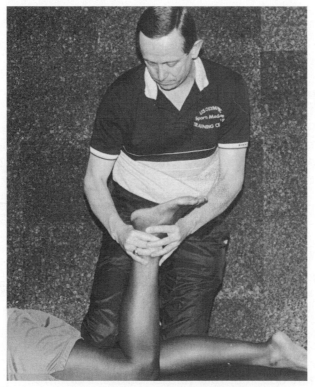

FIGURE 15-8

Apley distraction test to evaluate collateral ligament sprain or tear and/or capsular damage. (Photo by Joel Nichols, Greenwood, SC.)

sure by pulling upward while rotating the lower leg inward and outward. Pain with distraction or rotation may indicate collateral ligament and/or capsular damage.

Apley Compression Test of the Knee: Meniscus Cartilage Tear

In the Apley compression test (Fig. 15-9), with the athlete lying prone the examiner flexes the knee 90° and exerts downward pressure (compression) on the heel along the longitudinal axis of the lower leg while rotating the lower leg inward and outward. Pain with compression or rotation may indicate a meniscus cartilage tear.

McMurray Click Test of the Knee: Meniscus Cartilage Tear

In the McMurray click test (Fig. 15-10), with the athlete lying supine the examiner places one hand over the anterior joint line at the knee and grasps the plantar surface of the heel firmly with the other hand. The examiner passively moves the leg into full hip and knee flexion and slowly extends and flexes the knee while circumducting the lower leg. A reproducible palpable click in the knee as it is flexed or ex-

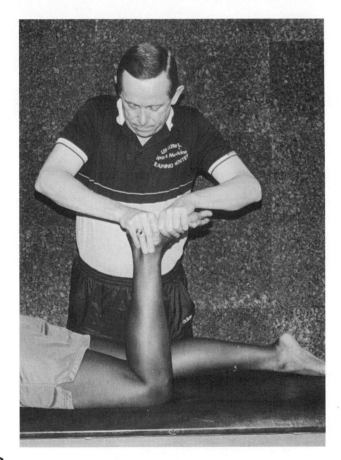

FIGURE 15-9

Apley compression test to evaluate meniscus cartilage tear. (Photo by Joel Nichols, Greenwood, SC.)

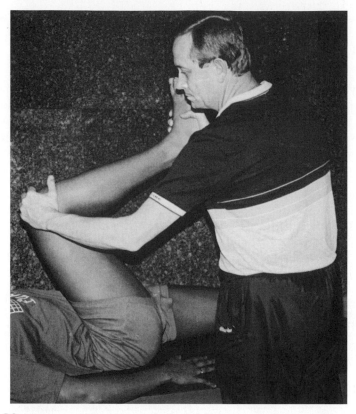

FIGURE 15-10

McMurray click test to evaluate meniscus cartilage tear. (Photo by Joel Nichols, Green-wood, SC.)

tended may indicate a torn meniscus cartilage. This test is most useful for identifying old tears in which the torn portion has begun to lose its plasticity.

Anterior Drawer Test of the Knee: Anterior Cruciate Ligament Sprain or Tear

In the anterior drawer test (Fig. 15-11), with the athlete lying supine the examiner passively flexes the knee to 90°. While supporting the foot, the examiner places his or her hands on either side of the knee with the fingers grasping the back of tibia and the thumbs on either side of the tibial tubercle. The examiner applies anterior force to the lower leg in an attempt to pull the tibia forward, away from the femur. Abnormal instability may indicate an anterior cruciate ligament sprain or tear.

Lachman Test of the Knee: Anterior Cruciate Ligament Sprain or Tear

In the Lachman test (Fig. 15-12), with the athlete lying supine and the knee in full extension the examiner lifts the leg by placing one hand under the lower leg just below the knee. The lower portion of the lower leg may be cradled between the ex-

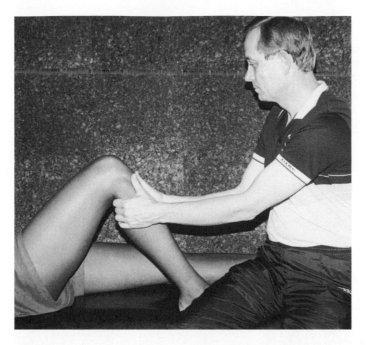

FIGURE 15-11

Anterior drawer test to evaluate anterior cruciate ligament sprain or tear. (Photo by Joel Nichols, Greenwood, SC.)

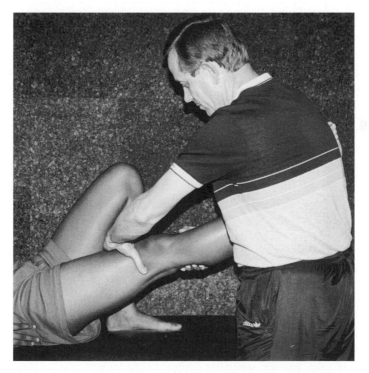

FIGURE 15-12

Lachman test to evaluate anterior cruciate ligament sprain or tear. (Photo by Joel Nichols, Greenwood, SC.)

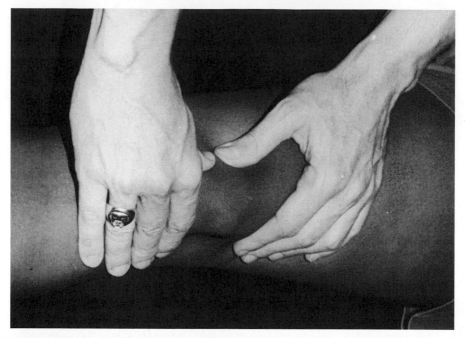

FIGURE 15-13

Overhead view of the patella apprehension test to evaluate chronic patellar subluxation. (Photo by Joel Nichols, Greenwood, SC.)

aminer's upper arm and body. The examiner's second hand is placed on the thigh just above the knee. While the upper hand applies firm pressure to stabilize the thigh, the lower hand applies upward force in an attempt to pull the tibia forward away from the femur. Abnormal instability may indicate an anterior cruciate ligament sprain or tear.

Patella Apprehension Test of the Knee: Chronic Patellar Subluxation

In the patella apprehension test (Fig. 15-13), with the athlete lying supine and the quadriceps and hamstrings completely relaxed, the examiner uses the fingers of both hands to move the patella gently laterally and medially, gradually increasing the degree of excursion out of the femoral groove. While forcing the patella farther across the lateral femoral condyle, the examiner closely observes the reaction of the athlete. Noticeable apprehension (e.g., facial grimace, sudden contraction of quadriceps and hamstrings) may indicate chronic patellar subluxation.

Noble's Test of the Knee: Iliotibial Band Friction Syndrome

In Noble's test (Fig. 15-14), with the athlete lying supine the examiner passively flexes the knee to 90°. With one hand on the knee and the thumb directly over the lateral femoral epicondyle, the examiner passively extends the knee. As the knee passes through 30° to 40° of flexion, the iliotibial band slides across the lateral femoral epicondyle. Pain as the iliotibial band crosses the epicondyle is generally as-

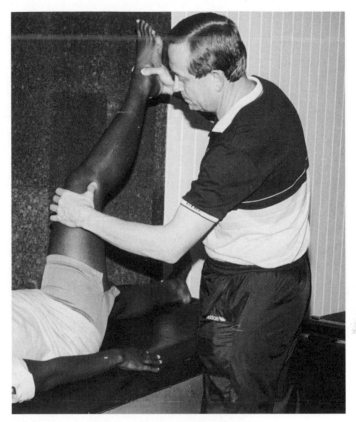

FIGURE 15-14

Noble's test to evaluate iliotibial band friction syndrome. (Photo by Joel Nichols, Green-wood, SC.)

sociated with iliotibial band inflammation resulting from chronic iliotibial band friction.

Renne's Test of the Knee: Iliotibial Band Friction Syndrome

Renne's test (Fig. 15-15) is similar to Noble's test in that the diagnostic mechanism entails placing the iliotibial band directly over the lateral femoral epicondyle. The athlete stands with all weight on the affected leg and lowers the body until the knee is at 30° to 40° flexion. The examiner exerts pressure by placing the thumb directly over the lateral femoral epicondyle. Pain resulting from pressure in this position may indicate iliotibial band inflammation resulting from chronic iliotibial band friction.

Lasèque's Test of the Lower Back: Sciatic Nerve Root Irritation

In Lasèque's test (Fig. 15-16), with the athlete lying supine, the knee fully extended, and the ankle dorsiflexed, the examiner passively lifts into full hip flexion the leg on the affected side. Pain that radiates down the back of the affected leg indicates sciatic nerve root irritation. The test may be repeated with the leg on the unaffected side; pain in the low back and down the back of the affected leg is additional evidence of nerve root irritation.

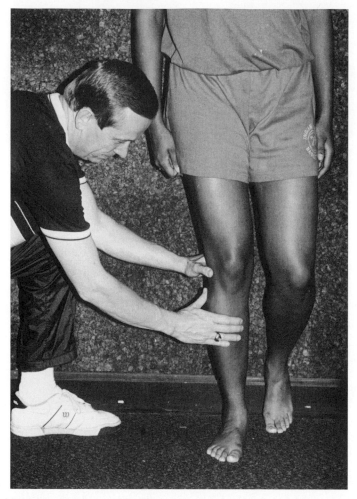

FIGURE 15-15

Renne's test to evaluate iliotibial band friction syndrome. (Photo by Joel Nichols, Greenwood, SC.)

Bowstring Test of the Lower Back: Sciatic Nerve Irritation

In the bowstring test (Fig. 15-17), with the athlete lying supine, the knee fully extended, and the ankle dorsiflexed, the examiner passively raises the leg on the affected side until pain is felt. The examiner gradually flexes the knee until the pain dissipates. The examiner then uses the thumbs to apply pressure in the popliteal fossa. Pain on palpation indicates sciatic nerve irritation.

Sacroiliac Compression Test of the Lower Back: Sacroiliac Strain

In the sacroiliac compression test (Fig. 15-18), with the athlete lying on the unaffected side the examiner exerts downward pressure on the iliac crest, compressing the sacroiliac joint. Pain indicates sacroiliac strain.

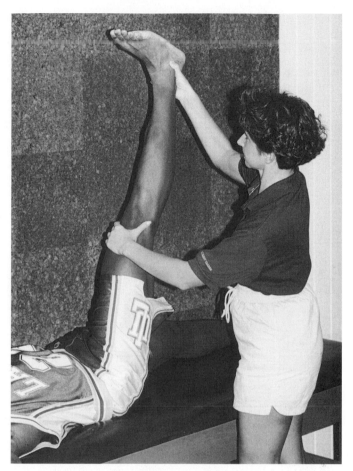

FIGURE 15-16

Lasèque's test to evaluate sciatic nerve root irritation. (Photo by Joel Nichols, Green-wood, SC.)

Glenoid Labrum Click Test of the Shoulder: Glenoid Labrum Tear

In the glenoid labrum click test (Fig. 15-19), with the athlete seated or standing, the examiner abducts the affected shoulder to 90° and flexes the elbow 90°. With one hand over the glenohumeral joint, the examiner passively moves the shoulder into external rotation. A palpable click as the shoulder moves into external rotation may indicate a glenoid labrum tear.

Drop Arm Test of the Shoulder: Supraspinatus or Rotator Cuff Tear

In the drop arm test (Fig. 15-20), with the athlete standing the examiner passively moves the affected arm, elbow fully extended, into abduction, slightly higher than 90°. The examiner instructs the athlete to lower the arm slowly to his or her side.

(text continues on page 520)

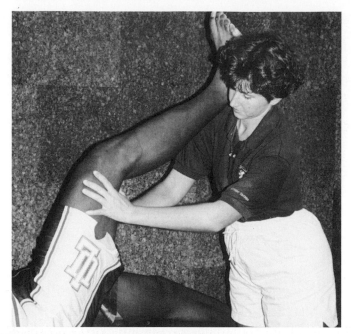

FIGURE 15-17

Bowstring test to evaluate sciatic nerve root irritation. (Photo by Joel Nichols, Greenwood, SC.)

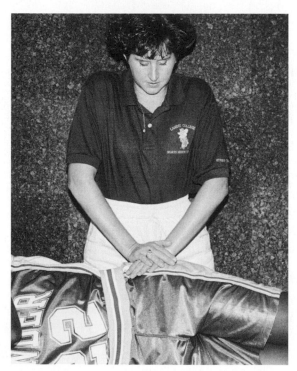

FIGURE 15-18

Sacroiliac compression test to evaluate sacroiliac strain. (Photo by Joel Nichols, Greenwood, SC.)

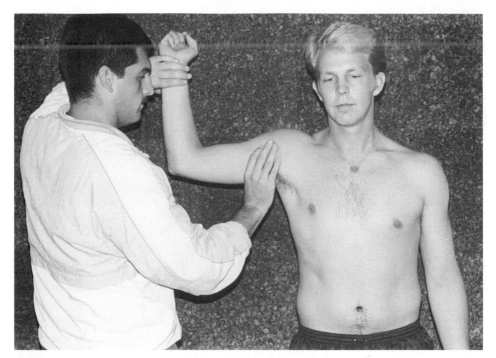

FIGURE 15-19

Glenoid labrum click test to evaluate glenoid labrum tear. (Photo by Joel Nichols, Greenwood, SC.)

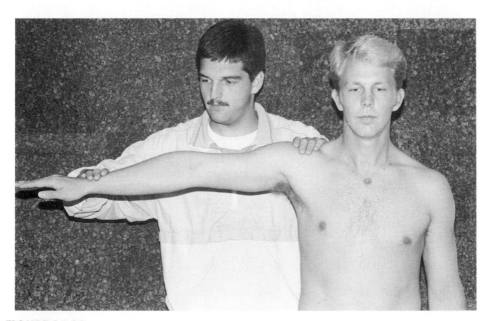

FIGURE 15-20

Drop arm test to evaluate supraspinatus or rotator cuff tear. (Photo by Joel Nichols, Greenwood, SC.)

The inability to lower the arm smoothly (irregular or quick drop) because of pain or weakness may indicate injury to the rotator cuff (primarily the supraspinatus muscle). If the arm can be held steady at 90° abduction, a mild tap or mild downward pressure at the wrist may cause the arm to drop, indicating rotator cuff injury.

Empty-Can Test of the Shoulder: Supraspinatus or Rotator Cuff Tear

Similar to the drop arm test, the empty-can test (Fig. 15-21) isolates the supraspinatus muscle. With the athlete standing, the examiner passively moves the affected arm, elbow fully extended, into 90° abduction and slight (30°) horizontal flexion. With the shoulder inwardly rotated (thumb down in the empty-can position), the examiner exerts mild downward pressure at the wrist. Noticeable weakness or sudden drop of the arm may indicate a tear in the rotator cuff (primarily the supraspinatus muscle).

Apley Scratch Test of the Shoulder: Inflexibility or Early Adhesive Capsulitis

In the Apley scratch test, the athlete, seated or standing, reaches down the back (arm in abduction and external rotation) as far as possible, as if scratching the upper back (Fig. 15-22). Measurable range-of-motion deficit compared with the unaffected shoulder may indicate early adhesive capsulitis or simply potentially problematic inflexibility. The athlete next reaches up the back (arm in adduction and internal rota-

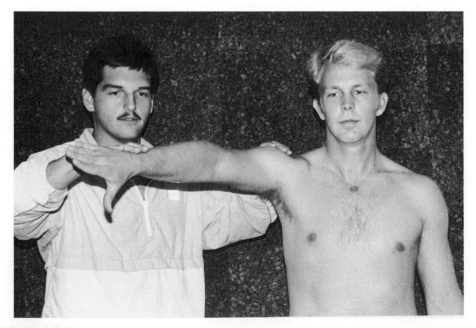

FIGURE 15-21

Empty-can test to evaluate supraspinatus/rotator cuff tear. (Photo by Joel Nichols, Greenwood, SC.)

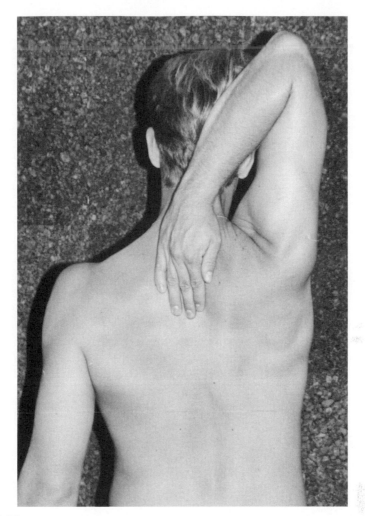

FIGURE 15-22

First position for the Apley scratch test to evaluate inflexibility or early adhesive capsulitis. (Photo by Joel Nichols, Greenwood, SC.)

tion) as far as possible (Fig. 15-23). Again, measurable range-of-motion deficit may indicate early adhesive capsulitis and/or potentially problematic inflexibility.

Glenohumeral Apprehension Test of the Shoulder: Chronic Anterior Glenohumeral Dislocation

In the glenohumeral apprehension test (Fig. 15-24), with the athlete lying supine and the affected shoulder free of support from the table the examiner abducts the affected shoulder to 90° and flexes the elbow to 90°. The examiner next passively moves the shoulder into external rotation as far as the athlete will permit. Noticeable apprehension on the part of the athlete (e.g., facial grimace, sudden muscle contraction) may indicate a history of chronic anterior glenohumeral dislocation.

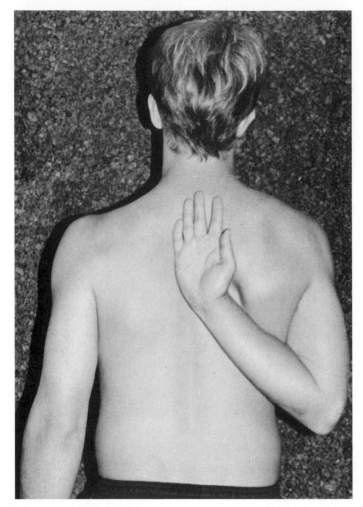

FIGURE 15-23

Second position for the Apley scratch test to evaluate inflexibility or early adhesive capsulitis. (Photo by Joel Nichols, Greenwood, SC.)

Medical Diagnostic Procedures

Injuries often require evaluation and definitive **medical diagnosis.** These procedures are often necessary to verify the findings of the athletic trainer's initial assessment or to determine the precise nature and severity of an injury when initial assessment was deemed not feasible or inappropriate. In such cases the attending physician may use a variety of diagnostic procedures. From a measurement and evaluation perspective, these procedures are particularly valuable because their validity, reliability, and objectivity have been well established through rigorous scientific research. It is important for the athletic trainer to develop a basic knowledge of advanced diagnostic procedures so that he or she may effectively communicate with physicians and other medical personnel and counsel injured athletes concerning the nature of and need for these tests.

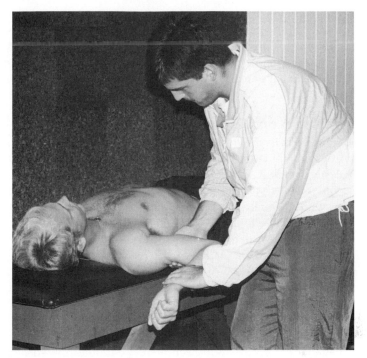

FIGURE 15-24

Glenohumeral apprehension test to evaluate chronic anterior glenohumeral dislocation. (Photo by Joel Nichols, Greenwood, SC.)

> Medical diagnosis is identification of the nature and severity of an injury or illness by
> a physician.

Conventional Radiography

Conventional radiography (also known as plain-film radiography) is the use of x-rays
to evaluate a suspected injury. X-rays are most commonly used to detect bony
changes (e.g., fractures) and articular disruptions (e.g., suspected dislocations). In
addition to bone evaluation, radiographs often reveal soft signs, or abnormal shad-
ows that indicate fluid accumulation in the area of a bony structure. In the absence
of known inflammatory disease (e.g., arthritis), such fluid accumulation may indicate
a stress fracture, which may not directly show up on a conventional radiograph. If
x-ray examination fails to confirm a suspected fracture, the procedure is often repeated in 10 to 14 days, since bony changes are often not detectable before this
time.

Stress Radiography

Stress radiography is the process of applying physical stress to a joint to produce suspected articular derangement and taking a radiograph of the stressed joint. This procedure is most helpful in diagnosing injuries that are difficult to detect when the
joint is not under stress. For example, stress radiography of acromioclavicular

sprains (separations) requires the injured athlete to hold a 5- to 10-lb weight to reproduce separation. Stress radiography of skier's thumb or gamekeeper's thumb (disruption of the ulnar ligament) requires manual radial deviation stress to demonstrate the articular disruption. While the structure is under stress, radiography reveals the extent of ligament damage.

Contrast Radiography: Arthrography

Contrast radiography entails the injection of a contrast medium (dye) into a joint, followed by vigorous manipulation and x-ray examination of the joint. Dye leakage, which can be easily detected on the film, indicates soft-tissue injury. In the past this technique was often used to diagnose soft-tissue injuries of the knee (e.g., meniscus tears). However, with the emergence of magnetic resonance imaging (MRI) as a primary diagnostic tool for knee injuries, arthrography is now more likely to be used to verify knee injuries that have been diagnosed through other procedures. However, arthrography is still preferred by many physicians for the diagnosis of shoulder injuries (e.g., rotator cuff tears) and wrist injuries.

Computed Tomography

Computed tomography (CT) uses multiple x-ray films of a structure taken from various angles throughout the entire 360° circumference around the structure. The patient is placed in a large cylinder as multiple radiographs are taken. Computerization of the information produces images of multiple thin cross-sectional slices of the structure being evaluated. This procedure is often used for the specific diagnosis of certain types of ankle and wrist fractures and a variety of nonorthopaedic conditions, including unexplained headaches, cerebral hemorrhage, and subdural hematomas.

Skeletal Nuclear Imaging: Bone Scan

Bone scans entail the injection of a radioactive contrast medium into a vein where it can be targeted to a specific type of body tissue (in this case, bone). The contrast medium is incorporated into the bony tissue, where structural activity, such as that associated with postfracture remodeling, can be detected with a special camera. Bone scans allow the physician to diagnose possibly serious skeletal injuries (e.g., stress fractures, epiphyseal disruptions, and nondisplaced carpal navicular fractures) that may not be detectable with conventional radiography.

Magnetic Resonance Imaging

MRI is rapidly becoming the diagnostic procedure of choice for soft-tissue injuries of the knee, shoulder, and other body structures. The injured body part is placed in a cylinder where it is introduced to a supercooled magnetic field. A series of radio frequency pulses is introduced, and the magnet senses the return pulses generated by the nuclei of the water molecules in the structure. The images are visually reproduced by a computerized process similar to the one used in CT. MRI allows the physician to see soft-tissue structures (e.g, fat, bone marrow, cartilage, tendons, and ligaments) that cannot be visualized with conventional radiography.

Arthroscopy

Diagnostic arthroscopy is a valuable tool for orthopaedic evaluation because it allows direct visualization of specific joint structures but is less invasive than conventional exploratory surgery. Most arthroscopic procedures involve three or more small incisions (portals) through which the arthroscope with fiberoptic light source, saline infusion apparatus, and surgical implements is placed. Visualization may be direct, through an eyepiece, or indirect, via projection from the arthroscope to a video monitor. Diagnostic arthroscopy is most commonly used to identify the nature and extent of injuries to the knee, shoulder, and ankle.

Compartment Pressure Monitoring

When injury or inflammation occurs in a closed muscle compartment (e.g., anterior compartment of the lower leg, femoral compartment), the result may be permanent damage to neuromuscular and/or neurovascular structures. Therefore, when excessive compartment pressures are suspected, compartment pressure may be monitored. Placing a needle directly into the compartment allows a wick catheter to be inserted. This catheter, attached to a pressure sensor, can measure the intracompartmental pressure. Excessive compartment pressure may warrant surgical release to relieve the pressure.

Chapter Summary

The importance of accurate and timely assessment of physical activity injuries cannot be overstated. Failure to identify or incorrectly identifying a possibly serious injury not only threatens the health and well-being of the injured person but may result in incomplete or improper care and/or rehabilitation. Therefore, it is imperative that the selection and use of injury assessment procedures be based upon a thorough understanding and application of the critical measurement and evaluation concepts of validity, reliability, objectivity, and freedom from assessment bias. This chapter explains how these concepts can be applied to effective assessment of sport- and exercise-related injury. It presents key concepts and a recommended process for systematic injury assessment. Also discussed are (*a*) signs and symptoms, (*b*) specific orthopaedic tests, and (*c*) medical diagnostic procedures.

SELF-TEST QUESTIONS

1. Which of the following criteria evaluates the extent to which a specific assessment technique (e.g., drawer test for the ankle) is effective in identifying the relevant condition (e.g., anterior talofibular ligament rupture)?
   A. Objectivity
   B. Subjectivity
   C. Reliability
   D. Validity

2. Which of the following is *not* a recommended principle of effective injury assessment?
   A. The athletic trainer should have a thorough working knowledge of human anatomy and physiology.

B. The athletic trainer should examine injuries as soon as possible.

C. The athletic trainer should develop a systematic strategy or plan for assessing all injuries.

D. If the nature of an injury is not immediately apparent, the athletic trainer should wait until symptoms (e.g., edema, loss of function) are present before conducting an examination.

3. Which of the following steps of the recommended injury assessment plan is the first to involve hands-on examination of an injury?

A. See

B. Ask

C. Observe

D. Test

4. Which of the following may result in joint edema?

A. Fracture

B. Sprain

C. Strain

D. All of the above

5. Which of the following specific signs demonstrates the inability of an athlete who has sustained a blow to the head to maintain balance while standing erect with the eyes closed?

A. Battle's sign

B. Cullen's sign

C. Kehr's sign

D. Romberg's sign

6. What specific knee injury is suspected when the drawer test is performed?

A. Anterior cruciate ligament sprain or tear

B. Medial collateral ligament sprain or tear

C. Medial meniscus cartilage tear

D. Patellar tendinitis

7. Which of the following diagnostic techniques entails the injection of dye into a joint prior to performing a radiograph?

A. Conventional radiography

B. Contrast radiography

C. Stress radiography

D. CT

8. Which of the following diagnostic techniques allows a physician to view directly the specific structures of a joint?

A. Arthroscopy

B. CT

C. MRI

D. Skeletal nuclear imaging

9. Which of the following injury assessment techniques should be performed only by a physician or other medical specialist?

A. Apley distraction test

B. Compartment pressure monitoring test

C. Glenohumeral apprehension test

D. Renne's test

10. Although anorexia nervosa and bulimia may produce similar symptoms, which of the following symptoms is more indicative of bulimia?
    A. Preoccupation with body image and diet
    B. Preoccupation with increasing exercise frequency and intensity
    C. Exaggerated fear of being overweight even though thin
    D. Recurrent binge eating without expected weight gain

ANSWERS

1. D   2. D   3. C   4. D   5. D
6. A   7. B   8. A   9. B   10. D

DOING PROJECTS FOR FURTHER LEARNING

1. If you are not familiar with athletic training services, make arrangements to visit the athletic training facilities of a nearby college or high school. Ask if you can observe while a trainer evaluates the rehabilitation of a recently injured athlete. Ask the trainer about the assessment procedures he or she employs.

2. Similarly, you might benefit by a visitation to a local sport medicine clinic. Ask the physical therapists and athletic trainers who work there about their use of tests to assess injuries from athletic endeavors, auto accidents, and work-related accidents.

SUGGESTED READING

The following sources are recommended to the student who is interested in learning more about the assessment of athletic injuries.

Arnheim, D.D., and Prentice, W.E.: Principles of Athletic Training. 9th ed. St. Louis, Mosby–Year Book, 1997.

Bloomfield, J., Fricker, P.A., and Fitch, K.D. (eds.): Textbook of Science and Medicine in Sport. Champaign, IL, Human Kinetics, 1992.

Fahey, T.D.: Athletic Training: Principles and Practice. Mountain View, CA, Mayfield, 1986.

Hartley, A.: Practical Joint Assessment Upper Quadrant: A Sports Medicine Manual. St. Louis, Mosby–Year Book, 1994.

Hawkins, J.D.: The Practical Delivery of Sports Medicine Services: A Conceptual Approach. Canton, OH, PRC, 1993.

Hunter-Griffin, L.Y. (ed.): Athletic Training and Sports Medicine. Rosemont, IL, American Academy of Orthopaedic Surgeons, 1991.

Kuland, D.N.: The Injured Athlete. Philadelphia, PA, Lippincott-Raven, 1988.

Roy, S., and Irvin, R.: Sports Medicine: Prevention, Evaluation, Management, and Rehabilitation. Paramus, NJ, Prentice Hall, 1983.

Thibodeau, G.A., and Booher, J.M.: Athletic Injury Assessment. 4th ed. St. Louis, Mosby–Year Book, 1999.

Webster. D.L., Mason, J.C., and Keating, T.M.: Guidelines for Professional Practice in Athletic Training. Canton, OH, PRC, 1993.

Williams, J.C.P.: Diagnostic Picture Tests in Injury in Sport. St. Louis, Mosby–Year Book, 1988.

CHAPTER 16

Assessing Risks in Sport and Recreation Facilities

Todd L. Seidler

As with all areas in the study of sport, measurement and evaluation are important tools for sport management. These tools can be extremely helpful to managers of sport and physical activity programs in many of their job functions. Some examples include formal evaluation of coaches, studying the demographics and psychographics of current and potential spectators, profiling athletes' fitness levels, and even tracking game statistics.

Managers of sport and physical activity programs have a number of legal duties. In part because of the expansion of programs, an increase in the number of participants, and the proliferation of personal-injury lawsuits, safety has become one of the most important concerns for today's sport manager. The establishment of a good, effective, formal risk management program has become the expected standard of practice. A good **risk management** program takes all reasonable precautions to ensure the provision of safe programs and facilities for all participants, spectators, and staff.

> Risk management is the formal process of assessing exposure to risk and taking whatever actions are necessary to minimize its effect.

A claim of unsafe facilities is one of the most common allegations made in negligence lawsuits in sport and physical activity programs. The best method of ensuring the safety of a facility is through the development of a facility risk review. This chapter discusses the steps involved in performing a sport facility risk review, that is, performing a formal evaluation of the safety of a sport facility.

As you read this chapter, watch for the following keywords:

Documentation	Risk management
Foreseeable hazard	Risk treatment

529

Legal Duties of the Sport Facility Manager

When determining the conduct expected of facility managers, courts have ruled that they are to be held to the standard of a reasonably prudent and careful manager. More specifically, the facility manager must perform the following five duties to be considered reasonably prudent and careful:

Keep premises in safe repair.

Inspect premises to discover obvious and hidden hazards.

Remove hazards or warn of their presence.

Anticipate foreseeable uses and activities by patrons and take reasonable precautions to protect them from foreseeable dangers.

Conduct operations on the premises with reasonable care for the safety of all.

If someone is injured in a facility and sues, claiming that the injury was caused by a situation the facility manager should not have permitted, the court will partially base its findings of liability on the concept of the **foreseeable hazard.** Was it foreseeable that the situation in question was likely to cause an injury? If the court determines that a reasonably prudent facility manager would have recognized it as a danger and acted to reduce or eliminate the hazard, there is a strong chance that the court will find liability. However, if it is determined that a reasonably prudent facility manager probably would not have identified the situation as likely to cause an injury, the potential for liability is greatly reduced. It is the legal duty of facility managers and program directors to address or treat all foreseeable risks in one way or another. Do you find a foreseeable hazard in Figure 16-1?

> A foreseeable hazard is a condition that is obvious enough that a reasonably prudent facility manager would recognize and correct it before someone is injured.

What Do YOU Think?

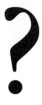

A high school gymnasium's wooden floor on the main basketball court was about 20 years old, and it began to develop problems. A few of the boards in the key area began to come loose and stick up about a quarter of an inch. Every few weeks one of the maintenance men would screw the boards back down, but as the floor was used, the boards would work back up again. This went on for some time causing players to trip occasionally but with no serious injuries. Eventually a player tripped and sustained a serious knee injury requiring surgery. He filed suit against the school, claiming that it had a responsibility to fix the floor permanently as soon as it knew it was a problem. You are a member of the jury. Do you think it was foreseeable that the protruding boards were dangerous and likely to cause a serious injury? If it was foreseeable, did the facility manager have a legal duty to fix it once and for all and eliminate the danger? What do YOU think?

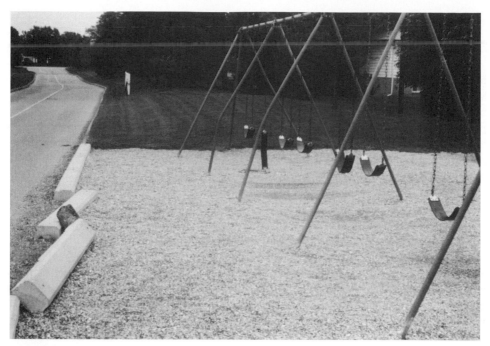

FIGURE 16-1

Hazard on an elementary school playground. Where will the kids land if they jump out of the swings—on the gravel, on the concrete blocks, or in the street beyond? (Photo by Dr. Todd L. Seidler, University of New Mexico, Albuquerque, NM.)

The Basis for Hazards

Safety problems in facilities can usually be traced to one or two primary causes:

Poor facility planning and design
Poor management

Poor design can typically be attributed to a failure by the planning and design team before the facility was constructed. It is not uncommon for a sport, physical education, or recreation facility to be designed by an architect with little or no experience with that type of building. Those without the proper background and understanding of the unique properties of sport and recreation facilities are likely to make mistakes that may lead to problems with safety, operations, and staffing.

Design problems commonly seen in activity facilities include inadequate safety zones around courts, poor planning for pedestrian traffic flow through activity areas, lack of proper storage space, and use of improper building materials, such as putting a slippery floor in the shower room. It may seem hard to imagine, but I have also seen many facilities built with major design flaws, such as a high school gymnasium that was constructed without a girls' locker room, a varsity football field only 80 yards long, a competitive swimming pool only 3 feet deep under the starting blocks (which cannot be used at that depth), a gymnasium with large, standard glass windows on the wall behind one basket of the main basketball court, and an international track and field stadium in which more than 40 percent of the seats did not have a view of the finish line!

It is essential that sport and recreation facilities be planned and designed by professionals with activity-related knowledge and experience. Often safety problems related to design are difficult, expensive, or impossible to fix once the facility has been built. On the other hand, the fact that a facility was constructed with built-in safety problems does not absolve the facility manager of responsibility for safety, nor does it mean that there isn't anything that can be done about them. Good management can often alleviate or at least lessen safety problems that are the result of poor planning.

Safety problems attributed to poor management are also a source of great concern. It has been estimated that negligent maintenance is the single most common allegation of the cause of injuries in facility-related claims. Typical examples of poor management include water or dirt on floors, equipment left out or poorly maintained, and inadequate supervision. Management practices that promote facility safety include performing a facility risk review, developing a safety checklist and applying it through periodic inspections, establishing a good preventive maintenance program, and teaching staff about safety and risk management. A conscientious facility manager inspects, identifies, and properly treats hazards as they are discovered. Although there are innumerable hazards in sport and recreation facilities, some are more common than others. Figure 16-2 provides examples of commonly occurring hazards that result from poor planning and/or poor management.

Facility Risk Review

One of the most effective methods of managing risk is the facility risk review. This may be performed either by a single person or a team of inspectors, and it begins with a check of the entire facility. The facility risk review is broken down into three major phases:

> Initial inspection
> Risk treatment
> Periodic inspection

Phase 1: Initial Inspection

The initial inspection begins with formation of a facility risk management committee. This committee may be one person or as many as feasible. Typically, the larger and more complex a facility is, the larger the risk management committee. While it may be feasible for one person to inspect a high school gymnasium, it may take a team of six or eight to inspect a large arena. Committees with several people are usually made up of the facility manager and others such as the athletic director, one or more coaches or teachers, the director of maintenance, security personnel, and a user of the facility, such as a club member or student.

Once the risk management committee has been established, it is time to determine who will be part of the initial inspection team. This may include any or all members of the risk management committee, but it may also be advantageous to include others. It is important to get input from as many points of view as possible. A

Indoors

Inadequate safety zones around courts
Improper storage of equipment
Traffic patterns routed through activity areas
Improper building materials
Weight machines not properly maintained
High-risk areas or equipment left unsupervised
Poor control of access
Improper maintenance of facilities and equipment
Non–safety glass in activity areas
Slick floors in locker and shower rooms

Outdoors

Overlapping fields
Improper storage of equipment
Uneven playing surface
Baseball team benches exposed to batted balls
Improper surface material on playground
Soccer goals not anchored or stored properly
Slippery pool deck
No warning track on baseball field
Unsafe bleachers
Improper fences for activity

FIGURE 16-2

Common safety hazards in sport and recreation facilities resulting from poor design and/or management practices.

custodian is likely to identify hazards that are different from those observed by the head of security. In this early stage of the risk review, input from many people is desirable.

Once the inspection team has been established, its primary task is to conduct the initial inspection. This begins by identifying as many risks or hazards as possible. Any hazard that could possibly cause an injury, from minor incidents to major catastrophes, must be noted and written down. At this point it is important to consider all situations with potential for injury. The initial inspection should include all inside areas (e.g., gymnasia, locker rooms, hallways, lobbies, pools) and outside areas (e.g., fields, sidewalks, parking lots, fences) as well as other areas associated with the main building. Each inspector should independently tour the entire facility and make a list of hazards.

The individual lists are then compiled into one comprehensive list of hazards. The risk management committee must assign priorities to this comprehensive list. The more likely a hazard is to cause an injury and the more serious the possible injury, the higher the priority assigned to that hazard. This priority list establishes the order in which the hazards are to be addressed. Following completion of the priority list, each hazard must be discussed and the best method of treating it determined.

Phase 2: Risk Treatment

Once the risks in the facility have been identified and assigned priority, it is time to treat the risks to (*a*) eliminate them or (*b*) make the situation as safe as possible. Decisions about the best method of **risk treatment** rely on the collective best professional judgment of the risk review committee. As each hazard is dealt with, the next one on the list can be addressed. This does not mean that items with a low priority on the list must wait until the ones before have been treated. If an item cannot be treated immediately, do not wait to go to the next hazard on the list and deal with it. Many situations can be quickly and easily treated and removed from the list; others take more time.

> Risk treatment entails determining the best method (*a*) to eliminate a hazard or (*b*) to make the situation as safe as possible.

There are two primary ways to treat or deal with a facility hazard:

Eliminate the hazard. This means make repairs or fix the problem so that it is no longer a hazard. If there is a broken basketball rim, replace it. If it cannot be fixed immediately, put it out of action until proper repairs can be made.

Reduce the hazard and compensate for it. This means make the situation as safe as possible and then determine ways to reduce the risk further. This may include warning of the situation or changing the rules slightly to reduce the hazard as much as possible.

With some hazards it is obvious how best to remedy the situation. For example, if there is a wet spot on the gymnasium floor, the obvious course of action is to dry it immediately and determine its source. If it was caused by a one-time accident, no more concern is necessary. If, however, the wet spot was caused by something that is likely to happen again, such as a leaky drinking fountain, the fountain should be fixed as soon as possible. If it will take some time to arrange for the required repairs, it may be necessary to warn patrons of the hazard and rope off the area until the problem can be properly addressed.

The treatment of some hazards is not so obvious or easy. If it is determined that it is not feasible to repair or eliminate the hazard, it will be necessary to determine another way to compensate for the problem to reduce the risk as much as possible. An example is a gymnasium built with inadequate space between the end line of the basketball court and the wall (Fig. 16-3). A mistake commonly made by facility managers is thinking that nothing can be done with a too-small safety zone. Although it is not feasible to move the walls, there are almost always other ways to compensate for and reduce the risk. In this situation it may be appropriate to shorten the court by moving the goals and end lines a few feet. It is more reasonable to shorten the court than to ignore a dangerous situation. It is also reasonable to hang pads on the wall under the baskets where players are most likely to hit if they to lose control while going out of bounds.

When compensating for a hazard, it is also appropriate to place signs warning of the remaining hazard so that all participants are well aware of the differences between this situation and a normal one. If they are aware of the risks associated with the facility, it is up to them (or their parents or legal guardians) to decide whether they want to assume those risks and participate anyway.

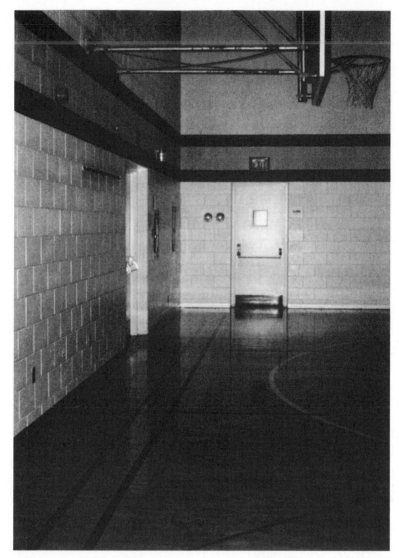

FIGURE 16-3

Facility with inadequate safety zone between the end line of the court and the wall and an access door along the baseline. Also, there are no pads on the wall. (Photo by Dr. Todd L. Seidler, University of New Mexico, Albuquerque, NM.)

Phase 3: Periodic Inspections

Once the hazards identified in the initial inspection have been treated, a checklist for periodic facility inspections should be developed. This checklist should be custom-designed for the specific facility. All too often facility managers borrow a checklist from another facility, put their facility's name and logo on it, and use it for their own building. This is not an effective practice. Every facility and situation is different. Therefore, every checklist should be customized. It can be very helpful to look at checklists from other facilities and borrow ideas from them, but it is essential that each item be appropriate and nothing overlooked.

It is important to keep the periodic inspection checklist relatively straightforward and simple. If it is too long and complex, it probably will be done poorly or not at all. On the other hand, all items of importance must be included.

The periodic inspection checklist should include the following items:

Name of the organization
Inspector's name (printed)
Date of inspection
Location of inspection if needed
Inspector's signature
Problems discovered

Two partial checklists for a hypothetical facility are given in Figures 16-4 and 16-5. The checklists for the main gymnasium and the fitness pool are specific to those areas.

Next an inspection schedule should be established. The frequency of inspections depends upon the type of facility and programs involved. In a spectator facility it may be appropriate to perform an inspection immediately prior to each event. However, in an activity facility it might be effective to establish a regular timetable for inspection, such as biweekly. The facility risk management committee must determine what is appropriate for each situation. Figure 16-6 shows a hazard that should be identified during a periodic inspection of a college weight training room.

Administrative Feasibility, Psychometric Qualities, and Documentation of Risk Reviews

A facility risk review has much in common with other measurement and evaluation tools. Like other tools, risk review procedures and checklists must be designed to be both administratively feasible and psychometrically sound.

Administrative Feasibility

The administrative feasibility of risk reviews is enhanced by development of procedures and checklists that are clear and straightforward. As already mentioned, if procedures or checklists are excessively long or unreasonably complex, it is highly unlikely that the risk review will be performed correctly and on time. Many of us tend to put off tasks that we find time-intensive and difficult. And of course time is money. Unless the inspection can be performed in a relatively speedy and efficient fashion, other tasks may soon take precedence.

A good way to evaluate the feasibility of risk review procedures and checklists is to ask a colleague to conduct a review using your materials. Using a step-by-step list of procedures and blank copies of checklists, this person should conduct the inspection. When the review is complete, sit down with the colleague and discuss what was found. Ask him or her about any questions or difficulties that came up during the inspection. When appropriate, edit the procedure guidelines and/or checklists accordingly.

ABC Recreation Center
Safety Inspection Checklist

Inspector's Name _____Paula Edwards_____ Date ___2/17/00___

Location of Inspection _____Fitness Pool_____

Inspector's Signature _____

Instructions for Inspector:
1. Inspect and complete all items.
2. Include comments on all "NO" responses.
3. Fill-out and report problems on completion of inspection.

#	POTENTIAL HAZARD	YES	NO	COMMENTS
1.	Deck clear of obstacles and debris	✓		
2.	All equipment properly stored	✓		
3.	Emergency procedures clearly posted	✓		
4.	Clear of standing water		✓	Drain in N.E. corner backed up
5.	Deck drains secure and unbroken	✓		
6.	Ground fault circuit interrupters (GFCI) have been installed on all electrical outlets	✓		
7.	All pool ladders, guard chairs, railings and other equipment tightly secured		✓	Ladder in deep end loose
8.	Decks are clean, disinfected, and algae-free	✓		
9.	Emergency telephone located on pool deck	✓		
10.	Emergency phone numbers and directions to facility are posted by the phone	✓		
11.	Pool rules and warning signs posted	✓		
12.	Starting blocks removed or covered to prevent use	✓		
13.	Rescue equipment including ring buoys, extension poles, and shepherd's crooks in good repair and in proper place		✓	Extension pole missing
14.	Access doors opened or locked as appropriate	✓		
15.	Bleachers secure and in good repair	✓		
16.	Backboard, rigid cervical collar, head support in good repair and in proper place	✓		
17.	Other			

FIGURE 16-4

A fitness pool inspection checklist.

ABC Recreation Center
Safety Inspection Checklist

Inspector's Name _____ Kevin Finn _____ Date _____ 2/17/00 _____

Location of Inspection _____ Main Gym _____

Inspector's Signature _____

Instructions for Inspector:
1. Inspect and complete all items.
2. Include comments on all "NO" responses.
3. Fill-out and report problems on completion of inspection.

#	POTENTIAL HAZARD	YES	NO	COMMENTS
1.	Floor clear of obstacles and debris	✓	___	_____
2.	Floor clear of standing water	✓	___	_____
3.	All standards, mats & goals properly stored	✓	___	_____
4.	All other equipment properly stored	✓	___	_____
5.	Gym rules clearly posted	✓	___	_____
6.	Warning sign on bleachers clearly visible	✓	___	_____
7.	All lights undamaged and working	___	✓	Light over center court is out
8.	Emergency procedures clearly posted	✓	___	_____
9.	Emergency telephone located in equipment room	✓	___	_____
10.	Emergency phone numbers and directions to facility are posted by the phone	✓	___	_____
11.	Rims unbroken, straight, & in good shape	✓	___	_____
12.	Backboards unbroken—no loose bolts & in proper position	✓	___	_____
13.	Access—Ingress and egress points opened or locked as appropriate	___	✓	N.E. outside door open
14.	Supervisor present	✓	___	_____
15.	Bleachers secure and in good repair	✓	___	_____
16.	No unsupervised children present	✓	___	_____
17.	Other	___	___	_____

FIGURE 16-5

A main gymnasium inspection checklist.

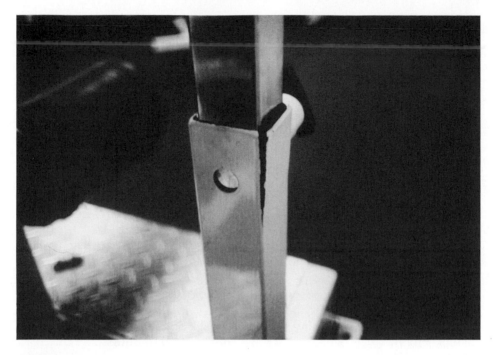

FIGURE 16-6

The broken seat of a weight machine in a college weight room should be discovered during a periodic risk inspection. Is it foreseeable that the seat may break during a lift, causing an injury? (Photo by Dr. Todd L. Seidler, University of New Mexico, Albuquerque, NM.)

It is also a good idea to record the time it takes to complete the risk review. Is it as efficient as possible? It is often helpful to plan and follow a set order for conduct of the review, following a logical pathway for movement through all areas of the facility. The checklist items should also be logically ordered within each particular area.

When reviewing a large facility, it may be helpful to space the review over 2 or 3 days. Another possibility is to divide up the facility and assign different areas to two or more staff members.

Psychometric Qualities

To be psychometrically sound, a risk review must be valid, reliable, objective, and free from assessment bias. How can one know whether or not these criteria are achieved?

To be valid, a risk review must measure what it claims to measure (see Chapter 3). Since a risk review is a criterion-referenced instrument, it must accurately classify as present or absent all foreseeable hazards in the facility. Omissions of areas or of concerns within an area are the greatest detractors from validity of risk assessments. A risk management think table (Fig. 16-7) can help ensure development of a comprehensive review for a sport or recreation facility that avoids inadvertent omissions. Instructions for the think table direct the user to select one area from the left-

Area	Concern
Gymnasium	**Dimensions**
Auxiliary gymnasium	Floor area
Other gymnasium	Adequate safety zone around courts
Wrestling	Adequate ceiling height for activities
Dance	**Surfaces**
Racquetball courts	Floors, walls, ceiling
Natatorium	Proper material for activity
Weight area	Foreign substance on floor (e.g., water, dust, glass)
Fitness area	Padding for walls, poles, protrusions
Fields	Breakable glass in or near activity area
Classroom	**Security**
Storage	Is access to area controlled adequately?
Offices	Do pedestrians have to walk through activity area?
Locker room	Are there provisions for supervision?
Shower area	**Storage**
Drying area	All equipment stored properly
Varsity team room	Storage areas locked
Visiting team room	**Warning signs** for high-risk activities
Staff locker room	**Emergency provisions and procedures**
Training room	Lighting
First aid	Egress: exit doors marked, not locked or chained
Laundry	Information signs
Equipment issue	Phone
Lobby	**Spectator seating**
Ticket booth	Proper handrails
Concessions	Nonskid steps
Maintenance areas	In good condition
Public rest rooms	**Electrical**
	Exposed wires
	Control boxes
	Ground fault circuit interrupter outlets in all wet areas
	Equipment
	Worn parts
	Loose parts
	Secure when not in use

Instructions: Select one **area** from the first column. Then go down the second column and consider each of the appropriate **concerns** for that area. Repeat for each area in your facility.

FIGURE 16-7

Risk management think table.

hand column and then consider each applicable concern in the right-hand column. The think table is designed to provide a starting point in the development of a facility risk review. It is meant to stimulate thought and should by no means be considered complete. Once again, every facility is unique and checklists should be customized.

The key to a reliable risk review is its consistency in identification of hazards. A reliable measurement tool is not affected to any significant degree by random errors that might improve the risk review one day but hurt it on another day. For example, the procedures and checklists must not be affected by seasonal variations or any other such factor that would cause a hazard to be overlooked. Consistency is also enhanced by standardization of procedures, as discussed earlier.

Similarly, objective risk review procedures and checklists can be used by different persons to derive the same essential assessment. In other words, subjective judgments are eliminated to the extent possible. Again, specificity in the design of the procedures and checklists increases objectivity. Interrater objectivity can be assessed by comparing independently conducted risk reviews by two or more trained persons. Any areas of disagreement may indicate that procedures and/or checklist criteria should be examined to see whether they can be clarified to reduce subjectivity.

Do be aware, however, that the background of a rater may affect his or her evaluation of a facility. If the evaluator lacks knowledge about the activities that take place in a particular area, he or she is more likely to overlook lurking hazards that someone more knowledgeable would catch. For example, a person who is unfamiliar with competitive swimming may not notice a hazard in the pool area, just as someone who has no experience in athletic training may miss problems in the training room. Similarly, a male rater may not notice problems in the women's locker room and vice versa. All persons participating in risk reviews must be knowledgeable about activities that take place in each area; knowledge increases their ability to foresee problems before they actually arise.

Assessment or test bias, the last of the traditional psychometric concerns, is not likely to be a serious problem in a facility risk review. Since a sport facility is an inanimate object, the procedures and checklists for a risk review are unlikely to be colored significantly by factors relating to gender, race, age, and so on. Be aware, however, of the potential for assessment bias. Some younger inspectors may underestimate abilities of the frail elderly.

Documentation

A well-organized, thorough, consistent method of documenting facility safety programs is an integral part of any risk management program. If litigation over an injury occurs, the courts will want to see evidence of the facility manager's efforts to ensure the safety of the participants, spectators, and staff. Keeping good records is essential in case one has to demonstrate in court that safety inspections and preventive maintenance were done. The facility manager may have done a great job of inspection and maintenance, but if there is no **documentation** to show it, why should the court take the manager's word for it? The old adage "If it wasn't written down, it didn't happen" is a great one to apply to a risk management program. It is important to keep copies of all periodic inspection reports, accident reports, preventive maintenance programs, repair work orders, staff training, and so on. It is necessary to document and save everything done that relates to safety.

Documentation is a written record. (If it isn't written down, it didn't happen!)

Final Thoughts

Understanding the fundamentals of measurement and evaluation can greatly enhance the sport manager's ability to perform job functions. This chapter presents one example of how knowledge of these fundamentals can help to ensure safe facilities, one of the primary legal duties of managers of sport, physical activity, and recreation programs. As part of this, managers must truly believe that the safety of patrons, spectators, and staff is a top priority. A good facility risk management program can usually be achieved through effort and for the most part without great expense. Most hazards, once identified, take little time or money to repair, remove, or compensate for when facility managers use their imaginations. The key to a quality facility risk review is caring enough to recognize hazards and deal with them before they become problems.

Chapter Summary

This chapter explains how to conduct a sport facility risk review so that the review is administratively feasible and psychometrically sound. The chapter begins with an explanation of the legal responsibility of the sport manager to protect participants, spectators, and staff from injuries from foreseeable hazards. Also explained are the two main causes of safety problems in sport and recreation facilities: poor design of facilities and poor management practices. Example checklists designed for risk reviews of a main gymnasium and a fitness pool in a hypothetical facility are included.

SELF-TEST QUESTIONS

1. Which of the following is *not* one of the legal duties of a sport facility manager?
   A. To keep the premises in safe repair
   B. To inspect the premises to discover obvious and hidden hazards
   C. To ensure that the facility is completely safe
   D. To remove the hazards or warn of their presence

2. Almost all facility hazards can be traced to which of the following?
   A. Poor facility planning and design
   B. Poor management
   C. Both A and B
   D. Neither A nor B

3. A checklist that measures what it claims to measure has which quality?
   A. Reliability
   B. Validity
   C. Bias
   D. Objectivity

4. The formal process of assessing exposure to risk and taking whatever action is necessary to minimize its effect is known as:
   A. Risk assessment

    B. Risk aversion

    C. Risk treatment

    D. Risk management

5. What are the three major parts of a facility risk review?

    A. Daily inspection, monthly inspection, annual inspection

    B. Initial inspection, risk treatment, periodic inspection

    C. Foreseeability, hazards, safety

    D. Initial investigation, risk assessment, periodic adjustment

ANSWERS

1. C   2. C   3. B

4. D   5. B

DOING PROJECTS FOR FURTHER LEARNING

1. Do an inspection tour of a sport or recreation facility near you. Make a list of all hazards you see. Next, for each of the hazards on the list, write down a recommendation for treatment.

2. Following the guidelines in the chapter, develop a checklist for a periodic inspection of the facility. Administer the checklist and determine whether you think its administrative feasibility and psychometric qualities meet with your approval.

3. Set up an interview with the facility manager. Discuss what is being done to manage the risks in the facility. If appropriate, offer to show him or her your hazard list, suggested treatments, and checklist. Ask for comments or feedback.

SUGGESTED READING

The following sources are excellent references for learning more about risk reviews:

Appenzeller, H.: Equipment and facilities. In H. Appenzeller (ed.): Managing Sports and Risk Management Strategies. Durham, NC, Carolina Academic Press, 1993.

Berg, R.: Unsafe. Athletic Business, 18(4):43, 1994.

Borkowski, R.P.: Checking out checklists. Athletic Management, 9(1):18, 1997.

Cotten, D.J., and Wilde, T.J.: Sport Law for Sport Managers. Dubuque, IA, Kendall/Hunt, 1997.

Gjertsen, L.A.: Stadiums spawn risk management challenges. National Underwriter/Property & Casualty Risk & Benefits, 102(32):7, 1998.

Hart, J.: Locker room liability. Strategies, 3(3):33, 1990.

Maloy, B.P.: Legal obligations related to facilities. Journal of Physical Education, Recreation, and Dance, 64(2):28, 1993.

Page, J.A.: The Law of Premises Liability. Cincinnati, Anderson, 1988.

Seidler, T.L.: Elements of a facility risk review. In H. Appenzeller (ed.): Management in Sport: Issues and Strategies. Durham, NC, Carolina Academic Press, 1997.

van der Smissen, B.: Liability and Risk Management for Public and Private Enterprises. Cincinnati, Anderson, 1990.

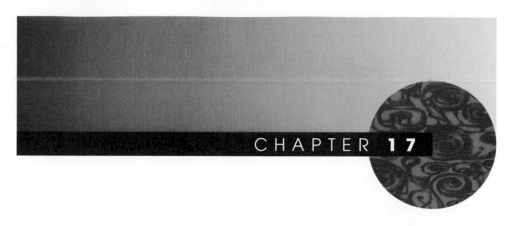

Written Knowledge Testing

Rosemary McGee

Human beings are born to move, feel, and think. When we step onto the basketball court, dance floor, or jogging trail, we do so as more than mere physical entities. It is essential that sport and exercise professionals learn to assess their clients' knowledge and understanding of physical performance. Assessing the thoughts, ideas, and perceptions of movers can broaden our professional understanding of movement and thereby guide the development of more effective and meaningful physical education and sport programs and services.

This chapter discusses valid and reliable assessment of cognitive knowledge and the development of good written tests. It also shows how to evaluate written tests developed by others. As you become more discerning about written tests, you are likely to develop some insights that will make you a better test taker yourself (Fig. 17-1). This chapter, which was originally written for the fourth edition of this textbook (1), is included here with minor modifications to update some of the content.

As you read this chapter, watch for the following keywords:

Analysis	Distractor (foil)	Knowledge
Application	Evaluation	Stem
Choice	Function	Synthesis
Comprehension	Index of discrimination	Table of specifications
Difficulty rating	Item analysis	

Functions of Tests

Whether taken orally, in a traditional paper-and-pencil format, or at a computer screen, knowledge tests can serve several functions. Among the common functions of tests are the following:

To Assess Achievement. The most prevalent use of tests is to assess achievement. Pretests are given at the beginning of a unit of study. At the completion of a unit, students are tested to see how much information and meaning they have assimilated. Unit tests should be consistent with the unit plan in terms of emphasis and

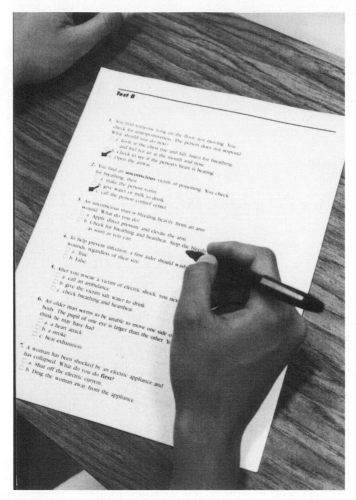

FIGURE 17-1

Written test.

general content. In many schools, written test performance becomes part of the final course grade and a requirement for promotion and graduation.

For Certification. Tests are also commonly used for certification, where certification depends upon performance on both practical and written examinations. The certification examinee is certified or not according to his or her score relative to a predetermined standard of mastery. Figure 17-2 lists several examples of certifications that include written knowledge testing.

For Learning. Tests should be learning experiences. Too often there is little or no follow-up after tests, resulting in missed learning opportunities. Teachers who are concerned about feedback may have students check papers immediately upon finishing. An accounting of the number of students who miss each question can give the teacher direction for a follow-up discussion of the test content during the next class period. False information and misconceptions can be clarified if students have

Certification	Certifying Organization
Exercise test technologist	American College of Sports Medicine
Athletic trainer	National Athletic Trainers Association
Physical education teacher	National Teachers Examination
Aerobic dance instructor	International Dance Educators of America
Weight training instructor	National Strength & Conditioning Association
Basketball officiating	National Collegiate Athletic Association
Cardiopulmonary resuscitation	American Heart Association
First aid	American Red Cross
Lifeguard	American Red Cross

FIGURE 17-2

Examples of certifications requiring written examinations.

the opportunity to study their incorrect answers along with the correct ones. Knowledge of correct information is, after all, the ultimate objective, even if it has to be learned after the test!

To Motivate Learners. Tests are powerful motivators for some learners. Unit tests are often motivational if students realize the uses to be made of the results. They should know the weighting of the unit test in the overall grade, the type of test, and the content areas. Plans should be made to go over test papers to discuss questions and misunderstandings. Such follow-up discussions are helpful to the instructor when test revisions are made. And if the test and its results are used in meaningful ways, students are motivated to learn.

To Diagnose Misunderstandings. Once or twice during a unit, a short test or quiz can be given to encourage students to keep up with the content of the unit. Short tests on scoring in tennis, on positions and marking in soccer, on the physiological aspects of weight training, or on terminology in golf are a few examples of this application. This serves a diagnostic purpose as well as a motivational one and tends to keep participants on their toes. This type of test usually covers only one content area and consequently should play a small part in the overall unit grade.

Whether for grading, for encouraging learning, for detecting weak areas, or for some other purpose, it is well for the exercise and sport professional to remember that written knowledge tests are part of the total assessment program. Remember that we are working with whole persons and must be concerned with their mental as well as their physical, social, and emotional accomplishments.

What Do YOU Think?

Lord Kelvin, a 19th-century British physicist, mathematician, and inventor, believed that "measurement is the basis for all knowledge." Was he correct? Is measurement essential to some—or all—types of knowledge? What can be learned through the process of measurement? What do YOU think?

Types of Written Tests

The six types of tests presented here have various qualities that are not mutually exclusive. For example, a criterion-referenced test can be either standardized or made by the practitioner. Knowing the qualities and characteristics attributed to each kind of test enables the reader to better evaluate and construct tests.

Standardized Tests

Standardized tests have been scientifically constructed and are usually accompanied by norms. The validity and reliability of standardized tests have been established, but often the value of the norms is questionable except for gross comparisons. This is because norms are computed from data derived from a particular unit of a certain length with a specific content presented to a certain age group. These factors vary so greatly that norms for knowledge tests are often inappropriate for use with other groups. Standardized tests are carefully developed and usually can be borrowed or bought. Relatively few knowledge tests in physical education are available commercially, but this is one area in which measurement progress undoubtedly will be made. Standardized tests have the following characteristics:

- They usually provide psychometrically sound measures of knowledge.
- They evaluate the content areas and cognitive levels reflected in the test as well as the degree of difficulty applied to various groups.
- They may be used when practitioners do not have the time or skill to construct their own tests.
- They can be written to assess knowledge in a wide variety of content areas.
- They serve as examples for format and content balance.
- They are usually in print somewhere for distribution. However, not all tests in print are standardized. The sample tests in college activities handbooks, courses of study, and state syllabi usually are not standardized.

Practitioner-Designed Tests

Most prevalent are tests designed by the local practitioner, that is, teacher, coach, or trainer. These tests are designed and used for local purposes. Their characteristics:

- They fit the unit for which they are planned in content and difficulty.
- They may or may not be scientifically constructed, depending on whether the practitioner has ascertained their psychometric qualities. The fact that a test has not been analyzed does not mean that it is invalid. If the test coincides with the unit of instruction, it has curricular validity.
- They may or may not be accompanied by local norms, depending on whether the practitioner has collected test scores year after year and prepared norms.
- They typically are prepared quickly and consequently usually are not as well constructed as standardized tests.
- They generally are used only locally.

Essay Tests

Essay tests require a written response by the student that entails the organization of information in paragraph form. Essay questions are usually general, designed to test the ability of the student to work with the material covered. Factors characteristic of essay tests:

- They usually are limited to only five or six questions and thus test only a limited sample of the subject content.
- They may be constructed quickly.
- They are efficient for small-scale testing.
- They usually require more time to answer and to grade than objective tests.
- They are difficult to grade reliably and objectively.
- The student's time is spent thinking and then writing the response.
- They favor the verbally inclined student (2).
- They test ability to compose in prose, which may *not* be one of the purposes of the test.
- They may test general explanations, interpretations, and problem-solving concepts that are difficult to measure in isolated questions of an objective test.
- They are not appropriate for testing simple knowledge and comprehension; they are most suitable for questions that require synthesis and judgments.
- Traditionally they have been considered more academically challenging than objective tests because they enable the student to focus and elaborate on a particular question, promoting critical thinking and development.
- They promote good study habits (2).
- They are usually good for creative and exploratory testing.
- Essay items can be used to provide students with opportunities to express their feelings about physical activity. These responses should not be used in assigning grades.

Objective Tests

Objective tests require brief responses to questions encompassing smaller chunks of information. Key characteristics of objective tests:

- It is difficult and time-consuming to prepare them well.
- They may be quickly, efficiently, and objectively graded.
- They can be validated and revised to improve validity.
- They can be highly reliable (2).
- They may test for many types of information, such as rules, strategy, techniques, terminology, and history of any activity.
- They too frequently measure only superficial and trivial facts.
- They can cover an extensive amount of the subject content.
- They lend themselves to follow-up lessons to correct errors and misconceptions.
- They can accurately rank students according to their overall knowledge of a content area.
- They may encourage guessing (2).
- They clearly define the task to be done, so they eliminate bluffing and evasion of an issue (2).

- The answer must be selected by the student from those given on the test.
- The student's time is spent reading, thinking, and then selecting the desired response.

Although some critics believe that objective tests examine only superficial information, a well-constructed objective test can be a challenging mental exercise that assesses insights, understandings, interpretations, and judgments. Too frequently, however, objective tests are prepared quickly and almost exclusively cover rote information. Such poorly designed tests are justifiably criticized, and it is hoped they are being used less frequently in physical education and sport settings.

Although most knowledge testing in physical education and sport uses the objective test format, it is to the advantage of the student if both objective and essay formats are used from time to time. Some students perform better on essay tests, and others perform better on objective tests. Alternating or mixing formats provides a fairer assessment of the student. With care, both kinds can be constructed to reap valid and reliable measures, even though they serve somewhat different functions.

Norm-Referenced Tests

Norm-referenced tests are used to interpret a student's score by comparing it with scores of other similar students. Norm-referenced tests are characterized in these ways:

- They reflect individual differences in the amount learned.
- They are used when the amount of content learned varies but the amount of time allotted for learning is set.
- They produce a scale of scores anchored in the middle of the distribution; interpretations are made in relation to achievement above and below the average.
- They reflect the proportion of students who learned less than or more than the norm (percentile ranks).
- They are useful when fixed quotas have been set and decisions have to be made about who is to be admitted to the next level, to the team, and so on.
- They require a wide range of scores to make the proper statistical applications and interpretations.
- They can be useful for testing complex material and a broad coverage of content.
- They can reveal maximum achievement in a content area.
- They are often used for summative evaluation at the completion of a unit of instruction.

Criterion-Referenced Tests

Criterion-referenced tests are used to interpret a student's score by comparing it with some predetermined standard. They are also known as mastery tests, domain-referenced tests, and universe-defined measurements. Criterion-referenced tests are unique in various aspects of their function and construction:

- They are useful for testing a high degree of comprehension on limited content.
- They are usually confined to relatively small units of instruction (3).
- They are used when the amount of content to be learned is set but the amount of time needed to learn it varies from student to student.
- They require a detailed statement of objectives that in itself enhances the precision of the measurement.
- Scores on criterion-referenced tests are anchored at the top of the distribution and indicate mastery. Scores below the cutting level indicate nonmastery.
- Scores cluster within a small range toward the top of the distribution. Consequently, the statistical analyses used for norm-referenced tests are not appropriate for criterion-referenced tests.
- They indicate whether specific areas of the curriculum have been learned to the level of mastery.
- They establish minimum acceptable learning essentials in a content area.
- They reflect the proportion of what could or should have been learned (percentages).
- They can be used in formative evaluation settings so subsequent instruction can be provided to help learners achieve mastery standards.
- They tend to encourage closed, convergent thinking.
- They are applicable for individualized instruction, and they help identify the kinds of learning activities to be prescribed.
- They are common in elementary school programs and in certification programs such as in sports officials training.

An increase in the use of criterion-referenced measures has been stimulated by individualized instruction and other student-centered educational trends. Measurement theorists consider criterion-referenced measures a supplement to, not a substitute for, norm-referenced measures (4, 5). The establishment of the criterion standard is crucial; the standard must be based partially on what students reasonably can be expected to attain. Experience, conventional wisdom, and norm-referenced information must be used to help decide on the cutting point indicative of mastery. It may not be possible to distinguish between test items used in criterion-referenced tests and those used in norm-referenced tests. The difference comes in judging the performance of the students, one by comparing a score with an ideal criterion and the other by comparing a score with the scores of similar students (6). Ideally, both norm-referenced and criterion-referenced measures could and should be used, because they can both inform decisions about the education of students.

Cognitive Taxonomies

The test developer should be able to show both the content (discussed later in the chapter) and the cognitive levels that go into a test. Otherwise there is no clear-cut information about whether the test is a beginning-level tool assessing only the basic knowledge of an activity or a more advanced instrument covering some of the higher levels of the cognitive taxonomy, such as the analysis and synthesis concepts of a sport activity.

This chapter presents two cognitive systems so that you can compare them and apply the appropriate one to a given situation.

Bloom's Taxonomy

Bloom and associates (7) classified the cognitive domain into six levels: knowledge, comprehension, application, analysis, synthesis, and evaluation. Knowledge and comprehension are the bases for cognition, and beyond them are the higher intellectual abilities and skills. A hierarchical arrangement from the simple to the more complex in these cognitive processes is shown in Figure 17-3.

Knowledge is defined as awareness of specific facts, universals, and information; it entails remembering and the ability to recall. The most common facts, universals, and information in the cognitive domain of sports, exercise, dance, and related activi-

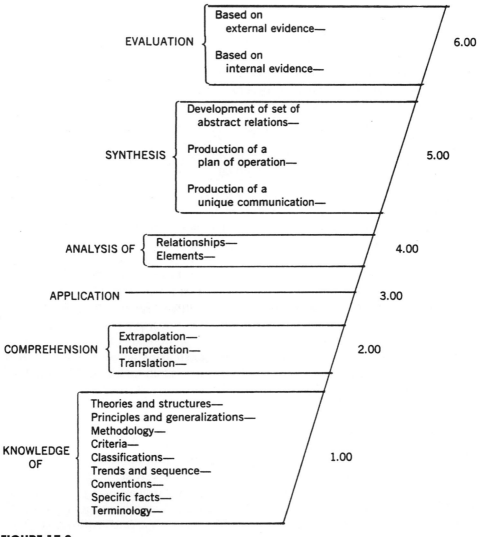

FIGURE 17-3

Bloom's taxonomy continuum for the cognitive domain. (Adapted from Bloom, B.S., and Krathwohl, D.R.: Taxonomy of Educational Objectives Handbook I: Cognitive Domain. White Plains, NY, Longman, 1984.)

ties are as follows: (*a*) terminology, (*b*) rules, (*c*) techniques, (*d*) historical background, (*e*) strategy, (*f*) equipment and facilities, and (*g*) courtesies and etiquette.

> Knowledge is awareness of specific facts, universals, and information; it requires remembering and the ability to recall.

Verbs used to write questions at the knowledge level of cognition are *recognize, recall, identify, define.* Knowledge items test the ability to bring to mind small pieces of material. Very little if any alteration of the material is required.

EXAMPLE

Which set of badminton terms can be most closely identified with court coverage systems?

A. Up and back, parallel, rotation
B. Horizontal, random, ad lib
C. Right-left, front face, rotation
D. Side-by-side, diagonal, freelance

Comprehension, the lower level of understanding, implies the ability to interpret knowledge and to determine its implications, consequences, and effects. An example of comprehension is knowing the facts and principles concerning the effect of exercise on the heart and circulatory systems and understanding the necessity of exercise for survival.

> Comprehension is the ability to interpret knowledge and to determine its implications, consequences, and effects.

Verbs for writing comprehension items are as follows: *translate, interpret, extrapolate, summarize, paraphrase, transform, give in one's own words, illustrate, represent, rephrase, restate, reorder, extend.* Comprehension items test the ability to redefine literal meaning, not just rote memory.

EXAMPLE

What is another badminton term that relates closely to the rotation system of court coverage?

A. Circular
B. Counterclockwise
C. Clockwise
D. Round

Application is a higher-level cognitive process that enables the learner to use knowledge and understanding in a particular concrete situation. It is possible to know and understand the facts but not be able to apply them.

> Application is the ability to use knowledge and understanding in a particular concrete situation.

Verbs used to write application level test items are as follows: *apply, use, generalize, relate, employ, transfer*. Application items test the ability to use abstractions such as general ideas, rules, and principles.

EXAMPLE

When is the badminton rotation system used most advantageously?

A. When the partners have equal ability
B. When the players are quick
C. When the partners are playing mixed doubles
D. When the opposition is using an up-and-back system

Analysis is a higher-level cognitive process than application. It is based on knowledge and understanding but implies the ability to identify the elements or parts of the whole, to see their relationships, and to structure them into some systematic arrangement or organization.

> Analysis is the ability to identify the elements or parts of the whole, to see their relationships, and to structure them into some systematic arrangement or organization.

Verbs used to write questions at the analysis level include *classify, identify elements, detect parts, distinguish, discriminate, categorize, compare, contrast, analyze, separate into parts, draw relationships*. Analysis items test the ability to break down material into its parts so the relations among the components can be seen.

EXAMPLE

Which factor seems most crucial to the success of the rotation plan of court coverage in badminton?

A. Quickness
B. Communication
C. Backhand strength
D. Stamina

Synthesis entails a process similar to that of analysis, but it is the reverse procedure. As a process it moves from the specific elements or parts to form the whole. Once again, knowing and understanding are the basis from which facts and information are combined into wholes or patterns that are different from and larger than any single part.

> Synthesis is the ability to structure a whole from understanding of the relationships among specific elements or parts.

Verbs used for synthesis items are as follows: *design, integrate, formulate, propose, plan, produce, originate, synthesize, develop, modify, combine, structure*. Synthesis items test the learner's ability to put together parts to make a whole. The process may result in a new whole, so it is a creative process.

> **EXAMPLE**
>
> Which set of combined elements seems most important to the successful use of the rotation plan of court coverage in badminton?
>
> A. Strong forehand, short serve, and clear
> B. Quick movements, talking, and execution
> C. Good footwork, backhand, and hairpin drop shot
> D. Lasting stamina, practice, and perseverance

Evaluation is the highest level of Bloom's cognitive domain because it is used to form judgments with respect to the value of information made available through the other cognitive processes.

> Evaluation is the ability to form judgments with respect to the value of information.

Verbs used to test evaluation ability are as follows: *judge, decide, compare with a standard, assess, argue, validate, appraise.* Evaluation items test the ability to make judgments and decisions.

> **EXAMPLE**
>
> You are accepting a challenge for a mixed-doubles badminton match with the city champions. They are well known for their dexterity, shrewdness, and thinking game. Which kind of court coverage would you be wise to select for the best defense?
>
> A. Parallel
> B. Up and back
> C. Rotation
> D. Diagonal

It is hoped that you can see how test items can tap various levels of cognition by the learners. Most tests probably should include a range of items assessing facility with the content at various levels of the taxonomy. Beginner-level tests usually include items predominantly at the knowledge, comprehension, and application levels. Intermediate and advanced tests usually have fewer items at these levels, concentrating on items of analysis, synthesis, and evaluation. The higher the item is on the taxonomy scale, the more difficult it is to construct. The payoff, however, is a better test by which to assess the cognition of students.

Table 17-1 makes use of Bloom's taxonomy for analysis of an intermediate tennis test. Item numbers are located on the two-way table to see the placement of items on both content and taxonomic axes. Table data show that 39% of the points on the test cover skill and techniques, and 26%, strategy, which seems appropriate for an intermediate test. Likewise, the row on the table for percent of points shows that only 13% of the test items were judged to be at the two lowest levels of the cognitive taxonomy. This provides further evidence that the designation of the test as an intermediate test is fitting.

TABLE 17-1 Two-Way Table of Specifications for an Intermediate Tennis Test Using Bloom's Taxonomy

							TOTALS		
CONTENT AREA	KNOWLEDGE	COMPREHENSION	APPLICATION	ANALYSIS	SYNTHESIS	EVALUATION	NUMBER OF ITEMS	NUMBER OF POINTS	PERCENT OF POINTS
Rules			25, 26, 27, 28, 29, 30 31, 32, 33, 34				10	20	23%
History	3, 36, 39 41, 42						5	6	7%
Skill and technique		5	1	8, 9, 10, 23, 24, 43, 44	17, 18 21, 22	13	14	34	39%
Equipment and facilities	35, 38, 40	37					4	4	5%
Strategy			4, 11 15, 20			2, 6, 7, 12 14, 16, 19	11	22	26%
TOTALS									
Number of items	8	2	15	7	4	8	44		
Number of points	9	3	30	20	8	16		86	
Percent of points	10%	3%	35%	23%	9%	19%			100%

Point breakdown
Questions 1–34, 2 points each.
Questions 35–42, 1 point each.
Questions 43–44, 5 points each.
Prepared by Pamela A. Reynolds.

A table of specifications is a two-way table used to depict the content emphasis and the cognitive taxonomic placement of items on a test of knowledge.

Educational Testing Service Taxonomy

The taxonomy in Figure 17-4 was developed by the Educational Testing Service (ETS), an institution well known for its expertise in test construction. ETS recommends this taxonomy for practitioners developing their own knowledge tests (8). The taxonomy has beneficial simplicity along with a graduated precision that reveals a clear picture of the cognitive levels included in a test.

ETS uses three major categories—remembering, understanding, and thinking— but also uses secondary words or phrases for clarification. No vertically hierarchical meanings are claimed. There is, however, value in horizontal development of levels. For example, a student who can reproduce something should next be able to translate it and finally to evaluate it, although a description of a test is reported only according to the number of items in the remembering, understanding, and thinking levels, respectively. Table 17-2 shows the ETS taxonomy for the intermediate tennis test analyzed according to the Bloom taxonomy.

Figure 17-5 provides sample questions from the intermediate tennis test that was analyzed by both the Bloom and ETS taxonomies. After each question, both the Bloom and ETS taxonomic classifications are given in parentheses. You may notice that Bloom's knowledge is roughly equivalent to ETS's remembering. Bloom's comprehension, application, and analysis are roughly equivalent to ETS's understanding. Similarly, a question that is classified by Bloom as synthesis or evaluation would be classified by ETS as thinking.

Construction of Objective Knowledge Tests

Figure 17-6 lists several computerized knowledge tests available through the SOFT-SHARE catalog (9). Comparatively speaking, however, there are relatively few knowledge tests for physical education and exercise and sport studies (ESS) in the published literature or available for purchase, so most tests must be developed locally. Acquisition of cognitive abilities is one of the objectives of our learning programs. Consequently, assessment of cognitive ability should be as accurate as possible. It is our responsibility to develop knowledge tests that are valid, reliable, and patterned to fit specific units of instruction. Once such professional skills are acquired, the practitioner begins to build a collection of good knowledge tests. Soon a

(text continues on page 563)

Remembering	Understanding	Thinking
Recall of facts, rules, procedures	Classification	Analysis
Routine manipulation	Application	Generalization
Reproduction	Translation	Evaluation

FIGURE 17-4

ETS taxonomy for the cognitive domain.

TABLE 17-2 Two-Way Table of Specifications for an Intermediate Tennis Test Using the ETS Taxonomy

CONTENT AREA	REMEMBERING	UNDERSTANDING	THINKING	TOTAL		
				NUMBER OF ITEMS	NUMBER OF POINTS	PERCENT OF POINTS
Rules		25, 26, 27, 28, 29, 30, 31, 32, 33, 34		10	20	23%
History	3, 36, 39 41, 42			5	6	7%
Skill and Technique		1, 5, 8, 9, 10, 23, 24, 43, 44	13, 17, 18, 21, 22	14	34	39%
Equipment and Facilities	35, 38, 40	37		4	4	5%
Strategy		4, 11, 15, 20	2, 6, 7 12, 14, 16, 19	11	22	26%
TOTALS						
Number of Items	8	24	12	44		
Number of Points	9	53	24		86	
Percent of Points	10%	62%	28%			100%

Point breakdown:
Questions 1–34, 2 points each.
Questions 35–42, 1 point each.
Questions 43–44, 5 points each.
Prepared by Pamela A. Reynolds.

OBJECTIVE KNOWLEDGE TEST FOR INTERMEDIATE TENNIS
by Pamela A. Reynolds

PART I—MULTIPLE CHOICE (2 points each)

Directions: Read each of the following items and select the best response. Place an X beside the number on the answer sheet under the letter that you choose. All of the items refer to right-handed players.

1. What is the best return of service in doubles?
   A. Cross-court shot*
   B. Drop shot
   C. Lob
   D. Alley shot   (Application; Understanding)

2. What is the best serve to use when seving to someone with a weak back-hand?
   A. Topspin
   B. Reverse twist
   C. Flat
   D. Americn twist*   (Evaluation; Thinking)

4. What is the best shot to make against a player at the net?
   A. Drop shot
   B. Deep lob*
   C. Down the line
   D. Shot to the backhand of player   (Application; Understanding)

5. Which forehand grip is the best and why?
   A. Continental—because the open-racket face allows one to lift the ball
   B. Continental—because one may use this same grip for the backhand also
   C. Eastern—because this position of the hand is more natural*
   D. Eastern—because the closed-racket face allows one to handle the high bounce of the ball   (Application; Understanding)

6. What is the advantage of playing an Australian formation in doubles?
   A. Prevents cross-court shots*
   B. Allows for better net coverage
   C. Forces the opponents to lob
   D. Intimidates the opponents   (Evaluation; Thinking)

FIGURE 17-5

Excerpts from an intermediate tennis test for the high school level. Correct answers are indicated by an asterisk, and Bloom and ETS taxonomic classifications are given in parentheses following each question. (Used with permission of Pamela A. Reynolds.) Continued

7. What is the best strategy against a player with a good serve and volley game?
   A. Force your opponent back by hitting deep lobs*
   B. Go to the net after receiving the ball
   C. Hit drop shots
   D. Hit strong forehand drives   (Evaluation; Thinking)

8. What path will the ball take if one uses an open-racket face?
   A. The ball will go directly into the net
   B. The ball will go in a straight path just clearing the net
   C. The ball will go high*
   D. The ball will barely clear the net and then immediately drop
                                              (Analysis; Understanding)

. . .

17. What corrections should you consider if your serve consistently goes into the net?
   (1) Toss the ball higher
   (2) Extend your racket arm more
   (3) Toss the ball closer to your body
   (4) Keep your weight on your back foot
   (5) Contact the ball at a higher point
   A. 2, 3
   B. 1, 5
   C. 2, 3, 4
   D. 1, 3, 5*   (Synthesis; Thinking)

. . .

19. What are the advantages of serving to a player's backhand in doubles?
   (1) Causes a weaker return
   (2) Reduces down-the-alley percentage shots
   (3) Pulls the player out of position in the ad court
   (4) Allows the server to approach the net sooner
   (5) Prevents the receiver from hitting effective lobs
   A. 1, 3, 4
   B. 2, 4, 5
   C. 1, 2, 3*
   D. 3, 4, 5   (Evaluation; Thinking)

FIGURE 17-5

Excerpts from an intermediate tennis test for the high school level. Correct answers are indicated by an asterisk, and Bloom and ETS taxonomic classifications are given in parentheses following each question. (Used with permission of Pamela A. Reynolds.) Continued

24. Which diagram below shows the path of the ball for the American twist serve?

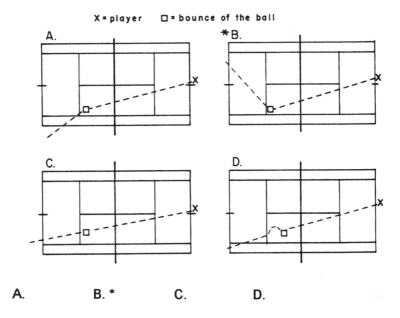

(Analysis; Understanding)

PART II—CLASSIFICATION (2 points each)

Directions: Read each of the situations and decide what the ruling would be from the selection of choices below. Place an X beside the number on the answer sheet under the letter you choose.,

Rulings
A. Point receiver
B. Point server
C. Let

. . .

26. Player A and player B are playing a match. Player A serves. In the middle of a rather long point, a string breaks in the racket of player A. Immediately, player A walks off the court for another racket. Player B puts the ball away with a drop shot. What is the decision?

    A*   (Application; Understanding)

FIGURE 17-5

Continued

27. Team A and team B are playing doubles. Team A is serving. After several hits, a player on team A contacts the ball so that it passes on the outside of the net posts and much below the top of the net, but somehow lands good down the alley. Team B fails to return the ball. What is the decision?
    B*   (Application; Understanding)

. . .

29. Player A and player B are playing a singles match in a local tournament. Player A is serving. In the middle of a very long point, a dog walks onto player B's side of the court. This obviously distracts both players. Player B stops the play and requests a let. What is the decision?
    C*   (Application; Understanding)

. . .

PART III—TRUE-FALSE (1 point each)

Directions: Read each statement below and decide whether it is true or false. If the statement is *true,* mark an X beside the number under column A on the answer sheet. If the statement is *false,* mark an X beside the number under column B on the answer sheet.

35. Composition-surfaced courts cause the ball to bounce more slowly than hard-surfaced courts.
    A*   (Knowledge; Remembering)

36. Wightman Cup competition is principally for men.
    B*   (Knowledge; Remembering)

37. Beginning players should string their rackets at about 65 pounds of pressure.
    B*   (Comprehension; Understanding)

. . .

42. The International Tennis Hall of Fame is located in Newport, Rhode Island.
    A*   (Knowledge; Remembering)

. . .

FIGURE 17-5

Excerpts from an intermediate tennis test for the high school level. Correct answers are indicated by an asterisk, and Bloom and ETS taxonomic classifications are given in parentheses following each question. (Used with permission of Pamela A. Reynolds.) Continued

Computerized Knowledge Tests

PHYSIO-QUIZ Contains advanced questions about the cellular and molecular mechanisms of muscles, nerves and the immune system. (MAC)

EXCEPTIONAL HEALTH EXAM 100 computerized health questions with multiple choice, true-false and matching. The computer evaluates the questions and posts a final score. Designed for high school level. (MAC)

SPORTS TRIVIA Contains 300 questions. For one to four players. A spinner selects a category from 17 choices and then provides a question. Scores are determined by correct answers and time. (IBM)

ZUPER SKELETON Easy way to learn major bones of the body. Click on a part of a skeleton and a lengthy list of bones appears. Select the correct name. (IBM)

FOOD PYRAMID GUIDE An easy-to-use program on the USDA food pyramid. Includes information about each group, reading food labels, recommended calorie levels and a quiz. (MAC)

ALL AMERICAN SPORTS TRIVIA & GUESSERS 100 multiple choice questions pertaining to pro football along with a football pool stats program. (MAC)

EKG A menu driven program which does the following: reviews the anatomy of the heart, reviews the electrical system of the heart, illustrates the waves made by an ECG tracing, illustrates the placement of the ECG electrodes and provides 13 tracings with their interpretations. A short quiz follows each section. (IBM)

DR. RUTH'S SEX TEST A definite adult program that is quite informative. Provides multiple choice questions on human sexuality and individuals compete against their own score or each other. (IBM)

ARE YOU READY FOR CALCULUS A review and quiz on all sections of algebra and trig which are essential for calculus. Also helpful for students planning to do biomechanic calculations, exponents, functions and equations, inequalities, curves and more. (IBM)

FIGURE 17-6

Selected shareware for knowledge tests available from SOFTSHARE.

nucleus of tests in which the instructor has confidence is available. Revisions must be made from time to time, but the basic structure of the tests remains the same.

Two pitfalls in test construction seem to have plagued the ESS practitioner in the past. One is the quickly constructed test that is composed of either essay questions or a short collection of ambiguous true-false statements. The other weakness is overemphasis on the inclusion of questions dealing with rules to the exclusion of questions on technique and strategy. Good tests should reflect the content of the unit of instruction, should be prepared carefully, and should be reanalyzed and updated on a regular basis.

In addition, the reading level of the test is important. The vocabulary level and sentence construction should be appropriate for the reading skills of the group taking the test. Formulas and computer programs are available to determine reading levels of tests and test questions (10).

Content Balance

The author of the test should itemize the areas of information to be covered and assign them certain proportional weights in the overall content. These weights should parallel the weight each area received in the instructional work. Figure 17-7 shows an example of content balance for a sport knowledge test at the beginning level.

The suggested content balance changes from unit to unit and from activity to activity. In most cases, however, rules and terminology should constitute no more than one-quarter of the point value of the total test. Emphasis should be on the execution of skills and how to apply them. Some basic facts concerning equipment, the historical background of the activity, and special terms seem appropriate. In some physical activities, safety is an important aspect and is worthy of some content emphasis in a test.

Content Area	Percentage
Rules and terminology	25
Etiquette and procedures	10
Technique and skills	30
Strategy and tactics	25
History and equipment	5
Safety	5

FIGURE 17-7

Example of content balance for a beginning level sport knowledge test.

Questions of fact and definitions covering rules and terminology are fairly simple to construct. They typically measure the lower levels of understanding. Questions covering the application, analysis, and synthesis of skills and strategies are more difficult to construct. How well students know a physical activity is better measured by how well they can apply understanding than by how well they can recall facts. Thus, the precision of the test instrument and the skill required to construct it are a reflection of how well the teacher is able to test for the depth of concepts about a particular activity.

Sources of Items

Good test questions can be gleaned from many sources. The practitioner should be alert for such questions and collect them as they appear. Ideas for original questions must come first and then be developed. The practitioner's own creativeness and intellectual endeavors provide many questions. Textbooks, rule books, and sport books are good sources. The questions that students ask during classes often bring out excellent ideas, and their wording is also worthy of note for future application to test questions. Sample tests from books and research reports supply good ideas for questions and formats. Colleagues can help by sharing written tests. And collections of test questions for activities are available both in hard copy and on computer (9, 11, 12).

When a practitioner uses a test developed by someone else, it is seldom appropriate to use the test exactly in its original form. It usually has to be adapted to fit a particular unit in content, difficulty, format, and the like. Although it is seldom possible to borrow a test in its entirety, it does give the practitioner a beginning on which to build.

Types of Items

There are several types of questions for objective tests. Each has certain applications and particular rules for construction.

Alternative-Response Questions

Alternative-response questions include true-false, yes-no, right-wrong, and same-opposite formats. Variations include true-false and tell why, true-false and correct if wrong, and true-false or sometimes. Plain true-false is the most prevalent of this style of question.

- Alternative-response questions permit a wide range of content coverage in limited space and time.
- Alternative-response questions are usually constructed quickly, although designing good questions may require a good deal of time.
- Alternative-response questions frequently test for trivial information.
- Alternative-response questions encourage guessing, although guessing can be minimized if students are told that the questions will be scored by deducting the number wrong from the number correct (number right minus number wrong equals score). Guessing can also be minimized by using other scoring methods, such as subtracting the percentage wrong from the number right or subtracting half the number wrong from the number right. The selection of the scoring method depends on how severely the teacher wants to penalize for guessing.

EXAMPLES OF POOR TRUE-FALSE STATEMENTS

Statement: The lines on a tennis court may be no more than 2 inches wide.
Correction: *This statement tests trivial information.*

Statement: The maximum number of sets in a match shall be 5, or when women take part, 3.
Correction: *Alternative-response statements are best used when only two responses are possible, and when only a single concept is to be judged.*

Statement: A freestyle swimmer should not do more than 3 strokes without taking a breath.
Correction: *The statement should be stated in positive terms unless the negative word is emphasized by underlining, capital letters, or italic type.*

Statement: A person engaged in strenuous activity should refrain from drinking water.
Correction: *False statements should not be stated in negative terms.*

Statement: There are several recognized systems of court coverage in badminton.
Correction: *The statement should be stated in specific quantitative terms instead of vague qualitative terms such as some, few, and several.*

Statement: The object rallied in badminton is called a birdie.
Correction: *The statement should **not** be tricky.*

Statement: The sidestroke is always used as a speed style of swimming.
Correction: *Cue words such as always and never should **not** suggest the correct answer.*

Additionally, questions of opinion should be avoided unless the authority is stated. Answers should not follow a pattern or sequence, and there should be approximately the same number of true-false, yes-no, and same-opposite statements.

EXAMPLES OF GOOD TRUE-FALSE STATEMENTS

Golfers who have holed out may repeat their putts for practice.

Trimming a canoe is a matter of balancing the weight of occupants and duffel.

One of the chief causes of accidents in rowboats and canoes is occupants exchanging positions.

Left-handed field hockey players may hit the ball on the rounded part of the stick.[1]

A goal may not be scored off the stick of a defense player unless it was first touched by the stick of an attacker within the striking circle.[2]

It is best to rest a sore muscle until the soreness is gone.[3]

EXAMPLE OF GOOD ALTERNATIVE-RESPONSE STATEMENT

Atherosclerosis causes (*a*) an increase in blood pressure or (*b*) a decrease in blood pressure.

Figure 17-8 shows two more examples of alternative-response items. These items are from a movement exploration knowledge test for first grade.

Multiple-Choice Questions

The multiple-choice question is held in high esteem by test developers. They consider it capable of assessing knowledge at all cognitive levels. The preliminary statement or question is the **stem**. The alternatives listed are **choices**; incorrect choices are **distractors** or **foils**.

A stem is the preliminary statement or question in a multiple-choice item.

A choice is a possible response to a multiple-choice question.

A distractor (foil) is an incorrect response to a multiple-choice question.

- Multiple-choice items are difficult to construct because skill is required to develop plausible distractors.

---

[1] Used by permission of Paula Drake.
[2] Used by permission of Paula Drake.
[3] Used by permission of Cindy Kennedy.

MOVEMENT EXPLORATION
Knowledge Test for First Grade

The teacher will give directions, read each question, and wait for each child to make the appropriate mark or response on his paper.

1. Draw a circle around the children who are in a scattered formation.

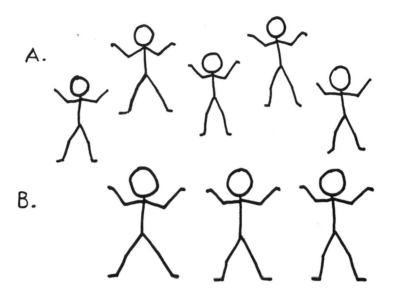

2. Draw a cross mark on the child who is landing softly from a jump.

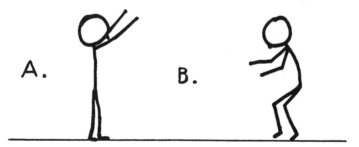

FIGURE 17-8

Alternative-response questions from movement exploration knowledge test for first grade. (Used with permission of Virginia Hart.)

- The stem should be a complete statement or question. The problem should be simply and concisely presented in the stem.
- Each choice should be plausible and should follow a parallel structure that is grammatically consistent.
- All choices should be about the same length.

- Multiple-choice items may be very easy or very difficult, depending on the closeness or homogeneity of the choices.
- Multiple-choice questions require discriminatory thinking on the part of the respondent.
- The multiple-choice format is inappropriate if only two choices are possible.
- Four plausible choices are adequate in most situations.
- Each multiple-choice question should have the same number of choices if possible. However, having few choices that function is better than having more just for the sake of consistency in format.
- Multiple-choice tests require no adjustment in scoring for guessing.
- Correct answers should follow no pattern.
- Questions are usually stated in the third person, although use of the second person (you) is sometimes advantageous because it puts the test taker in the setting of the question.
- Multiple-choice questions sometimes offer a choice of any, all, or none. Great care should be taken when using such a choice; they are overused. If such a choice is used at all, it should be used both when correct and when incorrect.
- Terminology used in the stem should *not* be repeated in the choices.
- Negatively stated questions should be avoided when possible, and it is important to emphasize the negative words with italics, underlining, or capital letters.
- It is important to ensure that a question does *not* give a clue to the answer of some other test question. Each item should be independent.

The multiple-choice format has several variations. One is the correct-answer form, in which one answer is correct and the others, while plausible, are definitely incorrect. Questions on rules often have this format because they are statements of facts and thus not debatable.

EXAMPLE

These are correct-answer multiple-choice questions:

1. Volleyball team A serves at the beginning of the match. Team B serves at the beginning of the next match. The score is tied 1 game to 1 game. Which team serves first in the final game of the match?[4]
   A. The team that served first in the first game
   B. The team that won the second game
   C. Decided by a coin toss
   D. The visiting team
2. Which condition causes a person to drown?
   A. Unconsciousness
   B. Shock
   C. Panic
   D. Suffocation

---

[4] Used by permission of Carolyn Littlejohn.

Another variation is the best-answer multiple-choice item. In a best-answer question one choice is definitely preferable and other choices have a degree of correctness but are not the best possible response. Questions on strategy and skill technique are suitable for this format because judgment is necessary to select the one best response.

EXAMPLE

These are best-answer multiple-choice questions:

1. What is the most important factor in determining the height and distance of the flight of a golf ball?
   A. The length of the shaft of the club
   B. The angle of the club's face
   C. The weight of the club's head
   D. The strength of the player
2. You are positioned behind your racquetball doubles partner, who swings at the ball and misses. Both of your opponents are in the front court. Which shot should you use?[5]
   A. Kill shot
   B. Cross-court pass
   C. Back-wall shot to either corner
   D. Ceiling shot

The cluster item, a variation of the best-answer multiple-choice format, is useful for analysis and synthesis questions that involve combinations of factors.

EXAMPLE

These are examples of cluster format multiple-choice questions:

1. Which combination of elements should a person have to be considered a conditioned person?[6]
   a. Agility
   b. Strength
   c. Flexibility
   d. Weight loss
   e. Muscular endurance
   f. Fast recovery rate
   g. Increased muscle bulk
   h. Decreased heart rate
      1. a, b, c, d
      2. b, d, f, g
      3. c, e, f, h
      4. d, e, g, h

---

[5] Used by permission of Byron Petrakis.
[6] Used by permission of Cindy Kennedy.

2. In which skills will a volleyball player increase efficiency by jumping?
   a. Spike
   b. Offensive volley
   c. Bump
   d. Overhand serve
   e. Block
      1. a, b, d, e
      2. b, c, d
      3. a, b, e
      4. a, b

For multiple-response items there is at least one correct answer and may be more. Two answer keys are necessary; one is used to check that all correct answers were selected; the other is used to see that no incorrect answers were selected. Each statement is scored. It is a mistake to choose an incorrect answer just as it is to omit a correct one.

EXAMPLE

Examples of multiple-response multiple-choice questions:

1. What are the functions of the round-the-head stroke in badminton?[7]
   A. To keep the court well covered
   B. To cover the weak backhand
   C. To retain the attack for the hitter
   D. To provide deception when returning
2. Which square dance calls are examples of the couple visitor figure?
   A. Birdie in the cage
   B. Texas star
   C. Rip and snort
   D. Form a star with a right-hand cross
   E. Inside arch and outside under

Matching

Matching items are useful for assessing knowledge of definitions, personalities, and rules. Several variations are possible on matching questions, including the following: (*a*) *Perfect* matches have the same number of responses as items to be matched. This practice is not recommended because some answers can be determined by the process of elimination. (*b*) *Imperfect* matches have more choices than are needed. At least two extra choices should be included. (*c*) *Multiple* matches have two columns of responses, and each item to be matched must be answered by one response from each column.

- Matching questions should be homogeneous in content. Terms should not be mixed with personalities in the same question. It is better to have two short matching sections than one longer one containing a mixture of content.

---

[7] Used by permission of Gwendolyn Davis.

- Matching questions are likely to measure only memory in contrast to comprehension and understanding.
- Matching questions are likely to include clues to the correct response.
- The response column should be arranged in some systematic order, such as alphabetically or chronologically (13).
- All of the parts of the question should be on one page (13).
- Matching questions should probably include at least 5 and probably not more than 15 items (13).
- More responses should be listed than items to be matched.
- Responses should be in the right-hand column.
- At least two plausible answers for each question should be included in the response column (13).

EXAMPLE

Match each term with the best definition. Indicate the letter of the correct response in the first set of brackets on the answer sheet.

1. Down	a. A stroke that makes a return possible
2. In	b. Lost service for the first server in doubles
3. Kill	c. The receiving side
4. One down	d. A fault
5. Out	e. A stroke that initiates each rally
6. Serve	f. A toss
	g. Shuttlecock
	h. The serving side
	i. The long service area
	j. Loss of service through failure of the serving side to score

---

Classification

Classification is a type of matching question with fewer choices. A choice may be used more than once. Classification questions lend themselves to assessment of the ability to organize information and understand the relation of small items to larger concepts.

- The content should cover material of similar nature.
- The format is opposite from that of matching categories. The short list of classifications usually is given either at the top or on the right-hand side, and the situations are listed in the left-hand column.
- It is important to be sure each entry fits into one of the categories.

EXAMPLE

This is a classification item for volleyball[8]

Situation	Ruling
1. Team B serves the ball. The center forwards on both teams jump up to get the ball, and the ball is held simultaneously. What is the correct ruling?	A. Point B. Side out C. Double fault D. Play continues

---

[8] Used by permission of Carolyn Littlejohn.

EXAMPLE

This is a classification item for a fitness class.[9]

Activity   Type of Activity

  1. Swimming   A. Aerobic
  2. Gymnastics   B. Anaerobic
  3. Tennis
  4. Jogging
  5. Softball
  6. Weight training
  7. Sprint
  8. Cycling

Rearrangement

Rearrangement questions emphasize the order of things. The sequence of a skill execution and the chronological order of sporting events are examples of content appropriate for rearrangement testing.

- The order provided should be well scrambled.
- The unraveled order of each question should follow no pattern.
- Care should be taken in scoring decisions, because an incorrect choice of the first answer may make the succeeding answers incorrect even though in logical order.
- Probably each question should have only a single value. Any error in the sequence means a missed question. If a sequence question with 5 parts is allotted 5 points, the weightings in the content balance are likely to be distorted.

EXAMPLE

This is a rearrangement item for diving:
Arrange in logical order the following steps in learning to dive.

  A. One-leg dive
  B. Crouched dive
  C. Standing dive
  D. Sitting dive
  E. Kneeling dive

Special Formats

Sometimes a high cognitive level can best be measured if diagrams, charts, stick figures, symbols, or other graphics are used. Examples may be seen in Figures 17-5 and 17-8. A diagram may be referred to for the answers to several questions. Strategy questions on court placements are appropriate for this format. Musical symbols and baseball scoring symbols have been used effectively in tests. Stick figures are effective for stunts, tumbling, and sports technique questions. Scoring lines in bowling and golf are examples of the use of graphics in the construction of test questions. Often rules questions can be placed at the application level instead of the basic

---

[9] Used by permission of Cindy Kennedy.

knowledge level by using diagrams of various kinds. Special formats permit a type of question that might otherwise be difficult to structure. They also add variety to the test, and they are challenging to construct.

Final Test Format

While the hardest part of writing a test is composing the individual items, consideration must also be given to how the items are to be ordered and formatted. The following are general guidelines for the final test format:

- Items should be ordered in a logical fashion. It is recommended that you begin a test with several easy items that most test takers are likely to answer correctly. This tends to give students a good start and build confidence.
- The test should be typed carefully, proofread, and duplicated. A double column of questions saves space; this is accomplished easily with today's word processing programs.
- A double space should be left between questions.
- All parts of a question should be on the same page of the test.
- The test should be titled.
- Directions for answering the questions should be stated carefully and thoroughly on the test paper.

EXAMPLE

These are directions for objective knowledge test items.

True-false: Read each question carefully. If the statement is entirely true, put an X in the first set of brackets on the answer sheet; if the statement is wholly or partly false, put an X in the second set of brackets.

Multiple choice: Read each statement carefully. The questions are worded for right-handed players. Decide which is the one *best* answer and place an X in the brackets on the answer sheet corresponding to the number of the response.

Matching: Indicate the letter of the correct response in the first set of brackets on the answer sheet.

Rearrangement: Arrange in logical sequence the correct order for each statement. Place the number representing the first factor in the first set of brackets on the answer sheet, the number of the second point in the sequence in the second set of brackets, and so forth.

Length of Test

Psychometricians have discovered that long tests tend to be more reliable than short ones. Therefore, the number of test questions should be sufficient to ensure some degree of reliability, but there should not be so many that few students can complete the test in the allotted time. A good rule of thumb is 50 questions, especially if most of the questions are multiple-choice items. It has been estimated that on the average, multiple-choice items require about 45 seconds to complete. Thus, a 50-item multiple-choice test takes about 35 to 40 minutes to complete. Alternative-response items require about 30 seconds each.

Many test writers are enamored with a test value of 100 points. They arrive at this number either by writing 100 questions or by assigning each question a numerical value. For example, multiple-choice questions might be worth 2 points each and true-false questions worth only 1 point. This practice is questionable because it tends to distort the content emphasis intended for the test. If the rules area is to cover only one-fourth of the test and each rules question is given a double value, it is possible, depending on the weightings given other questions, to put undue stress on this area of the content. Tests of 43 questions or of 61 questions, for example, are perfectly acceptable. You may, however, wish to scale the final scores in relation to the total number of points on the test. There is no magic in the 100-point test except for easy computation. A test composed of 54 good questions is a far better measuring tool than one with 100 questions that is prepared less thoughtfully.

Answer Sheets and Keys

Most types of questions can be answered on an answer sheet. The use of answer sheets is recommended for several reasons:

- They facilitate scoring.
- They are economical in time and money.
- They permit the reuse of the test papers.
- They permit a mark showing the correct answer for later study of the test by the students.
- They are convenient to use when doing an item analysis of the test. (Item analysis is discussed later in this chapter.)

Students must be taught to use an answer sheet; it is not as obvious as one might think. For example, suppose a form answer sheet has space for 5 responses while a test question has only 4 choices. Deciding the correct answer is the last one, the student may mark the fifth spot on the answer sheet and miss the question. The student should be cautioned about such practices. The use of an answer sheet may also require a little more test time because the student must shift attention back and forth between the test paper and the answer sheet.

Scoring keys for efficient hand grading can be made. Stencil keys, which have the correct answer cut out, are superimposed on the answer sheet. The grader can mark the correct answer, if not already indicated, so the student knows what it should have been when going over the test paper later. Strip keys are placed adjacent to the answers. Comparisons are necessary as the grader works down the column. When using a strip key, the grader should designate the correct answers for any questions missed.

Computerized answer sheets can be read, scored, and analyzed electronically by various types of optical scanners (14). If such equipment is available in the school or school system, it should be used for all large classes. And for a couple of decades now, it has been possible to take a test via computer (15). Now available from SOFT-SHARE is a shareware program, Create a Quiz, that helps practitioners generate their own on-screen interactive quizzes (9). The paper-and-pencil test is becoming outdated!

Construction of Essay Tests

Essay tests are often criticized for their low reliability and the inordinate amount of time required for reading and grading. However, the disadvantages of essay tests can be minimized if the test is carefully prepared.

Content

The content balance of an essay test should be similar to that for an objective test. It should parallel the emphasis given to various aspects of the content during instruction. It is likely, however, that the content at the knowledge, comprehension, application, and analysis levels can be more efficiently measured by an objective format. At the higher cognitive levels of the taxonomy, the essay format is especially useful.

Types of Items

There are three basic essay test item formats, each varying in the length of the response the student is asked to write.

Completion

The completion question requires a response of two to three words at the most. Longer responses result in less objective and more time-consuming grading. Suggestions for writing good completion questions:

- Omit only key significant words.
- Include only one or two blanks in any one statement.
- Locate the blank or blanks toward the end of the statement.
- All acceptable answers should be noted on the answer key before the test is given. Giving credit for only one certain word promotes rote learning that may be accompanied by little true understanding.

EXAMPLE

This is a poor completion item:
_____ and _____ are two important concepts in the definition of _____.

EXAMPLE

These are good completion items:

1. Two important concepts in the definition of first aid are _____ and _____.

2. Racquetball is more closely related to handball than to _____.[10]

Short-Answer Questions

The short-answer format requires a response of only one or two sentences. It is useful when a restatement of a rule or a brief explanation of some point is desired. Responses can be graded rather objectively because the key points are evident. (Be sure to leave plenty of room for the answer.)

---

[10] Used by permission of Byron Petrakis.

These are short-answer items.

1. Write in your own words the rule for a foot fault in tennis.
2. Explain how the factor of distance influences the application of the obstruction rule in field hockey.[11]

Long Answer: Essay Questions

The response to the long-answer or essay item, as it is traditionally called, can vary in length from a paragraph to several pages. Construction tips for the essay item are:

- Clearly define the aim of the question by using specific verbs. *Discuss* and *explain* are usually too general and do not help the student know the exact treatment of the information desired. (This is true especially if that student is Calvin [Fig. 17-9].) More helpful verbs: *define, describe, outline, select, illustrate, compare, contrast, classify, summarize, give reasons for, explain how, what factors contribute to, differentiate, criticize, predict what would happen if, give original examples of.*
- Indicate the point value of each question to help the student understand the depth of treatment desired.

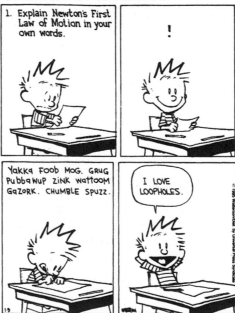

FIGURE 17-9

Essay questions must be worded carefully. (Used with permission of United Press Syndicate, Watterson/Dist., Calvin & Hobbes, 1/9/1995.)

---

[11] Used by permission of Linda Turkovich.

- Prepare the answer key carefully before administering the test. Preparation of the key sometimes helps the test writer identify the expected response, and this assists the writer in refining the essay item.
- Include several shorter questions instead of only one or two long items.
- Give all students the same items. If the grades are to be used to compare the performances of students (i.e., for a norm-referenced test), no choices should be allowed. That is, do not say, "Answer any two of the following five questions."
- State the ground rules. Approximate length is helpful and is usually correlated with the point value of the item. For instance, "In no more than one paragraph," or "Use a half page to." Indicate whether spelling, handwriting, and grammar will be considered in grading.
- Grade the papers anonymously if possible.
- Score all students on one question before proceeding to another item.

EXAMPLE

These are essay questions:

1. Outline the factors you would consider in analyzing your tennis serve if it consistently goes long. Include at least five factors. (15 points) [12]
2. Explain how composition-surfaced and hard-surfaced tennis courts differ in relation to the play of the ball specifically and to the game in general. Include at least four factors related to each type of surface. (16 points) [13]
3. Summarize the major differences in the principles of strategy that should be used in singles and doubles games of badminton. Indicate at least five factors for each type of game. (20 points) [14]

Evaluation of Objective Knowledge Tests

The evaluation of objective tests is a procedure that practitioners can learn and apply. As the practitioner builds a collection of written tests, revisions are under way continually; some revisions are only minor and some are major in scope. The revision of only one or two tests a year is certainly feasible. The work involved in test revision, however, prevents such a practice for every test. Other phases of teaching and testing would suffer from such overemphasis on written tests. The practitioner learns to save and label sets of answer sheets so they will be available whenever a test revision is anticipated.

Editing

Editing revisions come from close scrutiny of a test. Reading and rereading each question suggests changes in the structure of the item, in the choices, in the word order, and in the statements that changes in rules and strategy have altered. Feedback from test takers may also suggest better wordings for items and choices.

---

[12] Used by permission of Pamela A. Reynolds.
[13] Used by permission of Pamela A. Reynolds.
[14] Used by permission of Gwendolyn Davis.

A study of the unit outline can suggest ideas for new questions and the deletion of others. A review of the test by a colleague can be helpful. The study of other tests can suggest changes in question format that will improve the question. A growing knowledge of test construction and awareness of the fine points of item construction can make the practitioner more and more confident about test editing.

There are some differences in the validity and reliability procedures appropriate for norm-referenced and criterion-referenced tests. The former rely on a spread of scores, and the latter depend on a clustering of scores at the top. Consequently, different statistical procedures are indicated. The validity and reliability of each type of test are discussed separately.

Validity of Norm-Referenced Knowledge Tests

The validity of a written test is the same in concept as the validity of a performance test. A measure of the truthfulness and honesty of the test is indicated. At least two types of validity should be considered for the knowledge test.

Content Validity

Content validity is determined by the extent of agreement between the content of the test and the unit of instruction. The table of specifications for the test (similar to those shown in Table 17-1 and Table 17-2) is very helpful in analyzing content validity. The test may be studied by several authorities, who consider its contents in relation to what they consider such a unit should include. Also, the test can be compared in content with the content of books covering the activity or knowledge area, and it can be compared in content balance with similar tests. If approximately parallel emphasis is evident in some or all of these methods, content validity is claimed. Once administered, however, and once answer sheets are available for analysis, a further validity check of the test can be made using statistical procedures.

Statistical Validity

Statistical validity, a more involved process, answers the more technical question of the internal ability of the test to distinguish between test takers who "know" and those who "do not know." The process of determining statistical validity, known as **item analysis,** operates on the premise that each test question should meet certain standards. An item is retained in a test only if it proves to be good. The inference is that if each item is good, the test as a whole will be valid.

> Item analysis is a process of examining students' responses to a test item to discern the level of difficulty and the discriminatory quality of the item.

The Flanagan Method. The Flanagan method of statistical item analysis is the best known and most widely used (16, 17). An item analysis reveals three qualities about each item on a test: (*a*) the difficulty of each item, (*b*) the power of each item to discriminate between the students who know the most about the subject and those who know the least, and (*c*) the function of each possible response. This last is done by noting the frequency with which each response is chosen.

The **difficulty rating** shows the proportion of students who answered each test question correctly. The higher the percent, the easier the question. If the question is answered correctly by more than 90% of the students, it is considered too easy. If answered correctly by fewer than 10% of the students, it is considered too difficult. Revisions are indicated for such questions. Items with difficulty ratings of 50% are most desirable because they also discriminate maximally. The average difficulty rating for the entire test should be approximately 50 to 60%.

> The difficulty rating for a test item is the numerical value based on the proportion of students who answered that item correctly.

The power of each item to discriminate among knowledge levels of the test takers is reflected by the **index of discrimination,** reported as a correlation coefficient. It shows the relationship between answering an item either right or wrong and scoring either high or low on the total test. The index of discrimination is calculated by finding the difference between the number of correct responses by the top 25% of rexaminees and the bottom 25% of examinees and dividing by the number of examinees that represent 25% of examinees. This index is considered acceptable if greater than .20. If the coefficient for an item is between .15 and .19, it is deemed questionable; if below .15, the question should be deleted or be revised. The average index of discrimination for all the items on the test should probably fall between .30 and .40. A negative index, e.g., −.38, means that more of the students who scored at the low end on the total test than at the high end answered this particular question correctly. Negative coefficients indicate items that definitely should be eliminated from the test or slated to undergo major revision.

> The index of discrimination for a test item is a correlation coefficient that reveals the relationship between students' overall performance on a test and their performance on the particular item.

Function is the third characteristic of an item that is analyzed. Each response choice should be appealing enough to be chosen by some of the test takers. Some authors indicate that at least 3% of the students should use each response; others say 2%. If no one selects a choice, it cannot help the item or the total test to distinguish between students who know the most and those who know the least about the topic. Revision of nonfunctioning or inactive choices is indicated.

> The function of a choice is the proportion of test takers who selected that choice as the correct answer.

Once all three pieces of information are known about each item, revisions can be made. The process of constructing, administering, analyzing, and revising tests then starts over. This process continues to refine tests and to strengthen the validity evidence.

Whereas formerly such analysis was done by tediously hand-tallying every response to every question, the practice now is to process item analyses on a computer. TESTAN is one computer program for item analysis (14). The use of computer programs for item analysis is recommended, but hand tallying is described here to help you understand how the computer generates item analysis statistics and to assist the person who has to hand-tally tests.

The ETS Method. The ETS method of item analysis requires limited computational work because it makes use of only the top 10 answer sheets and the bottom 10 answer sheets for a class (8, 18). It is recommended for use by practitioners. At least 20 answer sheets are needed. The procedures are the same, however, no matter how many answer sheets are available. The ETS method of item analysis calculates both an index of difficulty and an index of discrimination for each multiple-choice term. It gives no information about the functioning of choices, but this is also easily determined by eyeballing the patterns of responses. Very easy items usually have one or more choices that do not function.

The ETS system also investigates the time necessary to complete the test. The difficulty and discrimination reports can be distorted if some of the students did not have time to complete the test. However, in most physical education, exercise, and sport settings, the test is designed to be completed within one lesson period.

ETS ITEM ANALYSIS

Step 1. Prepare a data collection form that provides for five columns of numbers (Table 17-3).

Step 2. Spread out the 10 high-answer sheets so the number of students in the high group who answered each question correctly can be counted. Record the number correct for each item on the test in the H column. Error is possible, so it is important that the answer sheets be properly aligned when they are displayed. A recounting is a good double check for accuracy.

Step 3. Repeat the same process using the 10 answer sheets in the low group. Record the number of students getting each question right in the L column.

Step 4. Add the numbers in the H and L columns to complete the H + L column. This number reflects the difficulty of the item. ETS suggests a standard of acceptance between 7 and 17. If more than 17 of the 20 students responded correctly, the item is probably too easy. If fewer than 7 in the combined groups answered an item correctly, the item is too difficult. Since there are 20 papers, this range of 7 to 17 could be interpreted as equivalent to 35 to 75% as a satisfactory standard for accepting an item on the basis of difficulty level alone.

Step 5. Subtract the H and L columns and place the resulting number in the H − L column. *It is possible to have negative numbers.* The numbers in this last column represent the discriminating ability of the item. Ideally, more students in the

TABLE 17-3	Sample Data Collection Form for ETS Item Analysis			
ITEM NUMBER	H (10 PAPERS)	L (10 PAPERS)	H + L (DIFFICULTY: ACCEPT IF 7–17)	H − L (DISCRIMINATION: ACCEPT IF 3+)
1.	8	4	12	4
2.	6	3	9	3
3.	5	1	6	4
4.	10	8	18	2

high group than in the low group should get an item correct. ETS suggests a standard of 3 and above as an acceptable criterion for accepting the discrimination power of an item. If lower, the item should be revised, and if in the negative range (i.e., −2), the item is definitely in need of revision. Each item should contribute to the mission of the whole test. If an item has a negative index of discrimination, the item is detracting from the overall test discrimination.

Step 6. Summarize the results of the tally and identify the items that are satisfactory, those that should be revised, and those that should be discarded.

Comments. While there is some reluctance to use this system because it uses only 20 answer sheets, the calculations are easy and the results provide the practitioner with a good estimate of the worth of each test item. The ETS item analysis also provides information needed to proceed with revisions.

Some teachers like to involve students in item analysis. If anonymity of answer sheets can be ensured, this can be an efficient process and worthwhile for the students. Proceeding item by item, students are asked to raise their hands so the appropriate numbers can be recorded for the number of correct responses shown on the top 10 papers and on the bottom 10 papers. Class members are alerted to the questions that caused trouble and become participants in the discussion of content that should be clarified (18).

Reliability of Norm-Referenced Knowledge Tests

Reliability indicates the consistency with which a test can rank the students from good to poor. Reliability of written tests is affected by several factors. The length of the test or the number of items determines the reliability to a great extent. The more items, the greater the reliability, excluding such factors as fatigue, boredom, running out of time, and so on. Reliability is also affected by the ability of the items to discriminate. The testing situation plays an influencing role. The more closely the items measure knowledge in one area of information, the more likely that reliability is high.

If the test is too easy, reliability is low. For example, if a 50-item test has a mean score of 43, the reliability is low because all of the students cluster toward the top of the scale, preventing a normal distribution and a greater range of scores. The average difficulty level of an entire test should be approximately 50 to 60% of the number of items. When this is the case, the reliability coefficient gives a fair picture of the test's consistency.

Assumed Reliability

Many authors believe that a valid test is automatically reliable. They see no need for estimating statistical reliability. If the test has sufficient items, if its content is homogeneous, if its difficulty level is stabilized around 50 to 60%, and if its scores have a good range, it is probably safe to assume adequate test reliability.

Test-Retest Reliability

This method requires two administrations of the complete test to the same group. The two scores for each student are correlated, and a reliability coefficient is the outcome. The coefficient indicates the stability of the test results.

Sometimes, however, memory and learning factors have an undue influence on the test-retest coefficient. Some students are bored with the second administration.

They fail to be motivated to perform at their best because they consider the second testing senseless. It helps some if the items are ordered differently on the second test. The test-retest method of establishing reliability is probably more appropriate to various motor tests than it is to written tests. In any case, the time element and the motivation of the students must be carefully considered.

It is generally accepted that the square root of a reliability coefficient estimates the upper limit of a validity coefficient. It is evident, therefore, that the two concepts are interrelated.

Parallel Forms

The test developer can prepare two tests covering the same topic that are believed to be similar in content balance, length, difficulty, and discriminating power. Both forms are administered to the same group, and the two scores for each person are correlated to obtain the parallel forms estimate of reliability. The resulting coefficient indicates the *equivalency* of the two forms. This method rests on the assumption that the two forms are actually parallel. In practice such a quality is fairly difficult to achieve. The use of parallel forms of written tests by the average practitioner is rare.

Parallel forms of a test are more prevalent in standardized written tests. Officials' rating examinations and certification examinations are often prepared in two forms so a person may have a second chance if unsuccessful on the first attempt. Parallel forms can be used to measure progress from the beginning to the end of a unit. If the tests are measuring the same thing to the same degree, comparison of the two test scores is reasonable. It should be clear to you, however, that these applications do not provide estimates of reliability.

Kuder-Richardson Formula

The Kuder-Richardson formula can be used to estimate the reliability of norm-referenced knowledge tests (19). It is preferable to the test-retest, parallel forms, and odd-even (see Chapter 3) methods because it requires only a single administration of the test. This method does not require calculation of a correlation coefficient and so reduces the computations. It does, however, operate on the same assumptions as the Spearman-Brown prophecy formula (see Chapter 3) with regard to difficulty and discrimination. The Kuder-Richardson formula is considered to estimate the lower limit of the real reliability of a test. The Kuder-Richardson formula:

$$r_{tt} = \frac{n\,\sigma_t^{\,2} - \overline{X}(n - \overline{X})}{(n-1)\sigma_t^{\,2}} \qquad \text{Formula 17-1}$$

where r_{tt} is the reliability of the total test, n is the number of items in the test, $\overline{X}$ is the mean of the scores, and σ_t^2 is the standard deviation of the test scores squared. A Kuder-Richardson formula calculation:

If n = 55 items, mean = 30, and standard deviation = 8, then

$$r_{tt} = \frac{(55)(64) - 30\,(55 - 30)}{(55 - 1)(64)} = .802 \approx .80 \qquad \text{Formula 17-2}$$

The practitioner will want to know the mean and standard deviation of the test scores anyway. With this information available, the teacher can easily apply the

Kuder-Richardson formula to estimate the reliability of a norm-referenced knowledge test. Note, however, that neither the Kuder-Richardson formula nor any of the other reliability methods discussed here should be used to estimate the reliability of speed tests. The introduction of the speed factor is not compatible with the assumptions of the various formulas.

Figure 17-10 shows a form that can be used to summarize the item analysis for a norm-referenced knowledge test. While this form assumes use of the Flanagan

TEST ANALYSIS SUMMARY FORM

Name of Test _____ Groups Tested _____ Dates _____

Number of Answer Sheets Used in Analysis _____

Content
    Total Number of Items _____
        Multiple-Choice   _____
        True-False   _____
        Matching   _____
        Classification   _____
        Rearrangement   _____
        Completion   _____

Scores
    Test Mean _____
    Standard Deviation _____

Validity

Difficulty Rating	Number	Percent	Judgment
Above 90%	_____	_____	_____
Between 11–90%	_____	_____	_____
Below 10%	_____	_____	_____

Index of Discrimination	Number	Percent	Judgment
Above 90%	_____	_____	_____
Between .16–.19	_____	_____	_____
Below .16	_____	_____	_____

Functioning of Choices	Number	Percent	Judgment
All choices function	_____	_____	_____
Between .16–.19	_____	_____	_____
Below .16	_____	_____	_____

Reliability
    Method Used _____
    Coefficient _____

Comments

Date of Report _____ Test Analyzer _____

FIGURE 17-10

Summary table for analysis of norm-referenced knowledge tests using the Flanagan method of item analysis.

method, a similar form could be designed for use with an ETS analysis. This summary information should be filed with the analysis materials, a copy of the test, and the key, so it is available for reference when revisions are to be made.

Validity of Criterion-Referenced Knowledge Tests

The item analyses already discussed are not appropriate for evaluating criterion-referenced tests because the developer of a mastery test intends a high percentage of learners to answer most test items correctly. The following two methods have been proposed for establishing the validity of criterion-referenced knowledge tests.

Domain-Referenced Validity

Domain-referenced validity is similar to content validity (20) (see Chapter 3). In this case, however, the behavioral objectives are stated more clearly and more precisely, and they encompass smaller segments of the unit of instruction. Test items should parallel the stated learning objectives established for the unit. The test might contain several items to accommodate each behavioral objective. This is possible because criterion-referenced tests usually cover short units of instruction. A series of short tests may be used instead of one long one.

Construct Validity

The second method reflects construct validity. The test is administered both before and after instruction. Validity is claimed if there is significant improvement in the scores or if the predetermined level of mastery is achieved by a sufficient number of the class members. An estimate about the performance of subsequent groups on just the final test could be made on the basis of this information.

Crucial to the whole realm of criterion-referenced testing is the setting of the cutting point indicative of mastery. It should be set high enough to enable the student to learn effectively at the next stage of instruction. It should be a realistic standard. Usually, a cutting score of 80 to 85% is mentioned as reasonable (21). This allows for some measurement error and still assures enough mastery to indicate with some confidence that the student is ready to proceed. If, indeed, the student does perform successfully on related tasks in the future, validity can be inferred.

Reliability of Criterion-Referenced Knowledge Tests

Classic test theory does not apply to criterion-referenced reliability estimates because of the lack of variability in the scores (22). Reliability of a criterion-referenced test requires that the items be closely parallel to the detailed objectives and that there be a sufficient number of items (3 to 5) to measure each objective.

Lovett (23) has worked with an analysis of variance (ANOVA) statistic to estimate the reliability of criterion-referenced tests. In an early edition of her textbook Safrit (24) proposed the use of a kappa coefficient; she considered it superior to the ANOVA approach because it uses a contingency table similar to the chi square concept and corrects for chance factors that influence the placement of students in the cells of the contingency table. Even so, measurement theorists are not yet satisfied with the statistical methods available to estimate criterion-referenced reliability and are continuing to refine these procedures.

Thorndike and Hagen (25) suggested a procedure that could be used by the practitioner who does not have a high degree of sophistication in statistics. They refer to a percentage of consistent decisions. Two forms of a criterion-referenced test are administered to a group of students within several days after a unit of instruction. Decisions about the proportion of students who achieved mastery and those who did not should be in fairly high agreement between the two administrations. In other words, there is a consistency of agreement on the two administrations about the proportion of students who achieved the designated cutting point of mastery and the proportion who did not meet mastery. Thorndike and Hagen illustrated their method using two standards of mastery: a severe one (100%), and lenient one (75%). The idea is to have a high proportion of students receiving the same decision on both tests, whether it is mastery or nonmastery. Reliability is low when a student meets the standard on one test and fails on the other. Higher percentages of consistent agreement are possible when using the less severe standard. When the determination of mastery is not consistent from test to test, a reversal results. This means either that students are being incorrectly advanced because they are really nonmasters who by chance score in the mastery level, or that students are being incorrectly retained because they are masters who by chance score at a nonmastery level. Either reversal means an incorrect decision has been made about a student. The interpretation is that the test was not consistent enough to enable the teacher to make reliable decisions about students' mastery levels. Thorndike and Hagen reported that percentages of consistent agreement between test administrations from 70 to 85% are about as high as can be expected. They also cautioned that the shorter the test and the more severe the standard, the more reversals can be expected. They also point out that the less important the decision (for example, to proceed to intermediate level golf lessons versus being certified as a lifeguard), the more reversals can be tolerated. The appropriate cutoff is established at the level that reduces the number of incorrect decisions in either direction.

Chapter Summary

There are many types of tests, and knowledge testing serves many educational purposes. It is important that the practitioner learn to evaluate tests written by another person and also learn to construct tests. An essential tool for test evaluation and construction is the cognitive taxonomy, such as those developed by Bloom and by ETS. The taxonomy can be used to analyze the nature and level of cognitive function required by a certain type of test item. It is recommended that good tests include questions at all levels of the taxonomy. It is also recommended that test authors follow the guidelines presented for construction of objective and essay knowledge test items.

The concepts of validity and reliability were revisited and applied to the knowledge test. The information gained from procedures to establish the validity and reliability of tests, whether they are norm-referenced or criterion-referenced, provides the direction for item revisions. Tests must be continually examined, polished, and revised so that they become more and more accountable instruments for both practitioners and their clients.

1. Which of the following types of tests is most likely to have established norms?
   A. Criterion-referenced
   B. Practitioner-designed
   C. Standardized
   D. All of the above

2. Which type of test items encourage study for understanding?
   A. Completion
   B. Correct-answer multiple-choice
   C. Essay
   D. True-false

3. Which is the lowest of the following levels of cognitive ability?
   A. Analysis
   B. Application
   C. Comprehension
   D. Synthesis

4. Matching items usually measure at which cognitive level?
   A. Analysis
   B. Evaluation
   C. Knowledge
   D. Synthesis

5. Which quality is most likely to improve if a two-way table of specifications is used to construct a written test?
   A. Balance
   B. Efficiency
   C. Relevancy
   D. Specificity

6. Which ETS category of cognitive function is roughly equivalent to Bloom's category of synthesis?
   A. Remembering
   B. Understanding
   C. Thinking

7. Which type of written test item is probably the quickest and easiest to construct?
   A. Essay
   B. Matching
   C. Multiple-choice
   D. True-false

8. A student answered 40 items correctly and 10 items incorrectly on a true-false test. If the test were rescored using the standard correction for guessing, what is the corrected score?
   A. 30
   B. 35
   C. 38
   D. 75

9. Which type of multiple-choice question will probably require the most critical thinking on the part of the examinee?
   A. Alternative response
   B. Best answer
   C. Correct answer
   D. Matching

10. A written test includes 20 true-false items and 20 multiple-choice items. What is the estimated number of minutes this test should take to complete?
    A. 20
    B. 25
    C. 30
    D. 35

11. An item on a knowledge test is answered correctly by a larger number of poor students than good students. What is the characteristic of the item?
    A. High difficulty
    B. Low difficulty
    C. Positive discrimination
    D. Negative discrimination

12. At least 2 to 3% of examinees should select each response in a multiple-choice question. What is this part of item analysis?
    A. Difficulty
    B. Discrimination
    C. Function
    D. Power

13. The majority of objective items on a written test should range in difficulty between what two ratings?
    A. .00 and 1.00
    B. .10 and .90
    C. .20 and .80
    D. .30 and .70

14. A written test was taken by 200 examinees. If 150 people answered an item correctly, what is the item difficulty rating?
    A. .25
    B. .30
    C. .70
    D. .75

15. A written test was administered to 80 students; 15 of the upper 25% and 10 of the lower 25% answered a given item correctly. What is the index of discrimination?
    A. + .15
    B. + .25
    C. + .35
    D. + .45

16. What should the test author do with an item that has an index of discrimination of −.45?
    A. Keep it as is
    B. Keep it but make minor revisions

C. Keep it but make major revisions

D. Eliminate it

17. How will adding to the length of a multiple-choice test affect the test qualities?

A. Increase reliability

B. Decrease reliability

C. Increase objectivity

D. Decrease objectivity

18. What is the estimate of reliability for an 88-item test that has a mean score of 60 and a standard deviation of 10? (Use the Kuder-Richardson formula.)

$r \approx$ _____

ANSWERS

1. C	2. C	3. C	4. C	5. A	6. C
7. D	8. A	9. B	10. B	11. D	12. C
13. D	14. D	15. B	16. D	17. A	18. .82

DOING PROJECTS FOR FURTHER LEARNING

1. Try your hand at revising the following test items to eliminate possible problems. (Revision suggestions are given at the end of the questions.)

A. In trampolining, a minimum of _____ spotters are required.

B. In basketball it is considered poor performance to fail to step toward the basket and to have your shooting arm pass directly over your head while executing a hook shot in basketball. True or false?

C. If a volleyball ball touches a boundary line:

a. It is out-of-bounds

b. Is played over

c. Is good

d. Neither team scores

D. Safety factors for swimming places do not include

a. Good bottom

b. Clear runways and decks

c. Swimming areas should be large

E. What are the differences between men's and women's gymnastics?

Revision Suggestions

For A, place the blank at the end of the sentence. (Actually, you may wish to rewrite this item in another format. Because there is only one correct answer, it is not best in a completion format.)

A. In trampolining, the minimum number of spotters required is _____.

For B, split this into two items so only one concept is tested in each item; avoid the double negatives; and move the qualifying phrase to the beginning of the sentence.

B. When executing a hook shot in basketball, it is considered good performance to step toward the basket. True or false?

For C, complete the stem sentence and make the choices parallel in structure.

    C. What decision is made when the ball touches a boundary line?
       a. It is out of bounds.
       b. It is replayed.
       c. It is good.
       d. It is dead.

For D, underline the negative word for emphasis, make the choices parallel in structure and grammar, and make the stem a complete sentence.

    D. Which factor is *not* essential to a safe bathing place?
       a. Good bottom
       b. Clear runways and decks
       c. Spaciousness

For E, use a more specific verb, and indicate the point value and/or the ground rules for length.

    E. Summarize the major differences for competition in men's and women's gymnastics. Identify at least five differences.

2. Develop your own test of knowledge about a topic area you know well. Your test should consist of about 15 to 20 four-choice multiple-choice items. Be sure to title your test and identify point values. When completed, administer your test to at least 24 people. Then do an ETS item analysis. Also check on the function of each choice. Which items appear to be good? Which items need revisions? Which items should be eliminated?

REFERENCES

1. Barrow, H.M., McGee, R., and Tritschler, K.A.: Practical Measurement in Physical Education and Sport. 4th ed. Baltimore, Williams & Wilkins, 1989.
2. Green, J.A.: Teacher-Made Tests. Reading, MA, Addison-Wesley Educational, 1990.
3. Gronlund, N.E.: Preparing Criterion-Referenced Tests for Classroom Instruction. Paramus, NJ, Prentice Hall, 1973.
4. Ebel, R.L.: Essentials of Educational Measurement. 3rd ed. Paramus, NJ, Prentice Hall, 1990.
5. Mehrens, W.A., and Lehmann, I.J.: Measurement and Evaluation in Education and Psychology. 4th ed. Fort Worth, TX, Harcourt Brace College, 1991.
6. Ebel, R.A.: The paradox of testing. Measurement in Education, 7, Fall 1976.
7. Bloom, B.S., and Krathwohl, D.R. (eds.): Taxonomy of Educational Objectives Handbook I: Cognitive Domain. White Plains, NY, Longman, 1984.
8. Cooperative Test Division: Making Your Own Tests. Princeton, NJ, Educational Testing Service. Mimeographed, n.d.
9. Department of Kinesiology, California State University at Fresno: SOFTSHARE (catalog). Available from American Alliance of Health, Physical Education, Recreation, and Dance, Reston, VA, 1999.
10. Fry, E.: Graph for estimating readability. In Zenger, C. (ed.): Handbook for Evaluating and Selecting Textbooks. Columbus, Fearon Teacher Aids, 1976.
11. McGee, R., and Farrow, A.C.: Test Questions for Physical Education Activities. Champaign, IL, Human Kinetics, 1987.
12. Shick, J.: Written tests in activity classes. Journal of Physical Education and Recreation, 52(4):21, 1981.
13. Hopkins, K.D.: Educational and Psychological Measurement and Evaluation. 8th ed. Needham Heights, MA, Allyn & Bacon, 1997.
14. TESTAN, VAX-DOC1. Academic Computer Center, University of North Carolina at Greensboro.

15. McBride, J.R.: Computerized adaptive testing. Educational Leadership, October 1985, p. 25.
16. Flanagan, J.C.: Calculating Correlation Coefficients. Pittsburgh, American Institute of Research and University of Pittsburgh, 1962.
17. Flanagan, J.C.: Statistical method related to a test construction. Review of Educational Research, 11:109, 1941.
18. Diederich, P.B.: Short-Cut Statistics for Teacher-Made Tests. Princeton, NJ, Educational Testing Service, 1973.
19. Richardson, M.M., and Kuder, G.F.: The calculation of test reliability coefficients based on the method of rational equivalence. Journal of Educational Psychology, 30:681, 1939.
20. Cronbach, L.J.: Test Validation. In R.L. Thorndike (ed.): Educational Measurement. 2nd ed. Westport, CN, Greenwood, 1971.
21. Messkauskas, J.A.: Evaluation models for criterion-referenced testing: views regarding mastery and standard-setting. Review of Educational Research, 46:133, Winter 1976.
22. Popham, J.W.: Classroom Assessment: What Teachers Need to Know. 2nd ed. Needham Heights, MA, Allyn & Bacon, 1998.
23. Lovett, H.T.: Criterion-referenced reliability estimated by ANOVA. Educational and Psychological Measurement, 37:21, 1977.
24. Safrit, M.J., and Wood, T.M. Introduction to Measurement in Physical Education and Exercise Science. St. Louis, MO, Mosby–Year Book, 1995.
25. Thorndike, R. L., and Hagen, E.P.: Measurement and Evaluation in Psychology and Education. 4th ed. Paramus, NJ, Prentice Hall, 1986.

CHAPTER 18

Assessment for Physical Education Teachers

Mary Lou Veal

"I never stop thinking about how to do the job better. I never stop asking questions of myself, my students, and my peers. . . . I hope I'll never be accused of simply stopping in my tracks and letting a predictable routine take over the life of my classroom" (1, p. 292). This chapter outlines methods by which teachers can use assessment to improve psychomotor learning. The first point is to clarify a few important assumptions about learning in physical education. The assumptions of this chapter are as follows:

- Physical education is an important school subject consisting of skills and content that all students should learn.
- Students will learn the skills and content of physical education only when the teacher (*a*) creates a learning climate for students that includes sufficient practice at an appropriate level of difficulty, and (*b*) gives feedback to students about their progress.
- Teachers who wish to teach intentionally use ongoing assessment that is linked to the instructional process.

These assumptions are at the heart of this chapter, and they distinguish what I call real physical education from pretend physical education, in which teachers only roll out the ball and function as recreation supervisors rather than as teachers (2). In real physical education, teachers work hard to help students learn the skills and content that will enrich the rest of their lives.

As you read this chapter, watch for the following keywords:

Authentic assessment	Reflection
Formative assessment	Rubric

The Role of Reflection in Teaching

Teachers often become more effective when they reflect. I refer to Sebren (3), who defined **reflection** as "giving serious and persistent consideration to a subject in order to act deliberately and intentionally rather than routinely and impulsively" (p. 23). Teaching involves hundreds, perhaps thousands, of decisions each day. It is thought that professionals make those decisions most effectively when they are in a frame of mind that includes consideration of alternative decisions and actions rather than simply relying on actions that have worked in the past. Teacher, educator, and researcher John Smyth (4) put it this way: "When teachers themselves adopt a reflective attitude toward their teaching, actually questioning their own practices, then they engage in a process of rendering problematic or questionable, those aspects of teaching generally taken for granted" (p. 63).

> Reflection is "giving serious and persistent consideration to a subject in order to act deliberately and intentionally rather than routinely and impulsively" (3, p. 23).

When teachers are reflective, nothing they do is allowed to become routine, but every aspect of teaching is open to question, revision, and improvement. Reflection is more than just sitting down at the end of the day and casually thinking about what transpired. Reflection should be purposeful and should lead to action. Hellison and Templin (5) wrote: "Reflection pervades every aspect of teaching. The teacher becomes a problem solver, analyzing every situation that did not work well, as well as every situation that did. The goal is to gain as much insight into one's teaching as possible and to build on these insights" (p. 158).

Because reflection is so important to teaching, it is the cornerstone of many teacher education programs. It is beyond the scope of this chapter to discuss reflection in greater depth, but the reader who wants to learn more about reflection is referred to Clift and associates (6).

What the Reflective Teacher Does

This section addresses the outcomes of reflection by discussing what a reflective teacher does, especially in regard to the use of assessment. The reflective teacher:

- Behaves in ways that communicate earnest caring about student learning
- Searches for new ideas, alternative solutions to problems, and ways to help students learn
- Uses data about student learning to make instructional decisions

Cares About Student Learning

Reflective teachers continually ask questions about student learning and the effectiveness of instruction. Student learning begins with goals and objectives that specify what students will learn. Teachers who plan for students to learn certain skills, teach intentionally so that students will have a good chance of learning, and continually assess progress to see whether students are on track to meet the objectives are reflective practitioners. All teachers, including physical educators, need to accept personal responsibility for asking questions and seeking answers about teaching and learning. This commitment to excellence is the essence of good teaching

(5). Especially in physical education, where there is a temptation to assume all is well if students are well behaved and having fun, teachers must concern themselves with making a contribution to the overall school mission, thereby making physical education indispensable as a school subject and essential to the education of all students.

Searches for New Ideas to Help Students Learn

This means being willing to try new approaches to teaching, to experiment, and to search for alternative solutions to problems. The reflective physical education teacher engages in ongoing analysis of the physical education program. In addition, the reflective teacher continually seeks new information through workshops, additional course work, and reading the latest books and professional journals.

There is an endless number of reflective questions, such as, "I wonder what would happen if...?, or "Last time I taught it this way; what would happen if I changed it to...?" Reflective teachers may ask why only some students are excelling. They may also ask themselves, "Are my students learning what I am trying to teach them?"

Uses Data to Make Instructional Decisions

When questions about student learning are asked, the reflective teacher becomes obligated to use assessment to find answers. Only through the systematic collection of information about the effects of teaching can trustworthy answers be found. Linn (7) wrote, "A major purpose of assessment is to identify student learning needs and use this information in making instructional decisions" (p. 431). This notion of basing instructional decisions on data is a far cry from simply eyeballing students' progress or using the results of testing just to determine a grade!

Distinguishing Between Formative Assessment and Evaluation

Formative assessment, although a powerful tool used by reflective teachers, is often confused with evaluation. One way to understand the difference between formative assessment and evaluation is to think of them as occurring at different times during the instructional process. Chapter 1 defines assessment as subjectively quantifying or qualitatively describing an attribute of interest. Put more simply, **formative assessment** can be thought of as "the process of gathering evidence and documenting a child's learning and growth" (8, p. 10). Formative assessments occur while skills, knowledge, or attitudes are being formed. In other words, they occur *during* the instructional process. In fact, as discussed later in this chapter, formative assessments are an important part of the instructional process. The primary focus of this chapter is on formative assessment.

> Formative assessment refers to the process of gathering evidence of learning during the instructional process.

Evaluation is "the process of summarizing and interpreting evidence, and making professional judgments based on the information collected" (8, p. 12). Evaluation is usually a summative process, commonly undertaken at the end of a unit of

What Do YOU Think?

Thinking about your own experiences in school, especially in physical education classes, do you agree with Crooks (9) that "too much emphasis has been placed on the grading function of evaluation, and too little on its role in assisting students to learn?" (p. 468). Why or why not? What do YOU think?

instruction after teaching is complete. Evaluation is used to make judgments about how much students have learned. It is typically followed by reporting a grade that communicates the evaluation to students and parents or guardians.

After an extensive review of numerous studies, Crooks (9) concluded, "Too much emphasis has been placed on the grading function of evaluation, and too little on its role in assisting students to learn" (p. 468). I agree that assessment should be used primarily to promote learning. Good teaching means using various kinds of formative assessment on a regular basis throughout the school year. It enables teachers to answer questions about what students are learning and how well they are learning it. Formative assessment that is linked to teaching creates continuous feedback that can be used by both teachers and students to improve teaching and learning. In addition, formative assessment is distinguished by the fact that the primary purpose for any testing is to aid and improve learning rather than to evaluate and grade.

Chittenden (10) wrote, "Assessment is an attitude before it is a method" (p. 29). He explained that teachers must see themselves as assessors who take the following four basic steps on a regular basis. Teachers who want to use assessment well should (10):

- Keep track of students' progress and improvement, using students', peers', and teachers' records
- Check up on students both formally by means of tests and informally by means of observational records
- Find out how students are doing by collecting data
- Sum up by preparing reports of student achievement

Formative assessment consists of collecting data and recording observations, while evaluation consists of summarizing those data and basing judgments on the data. Table 18-1 presents a theoretical framework for student assessment (11).

Formative Assessment and the Instructional Process

Using formative assessment as a tool to collect data on students' progress requires that assessment be an integral part of the instructional process. This means that assessments must be matched to their specific context. In other words, they must be relevant to the students and appropriate to both the content and the way the content was taught. Some educators call this curriculum-based assessment. It means assessment is not separate from teaching; it is part and parcel of the teaching process. As Wolf (12) put it, assessment is best viewed as "an occasion for learning" (p. 215).

TABLE 18-1   Theoretical Framework for Student Assessment

PHASES	TYPE OF ASSESSMENT	SUBJECTIVE	OBJECTIVE	REASONS FOR ASSESSMENT
Planning	Preassessment	Observation	Tests Cumulative records	Groups or classifies, marks entry level, determines needs, develops teaching strategies
Teaching and learning	Formative	Self-test Teacher observation Anecdotal records Oral questions Rating sheets	Daily records Student-kept records Checklists Performance tests Written tests	Motivates students, charts improvement, determines needs, charts progress, pinpoints weaknesses, allows self-analysis
Evaluation	Summative	Pupil self-evaluation Teacher rating sheet Teacher checklist Rating of playing ability Peer evaluation	Written tests Performance tests	Grading, accountability, curriculum plans, record of student achievement, extent to which objectives have been met, verification of teacher's success

Reprinted with permission from Veal, M.L.: Pupil perceptions and practices of secondary teachers. Journal of Teaching in Physical Education, 7(4):330, 1988.

The National Association for Sport and Physical Education (NASPE) agrees. In a publication on standards and assessment, NASPE included the following definition of what it termed the new vision of assessment: "The primary goal of assessment should be seen as the enhancement of learning, rather than simply the documentation of learning.... Assessment should be a dynamic process that continuously yields information about student progress toward the achievement of the content standards in physical education" (13, pp. vi–vii).

When assessment is an authentic part of the instructional process, it has the following characteristics:

- Assessment information is used as feedback to both students and teachers; it provides a continuous loop of diagnosis and monitoring of learning.
- Information obtained from assessments is used to change teaching strategies and make teaching decisions.
- Various assessment techniques are used by students for assessing their own learning progress and diagnosing learning problems.
- Assessment allows students to demonstrate what they can do and accounts for improvement over time.

Assessment as Feedback

You have probably already learned about the importance of feedback in motor learning. Not only can feedback be in verbal form from the teacher; it can also come just as well from the student or a peer. The feedback can be about the *process* of the movement (KP, knowledge of performance), or it can concern the *outcome* of the movement (KR, knowledge of results) (14). Table 18-2 presents six basic categories

TABLE 18-2	Six Basic Types of Assessment	
SOURCE	**PRODUCT FEEDBACK (QUANTITATIVE ASSESSMENT)**	**PROCESS FEEDBACK (QUALITATIVE ASSESSMENT)**
Teacher	Administering a skill test for a grade Spot checking performance records	Reviewing videotapes of students' performance against preestablished criteria Using subjective ratings for skill components
Peer	Counting, measuring, or timing for a partner	Using a checklist for feedback (peer coaching)
Self	Practicing a skill test to improve personal best Checking progress in preclass activities Keeping records of achievement (e.g., weight training charts, basketball shot charts) Recording results of station work	Reviewing and analyzing videotape of performance

Reprinted with permission from Veal, M. L.: Assessment as an instructional tool. Strategies: A Journal for Sport and Physical Educators, 8(6):10, 1995.

or types of assessments that result from consideration of the source and the focus of feedback (15).

For peer feedback, students can be paired with one student practicing and the other watching for specific performance criteria (KP). Or the observing partner can record the outcome of the performance as a count, a measurement, or a time (KR). Figure 18-1 shows examples of some products that can be counted, measured, or timed by a peer.

Some researchers have argued that it is important to separate feedback from grading because when assessments "count significantly toward the student's final grade, the student tends to pay less attention to the feedback" (9, p. 457). Similarly, students tend to focus less on process feedback when only the product is being graded.

Assessment Resulting in Change

When a teacher checks on students' learning while the learning is taking place, there are opportunities to make changes that result in greater achievement. For example, suppose middle-school students are in the third week of a beginning volleyball unit and are playing a practice game to apply their new skills. While the students are playing the practice game, the teacher observes carefully and collects data on the success of each student during the game. The teacher in this example has defined a successful serve as one that goes over the net into the opponent's court. Table 18-3 shows what the teacher's data for one team might look like.

These sample data reveal that only Jennifer is having much success in serving the volleyball. The other players need to be retaught the serve and need more opportunities to practice, perhaps initially from a line closer to the net. A teacher who simply allows students to continue playing without checking on their success is unlikely to make any instructional changes. It is also unlikely that most students would learn to serve successfully.

Students Assessing Their Own Progress

One way to engage students is to structure opportunities for them to keep records of their own progress. Keeping written records encourages students to do their personal best each day and helps them know whether or not they are improving. One of the most effective methods of self-assessment is to develop a regular procedure for the beginning of classes that engages students in practice as soon as they enter the gymnasium. If you want students to show improvement on performance posttests, it makes sense for them to practice the skills that will be tested at the end of the unit. As shown in Figure 18-2, you can make a skill development card from an index card by printing it with the names of the tests. Spaces should be left for students to record their best performance each day.

Assessment to Document Improvement

It is extremely motivating for students to see evidence that they are getting better as they practice. As a reflective teacher, you will want to search for ways to document your students' improvement. In two studies (2, 11), teachers indicated the importance they attach to improvement as a component of assessment. But they often

Count It!
Measure It!
Time It!

Products that can be counted

Team

- Number of completed passes in soccer and basketball
- Total points scored (instead of wins & losses)

Individual

- Number of shots made in basketball (figure %)
- Number of successful serves in tennis, badminton, volleyball (figure %)
- Score in bowling, archery, riflery
- Batting average in softball

Products that can be measured

Team

- Cumulative long jumps
- Total distance of all team members' shot puts

Individual

- Long jump
- Softball and discus throw
- Long serve in badminton
- High and triple jump
- Distance run in a given time

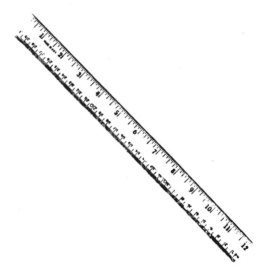

Products that can be timed

Team

- Total of all team members' times in any activity (e.g., wall handstands)

Individual

- 50-yard dash
- Mile run
- Relays
- Running the bases in softball
- Dribble around obstacles in basketball and soccer
- Amount of time standing on hands or holding headstand

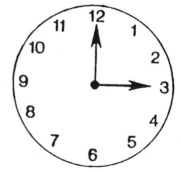

FIGURE 18-1

Products that can be counted, measured, or timed. (Reprinted with permission from Veal, M. L.: Assessment as an instructional tool. Strategies: A Journal for Sport and Physical Educators, 8(6):10, 1995 by the American Alliance for Health, Physical Education, Recreation and Dance, 1900 Association Drive, Reston, VA 22091.)

TABLE 18-3	Sample Serving Data for Students in a Beginning Volleyball Unit			
TEAM MEMBER	**SUCCESSFUL SERVES**	**UNSUCCESSFUL SERVES**	**TOTAL SERVES**	**SUCCESSFUL SERVES (%)**
Jim	//	////	6	33
Jennifer	///// //	/	8	88
Tom	/	/////	6	17
Tameka	/	////	5	20
José		///	3	0
Kim	/	///	4	25
Team Totals	12	20	32	38

struggle with how to use assessment and assign grades in ways that are fair to all students. One suggestion from an experienced teacher is to give lower-skilled students mainly credit for improvement and to weigh the evaluations of higher-skilled students more heavily on their skills. Highly skilled students may only be able to show a little improvement, but they do not need the extra credit for improvement because they already play well.

Table 18-4 shows sample scores on a badminton short-serve test whose criterion level for an A is 13 to 16 points. In this example James improved by only 4 points, but his final score is 5 points higher than Tyrone's score. If the teacher gives Tyrone extra credit for improvement, both boys may make an A on the test even though only James was at the A criterion level by the last day of practice.

Name _____		Period _____					
Station/Date	/	/	/	/	/	/	/
Wall Volley							
Short Serve							
Long Serve							
Overhead Clear							
Rally Tally							

FIGURE 18-2

A development card for practice of skill tests.

TABLE 18-4	Sample Scores on a Badminton Short Serve Test				
NAME	DAY 1	DAY 2	DAY 3	DAY 4	IMPROVEMENT
Tyrone	1	4	8	9	+8
James	10	11	11	14	+4

Does Formative Assessment Make a Difference?

Recently a group of teacher-researchers wanted to find out whether the use of formative assessment really helps students learn more (16). They conducted a study in a middle school with two classes of sixth- and seventh-graders. Prior to instruction students were tested on four badminton skills: the long serve, short serve, overhead clear, and wall volley. Two teachers taught an 8-week badminton unit to students who were divided within each class into an assessment group and a control group. Every Tuesday and Thursday the two groups received identical instruction, except that the assessment group took part in several kinds of formative assessments. To ensure that differences between the groups' posttest scores could be attributed to the assessments, the two teachers alternated the teaching of the two groups and took care to be sure that all students received quality instruction.

During the 8-week unit the assessment group completed the following formative assessments: (*a*) They kept written records on individual skill development cards while they practiced the four skill tests and had a rally tally at the beginning of every class period. (*b*) A partner completed a criteria sheet for the short serve. (*c*) They made a videotaped analysis and criteria sheet for the overhead clear. (*d*) They completed a quick quiz and a crossword puzzle. (*e*) They used scorecards during 2 days of tournament play.

In this research project students in the two groups practiced at the same four stations at the beginning of each class period. Figure 18-3 shows a student practicing the short serve. Students in the assessment group recorded their scores on a scorecard (Fig. 18-2); the control group merely practiced the skills. After students had practiced the four skill tests, a rally tally was held for both groups. Players and their partners attempted to keep the shuttlecock going back and forth. The assessment group counted and recorded their highest number of consecutive rallies, while the control group just practiced. The criteria sheets used with the short serve and overhead clear (Figs. 18-4 and 18-5) focused attention on important process criteria to help ensure that students were practicing the correct form of the movements. During the last 2 days of the badminton unit, a coed round-robin tournament was held for both groups. Tournament games lasted 6 minutes, and players changed partners after every two rounds. The assessment group recorded their scores (Fig. 18-6). The control group simply reported their wins and losses to the teacher.

After all students in the project completed their skill performance posttests, researchers analyzed the data. They concluded that the assessment group had scored significantly better on the individual badminton skills and were more successful at playing the game. The researchers saw other dramatic differences between the con-

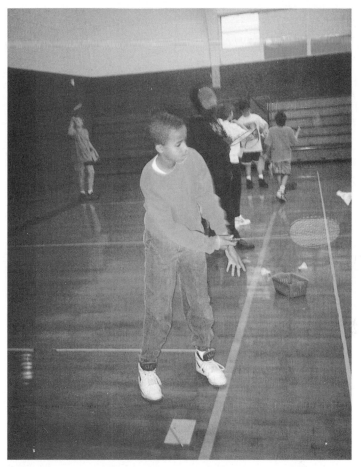

FIGURE 18-3

A student practices the badminton short serve. (Photo by Mary Lou Veal, Department of Exercise and Sport Science, University of North Carolina at Greensboro.)

trol and assessment groups during play. Although both groups were excited about playing in the tournament, the assessment group achieved significantly more playing time than the control group because they did not waste as much time between points. In addition, the research team noticed throughout the unit that the assessment group was better motivated to learn and stayed on task more consistently than the control group. They even came out of the locker room more quickly than the control group. Table 18-5 presents the results of the skills tests; Table 18-6 summarizes the game play analysis (16).

Other Research on Assessment and Student Learning

While one study does not prove conclusively that assessment helps students learn, it does suggest that researchers and teachers should continue to investigate the effects of assessment and evaluation on learning and motivation. Other studies, both from education and physical education, seem to support the badminton study findings.

Name _____ Period _____				
	TRIAL 1		TRIAL 2	
Things to Look For . . .	Yes	No	Yes	No
1. Feet are staggered and point toward the diagonal service court				
2. The shuttle is contacted low with racket head below the waist				
3. Racket sweeps forward smoothly				
4. Wrist does not snap forward				
5. Feet remain stationary				
Observer's Signature _____				

FIGURE 18-4

Process criteria sheet for the badminton short serve.

Name _____ Period _____				
	TRIAL 1		TRIAL 2	
Things to Look For . . .	Yes	No	Yes	No
1. Forward swing begins from the "backscratch" position				
2. Racket arm is fully extended when contacting shuttle				
3. Non-racket side is turned to the net in preparation for hitting the shuttle				
4. Results—The shuttle consistently travels high and deep to the back of the court				
Observer's Signature _____				

FIGURE 18-5

Process criteria sheet for the badminton overhead clear.

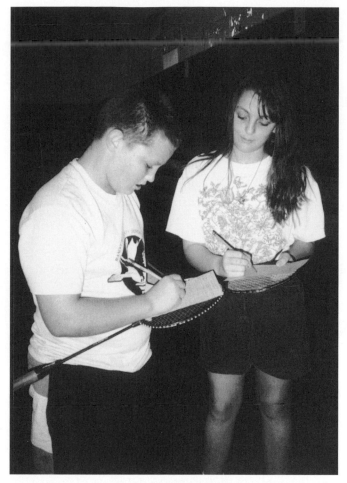

FIGURE 18-6

Assessment group students record their points during the badminton tournament. (Photo by Mary Lou Veal, Department of Exercise and Sport Science, University of North Carolina at Greensboro.)

For example, in one study researchers challenged students with specific individual goals for achievement and gave them feedback about their improvement in relation to these goals (17). Grades were based on a combination of achievement and improvement from the base score. Students in this study reported that they studied harder for quizzes and worked closer to their potential. A number of studies reviewed by Crooks (9) showed that evaluation has a strong effect on how students study.

Boyce (18) investigated the influence of teachers' grading practices on students' achievement. In her study students in nine physical education classes were taught a riflery unit with different grading methods. Boyce found that students learned most when the grade was based on 50% skill, 30% cognitive ability, and 20% participation. Students who were graded solely on participation improved erratically, but the group graded on a combination of factors improved steadily, and their final scores

TABLE 18-5	Skills Tests Analysis for Badminton Study		
	PRETEST	**POSTTEST**	**ADJUSTED**
LONG SERVE			
Treatment	7.73	12.27	12.97
Control	9.00	12.00	11.01
Male	12.42	11.79	8.19
Female	3.70	12.54	16.40[a]
OVERHEAD CLEAR			
Treatment	12.69	17.27	17.57[a]
Control	13.90	15.10	14.66
Male	14.88	16.13	14.97
Female	11.41	16.55	17.76[b]
WALL VOLLEY			
Treatment	23.92	47.19	48.36
Control	26.80	45.05	43.48
Male	30.29	55.83	50.59[b]
Female	19.59	35.81	41.48

[a]$p < .01$
[b]$p < .05$
Reprinted with permission from Veal, M.L., Bolt, B., Griffith, J.B., and Sluder, D.: The effects of formative assessment on learning. Academy Action, 4:11, 1996.

were significantly higher than the participation-only group. Boyce's study confirms the finding of Tousignant and Siedentop (19) that when there was a focus on motor skill development, recording of scores improved the rate of on-task behavior.

Although there is not a lot of research evidence to support the claim that assessment helps students learn, common sense suggests that when students are held accountable for learning, they are likely to be more successful. Some researchers who

TABLE 18-6	Game Play Analysis for Badminton Study		
TOURNAMENT PLAY: MEAN SHUTTLE AIRTIME (SECONDS)			
	6th Grade	**7th Grade**	**Combined**
Control group	56.31	76.30	66.30
Assessment group	71.45[a]	103.00[a]	87.68[a]
Average	63.88	90.10	

[a]$p < .05$.
Reprinted with permission from Veal, M.L., Bolt, B., Griffith, J.B., and Sluder, D.: The effects of formative assessment on learning. Academy Action, 4:11, 1996.

have studied the effects of accountability have concluded that (*a*) students learn more when teachers hold them accountable, and (*b*) there are many types of accountability (19–21). Assessment is only one type of accountability, but it appears to be a very powerful motivator for students and may also facilitate learning. Other positive forms of accountability include teacher monitoring, verbal checkups on progress, public recognition and rewards, and grading (21).

A good accountability system should communicate three important kinds of information to students: (*a*) a description of the task, (*b*) criteria or goals for successful completion of the task, and (*c*) how they will be held accountable for completing the task (22). Study the following example for serving in volleyball that uses these three steps in the design of an accountability system.

EXAMPLE

Description of the task: Serving and receiving serve in volleyball. Students play modified small-sided games of two-on-two volleyball, working on serve and serve reception. Each player serves 5 times in succession, and teams take turns serving and receiving. The object is to score as many points as possible.

Criteria for success: The serving team scores one point for a serve that goes over the net into the playing area. The receiving team scores one point for a pass that is caught by the receiver's partner (later the setter) before it touches the ground. The goal is to score at least 10 of the possible 20 points (i.e., each team can score a possible 10 points serving and 10 points receiving). This goal may be increased as players become better servers and receivers.

Accountability: Players earn a certain number of bonus points on their grade each day that they score at least 10 points in this game. Alternatively, the names of players who reach their goal are added to a recognition bulletin board.

Moving From a Testing Culture to an Assessment Culture

In the past many teachers thought the only way to see whether students were learning was to administer a test. Unfortunately, this might well be a rare event, possibly taking place only at the end of a unit of instruction. While many standardized skill tests are valid and reliable for research, they may not be appropriate for students in kindergarten through 12th grade. This is because the tests are often inefficient to administer or because teachers have found that they are not good predictors of game play. This does not mean that skill tests should never be used, but it explains why many teachers prefer to administer curriculum-based skill tests. However, no matter what type of test or alternative strategy is used, assessment must be an ongoing, regular event.

Authentic Assessment

A recent development in education is the concept of **authentic assessment,** sometimes called alternative assessment. For an assessment to be authentic, it must (*a*) measure essential skills and (*b*) "be scored in reference to authentic standards of performance, which students must understand to be inherent to successful performance" (23, p. 703).

Ryan (24) distinguished between authentic assessment and traditional standardized testing by noting, "Authentic assessments tell us how well students can apply their knowledge; standardized tests are more efficient for determining how well students have acquired basic facts."

> Authentic assessments (*a*) measure skills that are essential for successful performance, and (*b*) are scored according to real rather than arbitrary standards.

With these ideas in mind, one can conclude that authentic assessment in the psychomotor domain should be focused on how skills are used during game play or within a gamelike context. Assessing skills during game play is very different from using skill tests to determine achievement, because skill tests are designed to operate out of the context of the game. While skill tests are often highly reliable and valid for research, many teachers have found that they are not good predictors of game play (11). Recently several researchers have published suggestions for authentic assessment of game play (25, 26). These suggestions often include assessment of on- and off-the-ball skills and outcome measures, such as points scored.

Authentic assessments in physical education often take the form of culminating performances that require students to synthesize or analyze skills (Fig. 18-7). These assessments usually take place over several class periods as opposed to a single one.

For each of the examples in Figure 18-7, a **rubric** is used to assess the culminating performance. The rubric gives criteria for judging students' performance; it usually contains specific statements that define what the performance will look like at various levels of proficiency. Students are informed of the assessment criteria at the time they begin working on their culminating performances. Figure 18-8 is a rubric for assessing a culminating performance in a dance unit.

> A rubric is a set of criteria for judging quality of performance; it usually contains specific statements that define the performance at various levels of proficiency.

Authentic assessment represents a paradigm shift away from traditional measurement and evaluation. Because it places the individual child at the center of the curriculum, authentic assessment is different from both norm-referenced and criterion-referenced measurement and evaluation. Many educators believe that authentic assessment is more appropriate for use in classroom contexts.

Student Choice and Equity in Assessment

More and more in the future you, as a physical education teacher, will be asked to select and use authentic assessments in your classes. One of the things you should consider is the possibility of giving students choices in how they are assessed. An earlier section of this chapter discusses involving students in peer and self-assessments. Allowing assessment choices empowers students to demonstrate their strengths, testing them on what they have learned rather than what they have not learned. The idea of giving students assessment choices is a way of making your assessments more equitable for your students.

Type of Unit	Culminating Performance
Dance	Design and perform a dance routine.
Gymnastics	Design and perform a sequence of tumbling skills.
Tennis	Serve as an official for a match.
Badminton	Play in or provide commentary for an exhibition match demonstrating various strokes and strategy.
Basketball	Serve as a referee during a tournament.
Individual sport	Teach a younger student how to play the game.
Novel sport	Prepare a videotape on how to play the game.

FIGURE 18-7

Culminating performances for various physical education teaching units.

There is substantial evidence that educational assessment is becoming more qualitative, more subjective, and more likely to be teacher designed and curriculum based. As we recognize the role of both formative and summative assessment in helping students learn, we should also consider how assessment can be more equitable for all students. When I first began studying teachers' perceptions, I learned that many teachers approach assessment as an individualized process. Fairness is one of the important considerations when teachers use assessments (11). The teachers I interviewed did not use assessment to compare students with one another. Instead, they were concerned with the potential of each individual student. This keen interest in individualizing the physical education experience for students suggests the need for considering students' choice as a way of making assessment more equitable.

In traditional physical education skills have been tested at the end of a unit, with everyone taking the same tests. Is this equitable? Noddings (27), a teacher education researcher, claimed that equity is not synonymous with equality and even argued that requiring all students to take the same courses to achieve "equal" schooling is in itself inequitable. Applying Noddings's ideas to physical education, we might consider making assessment more equitable for students through assessment choices and by allowing students to select their best performance products. I am convinced of the worth of these ideas both by the arguments of Noddings and by those of Darling-Hammond (28), who said, "In order for assessment to support student learning, . . . it must allow for different starting points for learning and diverse ways of demonstrating competence" (p. 25). Darling-Hammond (28) also recommended use of "diverse and wide-ranging tasks that use many different performance modes and that involve students in choosing ways to demonstrate their competence" (p. 17).

Another critical feature of equitable assessment is that the teacher must establish criteria by which performance will be evaluated. These criteria may focus on either the process or the product, but either way students need to know the criteria that will be used to judge their performance. Figure 18-9 shows assessment choices that might be offered to secondary physical education students enrolled in volleyball, track and field, gymnastics, or dance.

RUBRIC FOR DANCE ROUTINE

Level 4: Gold
- 4 dance steps with smooth transitions
- 2 pieces of equipment that integrate object manipulation
- 2 locomotor skills with smooth transitions
- Active and effective group participation; provides leadership

Level 3: Silver
- 3 dance steps with smooth transitions
- At least limited use of 1–2 pieces of equipment
- 2 locomotor skills
- Active group participation; minimal leadership

Level 2: Bronze
- 2–3 dance steps
- At least limited use of one piece of equipment
- At least limited use of 1–2 locomotor skills
- Participates with group; no leadership

Level 1: Blue Ribbon
- 1 dance step
- At least limited use of 1 piece of equipment
- At least limited use of 1 locomotor skill
- Limited participation with group; no leadership

FIGURE 18-8

Rubric for assessing a culminating performance in dance unit. (Used with permission from Sue Bannister of Bowling Green, Kentucky, and Jeannette Askins of Western Kentucky University.)

If a battery of volleyball skill tests is used to assess skills, a teacher might allow students the choice of type of serve, a choice between passing or setting, plus either spike or drive. If students maintained a regular record of progress during the unit of instruction, they would be in a position to select and demonstrate their strongest skills on a performance test at the end of the unit. In a track and field unit, after all of the events had been taught, students could choose to perform their strongest event in each category in addition to being a member of a relay team. A class track meet might be used as a culminating event that would provide authenticity to class meetings devoted to practice time. Students could monitor their progress during the practice sessions, both as feedback for themselves and to help the teacher determine when additional instruction is needed. Eventually, the chosen events could be performed for a grade or the teacher could use the results of the track meet as a portion of the students' grades. Gymnastics students could choose to perform a tumbling combination of their choice, one type of vault, and either bars or beam. Choices within the gymnastics events can be designated with a difficulty level used

---

EXAMPLES OF ASSESSMENT CHOICES

Volleyball

Students may demonstrate their competence by choosing among the following tests:
- Underhand or Overhand Serve
- Setting or Passing
- Spiking or Driving

Track & Field

Students participate in an in-class track meet and choose:
- One Running Event (100 m, 200 m, or 400 m)
- One Throwing Event (discus, shot put, or softball throw)
- One Jumping Event (long jump, triple jump, or high jump)
- One Relay Team

Gymnastics

For the final performance assessment, choose one from each category:
- Tumbling Combination (designed by student)
- Valult (knee, pike, tuck, or flank)
- Parallel Bars, Uneven Bars, or Balance Beam (high or low)

Dance

For the performance assessment, choose one dance from each category:
- Folk Dance
- Line Dance
- Square Dance

FIGURE 18-9

Assessment choices for secondary physical education teaching units.

to adjust the scores up or down. In a folk dance unit, students could be graded on their performance of three of the dances taught during the unit. Another way to organize a dance unit is to group students according to their interests and allow them to teach dances to peers. Teaching dances to others could be designed as a culminating performance assessment, with a rubric to evaluate the performance.

Chapter Summary

The major premise of this chapter is that assessment is an instructional tool for effective teaching in physical education. Reflective teachers who engage in thoughtful examination of all aspects of their teaching benefit from using assessment data to inform their decisions. Formative assessment, distinguished from summative evaluation, is endorsed because it is invaluable in the development of effective instructional strategies. Research suggests that formative assessment also makes a real difference in student learning. Authentic assessment is offered as an alternative to traditional skill testing, especially when it allows students to choose their mode of performance. Student choice of assessments makes for equitable grading practices that focus on what students can do rather than on what they cannot do.

SELF-TEST QUESTIONS

1. A reflective teacher engages in all of the following behaviors *except* which one?
   A. Designing lessons to optimize practice opportunities
   B. Specifying learning goals prior to instruction
   C. Allowing students to practice skill tests before grading
   D. Using skill tests only for grading

2. Which of the following is *not* a justification for the use of formative assessment?
   A. To motivate students
   B. To verify the teacher's success
   C. To grade students
   D. To plan the curriculum

3. Which of the following examples represents authentic assessment?
   A. The teacher administers a serving test to students that requires them to place serves into optimal areas of the court.
   B. Students count how many times they can juggle a soccer ball.
   C. Students work at skill stations at the beginning of each class and record their progress.
   D. Students videotape their gymnastics routines and use a rubric to assess their peers' performances.

4. How is formative assessment different from summative evaluation?
   A. Formative assessment data are used to provide feedback to students, whereas summative evaluation data are used to sum up a student's achievement.
   B. There is no difference between these terms.
   C. Formative assessment takes place after learning is complete, whereas summative evaluation takes place during the learning process.
   D. Formative assessment is administered by peers, and summative evaluation is administered by teachers.

5. Viewing formative assessment as an occasion for learning means:
   A. Students are only learning when they are being assessed.
   B. Students should be assessed on a daily basis.
   C. An assessment task should provide feedback to learners that results in more learning.
   D. Learning in physical education can only be assessed using an authentic assessment.

6. Which of the following statements best distinguishes a testing culture from an assessment culture?
   A. In a testing culture, assessment occurs less often than in an assessment culture.
   B. In an assessment culture, assessment is ongoing.
   C. In a testing culture, skill tests are used as end-of-the-unit culminating events, while an assessment culture includes assessment as a continual aid to learning.
   D. All of the above.

7. Equity in assessment means that:
   A. Students do not have to demonstrate movement competence.
   B. Students should be able to choose their best performance for assessment.
   C. All students should receive an equal number of trials on a test.
   D. All students should be assessed on the same skills.

8. Which of the following statements about assessment research is true?
   A. Researchers have concluded that grades have no influence on students' learning.
   B. Researchers are convinced that assessment has a negative influence on students' motivation.
   C. A few studies seem to show that assessment plays a role in helping students learn.
   D. A few studies seem to show that grades in physical education based on participation and effort result in greater student learning.

ANSWERS

1. D	2. C	3. D	4. A
5. C	6. D	7. B	8. C

DOING PROJECTS FOR FURTHER LEARNING

1. Arrange a meeting with a physical education teacher in your community. Sit down together and talk about the role of assessment in his or her classes. How is assessment used? Refer to Table 18-1 and classify the assessments according to the framework categories. Pay particular attention to the reasons for assessment stated or implied by this teacher. In what ways is the use of assessment by this teacher consistent with the ideas promoted in this chapter? Explain.

2. For a sport or physical activity that you know well, design a teaching unit appropriate for either middle- or secondary-school learners. Specify how you will use both formative assessment and summative evaluation in the teaching unit. Use ideas from this chapter.

3. If you are particularly enthusiastic about assessment as an instructional tool and can work with students, please undertake the following action research project (29):

   Designate one class in which students are relatively cooperative and you feel comfortable about trying out new ideas. Plan a unit of 8 to 10 lessons and incorporate a feasible plan for assessing students' progress. (If you are a student teacher, work with your cooperating teacher to design something that is both informative and feasible.) You will have an opportunity in this project to use evidence of students' learning as a basis for formulating and evaluating your teaching (30). After you have collected baseline data, teach the 8 to 10 lessons aimed at improving students' psychomotor performance. As the lessons unfold, use the information you gain from tracking your students' progress to plan and revise instruction. Keep careful records of how you are adapting your instructional methods to students' learning.

   You are asked to:

   • Identify the unit goals you want students to learn.

- Devise a reasonably objective, valid, and reliable method of measuring that learning (e.g., performance test or analysis of form).

- Administer a preassessment to measure how much students already can do.

- Teach 8 to 10 lessons with ongoing formative assessment; use the assessment data to revise your teaching and make decisions about the lessons.

- Track students' progress and measure their improvement (formative assessment); records may be kept by either teacher or students.

- Use evidence of improvement at the end of the unit (summative evaluation) to evaluate the effectiveness of your teaching.

- Report your response and that of your students (and cooperating teacher) to the assessment project.

REFERENCES

1. Wigginton, E.: Sometimes a Shining Moment: The Foxfire Experience. Magnolia, MA, Peter Smith, 1993.
2. Veal, M.L.: The role of assessment in secondary physical education: a pedagogical view. Journal of Physical Education, Recreation, and Dance, 63(7):88, 1992.
3. Sebren, A.: Reflective thinking: integrating theory and practice in teacher preparation. Journal of Physical Education, Recreation, and Dance, 65(6):23, 1994.
4. Smyth, W.J.: Clinical Supervision: Collaborative Learning about Teaching. New York, State Mutual Book & Periodical Service, 1995.
5. Hellison, D.R., and Templin, T.J.: A Reflective Approach to Teaching Physical Education. Champaign, IL, Human Kinetics, 1991.
6. Clift, R., Houston, W.R., and Pugach, M.C.: Encouraging Reflective Practice in Education. New York, Teachers College Press, 1990.
7. Linn, R.: Essentials of student assessment: from accountability to instructional aid. Teachers College Record, 91(3):422, 1990.
8. Hill, B.C., and Ruptic, C.: Practical Aspects of Authentic Assessment: Putting the Pieces Together. Norwood, MA, Christopher-Gordon, 1994.
9. Crooks, T.J.: The impact of classroom evaluation practices on students. Review of Educational Research, 58:438, 1988.
10. Chittenden, E.: Authentic assessment, evaluation, and documentation of student performance. In K. Jervis, E. Chittenden, V. Perrone, and C. Hill (eds.): Expanding Student Assessment. Alexandria, VA, Association for Supervision & Curriculum Development, 1991.
11. Veal, M.L.: Pupil perceptions and practices of secondary teachers. Journal of Physical Education, Recreation, and Dance, 59(7):32, 1988.
12. Wolf, D.P.: Assessment as an episode of learning. In W.C. Ward and R.E. Bennett (eds.): Construction Versus Choice in Cognitive Measurement: Issues in Constructed Response, Performance Testing, and Portfolio Assessment. Mahwah, NJ, Lawrence Erlbaum, 1993.
13. NASPE: Moving into the Future: National Physical Education Standards: A Guide to Content and Assessment. Reston, VA, American Alliance of Health, Physical Education, Recreation, and Dance, 1995.
14. McGee, R.M.: Evaluation of processes and products. In B. Logsdon et al. (eds.): Physical Education for Children: A Focus on the Teaching Process. 2nd ed. Baltimore, Williams & Wilkins, 1984.
15. Veal, M.L.: Assessment as an instructional tool. Strategies, 8(6):10, 1995.
16. Veal, M.L., Bolt, B., Griffith, J.B., and Sluder, D.: The effects of formative assessment on learning. Academy Action, 4:11, 1996.

17. McIver, D.J., and Reuman, D.: Giving their best: grading and recognition practices that motivate students to work hard. American Educator, 17(4):24, 1993.

18. Boyce, A.: Grading practices: How do they influence student skill performance? Journal of Physical Education, Recreation, and Dance, 61(6):46, 1990.

19. Tousignant, M., and Siedentop, D.: A qualitative analysis of task structures in required secondary physical education classes. Journal of Teaching in Physical Education, 3:47, 1983.

20. Hastie, P., and Saunders, S.: Accountability in secondary school physical education. Teaching and Teacher Education, 7:373, 1991.

21. Lund, J.: Assessment and accountability in secondary physical education. Quest, 44:352, 1992.

22. Lund, J., and Veal, M.L.: Make students accountable. Strategies, 9(6):26, 1996.

23. Wiggins, G.: A true test: toward more authentic and equitable assessment. Phi Delta Kappan, 70:703, 1989.

24. Ryan, C.: Authentic Assessment. Westminster, CA, Teacher Created Materials, 1994.

25. Grehaigne, J., and Godbout, P.: Formative assessment in team sports in a tactical approach context. Journal of Physical Education, Recreation, and Dance, 69(1):46, 1998.

26. Schincariol, L., and Radford, K. Checklists and rubrics: an alternative form of assessment in a university volleyball activity course. Journal of Physical Education, Recreation, and Dance, 69(1):25, 1998.

27. Noddings, N.: The Challenge to Care in Schools: An Alternative Approach to Education. New York, Teachers College Press, 1992.

28. Darling-Hammond, L.: Performance-based assessment and educational equity. Harvard Educational Review, 64(1):5, 1994.

29. Veal, M.L., Russell, M., and Brown, J.: Practical assessment for physical education teachers. Journal of Physical Education, Recreation, and Dance, 67(9):21, 1996.

30. Anderson, W.G.: Analysis of Teaching Physical Education. St. Louis, MO, Mosby–Year Book, 1980.

CHAPTER 19

Assessment of Special-Needs Populations

Sue Combs

There are many reasons to test those with special needs (Fig. 19-1). Listed below are some of the reasons that are most important to physical education and recreation specialists:

- Assessment data can be used to place students in programs that will optimize their learning.
- Assessments can identify students' strengths and weaknesses.
- Assessment data can determine whether students need further testing.
- Assessment can guide the development of program goals and objectives.
- Assessment can help determine the effectiveness of program instruction.
- Assessment can suggest strategies that will be effective with certain learning styles and behaviors.
- Assessment can identify those who wish to participate in sport so as to ensure equitable competition.
- Assessment can build relationships by encouraging communication among parents and guardians, school officials, and others.
- Assessment of those with special needs is required by law.

Assessments play a critical role in determining worthwhile physical education and sport programs for those with special needs. But first the practitioner must understand how to sort out information generated by such testing. This chapter presents and discusses an array of assessment instruments that fall within four major categories defined by their intended use by the practitioner: (*a*) screening, (*b*) diagnosis and placement, (*c*) instruction and student progress, and (*d*) sport and activity classification.

No single test can meet the needs of all persons. Therefore, each of the tests in this chapter should be scrutinized carefully. Try to understand the characteristics of each test, noting the stated purpose, standardization, program applications,

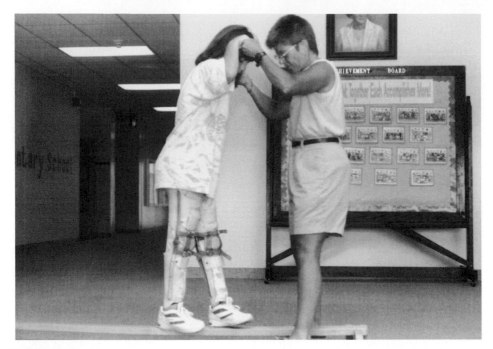

FIGURE 19-1

Testing a person with special needs. (Photo by Dr. Sue Combs, Department of Health, Physical Education, and Recreation, University of North Carolina at Wilmington.)

strengths, and weaknesses. How and why a test is used is ultimately what counts. Unfortunately, too many practitioners fail to realize this.

As you read this chapter, watch for the following keywords:

Diagnosis   Screening
Due process (procedural safeguards)   Special-needs populations

Defining Special-Needs Populations

Defining special needs and levels of needs is difficult because human beings do not fit neatly into categories. Terms such as *exceptional*, *special*, *impaired*, *disabled*, and *handicapped* have been used to describe those with special needs for learning and/or performance. In school settings these terms have been used to describe students whose physical, mental, and/or emotional characteristics interfere with their optimal development through regular educational offerings. **Special-needs populations** is a broad term that includes both special-needs students and other special-needs persons who are younger or older than the traditional-age student. *Special-needs programs* include a wide variety of school- and community-based programs that serve persons of varying ages who have special needs for their optimal learning and/or performance. Included among these programs are adapted physical education programs, wheelchair basketball leagues, and programs such as the Paralympics and the Special Olympics.

Special-needs populations are composed of individuals whose physical, mental, and/or emotional characteristics interfere with their optimal development and/or performance.

While the traditional classification system for special populations has been successful in identifying the need for special programming, the system has not guaranteed the development of *appropriate* programs. This is where we turn to assessment, a critical component in developing appropriate programming for special-needs populations.

Legal Requirements for Assessment

Assessment is mandated by federal Public Law (PL) 94-142, the Education for All Handicapped Children Act. It requires that appropriate, individualized educational and related services must be provided to all children after proper assessment. Although this has been the law of the land since its passage, it appears that compliance is far from universal. It has been estimated that approximately 12 to 15% of school-aged children have special needs, yet this population often receives improper or no assessment (1).

If assessment is not occurring because practitioners are unaware of or unable to select appropriate assessment tools, it is imperative that textbooks such as this one provide information to help practitioners learn to make informed decisions about assessment and programming for special-needs populations. While the provision of quality physical education services for special-needs students should not be justified solely on the basis of fulfilling a legal mandate, it is critically important that practitioners understand their legal responsibilities. Two areas, due process and standards, are discussed so as to clarify the intent of the law.

Due Process

In the area of special needs, **due process (procedural safeguards)** essentially means that parents or legal guardians must be informed of their rights and may challenge educational decisions if they consider that the process has been unfair to their child. Applied to assessment, due process requires the following:

- A parent's or guardian's permission to conduct assessments
- Translation and interpretation of assessment findings to parents or guardians
- Additional independent assessments if the parent or guardian wants them
- Mediation of results through a hearing if parents or guardians and the school system cannot agree
- Confidentiality of all results and recommendations

Due process (procedural safeguards) is the requirement that parents, guardians, and clients be informed of their rights and allowed to challenge decisions that they consider unfair.

Standards

PL 94-142 also mandates standards for assessing those with special needs. These standards address selection and administration of tests and characteristics and qualifications of test administrators. Test selection standards specify that the assessment must be focused on achievement level and/or abilities rather than on limitations of the person. Test selection standards also specify the use of both formal and informal tests. Standards for test administration require the measurement of abilities rather than communication skills and mandate adaptations to address a person's mode of communication. PL 94-142 also supports a multidisciplinary approach to assessment by requiring the involvement of several test administrators using several assessment tools.

Issues in Testing Special-Needs Populations

Several issues arise when planning for appropriate assessment of special-needs populations. Three of the most debated issues are (*a*) norm-referenced versus criterion-referenced testing, (*b*) general versus specific testing, and (*c*) process versus product testing.

Norm-Referenced Versus Criterion-Referenced Testing

As noted in the discussion of PL 94-142, tests administered to a person should not be all of one kind. They should not be all formal or all informal, nor should the tests be all norm-referenced or all criterion-referenced. Different types of tests provide different types of information. Norm-referenced tests allow for comparisons between the performance of the special-needs child and the performance of other children. Criterion-referenced tests are valuable for identifying level of performance relative to a defined standard. Results from both types of tests are important to decisions about special-needs programs.

Generality Versus Specificity

Effective use of the results of a test that measures general abilities rather than specific skills has recently been challenged. The challenge is based on the belief that tests that measure constructs such as general motor ability have limited usefulness and sometimes even provide misleading information. Practitioners are sometimes guilty of collecting information that cannot and should not be generated. Test results should provide *specific* data that are directly applicable to present levels of performance of specific skills.

Those who purport the benefits of specific motor skill tests for special-needs populations argue that assessments should focus on basic motor skills because they are the foundation of general motor abilities (Fig. 19-2). They also believe that motor skills that are specific to various environments should be assessed. In other words, all assessments of basic motor skills must be individualized to provide clear indications of the progress of individuals.

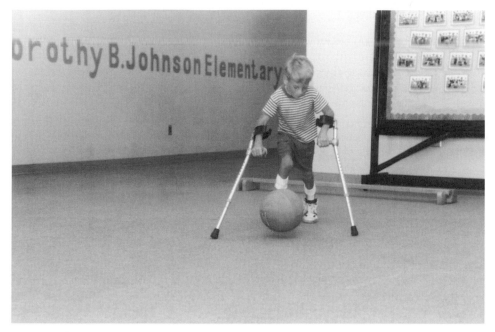

FIGURE 19-2

The kick is a basic motor skill that is commonly assessed. (Photo by Dr. Sue Combs, Department of Health, Physical Education, and Recreation, University of North Carolina at Wilmington.)

Process Versus Product Testing

One of the major reasons for assessment is to determine a person's level of performance. Product data offer an overview of a student's abilities and can be useful in comparing performances with those of other students. Product assessments can help to demonstrate a need for special programming. While product assessments can be used to identify a specific performance level, they will not tell the practitioner why or how the performance occurred. Product data may, for example, show that a person threw a ball 10 feet, but the score does not explain why the throw was only 10 feet. Process assessment uses a task analysis approach to provide information on the person's motor processes. For example, did the thrower use rotation, oppositional movement, follow-through? Product *and* process testing have roles in special-needs assessment.

Four Major Categories of Test Use

As previously noted, assessment should be done for specific purposes. Sherrill (2) wrote that assessment refers not only to data collection but also to interpretations and decisions based on the data. She further identified four major categories of tests that relate to the decision-making purpose of assessment. The four major categories of test use are (*a*) screening, (*b*) diagnosis and placement, (*c*) instruction and monitoring of students' progress, and (*d*) sport and activity classification (2).

Tests for Screening

Screening, a basic method of collecting information about possible special needs, can alert the service provider to the need for further testing. Screening tests are usually very efficient because they often are used during group observation and because they use simple yes-no, pass-fail scoring. Screening often occurs in a natural environment (e.g., a playground or classroom) and may be conducted by nonprofessionals (e.g., a parent, guardian, or classroom teacher). It should be clearly understood, however, that screening tests must be used with caution and that they should not be the sole basis for developing a diagnostic plan of intervention.

> Screening is the use of quick and simple tests or procedures to identify those who may have special learning and/or performance needs; screening tests are usually followed by more precise forms of assessment.

There are several useful motor skills screening tests. Practitioners working with children in or out of school benefit from being familiar with these instruments. Reviewed here are the Denver II (revision of the Denver Developmental Screening Test), the Sherrill Perceptual Motor Survey Checklist, and the Purdue Perceptual-Motor Survey.

Denver II: Revision of the Denver Developmental Screening Test (3)

Purpose

The purpose of this test is to screen for developmental delays in children from birth to 6 years of age in four areas of development: gross motor, language, fine motor-adaptive, and personal and social.

Description

The Denver II consists of 125 items that reflect developmental progressions in the areas of gross motor skills, including sitting, walking, jumping, and overall large muscle movement; language, including hearing, understanding, and use of language; fine motor-adaptive skills, including eye-hand coordination, manipulation of small objects, and problem solving; and personal and social skills, including getting along with people and caring for personal needs. Figure 19-3 shows how items in the four areas are sequentially addressed. Each item is norm-referenced, with a horizontal bar chart indicating the ages at which 25%, 50%, 75% and 90% of children can perform each specific task. Figure 19-4 indicates that 25% of the sample children walk well at approximately 11 months, 50% at 12.33 months, 75% at 13.5 months, and 90% at a little under 15 months.

Gross motor skills assessed in the Denver II deal primarily with postural control and basic motor skills. Examples of items assessing postural control include holding head up, bearing weight, rolling over, sitting with no support, stoop and recovering, and balancing for time. Basic motor skill items include walking, running, kicking, throwing, and jumping.

Scoring

Items are scored as pass, fail, refusal, or no opportunity to perform. Decisions about referrals for additional testing depend on numbers of recorded delays and cautions. A delay is recorded if a child fails an item that 90% of children the same age pass. A caution is recorded if a child fails an item that 75 to 90% of children the same age pass.

Validity

Final selection of the 125 items was based on eight criteria, and age placement of the items was guided by standardization data from more than 2000 children. Regression analyses were used to determine the ages at which the various percentages of children could perform each item. Content validity was demonstrated by recognition and acceptance of the test by professionals in child development all over the world (4).

Reliability

Interrater and test-retest reliability were reported to have mean percentage of agreement for most items at .99, with a range of .95 to 1.00.

Source

Available from Denver Development Materials, PO Box 6919, Denver, CO 80206–0919.

Comments

Criteria for performance of the test items are defined clearly in the test booklet. Age and maturity of the child determine time necessary for administration. This test is important for early identification of developmental problems and is an excellent way to provide appropriate intervention during a person's critical developmental period. There is an initial investment of time to become familiar with the procedures, but the Denver II provides an excellent opportunity for observing the whole child and comparing performances on a variety of basic motor tasks with performances of other children of the same age. While some professionals debate the need for elementary-school teachers to become proficient in working with children younger than 5 years of age, others consider increased knowledge of early childhood development to be clearly advantageous.

Sherrill Perceptual-Motor Screening Checklist (2)

Purpose

The purpose of the Sherrill Perceptual-Motor Screening Checklist is to identify perceptual-motor behaviors commonly associated with students who have learning disabilities.

Description

The Sherrill Perceptual-Motor Screening Checklist is composed of 46 statements that describe perceptual and/or motor behaviors (Fig. 19-5). Examples of statements: cannot name body parts or move them on command; has trouble crossing the midline of the body; confuses right and left sides; lacks body awareness; cannot imitate body postures and movements (Fig. 19-6).

Scoring

Items are scored by checking off behaviors. If 10 or more of the 46 statements are checked, the person should be referred for further testing for learning disabilities.

(text continues on page 624)

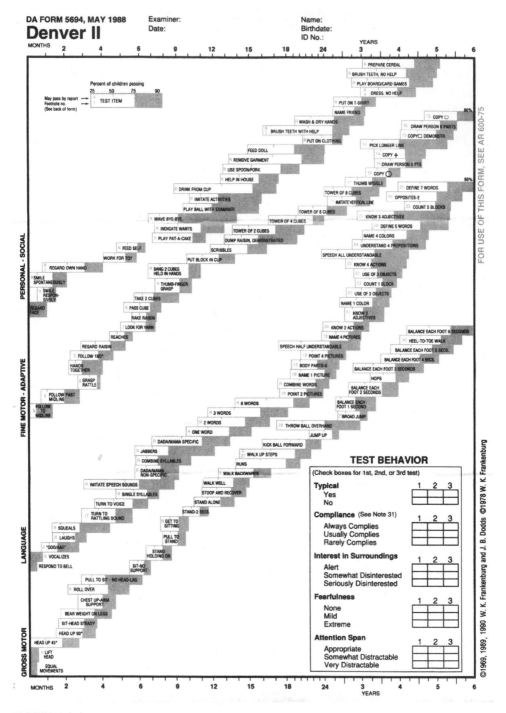

FIGURE 19-3

Sides 1 and 2 of score sheet for the Denver II . (Reprinted with permission of Denver Developmental Materials, Denver, CO.)

DIRECTIONS FOR ADMINISTRATION

1. Try to get child to smile by smiling, talking or waving. Do not touch him/her.
2. Child must stare at hand several seconds.
3. Parent may help guide toothbrush and put toothpaste on brush.
4. Child does not have to be able to tie shoes or button/zip in the back.
5. Move yarn slowly in an arc from one side to the other, about 8" above child's face.
6. Pass if child grasps rattle when it is touched to the backs or tips of fingers.
7. Pass if child tries to see where yarn went. Yarn should be dropped quickly from sight from tester's hand without arm movement.
8. Child must transfer cube from hand to hand without help of body, mouth, or table.
9. Pass if child picks up raisin with any part of thumb and finger.
10. Line can vary only 30 degrees or less from tester's line.
11. Make a fist with thumb pointing upward and wiggle only the thumb. Pass if child imitates and does not move any fingers other than the thumb.

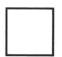

12. Pass any enclosed form. Fail continuous round motions.

13. Which line is longer? (Not bigger.) Turn paper upside down and repeat. (pass 3 of 3 or 5 of 6)

14. Pass any lines crossing near midpoint.

15. Have child copy first. If failed, demonstrate.

When giving items 12, 14, and 15, do not name the forms. Do not demonstrate 12 and 14.

16. When scoring, each pair (2 arms, 2 legs, etc.) counts as one part.
17. Place one cube in cup and shake gently near child's ear, but out of sight. Repeat for other ear.
18. Point to picture and have child name it. (No credit is given for sounds only.)
    If less than 4 pictures are named correctly, have child point to picture as each is named by tester.

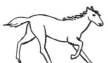

19. Using doll, tell child: Show me the nose, eyes, ears, mouth, hands, feet, tummy, hair. Pass 6 of 8.
20. Using pictures, ask child: Which one flies?... says meow?... talks?... barks?... gallops? Pass 2 of 5, 4 of 5.
21. Ask child: What do you do when you are cold?... tired?... hungry? Pass 2 of 3, 3 of 3.
22. Ask child: What do you do with a cup? What is a chair used for? What is a pencil used for? Action words must be included in answers.
23. Pass if child correctly places <u>and</u> says how many blocks are on paper. (1, 5).
24. Tell child: Put block **on** table; **under** table; **in front of** me, **behind** me. Pass 4 of 4. (Do not help child by pointing, moving head or eyes.)
25. Ask child: What is a ball?... lake?... desk?... house?... banana?... curtain?... fence?... ceiling? Pass if defined in terms of use, shape, what it is made of, or general category (such as banana is fruit, not just yellow). Pass 5 of 8, 7 of 8.
26. Ask child: If a horse is big, a mouse is __? If fire is hot, ice is __? If the sun shines during the day, the moon shines during the __? Pass 2 of 3.
27. Child may use wall or rail only, not person. May not crawl.
28. Child must throw ball overhand 3 feet to within arm's reach of tester.
29. Child must perform standing broad jump over width of test sheet (8 1/2 inches).
30. Tell child to walk forward, ⚬⚬⚬⚬➤ heel within 1 inch of toe. Tester may demonstrate. Child must walk 4 consecutive steps.
31. In the second year, half of normal children are non-compliant.

OBSERVATIONS:

FIGURE 19-3

Continued

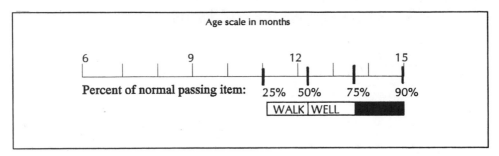

FIGURE 19-4

Norms for Denver II item "Walk Well." (Adapted with permission from Frankenburg, W.K., Dodds, J., and Archer, P.: Denver II Technical Manual. Denver, CO, Denver Developmental Materials, 1990.)

Validity

The validity of the Sherrill Perceptual-Motor Screening Checklist is not reported.

Reliability

The reliability of the Sherrill Perceptual-Motor Screening Checklist is not reported.

Comments

This screening test can be administered by parents or classroom teachers. Data collected may have limited applications but are very helpful in identifying a need for further testing. The nature of the checklist may enhance communication and collaboration among parents and classroom teachers.

Purdue Perceptual-Motor Survey (5)

Purpose

The purpose of the Purdue Perceptual-Motor Survey is to detect perceptual-motor problems among children in early elementary grades (6 to 10 years of age).

Description

The 30 items organized under five categories include balance and postural flexibility, body image and differentiation, perceptual-motor matching, ocular control, and form perception. The two categories *balance and postural flexibility* and *body image and differentiation* include aspects of laterality and directionality that are especially relevant to physical education. Each of these categories, shown in Figures 19-7 and 19-8 respectively, comprises several subskills. Listed under each subskill are descriptive statements of problems that should be watched for by the test administrator.

Scoring

For each subskill, 1 point is assigned for each observed performance problem. Therefore, a high score represents a poorer performance than a low score.

Validity

Criterion-related validity was reported to be .65.

SHERRILL PERCEPTUAL-MOTOR SCREENING CHECKLIST

____ 1. Fails to show opposition of limbs in walking, sitting, throwing.
____ 2. Sits or stands with poor posture.
____ 3. Does not transfer weight from one foot to the other when throwing.
____ 4. Cannot name body parts or move them on command.
____ 5. Has poor muscle tone (tense or flaccid).
____ 6. Uses one extremity much more often than the other.
____ 7. Cannot use arm without "overflow" movements from the other body parts.
____ 8. Cannot jump rope.
____ 9. Cannot clap out a rhythm with both hands or stamp rhythm with feet.
____ 10. Has trouble crossing the midline of the body.
____ 11. Often confuses right and left sides.
____ 12. Confuses vertical, horizontal, up, down directions.
____ 13. Cannot hop or maintain balance in squatting.
____ 14. Has trouble getting in and out of seat.
____ 15. Approaches new tasks with excessive clumsiness.
____ 16. Fails to plan movements before initiating task.
____ 17. Walks or runs with awkward gait.
____ 18. Cannot tie shoes, use scissors, manipulate small objects.
____ 19. Cannot identify fingers as they are touched without vision.
____ 20. Has messy handwriting.
____ 21. Has difficulty tracing over line or staying between lines.
____ 22. Cannot discriminate tactually between different coins or fabrics.
____ 23. Cannot imitate body postures and movements.
____ 24. Demonstrates poor ocular control; unable to maintain eye contact with moving objects; loses place when reading.
____ 25. Lacks body awareness; bumps into things; spills and drops objects.
____ 26. Appears tense and anxious; cries or angers easily.
____ 27. Responds negatively to physical contact; avoids touch.
____ 28. Craves to be touched or held.
____ 29. Overreacts to high-frequency noise, bright lights, odors.
____ 30. Exhibits difficulty in concentrating.
____ 31. Shows tendency to fight when standing in line or in crowds.
____ 32. Avoids group games; spends most of time alone.
____ 33. Complains of clothes irritating skin; avoids wearing coat.
____ 34. Does not stay in assigned place; moves about excessively.
____ 35. Uses either hand in motor activities.
____ 36. Avoids using the left side of body.
____ 37. Cannot walk sideways on balance beam.
____ 38. Holds one shoulder lower than other.
____ 39. Cannot hold a paper in place with one hand while writing with the other.
____ 40. Avoids turning to the left whenever possible.
____ 41. Cannot assemble puzzles that offer no difficulty to peers.
____ 42. Cannot match basic geometric shapes to each other.
____ 43. Cannot recognize letters and numbers.
____ 44. Cannot differentiate background from foreground in a picture.
____ 45. Cannot identify hidden figures in a picture.
____ 46. Cannot catch balls.

FIGURE 19-5

Sherrill Perceptual-Motor Screening Checklist. (Adapted from Sherrill, C.: Adapted Physical Activity. 6th ed. New York, McGraw-Hill, 1999.)

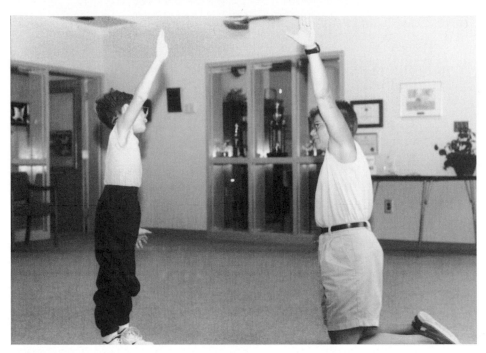

FIGURE 19-6

A young boy mirrors the arm position demonstrated by the test administrator. (Photo by Dr. Sue Combs, Department of Health, Physical Education, and Recreation, University of North Carolina at Wilmington.)

Reliability

Test-retest reliability has been reported in several studies. Seaman and DePauw (6) reported a reliability coefficient of .95 on 30 children, and Sherrill (2) reported test-retest coefficients ranging between .35 and .75 for specific subskills.

Source

The Purdue Perceptual-Motor Survey is available from Charles E. Merrill Publishing, 1300 Alum Creek Drive, Columbus, OH 43216.

Comments

Instructions for administration are very clear, but the examiner should practice administering the test to develop consistency in scoring. Data may contain red flags that suggest additional testing to verify whether certain perceptual-motor abilities are lacking. Test items are useful in detecting problems in neuromuscular differentiation that deal with laterality, body image, motor control, and rhythm.

Tests for Diagnosis and Placement

A second major purpose of assessment is to identify the present level of performance by gathering diagnostic information. **Diagnosis** is a comprehensive process that identifies strengths and weaknesses of the person to determine appropriate placement and intervention. Because of the comprehensive nature of assessment for

PURDUE PERCEPTUAL-MOTOR SURVEY
BALANCE AND POSTURAL FLEXIBILITY

1. Walking Board

Forward

Steps off board	_____	Comments
Pauses frequently	_____	
Uses one side of body more consistently than other	_____	
Avoids Balance:		
Runs	_____	
Long steps	_____	
Feet crosswise of board	_____	
Maintains inflexible posture	_____	Score _____

Backward

Steps off board	_____	Comments
Pauses frequently	_____	
Uses one side of body more consistently than other	_____	
Avoids Balance:		
Runs		
Long steps	_____	
Feet crosswise of board	_____	
Twists body to see where he is going	_____	
Must look at feet	_____	
Maintains inflexible posture	_____	Score _____

Sidewise

Unable to shift weight from one foot to the other	_____	Comments
Confusing or hesitation in shifting weight	_____	
Crosses one foot over the other	_____	
Steps off board	_____	
Performs more easily in one direction than the other	_____	
Right lead	_____	
Left lead	_____	Score _____

2. Jumping

Both feet

Cannot keep both feet together	_____	Comments
Uses one side of body only	_____	
"Ties" one side of body to the other	_____	Score _____

One foot

Postural shift not smooth	_____	Comments
Cannot keep opposite foot off the floor	_____	
Performance better on one foot than other		
Right	_____	
Left	_____	Score _____

Skip

Movement not free	_____	Comments
Hesitates after each step to determine which side	_____	
to use	_____	Score _____

Hop

Cannot remain in one spot while performing	_____	Comments
Cannot shift easily from side to side	_____	
Movements jerky and lack rhythm		
All patterns	_____	
Asymmetrical patterns only	_____	Score _____

FIGURE 19-7

Score sheet for Balance and Postural Flexibility from the Purdue Perceptual-Motor Survey. (Adapted from Roach, E., and Kephart, N.: The Purdue Perceptual-Motor Survey. Columbus, OH, Charles E. Merrill, 1966.)

PURDUE PERCEPTUAL-MOTOR SURVEY
BODY IMAGE AND DIFFERENTIATION

3. Identification of Body Parts

Show hesitancy in one or more responses	_____	Comments
Does not touch both member of paired parts	_____	
Must "feel around" to find parts	_____	
Makes more than one error in identification	_____	Score _____

4. Imitation of Movement

Does not mirror the patterns	_____	Comments
Not consistent (sometimes mirror, sometimes parallel)	_____	
Shows hesitation or lack of certainty	_____	
Makes abortive movements	_____	
Moves wrong limb	_____	
Does not recognize errors spontaneously	_____	
Recognizes errors after some delay	_____	Score _____

5. Obstacle Course

Going Over

Overestimates (steps too high)	_____	Comments
Catches foot on bar	_____	
Cannot correct on one repetition	_____	Score _____

Going Under

Knocks bar off	_____	Comments
Bends too low to clear bar	_____	
Cannot correct on one repetition	_____	Score _____

Going Between

Does not turn body	_____	Comments	Score _____

6. Kraus-Weber

Cannot raise chest and hold	_____	Comments
Cannot raise legs and hold	_____	Score _____

7. Angels-In-The-Snow

Must look from one limb to the other to identify	_____	Comments
Cannot identify by visual data alone	_____	
Requires tactual information to identify limbs	_____	
Taps or moves limbs on floor to identify	_____	
Abortive movements to get started	_____	
Hesitation at beginning of movement	_____	
Movements are hesitant and jerky	_____	
Overflow into other limbs than those called for	_____	
Movements do not reach maximum extension	_____	
Requests repetition of instructions	_____	
Cannot correct response on one repetition	_____	Score _____

FIGURE 19-8

Score sheet for Body Image and Differentiation from the Purdue Perceptual-Motor Survey. (Adapted from Roach, E., and Kephart, N.: The Purdue Perceptual-Motor Survey. Columbus, OH, Charles E. Merrill, 1966.)

diagnosis and placement, more than one test should be used to pinpoint specific strengths and weaknesses. Pinpointing specific performances reveals the level of performance and directly influences the setting of priorities for skills to be taught. Annual instructional goals and objectives can be developed from the data, and periodic review of these goals and objectives provides additional information about the appropriate placement of the student.

> Diagnosis is a comprehensive process that identifies strengths and weaknesses of the person to determine appropriate placement and intervention.

Various types of tests fall within this category of assessment. The Test of Gross Motor Development (TGMD) is a popular criterion-referenced test that provides valuable information about a student's level of gross motor performance (7). Collected data from this test lead to development of short-term behavioral objectives. The Physical Fitness Testing for the Disabled: Project UNIQUE and the newer test, the Brockport Physical Fitness Test, also assess level of performance (i.e., physical fitness), which in turn can provide valuable data for use in developing appropriate programs for the special-needs person (8, 9).

Test of Gross Motor Development (7)

Purpose
The TGMD, which qualitatively measures locomotor and object control gross motor skills, is designed for children aged 3 to 10 who appear to be delayed in certain areas of motor development.

Description
The TGMD assesses performance on 12 motor skills. The locomotor skills subtest includes running, galloping, hopping, leaping, horizontal jumping, skipping, and sliding. The object control skills subtest assesses two-handed striking, stationary bouncing, catching, kicking, and overhand throwing.

Scoring
Each skill has three or four stated performance criteria, and one point is awarded for each criterion met. There are 26 possible points for the locomotor skills subtest and 19 possible points for the object control skills subtest. The higher the score, the better the performance. Tables 19-1 and 19-2 present the score sheets for the locomotor skills subtest and the object control skills subtest respectively.

Validity
Content validity was established by having three content experts verify that the gross motor skills selected for the TGMD were skills that are frequently taught to children. Construct validity was established by (*a*) demonstrating that gross motor development improved significantly across age levels, and (*b*) demonstrating that children with mental disabilities scored lower than normal peers of similar ages (10, 11).

(text continues on page 634)

TABLE 19-1 **Test of Gross Motor Development Score Sheet for Locomotor Skills**

LOCOMOTOR SKILL	EQUIPMENT	DIRECTIONS	PERFORMANCE CRITERIA	FIRST	SECOND
Run	50 feet of clear space, masking tape, chalk, or other marking device	Mark two lines 50 feet apart Tell student to run fast from one line to the other Repeat for three trials	1. Brief period where both feet are off the ground 2. Arms in opposition to legs, elbows bent 3. Foot placement near or on a line (not flat footed) 4. Nonsupport leg bent approximately 90° (close to buttocks)		
Gallop	At least 30 feet of clear space, masking tape, chalk, or other marking device	Mark two lines 30 feet apart Tell student to gallop from one line to the other 3 times, leading with one foot and then the other	1. A step forward with lead foot followed by a step with trailing foot to a position adjacent to or behind the lead foot 2. Brief period when both feet are off the ground 3. Arms bent and lifted to waist level 4. Able to lead with right and left foot		
Hop	At least 15 feet of clear space	Tell student to hop three times, first on one foot and then on the other	1. Foot of nonsupport leg bent and carried behind the body 2. Nonsupport leg swings in pendular fashion to produce force 3. Arms bent, swing forward on takeoff 4. Able to hop on right and left foot		

LOCOMOTOR SKILL	EQUIPMENT	DIRECTIONS	PERFORMANCE CRITERIA	FIRST	SECOND
Leap	A minimum of 30 feet of clear space	Tell student to leap, taking large steps, from one foot to the other	1. Take off on one foot and land on opposite foot 2. A period when both feet are off the ground (longer than running) 3. Forward reach with arm opposite the lead foot		
Horizontal jump	10 feet of clear space, tape or other marking device	Mark a starting line Have the student start behind the line Tell student to jump far	1. Preparatory movement includes flexion of both knees with arms extended behind the body 2. Arms extended forcefully forward and up, reaching full extension above head 3. Take off and land on both feet simultaneously 4. Arms brought down during landing		
Skip	At least 30 feet of clear space, marking device	Mark two lines 30 feet apart Tell student to skip from one line to the other 3 times facing same direction	1. A rhythmical repetition of the step-hop on alternate feet 2. Foot of nonsupport leg carried near surface during hop 3. Arms moving in opposition to legs at waist level		
Slide	At least 30 feet of clear space, masking tape or other marking device	Mark two lines 30 feet apart Tell student to slide from one line to the other 3 times facing same direction	1. Body turned sideways to desired direction of travel 2. A step sideways followed by a slide of the trailing foot to a point next to the lead foot 3. A short period when both feet are off the floor 4. Able to slide to right and left		

LOCOMOTOR SKILL SUBTEST SCORE

TABLE 19-2 Test of Gross Motor Development Score Sheet for Object Control Skills

OBJECT CONTROL SKILL	EQUIPMENT	DIRECTIONS	PERFORMANCE CRITERIA	FIRST	SECOND
Two-hand strike	4–6-inch ball and plastic bat	Toss ball to student's waist Tell student to hit ball hard Only count tosses between student's waist and shoulders	1. Dominant hand grips above nondominant 2. Nondominant side faces tosser, feet parallel 3. Hip and spine rotate 4. Weight is transferred by stepping with front foot		
Stationary bounce	8–10-inch playground ball	Tell student to bounce ball 3 times using 1 hand Repeat for 3 trials	1. Contact ball with 1 hand hip height 2. Push ball with fingers (no slapping) 3. Ball contacts floor in front of foot on side of hand being used		
Catch	6–8 inch sponge ball, 15 feet of clear space, masking tape	Mark two lines 15 feet apart Student stands on one line; tosser stands on the other Ball is tossed underhand with a slight arc; student is told to catch with hands	1. In preparation phase elbows flexed and hands in front of body 2. Arms extend to contact ball 3. Ball is caught and controlled by hands 4. Elbows bend to absorb force		

OBJECT CONTROL SKILL	EQUIPMENT	DIRECTIONS	PERFORMANCE CRITERIA	FIRST	SECOND
Kick	8-10-inch plastic or slightly deflated ball, 30 feet clear space, masking tape	Place ball on line marked 20 feet from wall Student stands on line marked 30 feet from wall Tell student to kick ball hard toward wall	1. Rapid continuous approach to ball 2. Trunk inclined backward during ball contact 3. Forward swing of arm opposite kicking leg 4. Follow-through by hopping on nonkicking foot		
Overhand throw	Tennis ball, a wall, 25 feet of clear space	Tell student to throw ball hard at the wall	1. Downward arc of throwing arm initiates windup 2. Rotation of hip and shoulder so nondominant side faces wall 3. Weight transferred by stepping with foot opposite throwing hand 4. Follow-through beyond ball release diagonally across body toward side opposite throwing arm		
			OBJECT CONTROL SKILLS SUBTEST SCORE		

Reliability

Test-retest reliability coefficients for the 12 gross motor skills ranged from .84 to .99. Interscorer reliability estimates for the skills ranged from .79 to .98 for 10 raters (12).

Source

The TGMD is available from Pro-Ed, 5341 Industrial Oaks Blvd., Austin, TX.

Comments

The TGMD provides a detailed description of performance criteria for each skill. The score sheet offers a quick reference to the specific level of performance and may assist in developing appropriate programs if particular delays are found. The score sheet also provides directions for test administration, which ensures standardization in data collection.

The Physical Fitness Testing for the Disabled: Project Unique (8)

Purpose

The purpose of this test is to measure the body composition, flexibility, cardiorespiratory endurance, and muscular strength and endurance of students 10 to 17 years of age who have sensory (visual and hearing), orthopaedic (e.g., cerebral palsy, spinal cord), and developmental disabilities.

Description

The Project Unique Physical Fitness Test includes seven items that measure health-related or performance-related physical fitness. The fitness items assessed are skinfold, grip strength, 50-meter dash, number of sit-ups completed in 60 seconds, softball throw for distance, standing broad jump, sit and reach, and a long-distance run.

Scoring

Items are scored by the following descriptors of performance data.

Skinfold Measurement. Three independent skinfold measurements are taken at the triceps and subscapular sites. Measurements are recorded to the nearest millimeter; the three measurements are averaged for each site. The final score is the sum of the average skinfold for each of the two sites.

Grip Strength. With the subject seated in a straight-back chair, three trials for each hand on a hand-grip dynamometer are recorded to the nearest kilogram. The three trial scores are averaged, then summed to obtain a final grip score.

50-Meter Dash. Time is recorded in seconds for either 50 meters or 50 yards.

Sit-ups. The score is the number of bent-knee sit-ups, hands placed across chest, completed in 60 seconds.

Softball Throw. The throw is measured in feet and inches where the ball first lands. The average of three trials is recorded.

Standing Broad Jump. The distance jumped is recorded to the nearest inch. The average of three trials is recorded.

Flexibility. Using a sit-and-reach board, the distance reached is measured in centimeters. The average of two trials is recorded.

Long Run. The score is either (*a*) the time is takes to complete the prescribed distance (1 mile for 10- to 12-year-olds, 1.5 miles for 13- to 17-year-olds), or (*b*) the distance traveled in 9 minutes (for the younger group) or 12 minutes (for the older group). A yards-per-minute score is calculated for runners who do not cover the required distance. This is accomplished by dividing the distance covered in yards by either 9 minutes or 12 minutes.

Validity
The fitness battery has reported criterion and construct validity ranging from .53 to .95.

Reliability
Reliability coefficients for most test items for are reported in the .90s.

Comments
Several of the test items are similar to those used in the Prudential FITNESSGRAM, which emphasizes the importance of health-related fitness for everyone. The test offers adaptations for various test items depending on type and severity of disability. For example, guide wires can be used for the running tests for those with visual disabilities. Age, gender, and disability are considered when interpreting the results. Extensive research on each test item provides valid and reliable normative data. While fitness tests are limited in scope for use in placement decisions, the information they provide can be useful in evaluating the effectiveness of program instruction.

Tests for Instruction and Student Progress

Often assessment is conducted as pretest and posttest measurements of a student's skill development. Instead, assessment should be considered an ongoing process. Not only students' progress but effectiveness of instruction, which has paramount importance, could be measured. Assessment can provide a periodic review determining whether progress or behavioral change is occurring. Systematic analysis of students' progress also produces analysis and evaluation of the instructional process. Students' lack of progress is often due to inappropriate or ineffective teaching. The teacher's neglect to break down a skill into smaller steps, inconsistent prompting and reinforcing, and limited practice time are practices that may hinder learning. Integration of assessment, teaching, and learning is a very powerful instructional strategy.

Data-based assessment is especially important for providing appropriate educational programs for those with severe disabilities. Several tests for the severely disabled have built-in teaching and evaluation strategies. Two reviewed here are the OSU (Ohio State University) Data-Based Gymnasium Model and the Project TRANSITION Model (13–15).

OSU Data-Based Gymnasium Model (13)

Purpose
The purpose of this test is to use an ecological, data-based method of assessment to determine levels of performance of severely handicapped persons.

Description

The OSU Data-Based Gymnasium Model is a systematic assessment and curriculum tool developed for severely handicapped school-age students. It is a comprehensive guide that measures level of performance through behavior management. Assessment determines students' abilities related to movement concepts, skills found in elementary games, physical fitness skills essential for survival, and skills used in lifetime leisure pursuits. Task analysis, applied to all of the skills in the four areas, provides the teacher with terminal objectives, prerequisite skills, progressively arranged phases of the skills, and additional teaching ideas and materials. Both the assessment and teaching emphasize a systematic approach to cueing, reinforcing (reinforcers and punishers), shaping, fading, and chaining. This model is individualized and seeks to offer age-appropriate functional activities.

Scoring

Scoring is a comprehensive system that uses a clipboard concept. It includes the following:

- Weekly cover sheets that specify three to four motor programs to be practiced daily
- Language and consequence file sheets that list students' reinforcers
- Placement forms that list tasks with specific cueing and recommended trials for each task
- Motor skill sequence sheets that offer task analyses for terminal objectives of specific skills (Fig. 19-9)
- Program cover sheets that include summative information on items such as prompting, verbal cueing strategies, materials needed, and correction protocol (Fig. 19-10)
- Program data sheets with spaces to record correct and incorrect performance for 10 trials on each phase and step of a motor skill sequence (Fig. 19-11)
- Maintenance files for summative information on skills already learned

Validity

Validity of this test is not reported.

Reliability

Reliability of this test is not reported.

Source

This test is available from Pro-Ed, 5341 Industrial Oaks Blvd., Austin TX.

Comments

While the comprehensiveness of this model may be somewhat overwhelming at first to service providers who do not specialize in working with the severely disabled, the OSU Data-Based Gymnasium Model is an excellent tool for understanding the application of behavior management strategies in the psychomotor educational arena. The model provides instruction for teachers on topics such as gymnasium management, recording students' progress, training volunteers, and facilitating parents' involvement.

BASIC GAMES SKILLS

A. Underhand Roll

Terminal Objective: Student, from a standing position, will perform an underhand roll by swinging the arm backward and then forward, stepping forward with the opposite foot and releasing the ball at the end of the swing in the direction of the target.

Prerequisite Skills: Gross motor, DD; fine motor skills, A and G.

Phase I	Sitting in a chair, swing arm backward and then forward, releasing ball.
Phase II	Standing with knees bent, swing arm backward and then forward, releasing ball.
Phase III	Standing with one foot forward and one foot back, knees bent, swing arm backward then forward, releasing ball.
Phase IV	Standing with knees bent, swing arm backward and then forward, releasing ball while stepping forward with the opposite foot.

Teaching Notes:

1. For students in wheelchairs, the underhand roll can be performed with the student sitting in the wheelchair, eliminating the need for the prerequisite body positions.

2. Nonambulatory students who are not in a wheelchair can be taught ball rolling in a supported sitting position.

3. When students have problems with timing the step and throw, the teacher may physically assist and/or prompt the foot during the throw.

Suggested Materials: A tennis ball and a 3-foot × 3-foot target placed on the floor. Any type of ball may be used to facilitate learning.

FIGURE 19-9

Instructional progression for underhand roll from OSU Data-Based Gymnasium Model. (Adapted from Dunn, J.M., and Fait, H.F.: Special Physical Education: Adapted, Individualized, Developmental. 7th ed. Madison, WI, Brown & Benchmark, 1996.)

Project Transition Model (14, 15)

Purpose

The purpose of this test is qualitative and quantitative assessment of fitness and hygiene skills of those with severe disabilities.

Description

The Project Transition model tests five skills in fitness (upper body strength, cardiorespiratory endurance, abdominal strength, trunk flexibility, and grip

Pupil: John Q.	**Program:** Games skills, basic
Date started: October 3	A. Underhand roll
Date completed:	

Setting (nonverbal cue):	
Establish eye contact with John before delivering the cue.	**Materials:** Clipboard Pencil Chair Ball 3-foot × 3-foot target

Instructional process:	**Criterion:**
Verbal cue model	Three consecutive responses before
"John, roll the ball underhand."	moving to the next phase
Demonstrate if the response to the	
verbal cue is incorrect.	
Physical assistance	
Provide assistance if the response to	
the verbal cue and demonstration	
is incorrect.	

FIGURE 19-10

Example of a program cover sheet from the OSU Data-Based Gymnasium Model. (Adapted from Dunn, J.M., and Fait, H.F.: Special Physical Education: Adapted, Individualized, Developmental. 7th ed. Madison, WI, Brown & Benchmark, 1996.)

strength) and five skills in hygiene (face washing, teeth brushing, hand washing, deodorant use, and overall appearance). The tests are embedded in the curriculum, which means they offer strategies for teaching the skills based on the assessment.

Scoring

Test items have been task-analyzed, and scores yield qualitative data about the level of independence and quantitative data about the actual performance. The qualitative data yield two separate scores that assess the person's ability to complete a target skill independently. One score indicates the percent of the total number of steps a person can complete with only a verbal prompt. The second qualitative score is a single percentage score based on a total number of points acquired through the number of prompting steps (levels of independence) needed to perform the skill (Figs. 19-12 to 19-16).

Validity

The validity of this test is not reported.

Reliability

The reliability of this test is not reported

Comments

The test items are limited and some unique equipment is necessary, but the criteria performances are clear, with detailed task analyses. The strength of the model

(text continues on page 645)

Name: _John Q._   **Program:** _Underhand Roll_   _Underhand Roll_

X = correct   O = incorrect

Reinforcer	Phase	Step	Trials										Comments	Date
Social	I		O	O	X	X	X	O	O	X			Has trouble attending	3/8
Social	I		O	O	X	X	X	X	X				Seems to have the idea	3/9
Social	II		O	X	O	X	X	O	X	X	X		Needs help with backward swing	3/10
Social	II		X	O	X	X	X						Good day	3/11
Social	III		O	O	X	X	X	X	X	X			Has the idea	3/12
Social	IV		O	X	O	O	O	X	O	X	O		Has difficulty with step	3/15
Social	IV		X	O	X	X	X	X	O					3/15
Maintenance														

FIGURE 19-11

Program data sheet from the OSU Data-Based Gymnasium Model. (Adapted from Dunn, J.M., and Fait, H.F.: Special Physical Education: Adapted, Individualized, Developmental. 7th ed. Madison, WI, Brown & Benchmark, 1996.)

UPPER BODY STRENGTH/ENDURANCE

LEVELS OF INDEPENDENCE

NAME _____
DATE _____
SCORER _____
TEST _____

Abbreviated Curriculum Steps

STEPS	UO (0)	HI PHY+ (1)	MIN PHY+ (2)	HI V/M (3)	MIN V (4)	IND (5)	TOTAL INDEPENDENCE
1.1 Sit on mats	1.1							
1.2 Supine position	1.2							
1.3 Bar over mid-sternum	1.3							
2.1 One hand grasp	2.1							
2.2 Two hand grasp	2.2							
2.3 Lift	2.3							
2.4 Return	2.4							
3.1 Lift x 2	3.1							
3.2 Lift x 4	3.2							
3.3 Lift x 6	3.3							
3.4 Lift x 8	3.4							
Subtotals								

Scoring Key

Unobserved Will not attempt (0 points)

High Physical+ Constant physical prompt, in addition to verbal prompting w/modeling (1 point)

Minimal Physical+ Physical to initiate, in addition to verbal w/modeling (2 points)

High Verbal/Modeling Verbal and modeling (3 points)

Minimal Verbal Verbal direction throughout steps (4 points)

Independence Verbal direction to initiate (5 points)

- -

Total Independence Self initiation of skill, *not* to be considered in scoring.

___ *% Task Score* $\left(\dfrac{\text{\# Steps Ind.}}{11} \right) \times 100$

___ *Ave. Ind. Score* $\left(\dfrac{Sum\ Points}{55} \right) \times 100$

___ Performance Score

Observations: _____
_____
Reinforcer: _____
_____
Reinforcement Schedule: _____
_____

FIGURE 19-12

Score sheet for upper body strength and endurance from Project TRANSITION.

CARDIORESPIRATORY ENDURANCE

NAME _____
DATE _____
SCORER _____
TEST _____

Abbreviated Curriculum Steps

1.1 Run/walk 50 yards

1.2 Run/walk 100 yards

2.1 Run/walk 150 yards

2.2 Run/walk 200 yards

3.1 Run/walk 250 yards

3.2 Run/walk 300 yards

STEPS	UO (0)	HI PHY+ (1)	MIN PHY+ (2)	HI V/M (3)	MIN V (4)	IND (5)	TOTAL INDEPENDENCE
1.1							
1.2							
2.1							
2.2							
3.1							
3.2							
Subtotals							

LEVELS OF INDEPENDENCE

Scoring Key

Unobserved Will not attempt (0 points)

High Physical+ Constant physical prompt, in addition to verbal prompting w/modeling (1 point)

Minimal Physical+ Physical to initiate, in addition to verbal w/modeling (2 points)

High Verbal/Modeling Verbal and modeling (3 points)

Minimal Verbal Verbal direction throughout steps (4 points)

Independence Verbal direction to initiate (5 points)

- -

Total Independence Self initiation of skill, *not* to be considered in scoring.

____ *% Task Score* $\left(\dfrac{\text{\# Steps Ind.}}{6} \right) \times 100$

____ *Ave. Ind. Score* $\left(\dfrac{Sum\ Points}{30} \right) \times 100$

____ Performance Score

Observations: _____
_____

Reinforcer: _____
_____

Reinforcement Schedule: _____
_____

FIGURE 19-13

Score sheet for cardiorespiratory endurance from Project TRANSITION.

ABDOMINAL ENDURANCE

LEVELS OF INDEPENDENCE

NAME _____

DATE _____

SCORER _____

TEST _____

Abbreviated Curriculum Steps

1.1 Sit on mat

1.2 Sit, knees flexed, feet 12-18"

1.3 Arms extended

1.4 Negative to supine

2.1 Head, shoulders up

2.2 Trunk up

2.3 Sit-up complete

3.1 Cross arms over chest

3.2 Negative to supine

3.3 Head, shoulders up

3.4 Trunk up

3.5 Sit-up complete (30 sec)

3.6 Sit-up complete (45 sec)

3.7 Sit-up complete (60 sec)

STEPS	UO (0)	HI PHY+ (1)	MIN PHY+ (2)	HI V/M (3)	MIN V (4)	IND (5)	TOTAL INDEPENDENCE
1.1							
1.2							
1.3							
1.4							
2.1							
2.2							
2.3							
3.1							
3.2							
3.3							
3.4							
3.5							
3.6							
3.7							
Subtotals							

Scoring Key

Unobserved Will not attempt (0 points)

High Physical+ Constant physical prompt, in addition to verbal prompting w/modeling (1 point)

Minimal Physical+ Physical to initiate, in addition to verbal w/modeling (2 points)

High Verbal/Modeling Verbal and modeling (3 points)

Minimal Verbal Verbal direction throughout steps (4 points)

Independence Verbal direction to initiate (5 points)

- -

Total Independence Self initiation of skill, *not* to be considered in scoring.

____ % Task Score $\left(\dfrac{\# \ Steps \ Ind.}{14} \right) \times 100$

____ Ave. Ind. Score $\left(\dfrac{Sum \ Points}{70} \right) \times 100$

____ Performance Score

Observations: _____

_____

Reinforcer: _____

_____

Reinforcement Schedule: _____

_____

FIGURE 19-14

Score sheet for abdominal endurance from Project TRANSITION.

FLEXIBILITY

LEVELS OF INDEPENDENCE

NAME _____
DATE _____
SCORER _____
TEST _____

Abbreviated Curriculum Steps	STEPS	UO (0)	HI PHY+ (1)	MIN PHY+ (2)	HI V/M (3)	MIN V (4)	IND (5)	TOTAL INDEPENDENCE
1.1 Sit, legs straight, arms support	1.1							
1.2 Sit, feet against box	1.2							
2.1 Sit, feet against box, no arm support	2.1							
2.2 Shoulders forward	2.2							
2.3 Back rounded	2.3							
2.4 Hands on knees	2.4							
3.1 Arms extended, one hand on box	3.1							
3.2 Two hands on box (knee check)	3.2							
4.1 Hands overlapped, maximum reach (knee check)	4.1							
Subtotals								

Scoring Key
Unobserved Will not attempt (0 points)
High Physical+ Constant physical prompt, in addition to verbal prompting w/modeling (1 point)
Minimal Physical+ Physical to initiate, in addition to verbal w/modeling (2 points)
High Verbal/Modeling Verbal and modeling (3 points)
Minimal Verbal Verbal direction throughout steps (4 points)
Independence Verbal direction to initiate (5 points)

- -

Total Independence Self initiation of skill, *not* to be considered in scoring.

___ % Task Score $\left(\dfrac{\# \; Steps \; Ind.}{9} \right) \times 100$

___ Ave. Ind. Score $\left(\dfrac{Sum \; Points}{45} \right) \times 100$

___ Performance Score

Observations: _____
_____
Reinforcer: _____
_____
Reinforcement Schedule: _____
_____

FIGURE 19-15

Score sheet for flexibility from Project TRANSITION.

GRIP STRENGTH

LEVELS OF INDEPENDENCE

NAME _____
DATE _____
SCORER _____
TEST _____

Abbreviated Curriculum Steps

	STEPS	UO (0)	HI PHY+ (1)	MIN PHY+ (2)	HI V/M (3)	MIN V (4)	IND (5)	TOTAL INDEPENDENCE
1.1 Palm up	1.1							
1.2 Open palm	1.2							
1.3 Bulb in palm	1.3							
1.4 Close fingers	1.4							
1.5 Maximum contraction	1.5							
1.6 Repeat maximum contraction	1.6							
2.1 Palm up	2.1							
2.2 Open palm	2.2							
2.3 Bulb in palm	2.3							
2.4 Close fingers	2.4							
2.5 Maximum contraction	2.5							
2.6 Repeat maximum contraction	2.6							
Subtotals								

Scoring Key

Unobserved Will not attempt
  (0 points)
High Physical+ Constant physical
  prompt, in addition to verbal
  prompting w/modeling (1 point)
Minimal Physical+ Physical to initiate, in addition to verbal
  w/modeling (2 points)
High Verbal/Modeling Verbal and
  modeling (3 points)
Minimal Verbal Verbal direction
  throughout steps (4 points)
Independence Verbal direction to
  initiate (5 points)
- -
Total Independence Self initiation
  of skill, *not* to be considered in
  scoring.

____ % Task Score $\left(\dfrac{\text{# Steps Ind.}}{12} \right) \times 100$

____ Ave. Ind. Score $\left(\dfrac{\text{Sum Points}}{60} \right) \times 100$

____ Performance Score

Observations: _____
_____
Reinforcer: _____
_____
Reinforcement Schedule: _____
_____

FIGURE 19-16

Score sheet for grip strength from Project TRANSITION.

is the use of qualitative as well as quantitative assessments, which yield individualized data. Understanding the use of prompting levels when working with those with severe developmental delays can be a very valuable strategy, useful in developing a behavior management approach.

Tests for Sport and Activity Classification

Passage of federal legislation has brought about an emphasis on sport participation as well as physical education services for individuals with disabilities. Perhaps the most relevant law passed was PL 95-606, The Amateur Sports Act of 1978. One of the purposes of the legislation was to provide assistance to amateur athletic programs in offering meaningful participation for all individuals regardless of ability or disability. A major outcome of the law was to encourage meaningful and equitable competition. Classification systems have historically been used in sports for the nondisabled to promote equity in competition. It therefore stands to reason that classification systems for sport participants with disabilities is also necessary.

Sport and activity classification is used to provide equal competition by assigning individuals to a disability classification based on their medical or functional capacity (2). While there is some controversy as to the more equitable method of classification, it is important to understand the purpose each method serves. The medical classification system assigns individuals to competition based on their medical diagnoses. The functional classification system is modeled after sport competition systems for the nondisabled by matching competitors based on their sport performances. In other words, disabled persons are assessed on what they can or cannot do relevant to the requirements of the sport skills, then placed appropriately.

Most medical conditions have a primary sport organization that implements a classification system. Two sport organization medical classification systems are described here. They are the National Wheelchair Athletic Association (NWAA) medical classification and the United States Association for Blind Athletes (USABA) medical classification (16). The Strohkendl Basketball Function Test, a functional classification system, is also described (17).

What Do YOU Think?

Integration is often promoted as a strategy to eradicate injustices against minority groups based on race, gender, or other types of human differences. In wheelchair sports competitions, consensus about the effectiveness of this strategy has not been reached. In *Are We Winning Yet?* author Mariah Burton Nelson tells the story of a disabled swimmer who competed in the 1988 Paralympics in the Netherlands. The swimmer, like the handful of track athletes who now compete in the regular Olympics, stated that she felt like a real Olympian. Nelson poses the following question: "If integration becomes the goal, how many of the 4000 people who competed in the 1988 Paralympics will be invited to the Olympics—a festival already bursting at the seams from its unwieldy size? Would integration yield fewer opportunities?" (18). What do YOU think?

National Wheelchair Athletic Association Medical Classification (16)

Purpose

The purpose of this battery is to classify a person to a particular sport class as determined by the region of the spinal cord that has been injured.

Description

There are seven classifications for competition based on site of spinal cord injury, which correlates with functional ability. Members of classes IA, IB, and IC are those whose spinal cord injuries in the cervical region result in quadriplegia. The remaining classes, II through V or VI are for those whose injuries to the thoracic or lumbar region result in paraplegia.

Scoring

Figure 19-17 has descriptions of classifications.

Comments

This classification system does not address those whose degree of functioning differs from one side to the other, which precludes a true classification. It does, however, permit individuals with severe involvement to compete safely and under as normal and equitable conditions as possible. The increased interest in sport participation for persons in wheelchairs enhances the importance of providing fair competition.

United States Association for Blind Athletes Medical Classification (16)

Purpose

The purpose of this test is to classify a person to a particular sport class based on degree of visual acuity.

Description

Three levels of classification for competition include B1, for persons who are totally blind; B2, for those who can perceive hand shapes but whose visual acuity is less than 20/600; and B3 for those whose visual acuity is less than 20/200 but more than 20/600.

Scoring

Figure 19-18 describes sport classifications for blind athletes.

Comments

The development of this classification system has significantly increased both numbers participating and numbers of sanctioned sports for those with visual disorders. This is a very useful system for equalizing competition.

The Strohkendl Basketball Function Test (2, 17)

Purpose

The purpose of this test is to classify a person for basketball competition based on test performance of skills relevant to success in basketball.

Competitors Are Classified as Follows in Agreement With These Guidelines

Class 1A
All cervical lesions with complete or incomplete quadriplegia that have involvement of both hands, weakness of triceps (up to and including grade 3 on testing scale) and with severe weakness of the trunk and lower extremities interfering significantly with trunk balance and ability to walk.

Class 1B
All cervical lesions with complete or incomplete quadriplegia that have involvement of upper extremities but less than 1A with preservation of normal or good triceps (4 or 5 on testing scale) and with a generalized weakness of the trunk and lower extremities interfering significantly with trunk balance and the ability to walk.

Class 1C
All cervical lesions with complete or incomplete quadriplegia who have involvement of upper extremities but less than 1B with preservation of normal or good triceps (4 or 5 testing scale) and normal or good finger flexion and extension (grasp and release) but without intrinsic hand function and with a generalized weakness of the trunk and lower extremities interfering significantly with trunk balance and the ability to walk.

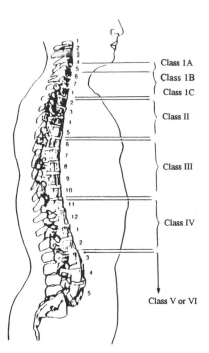

Class II
Complete or incomplete paraplegia below T1 down to and including T5 or comparable disability with total abdominal paralysis or poor abdominal muscle strength (0–2 on testing scale) and no useful trunk sitting balance.

Class III
Complete or incomplete paraplegia or comparable disability below T5 down to and including T10 with upper abdominal and signal extensor musculature sufficient to provide some element of trunk sitting balance but not normal.

Class IV
Complete or incomplete paraplegia or comparable disability below T10 down to and including L2 without quadriceps or very weak quadriceps with a value up to and including 2 on the testing scale and gluteal paralysis.

Class V
Complete or incomplete paraplegia or comparable disability below L2 with quadriceps in grades 3–5.

For Swimming Events Only

Class VI
Complete or incomplete paraplegia or comparable disability below L2.

Amputees

Unilateral amputee	Class VI	
Bilateral above knee	Class IV	Amputations above level of lesser trochanter
Bilateral above knee	Class V	Amputations below level of lesser trochanter
Above knee/below knee	Class V	
Bilateral below knee	Class VI	

FIGURE 19-17

National Wheelchair Athletic Association Medical Classification. (Adapted from Dunn, J.M., and Fait, H.F.: Special Physical Education: Adapted, Individualized, Developmental. 7th ed. Madison, WI, Brown & Benchmark, 1996.)

Classification	Description
B1	Totally blind, may possess light perception but unable to recognize hand shapes at any distance.
B2	Perceives hand shapes but visual acuity not better than 20/600 and/or less than 5° in visual field
B3	Visual acuity from 20/200 to 20/599 and/or more than 5° to 20° visual field.

FIGURE 19-18

United States Association for Blind Athletes Medical Classification. (Adapted from Dunn, J.M., and Fait, H.F.: Special Physical Education: Adapted, Individualized, Developmental. 7th ed. Madison, WI, Brown & Benchmark, 1996.)

Description

Three skills are measured for classifying individuals for wheelchair basketball competitions. These include sitting stability and rotation of trunk, forward and backward bending (flexion and extension) of trunk, and lateral flexion of trunk. Each skill has precise instructions and performance criteria that determine a pass or fail resulting in a classification.

Scoring

Figure 19-19 describes the standardization for assessing sitting stability and rotation of trunk. For assessment and standardization information for forward and backward bending and for lateral flexion of trunk, see *Adapted Physical Activity*, by Claudine Sherrill (2).

Comments

Horst Strohkendl has developed a useful functional assessment system in basketball for those who are in wheelchairs. This sport-specific functional system has most recently become the favored method of classifying sport participants who are physically disabled. The amount of training required to become competent in classifying athletes may limit the practitioner; however, the Strohkendl system provides an excellent means of describing level of performance and has the potential to be applied to other sports and other types of disabilities.

Concluding Thoughts

Practitioners in physical education, sports medicine, and sport management who offer programs for special-needs populations must take into consideration the following two facts. First, assessment results used alone seldom, if ever, provide complete answers or real understanding of individuals' problems, deficiencies, and weaknesses. The ingredients for making valid judgments about individual needs include observation, understanding of growth and development, background knowledge about the individual, *and* results from a variety of screening tests, diagnostic and placement tests, instruction and student progress tests, and sport and activity classification tests. Second, selective and judicious use of tests is an important and integral part of good teaching, but assessment is not all there is to good teaching. As-

---

Test 1: Assessment of Sitting Stability and Rotation of the Trunk

Purpose
To differentiate between class I and class II basketball players.

Instructions
Sit as straight as possible in your chair. Bounce and catch the ball with both hands at the same time while changing the side of the chair after each try. Rotate your trunk as far as possible to each side without losing your balance or leaning back in the chair.

Test Performance
Failure of test is characterized by poor balance and/or leaning back in the chair to prevent falling when reaching for the ball. Passing of the test is characterized by no loss of balance and/or demonstration of full range of arm motion and good arm and shoulder strength.

Performance Expectations

Level of Lesion or Comparable Disability	Performance	Classification
T7 and above, CP classes 1-3	Fail	I
T8 to L2, CP classes 4-6, and bilateral hip amputees	Pass	II
L3 & below, CP classes 7-8, and lower extremity amputees	Pass	III

Functional Profile of Class I
In wheelchair with high back. Poor to nonexistent trunk control and sitting balance. Limited range of motion in arm movements; cannot raise one or both arms above head. Functional limitations in pushing and steering chair; weak, short, choppy arm pushes.

FIGURE 19-19

Strohkendl Basketball Function Test for Wheelchair Basketball Players. (Adapted from Sherrill, C.: Adapted Physical Activity. 6th ed. New York, McGraw-Hill, 1999.)

sessing simply to get results to file away is a waste of everyone's time. Assessment results should be used to improve instruction and/or programming.

Chapter Summary

Special-needs populations are composed of individuals whose physical, mental, and/or emotional characteristics interfere with their optimal development and/or performance. There are many reasons for testing those with special needs. One of the reasons is that such testing is mandated by law. PL 94-142 guarantees that appropriate, individualized educational and related services must be provided to children through proper assessment. However, not all educators agree about the best way to go about special-needs assessment. I believe tests should be focused on specific motor skills, but the tests may be either norm-referenced or criterion-referenced and may yield either product or process data. This chapter presents many tests for special-needs populations. Each test is categorized by purpose as for screening, for diagnosis and placement, for instruction and progress, or for sport and activity classification.

SELF-TEST QUESTIONS

1. Which of the following is the *least* appropriate reason for testing a special-needs child?
   A. To determine whether further testing is needed
   B. To place him or her in an appropriate learning program
   C. To identify his or her abilities as a learner
   D. To identify his or her learning limitations

2. Approximately what percent of all school-aged children have special needs?
   A. 2 to 5%
   B. 5 to 12%
   C. 12 to 15%
   D. 15 to 22%

3. Which of the following legal principles requires that school officials receive parental permission before testing a special-needs child?
   A. Confidentiality
   B. Due process
   C. Intervention
   D. Standards

4. The best test for a person with a disability is:
   A. A norm-referenced test
   B. A criterion-referenced test
   C. A test that measures the movement product
   D. A test selected for the specific person

5. Which assessment purpose pertains mostly to prescribing ecologically valid sport activity and creating systems by which abilities of competitors are equalized so each has a fair chance of winning?
   A. Instruction
   B. Diagnosis
   C. Screening
   D. Sport classification

6. Which assessment purpose uses more than one test to pinpoint specific weaknesses?
   A. Instruction
   B. Diagnosis
   C. Screening
   D. Sport classification

7. Which test has the primary purpose of screening for developmental delays in gross motor, language, fine motor-adaptive, and personal-social development?
   A. Denver II
   B. Purdue Perceptual-Motor Survey
   C. Test of Gross Motor Development
   D. None of the above

8. Which test identifies children who are significantly behind their peers in the execution of gross motor skills?
   A. AAHPERD's Physical Best
   B. Project TRANSITION Model
   C. Sherrill Perceptual-Motor Screening Checklist
   D. Test of Gross Motor Development

9. Which test has the primary purpose of assessing, qualitatively and quantitatively, fitness and hygiene skills of those with severe disabilities?
   A. AAHPERD's Physical Best
   B. Project TRANSITION Model
   C. Sherrill Perceptual-Motor Screening Checklist
   D. Test of Gross Motor Development

ANSWERS

1. D	2. C	3. B	4. D	5. D
6. B	7. A	8. D	9. B	

DOING PROJECTS FOR FURTHER LEARNING

1. Using the Project TRANSITION Model format, select a motor skill, task-analyze the skill into a minimum of six steps, and develop a score sheet that will give average independence, percent task, and performance score.

2. Using the information given below, develop a score sheet for the following test items found in the Denver II:

TEST ITEM	Age When Given Percent of Standardization Sample Passed Item			
	25%	50%	75%	90%
Walk backward	12.3 mo	13.8 mo	15.2 mo	16.6 mo
Broad jump	2.4 yr	2.7 yr	2.9 yr	3.2 yr

3. Consider the four purposes of testing and identify one additional test that you are familiar with and that you think would fall within each category. Explain your reasons for the categorization. What category of purpose do you feel is the most relevant for writing individualized education plans? For placement in a swimming program? For determining fitness?

REFERENCES

1. Hastad, D.N., and Lacy, A.C.: Measurement and Evaluation in Physical Education and Exercise Science. 3rd ed. Needham Heights, MA, Allyn & Bacon, 1998.
2. Sherrill, C.: Adapted Physical Activity. 6th ed. New York, McGraw-Hill, 1999.

3. Frankenburg, W.K., Dodds, J., and Archer, P.: Denver II Technical Manual. Denver, Denver Developmental Materials, 1990.

4. Frankenburg, W.K., et al.: The Denver II: a major revision and restandardization of the Denver Developmental Screening Test. Pediatrics, 89, 1992.

5. Roach, E., and Kephart, N.: The Purdue Perceptual-Motor Survey. Columbus, OH, Charles E. Merrill, 1966.

6. Seaman, J.A., and DePauw, K.P.: The New Adapted Physical Education: A Developmental Approach. 3rd ed. Mountain View, CA, Mayfield, 1989.

7. Ulrich, D.A. The Test of Gross Motor Development. Austin, TX, Pro-Ed, 1985.

8. Winnick, J., and Short, F.: Physical Fitness Testing of the Disabled: Project UNIQUE. Champaign, IL, Human Kinetics, 1985.

9. Winnick, J.P., and Short, F.X.: The Brockport Physical Fitness Test Manual. Champaign, IL, Human Kinetics for the American Fitness Alliance, 1999.

10. Ulrich, D.A.: The reliability of classification decisions made with the objectives-based motor skill assessment instrument. Adapted Physical Activity Quarterly, 1:52, 1984.

11. Ulrich, D.A., and Ulrich, B.D.: The objectives-based motor skill assessment instrument: validation of instructional sensitivity. Perceptual and Motor Skills, 59:175, 1984.

12. Ulrich, D.A., and Wise, S.L.: The reliability of scores obtained with the objectives-based motor skill assessment instrument. Adapted Physical Activity Quarterly, 1:230, 1984.

13. Dunn, J.M., Morehouse, J.W., and Fredericks, H.D.: Physical Education for the Severely Handicapped: A Systematic Approach to a Data-based Gymnasium. Austin, TX, Pro-Ed, 1986.

14. Jansma, P., et al.: Project TRANSITION Assessment System. Ohio State University, Adapted Physical Activity, Columbus, 1987.

15. Jansma, P., et al.: A fitness assessment system for individuals with severe mental retardation. Adapted Physical Activity Quarterly, 5:223, 1988.

16. Dunn, J.M., and Fait, H.F.: Special Physical Education: Adapted, Individualized, Developmental. 7th ed. Madison, WI, Brown & Benchmark, 1996.

17. Strohkendl, H.: The new classification system for wheelchair basketball. In C. Sherrill (ed.): Sport and Disabled Athletes. Champaign, IL, Human Kinetics, 1986.

18. Nelson, M.B.: Are We Winning Yet? How Women Are Changing Sports and Sports Are Changing Women. New York, Random House, 1991.

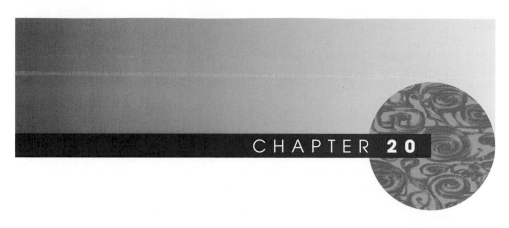

CHAPTER **20**

Assessment in Dance Education

Rayma K. Beal

Accountability is paramount in modern education. It is no longer sufficient for teachers to feel that students have learned particular intellectual and physical skills; rather, it is critical that teachers validly and reliably determine that students have indeed mastered concepts and skills. In some academic areas (e.g., mathematics and biology), learning criteria are relatively straightforward and easy to establish. In the arts, however, especially in dance, criteria for determining what is important and how to demonstrate mastery of skills are less easily established.

This chapter discusses a number of proposals to enable the dance teacher and program evaluator to assess dance learning. The assessment approaches of Ruth Murray, Mary Joyce, Maxine DeBruyn, Project Spectrum, and models from Britain and British Columbia are reviewed. Following this discussion, the U.S. National Standards for Dance are discussed. The chapter concludes with a brief discussion of several other concerns relevant to the assessment of dance.

While you are reading this chapter, pay special attention to the following keywords:

Aesthetic response	Portfolio
Elements of dance	Studio activities

Ruth Murray and Dance Education

Ruth Lovell Murray, chair of the Women's Department of Physical Education at Wayne State University for many years, was among the first to write about teacher education and dance education. Murray's primary interests were in teaching dance to children, student teachers, classroom teachers, and dance specialists. In response to requests from her graduate students during the 1950s, Murray began work on the first standards for dance performance. The result were performance standards for grades 1 and 2 (Table 20-1), grades 3 and 4, and grades 5 and 6 (1).

653

TABLE 20-1	Performance Standards for Grades 1 and 2: Basic Locomotor Movements (continues on page 655)

I. **Walk**: performing a natural walk. Students can create the following variations:
  A. In *space* pattern
   1. Changes in *direction*: In place, backward; sideways (step-together); turning around
   2. Changes in *level*: On tiptoe; with knees half bent; with knees fully bent
   3. Changes in *dimension*: Steps shorter than natural; steps longer than natural
  B. In *shape*
   1. Simple variations such as: Knees bent up high in front; body bent forward; hands on knees; arms high over head
  C. In *timing*
   1. Changes in *tempo*: Steps faster than natural; steps slower than natural
  D. In walking *with others*
   1. *With one other*: Side by side, inside hands joined, walking forward; facing, both hands joined, walking around in a small circle
   2. *With two others*: Side by side, inside hands joined, walking forward; in a circle, hands joined, walking around circle
   3. *With many others*: In a circle, hands joined, walking around circle; in a line with one child leading, hands joined, walking forward

II. **Run**: performing a natural run. Students can create the following variations:
  A. In *space* pattern
   1. Changes in direction: In place; turning around
  B. In *shape*
   1. Simple variations such as: Knees bent up high in front; arms extended forward or backward (Fig. 20–1*A*)
  C. In running *with others*
   1. *With one other*: Side by side, inside hands joined, running forward

III. **Jump**. Student can create the following variations:
  A. In *space* pattern
   1. Changes in direction: forward; turning around
   2. Changes in level: knees fully bent; knees half bent (Fig. 20-1*B*)
  B. In *shape*
   1. Simple variations such as landing with feet alternately apart and together, swinging arms out and in as feet jump apart and together

Murray's Concepts of Dance Assessment

Murray believed that after 2 years of studying dance skills, children should be able to meet the performance standards for grades 1 and 2. These young children should also be able to demonstrate rhythmic responses accurately and reliably (Fig. 20-1). Murray did not include the leap in the performance standards for grades 1 and 2 because it is so difficult to master in the first years of learning; Murray believed, however, that the leap should be taught and practiced during these grades. Similarly,

IV. Hop: performing a natural hop. Students can create the following variations:

 A. In *space* pattern

  1. Changes in direction: forward; turning around

 B. In *shape*

  1. Simple variations such as changing from one foot to the other after a certain number of hops; with arm on side of hopping foot extended sideways

V. Gallop: performing a natural gallop. Students can create the following variations:

 A. In galloping *with others*

  1. *With one other:* Side by side, inside hands joined, galloping forward; one in back of other, both facing forward, both hands joined, galloping forward

  2. *With two others:* One in front and two in back or vice versa, all facing forward, hands joined, galloping forward

VI. Slide: performing a natural slide. Students can create the following variations:

 A. In sliding *with others*

  1. *With one other:* facing, both hands joined, arms extended toward other person or extended sideways, sliding sideways

VII. Skip. Students can create the following variations:

 A. In *space* pattern (Fig. 20-1*C*)

  1. Changes in direction: turning around

 B. In skipping *with others*

  1. *With one other.* Side by side, inside hands joined, skipping forward; side by side, inside hands crossed and joined with outside hands, skipping forward; right or left hands joined, skipping in small circles; facing both hands joined, skipping in small circle

  2. *With two or three others*: Side by side, inside hands joined, skipping forward; in circle, hands joined, skipping around circle; in line, one child leading, hands joined, skipping forward

Murray believed that a formal response to accents should not be expected until the third grade.

Murray's grade-specific standards were based on children's rhythmic responses to nonlocomotor and locomotor movements. According to Murray, rhythmic skills are important to the overall assessment of children's dance skills. She identified three categories of rhythmic skills: (*a*) pulse beats, (*b*) music phrasing, and (*c*) rhythmic patterns. Each category included responses from children while they moved alone, while they moved with others, and during participation in rhythmic games.

According to Murray, assessment of performance standards would be valid only under certain conditions. She believed the following: (*a*) The dance room must be large enough to allow children to move freely. (*b*) Percussion instruments and/or a piano must be used for improvised accompaniment. (*c*) A pianist or a recording machine must be available to play the accompaniment. (*d*) Children must have at least two dance classes weekly. (*e*) Biweekly dance classes must be no shorter than 20 to 30 minutes each. (*f*) Each class must have fewer than 40 children unless an assisting teacher is present to help with the teaching and instruction (1).

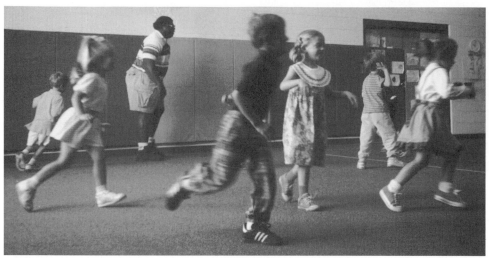

A

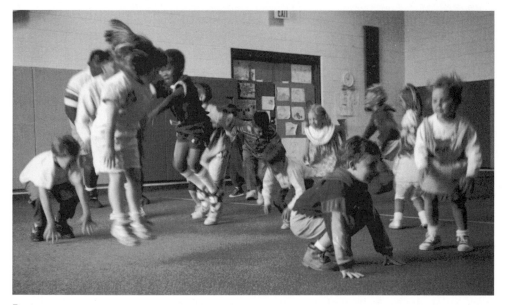

B

FIGURE 20-1

Students perform a natural run (**A**) while varying the shape by running with arms in a forward position. The jump pattern (**B**) is varied with changes in level. The skip (**C**) is varied in space with changes in direction. (Courtesy of Dr. Rayma K. Beal, Department of Health, Physical Education, and Recreation, University of Kentucky at Lexington.)

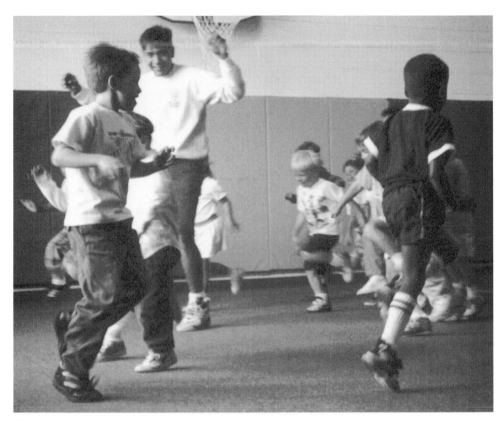

C

FIGURE 20-1

Continued

Reflections on the Ideas of Murray

Ruth Murray's performance standards addressed the problem of performing basic dance steps rhythmically with variations in space, time, and force. Ideas about student assessment of dance skills have evolved since Murray's contributions during the 1950s and 1960s. While Murray's analysis of dance movement skills remains developmentally appropriate, many newer ideas affect how dance skills are assessed today.

Murray also clarified the conditions necessary for valid assessment: a large room, accompaniment, assistance with teaching a large class, and two dance classes weekly. The last condition, biweekly dance classes, is uncommon in today's schools. If, however, all high-school students *could* perform the dance skills specified for Murray's sixth level of performance, they would likely be competent and confident movers.

Mary Joyce's Dance Assessment

In the 1970s Mary Joyce wrote a textbook on teaching creative dance to children. Her book was revised in the 1980s; the third edition of this popular book was published in 1994. The intent of each edition of Joyce's text was the same, that is, to teach the joy of dancing by providing a firm foundation in the elements of dance. She further believed that dance provides an opportunity for teachers and students to get to know each other in various ways, to establish respect for each other, and to learn to work together cooperatively.

Joyce's Assessment Concepts

Mary Joyce suggested that all dance lessons focus on an **element of dance** with a lesson theme that helps facilitate the idea of the lesson (2). The teacher assesses students' learning during the lesson by observing how the elements of dance and lesson theme were used by students (Fig. 20-2). Joyce noted that teachers must learn to observe closely to determine whether students are moving with "skill, conviction, and variety"; teachers must also learn to record their observations carefully. According to Joyce, by the end of the lesson students should be able to demonstrate all of the dance elements they practiced and describe each dance element and relate it to the world in which they live.

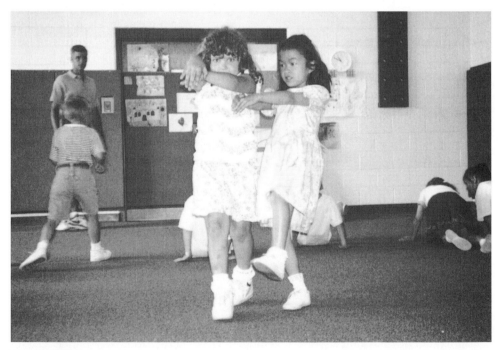

FIGURE 20-2

Joyce's approach to dance assessment entails observation of children as they demonstrate elements of dance within the context of a lesson theme. (Courtesy of Dr. Rayma K. Beal, Department of Health, Physical Education, and Recreation, University of Kentucky at Lexington.)

Elements of dance are variations in space, time, and force created by the move-
~~ments of the body~~

Table 20-2 shows Joyce's elements of dance. Space, time, and force are her central concepts. The elements of space include shape, level, direction, size, place,
focus, and pathway. Elements of time include beat, tempo, accent, duration, and pattern. Elements of force include attack, weight, strength, and flow. Joyce perceived
the body as the instrument by which space, time, and force are created with the
inner body parts (muscles, bones, heart, lungs) and the outer body parts (e.g., head,
shoulders, arms, torso, legs, feet). Body movements include nonlocomotors, such as
stretch, bend, twist, swing; the eight basic locomotor steps of walk, run, leap, hop,
jump, gallop, skip, slide (Fig. 20-3); and dance steps of two-step, step hop, schottis-
che, waltz, waltz-run, mazurka, grapevine, and polka.

Four occasions in a lesson allow the teacher to evaluate a student's understanding of an element of dance: (*a*) the exploratory section of the lesson; (*b*) the form
section, when performing the shape-movement-shape dance; (*c*) the section when
students describe "what moves like that"; and (*d*) the good-bye dance at the end of

TABLE 20-2		Mary Joyce's Elements of Dance
Body	Body parts	*Inner:* Muscles, bones, joints, heart, lungs (breath)
		Outer: Head, shoulders, arms, hands, back, ribcage, hips, teet, legs
	Body moves	Stretch, bend, twist, circle, rise, fall, swing,[a] sway,[a] shake, suspend,[a] collapse[a]
	Steps	Walk, run, leap, hop, jump, gallop, skip, slide
	Dance steps	Two-step, step hop, schottische, waltz, waltz-run, mazurka, grapevine, polka
Space	Shape	Body design in space
	Level	High, middle, low
	Direction	Forward, backward, sideways, turning
	Size	Big, little
	Place	On the spot, through space
	Focus	Direction of gaze
	Pathway	Curved, straight
Time	Beat	Underlying pulse
	Tempo	Fast, slow
	Accent	Force
	Duration	Long, short
	Pattern	Combinations
Force	Attack	Sharp,[a] smooth[a]
	Weight	Heavy, light
	Strength	Tight, loose
	Flow	Free flowing, bound, or balanced

[a]These are considered "qualities of movement."

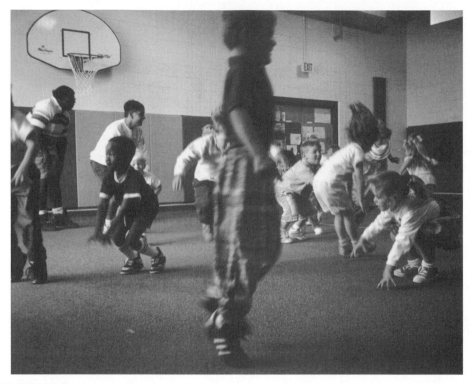

FIGURE 20-3

The jump is a basic locomotor step used in dance. (Courtesy of Dr. Rayma K. Beal, Department of Health, Physical Education, and Recreation, University of Kentucky at Lexington.)

the lesson. According to Joyce, the critical requirements for student assessment are (*a*) concentration while solving a movement problem, (*b*) challenging the body to create a variety of movements while communicating an idea, and (*c*) developing movement freedom while using the whole body.

While the primary goal of creative dance is to learn to use the elements of dance while moving with skill, conviction, and variety, Joyce (2) identified a secondary goal of dance education as effective personal and group interactions via development of the personal attributes of "respect, concentration, self-discipline, responsibility, and sensitivity." Joyce suggested that achievement of learning goals can be tracked by use of a chart. Students' names can be listed vertically, and dance elements and personal attributes can be listed horizontally. A star, sticker, or stamp can be used to signify achievement of an element or attribute. If a child does not do well on a skill, the teacher may draw a partial star with two or three lines. Joyce suggested that at least one line of a star should be awarded to a student who has attempted a skill.

Reflections on the Ideas of Joyce

Joyce believed that ongoing assessment affords benefits to both teachers and students. Students can observe their own progress toward the goals of demonstrating their dance skills physically and describing and relating them to their world. Teachers can assess their abilities in observation and guidance of students through effective communication. To explain verbally what we want from our students involves clear language with our eyes open to evaluate what they have accomplished and how far they have progressed in developing their dance skills.

Project Spectrum

Another example of an assessment plan for creative dance is the 1989 Project Spectrum Creative Movement Activity Scoring Procedure. Project Spectrum, designed for preschool children, was part of the Harvard University Project Zero research projects in the arts. Project Spectrum involved 15 creative dance activities, with scoring based on several components (Fig. 20-4). To understand the theoretical rationale for the Project Spectrum Creative Movement project, it is necessary to review Howard Gardner's work on multiple intelligences and Harvard University's Project Zero research findings.

Howard Gardner's Concept of Multiple Intelligences

Assessment in education has undergone many changes in recent years as a result of increased research on education, demands for major reform and accountability in education, and the changes and challenges in the global world of business. A major influence on our understanding of intelligence and education reform comes from

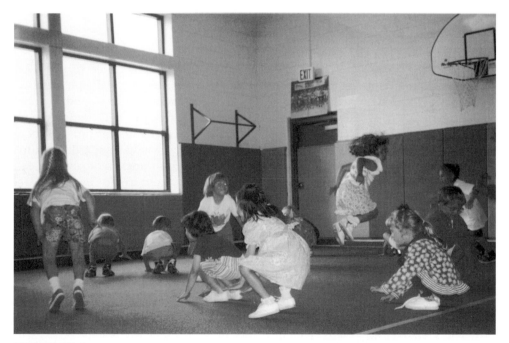

FIGURE 20-4

In Project Spectrum, components of 15 creative dance activities are assessed. (Courtesy of Dr. Rayma K. Beal, Department of Health, Physical Education, and Recreation, University of Kentucky at Lexington.)

the work of Gardner and his colleagues at Harvard University. Gardner worked on the Project for Human Potential in the early 1980s. His work described a large, comprehensive view of the human mind.

Gardner, as summarized by Johnson (3), suggested that "all human beings develop at least seven different ways of knowing the world." These ways of knowing were defined by Gardner as intelligences. According to Gardner, the mind is not one general-purpose organ; rather, it is composed of a number of content-specific information devices. Gardner identified seven specific intelligences in the human mind: the linguistic, the logical-mathematical, the musical, the spatial, the bodily-kinesthetic, the interpersonal, and the intrapersonal (Table 20-3).

Educational assessment in the United States has traditionally focused on the linguistic and logical-mathematical aptitudes as demonstrated by standardized tests such as the American College Test, Scholastic Achievement Test, and Graduate Record Examination. According to Gardner, because the other five aptitudes are not assessed, more than 70% of a child's mental abilities are not systematically developed during traditional schooling.

Gardner said further that some intelligences must be stimulated at optimal or critical periods. That is, there is a window of opportunity during which each child's intelligences are most amenable to stimulation and development. According to Gardner, most aptitudes must be developed early in life or the synapses associated with that intelligence may atrophy (4). The result is an underdeveloped intelligence that may be impaired for life. Gardner recommended that every student receive instruction in each of the seven intelligences from an early age.

Implications of Gardner's Work for Dance Assessment

Gardner's theory of multiple intelligences has implications for dance through the bodily-kinesthetic intelligence and the musical, spatial, interpersonal, and intrapersonal domains of intelligence. When we observe the general changes in educational assessment and reflect on how the dance profession struggles with defining new ways to assess and report students' learning, all of this seems to indicate that new methods of assessment are needed. While kinesthetic knowledge is not difficult for teachers to assess, writing a report to parents on students' kinesthetic abilities can be a struggle. Bucek (5) posited that in a good child-centered dance curriculum, reporting kinesthetic knowledge by traditional word and number systems is often ineffective. The research by Gardner and others is helping to define alternative ways for assessing and reporting kinesthetic knowledge.

Project Zero

Gardner has also been active with a consortium of researchers who study development and evaluation of intellectual competencies in the field. This Harvard-based program, called Project Zero, includes preschools through secondary schools in Boston, Pittsburgh, Indianapolis, New Haven, and Washington. All Project Zero schools share a common concept, that is, the development of student projects. Key factors to the student projects are that they must have depth and address several of the seven intelligences, and the student must have an investment in the outcome.

TABLE 20-3	Howard Gardner's Seven Intelligences

Through his theory of multiple intelligences, Howard Gardner has identified these seven intelligences:

LINGUISTIC

Characterized by Gardner as the "Poet," this embraces the capacity for language and its use beyond the mere ability to compose papers or paragraphs, It reflects the ability to see and develop patterns in language and to shape words and phrases that embody concepts and convey meaning.

LOGICAL-MATHEMATICAL

Characterized by Gardner as the "Scientist," this capacity for reasoning, logic, and problem solving is characterized by proficiency with categorization, classification, and understanding of abstract patterns and relations. It can include the ability to visualize relations between objects and the environment and how actions would alter the relations.

MUSICAL

Characterized as the "Composer," this reflects one's ability to discern sounds, melodies, pitches, rhythms, and timing. Gardner emphasizes pitch, rhythm, and timbre.

SPATIAL

Characterized as the "Sculptor" and "Sailor," the spatial aptitude encompasses the ability to imagine, sense environmental changes, solve mazes, and interpret locations using maps. The spatial intelligence, which relates directly to visual acuity, allows one to visualize how an object would look or feel from a different perspective.

BODILY-KINESTHETIC

Characterized as the "Dancer" or "Athlete," this reflects an ability to use the body to accomplish complex and intricate activities or manipulate objects with well-controlled finesse. Overt actions are not the sole reflections of the Bodily-Kinesthetic intelligence. Detailed movement, including dexterity, is the core of the Bodily-Kinesthetic aptitude.

INTERPERSONAL

Characterized by Gardner as the "Teacher" or "Salesman," this encompasses the ability to understand people's motivations, as well as skills in leadership, organization, and communication. The ability to comprehend aspects of character in other people is a primary feature of this intelligence.

INTRAPERSONAL

Gardner calls this the "One with Self-Understanding." This intelligence allows individuals to recognize their strengths and weaknesses, motivations and aptitudes. Intrapersonal intelligence allows an individual to assess situations in light of personal strengths and weaknesses and to determine the best approach to ensure successful resolutions.

Reprinted with permission from Gardner H.: Frames of Mind: The Theory of Multiple Intelligences. New York, Basic Books, 1983.

(See Gardner [4] or the Project Zero library for a detailed explanation of this program.)

Project Spectrum Creative Movement Activity

As mentioned earlier, the Project Spectrum Creative Movement Activity Scoring Procedure involves 15 dance activities, with scoring divided into six components: (*a*) rhythm sensitivity; (*b*) body control; (*c*) movement dynamics; (*d*) use of space;

(*e*) generates movement ideas; and (*f*) responsivity to music. The dance teacher scores each child on each target component while the child engages in a movement activity. A score of 1 (low-skill performance), 2 (medium-skill performance), or 3 (high-skill performance) is assigned on each component. A brief note written in the space provided can be used later to raise a child's score if appropriate. For example, the child who initially scored a 2 on the rhythm activity and later demonstrated a strong sense of rhythm in the free-dance section would be given a 3. Figure 20-5 describes in detail the Project Spectrum Creative Movement Activity Scoring procedures.

(text continues on page 668)

Scoring for the creative movement activity is divided into the six components, A to F. Each section of the creative movement activity focuses on a target component. As the experimenter proceeds through the activity, she scores (1, 2 or 3) the child on each target component.

A. **Rhythm Sensitivity.** Rhythm sensitivity refers to the child's ability to move in synchrony with rhythms. In the target activity, the focus is on the child's ability to repeat hand-clapping rhythm patterns initiated by the experimenter and tapping sticks to rhythm patterns set by the music.

____ 1. Child does not repeat rhythmic patterns correctly (e.g., child does not participate or claps or taps sticks off rhythm).

____ 2. Child repeats simpler patterns correctly but cannot properly repeat the more difficult ones (e.g., the first two patterns are repeated correctly, but the child cannot or does not repeat the last two); child has sense of simple (1-2, 1-2) rhythm of songs when tapping sticks together.

____ 3. Child repeats all patterns correctly (minor error is allowable); child has good sense of rhythm when tapping sticks together to music.

Notes:

Questions to consider:

Does child show an outstanding sense of rhythm when tapping sticks?

Does child try to tap out more complex rhythm patterns in music?

Does child bring out more complex rhythms than provided in the songs?

Other?

B. **Body Control.** Body control is defined as the child's ability to place his or her body properly, and isolate and use his or her body parts successfully and effectively toward a desired goal. Ability to keep one's balance also figures in this component. In the "mirror" activity, the child's sequencing and execution of movements initiated by the experimenter is the focus of observation.

FIGURE 20-5

Project Spectrum, SPFI Creative Movement Scoring Procedures, 1989. (Reprinted with permission from Jackie Chen at Project Spectrum, Arts Propel Project, Harvard Project Zero, 323 Longfellow Hall, Harvard Graduate School of Education, 13 Appian Way, Cambridge, MA 02138.)

____ 1. Child has difficulty isolating relevant body parts. Child generalizes movements (e.g., moves whole arm and side of body rather than just hand).

____ 2. Child has some success isolating body parts; successfully imitates gross gestures but demonstrates some difficulty with more subtle gestures (e.g., child has difficulty moving one finger at a time).

____ 3. Child shows almost perfect reproduction of the experimenter's gross and subtle movements. (Movements are imitated with exact isolation; child has good balance.)

C. **Movement Dynamics.**   Movement dynamics refers to the child's ability to change and diversify movements in accordance with the experimenter's request and change of music, rhythm, or tempo. In "Simon Says," movement dynamics are observed in the child's ability to diversify his or her movements at the experimenter's request that he or she simulate various things, animals, and ideas. The experimenter notes how much differentiation exists between the child's movements.

____ 1. Child demonstrates little variety with each movement request. An unvarying pattern of movement is prevalent (very little or no change in child's movements from one movement request to the other).

____ 2. Child demonstrates some variance in the movements he or she chooses (e.g., person walking very similar to person walking in mud, but these two differ greatly from tightrope walker).

____ 3. Child demonstrates great variance from one movement to another. He or she is attuned to nuances and various movement possibilities. (Each movement request brings out a quite different movement by child.)

D. **Use of Space.**   This component refers to the child's awareness of and ability to use the space around him or her, both laterally and vertically. The experimenter considers factors such as a child's standing tall, crouching down, spreading out, use of available floor space, and frequency of the child's use of these factors. "Simon Says" provides the opportunity to observe the child's use of space. (The free dance component provides another excellent opportunity to observe use of space. See below.)

____ 1. Child virtually plants feet in one area and rarely strays. Very little or no vertical movement is demonstrated.

____ 2. Child sometimes uses horizontal and/or vertical space but usually only when specifically called for ("Simon says be a tall tree blowing in the wind"; child stands tall).

____ 3. Child uses the bounds of designated area (experimenter may have difficulty keeping child within designated area). Child demonstrates a variety of vertical movements and positioning.

FIGURE 20-5

Continued

Notes:

Are other movement components apparent? Circle. Use an asterisk (*) if outstanding.

____ Body control

____ Generates movement ideas (suggests other possibilities on his or her own)

____ Other:

E. **Generates Movement Ideas.** This component focuses on the child's ability to invent interesting and novel movement ideas. Scoring is based on the child's ideas, either verbalized or demonstrated physically, not on the quality of execution. The child is observed during the second part of "Simon Says," when the experimenter asked the child to come up with movements or ideas to imitate.

____ 1. Child cannot generate original movement ideas on his or her own.

____ 2. Child generates one or two novel movement ideas.

____ 3. Child generates several novel movement ideas.

Notes:

Are other movement components apparent? Circle. Use an asterisk (*) if outstanding ability is noted.

____ Body control (good body control in execution of movements)

____ Use of space (movement ideas involve great use of space; child executes ideas making use of horizontal and vertical space)

____ Movement dynamics (ideas involve a variety of movements, which child demonstrates)

____ Other:

F. **Responsivity to Music.** Some children respond more to music than to a verbal idea or image. This category assesses children's responses to a variety of music through movement and expressiveness when asked to move to the music any way they wish in the free dance component. Because this is a free dance component, the experimenter should focus on *how* the child responds to the music, and the other five target areas might lend themselves to being noted during this activity.

____ 1. Child does not seem particularly responsive to music. Movement is limited and/or does not reflect differences in the music (e.g., child spins around on his or her buttocks for almost the entire song).

____ 2. Child reflects general differences in music through movements but does not respond to more subtle features in the music (e.g., child moves quickly

FIGURE 20-5

Project Spectrum, SPFI Creative Movement Scoring Procedures, 1989. (Reprinted with permission from Jackie Chen at Project Spectrum, Arts Propel Project, Harvard Project Zero, 323 Longfellow Hall, Harvard Graduate School of Education, 13 Appian Way, Cambridge, MA 02138.) Continued

or slowly, depending on the tempo, but uses the same type of movement for all music segments).

_____ 3. Child demonstrates many subtle movements in response to different features of music, such as tempo, rhythm, style, and mood (e.g., child moves fluidly and quickly; jaggedly and slowly; uses facial expressions).

Notes:

Do other components stand out? Circle. Use asterisk (*) if outstanding.

_____ Body control (Note "freeze": does child freeze successfully?)

_____ Movement dynamics (great variety in movement between songs)

_____ Use of space (child uses bounds of available space; much up and down movement)

_____ Rhythm sensitivity (child's movements focused on beat of music)

Other notes?

Totals:
A _____   D _____
B _____   E _____
C _____   F _____   CUMULATIVE _____

Date _____

Creative Movement Score Sheet

Name _____   D.O.B. _____
Experimenter _____   Scorer _____

				Score
Rhythm sensitivity	1	2	3	_____
Body control	1	2	3	_____
Movement dynamics	1	2	3	_____
Use of space	1	2	3	_____
Generates movement ideas	1	2	3	_____
Responsivity to music	1	2	3	_____
		Total Score		_____

Additional comments:

FIGURE 20-5

Continued

Reflections on Project Spectrum

The Project Spectrum Creative Movement Activity Scoring Procedure is a fully developed dance assessment for preschool children. It also has potential for use in kindergarten to third grade with slight revisions in the skill demonstration descriptors and rating scale. The scoring procedure assesses bodily-kinesthetic knowledge qualitatively, thus providing information for students and teachers to determine students' levels of development in Gardner's bodily-kinesthetic domain.

Maxine DeBruyn's Assessment Model

The exploration of dance assessment models has been a central topic of ongoing research by DeBruyn at Hope College in Michigan. In a presentation at the Dance and Child International Conference on applying concepts of the Arts Propel project to dance assessment, DeBruyn (6) reported that portfolios offer a valuable overall indication of progress in dance for students in grades 9 to 12 and college. She maintained that if dance students are encouraged to review their choreography and performances and to criticize their own works and those of others by observation, group discussion, individual analysis, and writing down of personal reactions, they will be more active participants in their own learning.

DeBruyn found that materials developed by Gardner and Project Zero were useful in developing portfolio components for dance assessment. DeBruyn also borrowed ideas from Seidel and Walters (7). DeBruyn determined that dance students should consider the following questions when analyzing and writing about dance activities for inclusion in their portfolios:

- Does my work show development?
- Have I effectively expressed myself and shared my knowledge of the skills involved?
- What problems and challenges have I worked on, and what strategies were used to complete them?

DeBruyn also believed that use of the dance portfolio as an assessment tool concomitantly developed another dimension; it became a representation of the student's skill and abilities beyond what a written or skills test could distinguish. In other words, the student portfolio says, "Here is my work. This is how I approached it. This is why I value it. This is what it tells me. I should work on this next" (8). Portfolios can accurately reflect strengths, weaknesses, skills mastered, and personal reflections of the student while learning a new skill or technique. Indeed, DeBruyn posited that portfolios can present a clear picture of students' accomplishments in dance. The process of portfolio development enables students to create and perform dance, to analyze, to think about dance in its many genres, and to develop critical analysis skills while viewing dance. Portfolios are discussed further later in this chapter.

Figure 20-6 shows a chart that DeBruyn developed to assess technique skills for beginning modern dance students. The major categories of movement are listed on the left side of the chart: technique while lying down or in a sitting position, standing, and traveling; and a short dance sequence or combination. Across the top of the page, the categories to assess while a student performs the technique are: alignment,

BEGINNING MODERN DANCE
EVALUATION OF KEY TECHNIQUE*

Technique 1–5 points Dance sequence 1–10 points (96 counts)	Alignment	Effective Approach	Effective Conclusion	Transitions	Rhythm Clearly Executed	Effective Use of Space (Shape)	Dynamics of Movement	Overall Impression	Total Points
TECHNIQUE									
Lying and sitting									
1. Chest arches									
1. Pull-ups									
3. Leg lifts									
4. Torso stretch and scoop									
5. Spinal flexion									
6. Side stretches									
7. Stretch leg and arch back									
STANDING									
1. Leg: Brushes									
Extensions									
Swings									
2. Pliés: Demi									
Grand									
Relevé									
3. Slow stretches									
4. Sustained curling movement									
5. Body rotation									
6. Body swings: Forward									
Sideways									

FIGURE 20-6

DeBruyn's modern dance technique evaluation form. (From DeBruyn, M.: Application of arts propel in dance. Conference Proceedings of the 1991 Conference: Dance and the Child International, Salt Lake City, July 1991.) Continued

Technique 1–5 points Dance sequence 1–10 points (96 counts)	Alignment	Effective Approach	Effective Conclusion	Transitions	Rhythm Clearly Executed	Effective Use of Space (Shape)	Dynamics of Movement	Overall Impression	Total Points
TECHNIQUE									
Traveling									
1. Leaps									
2. Skips and slide									
3. Triplets									
4. Two runs and leap									
5. Two triplets and three step turns									
6. Four skips and two slides									
7. Three runs, hop, step, leap									
DANCE SEQUENCE (*Smile Happy*)									
GRAND TOTAL									

(Done at the end of the technique unit or semester)

FIGURE 20-6

DeBruyn's modern dance technique evaluation form. (From DeBruyn, M.: Application of arts propel in dance. Conference Proceedings of the 1991 Conference: Dance and the Child International, Salt Lake City, July 1991.) Continued

effective approach, effective conclusion, transitions, rhythm clearly executed, effective use of space (shapes), dynamics of movement, and overall impression.

Another example of dance assessment that DeBruyn developed is a combined profile of the students' abilities (Fig. 20-7) that both the teacher and student fill out. On the left side of the chart the assessment begins at the highest level and ends at the did-not-do level. Across the bottom of the chart are the three categories technique, improvisation, and composition. Elements of technique are alignment, transitions, dynamics, effective use of space (defined shapes), and rhythm clearly demonstrated. Components of improvisation are discovery (take risks), willingness to explore (freedom), and ability to solve problems. Composition elements are kinesthetic literacy, aesthetics, create choreography worthy of presentation, and demonstrate knowledge of elements of dance. Rating all the factors, the teacher marks squares at the level that represents the student's achievement; the student marks circles at the level of his or her self-evaluation.

Squares = Teacher   Circles = Student

STUDENT PROFILE
(Grades 9–12 or college)

Name: Date: Class:

ASSESSMENT LEVEL													
Highest	10												
	9												
High	8												
	7												
	6												
Medium	5												
	4												
	3												
Low	2												
	1												
Did not do	0												
		1	2	3	4	5	1	2	3	1	2	3	4
		Alignment	Transitions	Dynamics	Effective use of space (defined shapes)	Rhythm clearly demonstrated	Discovery (take risks)	Willingness to explore (freedom)	Ability to solve problems	Kinesthetic literacy	Aesthetics	Create choreography worthy of presentation	Demonstrate knowledge of elements of dance

TECHNIQUE   IMPROVISATION   COMPOSITION

Comments by Teacher:
   (Do at end of units or semester)

FIGURE 20-7

DeBruyn's dance profile form. (From DeBruyn, M.: Application of arts propel in dance. Conference Proceedings of the 1991 Conference: Dance and the Child International, Salt Lake City, July 1991.)

DeBruyn's Dance Rehearsal Critique Sheet

A third assessment tool developed by DeBruyn is a dance rehearsal critique sheet (Fig. 20-8) that can be used to provide both individual and ensemble feedback on performance at selected points in a rehearsal. A description of the point in the rehearsal is indicated by counts, location, and dimension. Comments are made and plans for revision or further practice are included.

Reflections on the Ideas of DeBruyn

DeBruyn's assessment tools provide a comprehensive view of achievement in dance. A portfolio containing the technique chart, the student's profile, and the rehearsal critique sheet along with written analyses of choreography and performances provides a multidimensional, longitudinal picture that details the student's achievement in dance.

Location	Dimension	My (section's) performance	For Myself (my section)
Beg. Cts. 1–12 At end of first phrase	Weak shapes Alignment is off	Missed levels in technique and the accent is on ct. 4. I let my back take over my technique.	Relax more; too much tension at beginning. Work on technique for strength.

Location	Dimension	Ensemble's Performance	For the Whole Ensemble
Cts. 1–12 First phrase	Shapes Alignment	Other students had the same problem: transition from shape to shape needs work; also anticipate accent and hit levels with more force. My back really stands out.	We need practice before the next class and understand the feeling needed to strengthen the performance. Set up a daily practice schedule for strengthening my back.

FIGURE 20-8

Sample rehearsal critique sheet done by student after combination is taught. (From De-Bruyn, M.: Application of arts propel in dance. Conference Proceedings of the 1991 Conference: Dance and the Child International, Salt Lake City, July 1991.)

Dance Assessment in Great Britain

The focus of dance in Great Britain is on body management and control and the aesthetic development of movement. Although the British assessment of dance appears less comprehensive than either the Project Spectrum or DeBruyn models, it is worthy of inclusion here because it is embedded in the physical education curriculum and because it provides a viewpoint of dance assessment outside the United States.

British National Curriculum

In an article describing the British national curriculum, Smith (9) reported that strengthening teacher accountability, improving teacher preparation (preservice, or as the British call it, initial teacher education), and instituting student assessment have led to many improvements in physical education in Great Britain. Elements of the British physical education curriculum include five areas: athletic activities (track and field), dance, games, gymnastic activities, and outdoor adventure activities. If a school chooses, a sixth curricular content area of swimming may also be taught. Movement expectations for each area of activity are divided into four age levels, called stages: stage 1 is for students 5 to 7 years old; stage 2 is for students 7 to 11 years old; stage 3 is for students 11 to 14 years old; and stage 4 is for students 14 to 16 years old. During stage 1 the five basic areas must be taught. In stage 2, students must receive instruction in all five activities plus swimming, if it was not taught in stage 1. For stage 3, students must receive instruction in four activities, but games are a compulsory event each year. At stages 3 and 4, students who want to continue swimming can explore water skills in other activity areas (e.g., sailing or water polo as outdoor and game activities). In stage 4, general-education students must study at least two activities selected from one or two different areas or categories.

A working group of the Department of Education and Science and the Welsh Office justified inclusion of the six areas of activity by saying that they "offered different kinds of learning experience and reflected different characteristics" (10). Games engage students in competitive and cooperative experiences that use "skill and strategy to outwit the opposition." Dance and gymnastic activities focus on "body management and control" as well as the aesthetic development of movement. Athletic activities provide students with opportunities to "achieve individual excellence." Swimming is included for health and safety reasons and is a prerequisite for participation in other water-centered activities. Outdoor and adventure activities provide students with "opportunities to learn to travel safely and to adapt skills in challenging and stimulating environments." The dance activities prescribed in the British national curriculum are shown in Table 20-4.

To assess how well students meet the dance objectives of the British national curriculum, it was necessary to select certain aspects of the curriculum for assessment. The end-of-key statements (Table 20-5) delineate the expectations at physical performance for British students at ages 7, 11, 14, and 16. If students in key stage 1 are guided toward making dances with clear beginnings, middles, and ends, the basic actions (e.g., locomotor, nonlocomotor), contrasts of speed, tension, shape, and continuity performed with control, balance, and elevation can be paired with the following end-of-key stage statements:

(text continues on page 676)

TABLE 20-4	British Dance Curriculum

DANCE KEY STAGE 1 (FOR PUPILS 5 TO 7 YEARS)

Pupils should:

Experience and develop control, coordination, balance, poise, and elevation in basic actions, including traveling, jumping, turning, gesture and stillness

Explore contrasts of speed, tension, continuity, shape, size, direction, and level and describe what they have done

Work with a range and variety of contrasting stimuli, including music

Be given opportunities to explore moods and feelings through spontaneous responses and through structured tasks

Be helped to develop rhythmic responses

Experience and be guided toward making dances with clear beginnings, middles, and ends

DANCE KEY STAGE 2 (FOR PUPILS 7 TO 11 YEARS)

Pupils should:

Make dances with clear beginnings, middles, and ends involving improvising, exploring, selecting, and refining content, and sometimes incorporating work from other aspects of the curriculum, in particular music, art, and drama

Be given opportunities to increase the range and complexity of body actions, including step patterns and use of body parts

Be guided to enrich their movements by varying shape, size, direction, level, speed, tension, and continuity

In response to a range of stimuli, express feelings, moods, and ideas and create simple characters and narratives in movement

Describe and interpret the various elements of a dance

DANCE KEY STAGE 3 (FOR PUPILS 11 TO 14 YEARS)

Pupils should:

Be taught how to develop and use appropriate methods of composition, styles, and techniques to communicate meanings and ideas

Be guided to create and perform short dances showing sensitivity to the style of accompaniment

Be taught to perform set dances, showing an understanding of style

Be taught to support their own dance compositions with written and/or oral descriptions of their intentions and outcomes

Be taught to describe, analyze, and interpret dances, recognizing stylistic differences, aspects of production, and cultural and historical contexts

DANCE KEY STAGE 4 (FOR PUPILS 14 TO 16 YEARS)

Pupils should:

Be taught to perform complex and technically demanding dances accurately and expressively

Be given opportunities to create dances that successfully communicate the artistic intention

Be given opportunities to dance in a range of styles showing understanding of form and content

Be enabled to record the process of composition

Be guided to devise and design aspects of production for their own compositions

Be given opportunities to describe, interpret, and evaluate all aspects of dance, including choreography, performance, cultural and historical contexts, and production

TABLE 20-5	End-of-Key Stage Statements for Dance, Athletics, Games, Gymnastics, Outdoor Activities, and Swimming (British Dance Curriculum)

KEY STAGE 1 (FOR PUPILS 5 TO 7 YEARS)

By the end of this key stage, pupils should be able to:

- Plan and perform safely a range of simple actions and linked movements in response to given tasks and stimuli
- Practice and improve their performance
- Describe what they and others are doing
- Recognize the effects of physical activity on their bodies

KEY STAGE 2 (FOR PUPILS 7 TO 11 YEARS)

By the end of this key stage, pupils should be able to:

- Plan, practice, improve, and remember more complex sequences of movement
- Perform effectively in activities requiring quick decision making
- Respond safely, alone and with others, to challenging tasks, taking account of levels of skill and understanding
- Swim unaided at least 25 meters and demonstrate an understanding of water
- Evaluate how well they and others perform and behave against criteria suggested by the teacher and suggest ways of improving performance
- Sustain energetic activity over appropriate periods in a range of physical activities and understand the effects of exercise on the body

KEY STAGE 3 (FOR PUPILS 11 TO 14 YEARS)

By the end of this key stage, pupils should be able to:

- Devise and adapt strategies and tactics across appropriate activities within the programs of study
- Adapt and refine existing skills and develop new skills safely across the activities in the programs of study
- Practice and perform movement compositions devised by themselves and others in appropriate activities in the programs of study
- Understand and evaluate how well they and others have achieved what they set out to do, appreciate strengths and weaknesses, and suggest ways of improving
- Understand the short- and long-term effects of exercise on the body systems and decide where to focus their involvement in physical activity for a healthy and enjoyable lifestyle

KEY STAGE 4 (FOR PUPILS 14 TO 16 YEARS)

By the end of the key stage pupils should be able to:

- Show increased knowledge, improved competence, and safe performance in their selected activities
- Understand and undertake various roles in their selected activities
- Develop and apply their own criteria for judging performance
- Prepare, carry out, and monitor personal programs for a healthy and enjoyable lifestyle, considering the use of community resources where appropriate

- Did the students plan and perform a range of linked movements in response to a task or stimuli?
- Did the students practice and improve their performance of the dance?
- Could they describe what they and their peers were doing in the dance?
- Did they recognize the physical effects of dance in activity in their own bodies?

To complete the assessment, the teacher or test administrator must have determined a specific level of achievement before viewing students' dance performances. A scoring rubric (e.g., 1, low; 10, high) aids in the determination of how well the student performed the dance.

Reflections on the British National Curriculum

While the dance activities described in the British national curriculum give another view of appropriate dance activities, the procedures for assessment of these skills are not completely clear. The British national curriculum does, however, provide a glimpse into various world views of dance education. Additionally, it provides an example of how dance can effectively be part of a comprehensive physical education curriculum.

Dance Assessment in British Columbia

Van Gyn and O'Neill (11) described a project examining fine arts assessment in British Columbia, Canada. Their report on dance assessment in education was presented at the 1991 Dance and Child International Conference. They opined that the creative nature of dance education makes the task of systematic assessment very difficult. If the requirements of assessment are to be ongoing, self-referenced or criterion-based, and related to the goals of **aesthetic response** and artistic development, it is necessary to develop solid conceptual schemes to support professional opinion. Van Gyn and O'Neill stated that a critical beginning step is to reexamine what is taught in the dance curriculum and how teachers assess what dance students learn in class. Afterward, statements on effective dance education with the goals of aesthetic response and artistic development can be established.

An aesthetic response is movement that meets universal standards of beauty.

Van Gyn and O'Neill's Concept of Aesthetic Development in Dance

Van Gyn and O'Neill noted that while much has been written about aesthetic development, very little has been reported on how aesthetic abilities are developed and their role in overall learning. The authors maintained that in dance, aesthetic development should be part of the performance, composition, and appreciation and enquiry categories. They contended that the outcome of a quality dance program should be an "informed, aesthetic response" by the student. Two communication abilities help define the aesthetic development concept. The first is communication with the skillful use of the body, by expressing an idea, thought and/or feeling through performing and composing dance. The second is communication through written and spoken language by expressing ideas and thoughts about observation of dance performances.

While admitting that there may be certain elements of dance learning that are impossible to assess, Van Gyn and O'Neill maintained that a "key to determining what is to be assessed is to identify the knowledge to be learned" (11). Because the body is a closed system, they suggested that one can assess only human behavior (what students do), their thoughts as reflected in their movements, and/or their feelings as reflected in discussion of dance, writings about dance, and so on. The target of assessment then becomes twofold: what the student can demonstrate and the cognitive processes that the student used to reach the outcome. Van Gyn and O'Neill stated, "How well the product reflects the process is dependent on the instrumentation and the conditions of the assessment" (11).

Van Gyn and O'Neill developed the chart in Figure 20-9 to illustrate objectives of the dance education program and development of the aesthetic response. Each category on their chart includes ways to achieve aesthetic development and serves as a guide to short-term and long-term lesson planning.

Van Gyn and O'Neill suggested that assessment in dance be a combination of objective and subjective judgments. Subjective assessment may be more valuable to the learner, but it is critical that the assessor (i.e., teacher or other trained professional) be knowledgeable in dance and have highly developed observational skills. Furthermore, to maximize the outcomes of the process, Van Gyn and O'Neill recommended collaboration among the student learners, their peers, and the teacher.

Reflections on the Ideas of Van Gyn and O'Neill

Van Gyn and O'Neill concluded that the fundamental problem of assessment is to determine (*a*) what dance students need to know and (*b*) the stage of development when they should master the various dance concepts and skills (11). However, assessment is more difficult when student learners create and produce their own dance program. Van Gyn and O'Neill suggested that the models and choices of assessment must be preceded by careful analysis of philosophic ideals and program goals and delineation of an operational definition of aesthetic development. Their work provides another perspective on dance education outside the United States.

U.S. National Standards in Dance

The National Standards represent the current consensus of broadly identified dance competencies for grades 4, 8, and 12 in the United States. The standards are intended for use in evaluating dance education programs at local, state, and national levels.

The National Standards for Arts Education are comprehensive criteria in dance, music, theater, and visual arts (12). They ask that students know and be able to do the following five competencies by the time they have completed the 12th grade: (*a*) communicate in the four arts disciplines; (*b*) communicate proficiently in at least one art form; (*c*) develop and present basic analyses of works of art; (*d*) have an in-

Development of the Aesthetic Response

Aesthetic Production and Aesthetic Understanding

The learner will have the opportunity to:
  Perform dance
  Compose dances
  Engage in an enquiry to seek personal meaning of cultural and global meaning
    in dance

Knowledge Bases of the Aesthetic Response

Application of Learning Strategies
Remembering   Judging
Considering   Transforming
Solving   Elaborating
Analyzing   Creating

Performance Knowledge

Technical	*Expressive*
Understanding of and	Understanding of action
physical competency	symbols and physical
in action	competency in symbol
Action bases	making
Action in parts	Action in space
Action in place	Action in time
Action on the move	Action with energy

Composition Knowledge

Form	*Content*	*Style*
Motif (movement	Effective use	Personal
pattern)	of action	Group
Repetition	symbols	Period
Variety and contrast		Culture
Proportional balance		
Logical development		
Unity		

Knowledge of Dance History

Dance as culture   Dance as fine art

Knowledge of Dance Criticism

Own   Peer   Dance in
production   production   popular culture

Dance in   Dance in
multi cultures   high cultures

FIGURE 20-9

Objectives of the dance education program in British Columbia.

formed acquaintance with exemplary works of art; and (*e*) relate various types of arts knowledge and skills within and across the arts disciplines. The vision of the National Standards for Arts Education is captured by this quotation: "A future worth having depends on being able to construct a vital relationship with the arts" (12). To develop this vital relationship requires discipline and study.

The National Standards for Dance provide the dance discipline with broadly identified competencies at kindergarten to 4th grade, 5th to 8th grade, and 9th to 12th grade. Content standards specify what students should know and be able to articulate and perform in dance. The achievement standards (Table 20-6) specify the understandings and levels of achievement that students are expected to attain in dance at the end of grades 4, 8, and 12.

The National Standards for Dance are based on three premises, that there is objectively identifiable achievement in dance, that knowledge and skills in dance are important, and that mere dancing is different from dance education. The Standards affirm "that discipline and rigor are the road to achievement" (12). They assert that dance content and achievement standards can be measured by either numerical scales or informed critical judgment.

Other Useful Approaches for Assessment in Dance

The videotape, the portfolio, and checklists are also valuable tools for assessment of dance. They are discussed in the following sections.

TABLE 20-6	U. S. National Standards in Dance

GRADES K-4	GRADES 5-8	GRADES 9-12, PROFICIENT	GRADES 9-12, ADVANCED
Content standard 1	Identifying and demonstrating movement elements and skills in performing dance		
Content standard 2	Understanding choreographic principles, processes, and structures		
Content standard 3	Understanding dance as a way to create and communicate meaning		
Content standard 4	Applying and demonstrating critical and creative thinking skills in dance		
Content standard 5	Demonstrating and understanding dance in various cultures and historical periods		
Content standard 6	Making connections between dance and healthful living		
Content standard 7	Making connections between dance and other disciplines		

For each content standard there are achievement standards at grades K-4, 5-8, 9-12 proficient, and 9-12 advanced. See National Standards for Arts Education document for complete details.
The Standards book can be ordered from MENC Publication Sales, 1806 Robert Fulton Drive, Reston, VA, 22091, or call 800-828-0229.

Videotape

For teachers to guide students in the development of projects, additional procedures are needed to expand the usual paper-and-pencil process. Students may use video to record the presentation of their projects, documenting their project and their presentation skills. During the school year, three to four projects can be recorded on videotape, then stored at a central location in the school for reference by the students, teachers, and/or parents or guardians. Videotapes of dance projects facilitate evaluation.

Video technology provides students with direct feedback on their development of skills, records both formal and informal performances, and is a resource for both students and teachers to view dancing by others. When using video in the classroom, remember that videotape is a two-dimensional representation of a three-dimensional activity. Students often ask, "Do I really look like that?" At this point a reassurance that the video picture is a likeness rather than a perfect image is usually sufficient.

The Portfolio

As noted earlier in this chapter, the **portfolio** is a valuable assessment tool for dance. A portfolio that includes a student's profile, standardized tests, videotapes of the project performance, journal entries, and teachers' comments allows a valid evaluation of a student's dance education (7). That portfolio is a vehicle for students to describe themselves. It speaks to the students' abilities beyond what a multiple-choice test describes.

Bucek (5) also addressed the contents of a good dance portfolio. She explained that portfolios can document learning styles, conceptual ideas in dance, and planned and informal dance projects. Bucek also noted that drafts, critiques, and revisions that allow the reader to follow the development of a project are appropriate components of a portfolio. Table 20-7 lists portfolio contents suggested by Bucek. Portfolios provide the teacher and students with opportunities to think and assess work in dance produced over a grading period, a semester, or a year. Bucek concluded that dance portfolio assessment expands evaluation "beyond written and numerical forms" (5). She has found that portfolio assessment provides an objective standard, allows for a variety of interpretations, and ensures that both students' and teachers' voices are heard.

> The portfolio is a compilation of dance work intended to demonstrate the developing skills and knowledge of a student.

Checklists

Designing an assessment form to aid in the evaluation of students' abilities during a dance class is a perplexing task. Checklists can be an important aid to assessing dance abilities.

Figures 20-10 and 20-11 show checklists developed for essential skills for Kentucky for Dance. These forms have been used to document students' progress in the schools participating in the basic arts program. The level 1 checklist shows begin-

TABLE 20-7	Portfolio Contents Suggested by Bucek

Improvisations
Written reflections and journals
Sketchbook and illustrations
Guided, open-ended questioning
Quizzes and examinations
Individual critique of video or live performance
Photography
Song writing or instrumental compositions
Class discussions
Individual or group dances
Dance studies
Verbs, jot lists, idea maps
Collages
Playwriting
Class critique of dances
Audio or videotape rehearsals
Dance game structure
Costume, lighting, and set design
Peer interaction and exchange
Revisions of individual or group dances

ning or entry level of skills for students in kindergarten through second grade. Broad categories for assessment at level 1 include locomotor movements, nonlocomotor movements, space, time, force, and problem solving through creative expression. Figure 20-11 is a comparable checklist for level 4 students of dance who have had 3 to 5 years of creative dance. It includes the use and demonstration of advanced skills in dance. The major checklist categories for level 4 are locomotor movements, nonlocomotor movements, space, time, force, problem solving through creative expression, and appreciation. Coding for dance skills uses a 1 to 4 scale: 1, attempted; 2, needs work; 3, partial mastery of skill; 4, mastery of skill.

The Kentucky Dance Committee recommended that these checklists and teachers' observations be supplemented with other assessment methodologies, such as (*a*) videotaping of dance sequences and beginning compositions for students' observation and feedback, teachers' assessment, and group discussion; (*b*) oral discussions by students of observations from dance performances by professionals and classmates; and (*c*) student writings, such as journal entries on classwork, observations of dances by peers and professionals, and critical writing on live dance performances.

Final Considerations for Assessment in Dance

There are two final issues that must be considered for valid and reliable dance assessment. Discussed below are space considerations and types of dance assessment.

(text continues on page 684)

	LOCOMOTORS—Level 1		
NAMES	**Walk, run, hop, jump, gallop**	**Produces motion vs. stillness**	**Uses different directions with walks, runs, hops, etc.**

	NONLOCOMOTORS—Level 1	
NAMES	**Directional concepts: forward, backward, sideways, up, down**	**Bend, stretch, push, pull, twist, turn**

	SPACE—Level 1		
NAMES	**Maintains personal space**	**Uses general space**	**Varies size of movements**

	TIME—Level 1	FORCE—Level 1
NAMES	**Uses quick and slow while moving**	**Sustained and/or percussive qualities while moving**

	PROBLEM SOLVING THROUGH CREATIVE EXPRESSION—Level 1	
NAMES	**Observes and interprets moods and feelings in movement**	**Solves movement problems**

Scoring Code   1, attempted   3, partial mastery of skill
                 2, needs work   4, has mastered skill

FIGURE 20-10

Kentucky for Dance level 1 checklists for dance skills.

NAMES	LOCOMOTORS—Level 4		
	Combines locomotors; uses a variety of locomotors in creative dance	Performs structured and partner dances with ease	Moves efficiently while performing fitness dance

NAMES	NONLOCOMOTORS—Level 4	SPACE—Level 4	
	Combines nonlocomotors; uses a variety of non-locomotors in creative dance	Controls body while moving with others	Distinguishes levels, directions, size, and range movement

NAMES	TIME—Level 4	FORCE—Level 4
	Distinguishes short from long duration, accent, and tempo	Identifies and distinguishes force elements

NAMES	PROBLEM SOLVING THROUGH CREATIVE EXPRESSION—Level 4			
	Uses variety of dance steps	Keeps beat while moving	Creates patterns related to music	Creates dance using simple movements while communicating an idea

NAMES	APPRECIATION—Level 4	
	Recognizes several purposes of dance and its relation to cultures	Recognizes the value of creative work by self and others

Scoring Code   1, attempted   3, partial mastery of skill
2, needs work   4, has mastered skill

FIGURE 20-11

Kentucky for Dance level 4 checklists for dance skills.

Space

The physical dimensions of a room and its floor are crucial to success in dance and to valid and reliable assessment. Stinson (13) suggested that the size and even the shape of a room affect students' movement responses. Furthermore, she said that too much open space can be as much of a problem as too little. The flooring should be shock absorbent and resilient; a wood or marley-covered floor is most desirable. For bare feet to move safely, the floor has to be smooth, warm, uncluttered, and dry. Distractions in the dance room, such as toys and other materials, should be removed or made to look uninviting.

Types of Dance Assessment

Five further points should be considered in a dance assessment. These issues relate to what is assessed and how the assessment is performed. The most obvious issue is defining the conditions for demonstration of skill. Dance skill can be demonstrated through either performance or **studio activities.** To state the obvious, accurate assessment in dance requires that the student move. Dance can be performed in response to a prompt, or it can be rehearsed and presented. It can also be an ongoing studio activity in which students use their knowledge of dance to define problems, generate solutions, or create a dance as a summation of a semester's course work.

> Studio activities are structured tasks that require students to use their dance knowledge and skills in defining a problem, generating a solution, evaluating choices based on criteria, or demonstrating a final dance.

A second issue is using the mind, eyes, ears, and mouth to analyze and describe dance. There are three opportunities to do this form of assessment: (*a*) Problem solving can be done through pencil-and-paper assessment, individual movement demonstration, or development of an action plan by the individual or small group. (*b*) Structured discussions can produce a solution to a problem. (*c*) Dance description requires students to respond to video clips in either oral or written form.

Dance assessments should include multiple opportunities for students to demonstrate what they know about dance. The following five points should be considered when developing dance assessments:

Performance. Dance pieces are created in response to a prompt, or they are rehearsed.

Problem Solving. Problems in dance can be solved by movement demonstration or through paper-and-pencil activities to assess creative thinking, individual or group organizational skills, and development of an action plan.

Structured Discussion. This oral activity requires an answer and solution to a question or problem about dance.

Studio Activities. These structured tasks require students to use their knowledge and skills to define a problem, generate a solution, evaluate choices based on criteria, and/or demonstrate a final dance.

Description of Dance. Students respond in oral or written form to video clips of dance.

Chapter Summary

This chapter reviews and discusses a number of models and concerns for the assessment of dance. It identifies learning goals for dance and defines elements of dance for students across many grade levels and provides specific assessment tools, such as portfolios and checklists.

SELF-TEST QUESTIONS

1. Which of the following dance education pioneers designed the first evaluation standards for performance?
   A. DeBruyn
   B. Joyce
   C. Murray
   D. Van Gyn and O'Neill

2. Which of the following educators identified the primary goal of creative dance as learning to use the elements of dance while moving with "skill, conviction, and variety"?
   A. DeBruyn
   B. Joyce
   C. Murray
   D. Van Gyn and O'Neill

3. According to Gardner's theory of multiple intelligences, dance education is likely to develop which of the following "intelligences"?
   A. Bodily-kinesthetic
   B. Interpersonal
   C. Intrapersonal
   D. Spatial
   E. All of the above

4. According to British educators, the *primary* justification for the inclusion of dance in the school curriculum is that dance helps students develop

   _____.
   A. Body management and control
   B. Individual excellence
   C. Health and safety
   D. Skill and strategy

5. According to the British system, a 12-year-old child is in what stage?
   A. Stage 1
   B. Stage 2
   C. Stage 3
   D. Stage 4

6. Where does the development of aesthetic production and understanding receive the *most* emphasis in the school dance curriculum?
   A. British Columbia
   B. Great Britain
   C. United States
   D. All of the above

7. According to the U.S. National Standards for Arts Education, students should be able to communicate in which of the following arts disciplines?
   A. Dance
   B. Music
   C. Theater
   D. Visual arts
   E. All of the above

8. Which of the following is commonly included in a student dance portfolio?
   A. Journal entries
   B. Photographs
   C. Videotapes
   D. Written critiques
   E. All of the above

ANSWERS

1. C	2. B	3. E	4. A
5. C	6. A	7. E	8. E

DOING PROJECTS FOR FURTHER LEARNING

1. Locate an ongoing dance program at your own college or university, at an area public school, or at a community arts center, and ask the instructor to discuss dance assessment with you. How does he or she evaluate what dance students have learned? Ask the instructor for permission to observe one or more classes. While observing, practice use of one or more of the evaluation tools in this chapter. If the instructor is willing, discuss your observations and evaluations of students with him or her.

2. According to the U.S. National Standards for Arts Education, students who have completed high school should be able to "communicate proficiently in at least one art form." Survey your friends and classmates to determine the percentage of students who agree that they have achieved this standard. Write a short paper that summarizes what you learned about arts education in the United States.

REFERENCES

1. Murray, R.L.: Dance in Elementary Education: A Program for Boys and Girls. 3rd ed. Reading, MA, Addison-Wesley, 1975.
2. Joyce, M.: First Steps in Teaching Creative Dance to Children. 3rd ed. Mountain View, CA, Mayfield, 1994.
3. Johnson, C.M.: Howard Gardner: Redefining Intelligence. Cardinal Principles, 6:1. Louisville, KY, University of Louisville, 1991.
4. Gardner, H.: Frames of Mind: The Theory of Multiple Intelligences. New York, Basic Books, 1983.
5. Bucek, L.: Constructing a child-centered dance curriculum. Journal of Physical Education, Recreation and Dance, 63(9):39, 1992.

6. DeBruyn, M.: Applications of arts propel in dance. Conference Proceedings of the 1991 Conference: Dance and the Child International, pp. 33–39. Salt Lake City, July 1991.

7. Seidel, S., and Walters, J.: The Design of Portfolios for Authentic Assessment. Cambridge, MA, Harvard University School of Education, 1991.

8. New Modes of Assessment: Workshop Handouts. Skidmore College, July 1991.

9. Smith, M.D.: Physical education in the British national curriculum. Journal of Physical Education, Recreation, and Dance, 63(9):21, 1993.

10. Department of Education and Science and the Welsh Office: Physical Education for Ages 5 to 16: Proposals for the Secretary of State for Education and Science and Secretary of State for Wales. London, Her Majesty's Stationery Office, 1991.

11. Van Gyn, G.H., and O'Neill, D.V.: Assessment of dance in education: introduction to the year 2000. Conference Proceeding of the 1991 Conference: Dance and the Child International, pp. 40–47. Salt Lake City, July 1991.

12. Consortium of National Arts Education Associations: National Standards for Arts Education. Reston, VA, Music Educators National Conference, 1994. (The Standards book can be ordered from MENC Publication Sales, 1806 Robert Fulton Drive, Reston, VA, 22091; 800-828-0229.)

13. Stinson, S.W.: Dance for Young Children: Finding the Magic in Movement. Reston, VA, American Alliance of Health, Physical Education, Recreation, and Dance, 1988.

SUGGESTED READING

The following sources are recommended for the reader who would like to learn more about assessment in dance education.

Allen, B.: Teaching training and discipline-based dance education. Journal of Physical Education, Recreation and Dance, 59(9):65, 1988.

Blaine, V., and Bucek, L.: Creating a public image for K-12 dance education. Design for Arts in Education, Jan/Feb:38, 1988.

Bucek, L., and Yoder, L.: Columbus K-12 Dance Course of Study. Columbus, OH, Columbus Public Schools, 1991.

Department of Education and Science and the Welsh Office: National Curriculum Physical Education Working Group Interim Report. London, Her Majesty's Stationery Office, 1991.

Gardner, H., and Hatch, T.: Multiple intelligences go to school. Educational Researcher, 18(8):4, 1989.

Gilbert, A.G.: Creative Dance for All Ages. Reston, VA, American Alliance of Health, Physical Education, Recreation, and Dance, 1992.

Kornhaber, M., Krechevsky, M., and Gardner, H.: Engaging intelligence. Educational Psychologist, 25(3, 4):177, 1990.

Krechevsky, M.: Project Spectrum: an innovative assessment alternative. Educational Leadership, 48(5):43, 1991.

Krechevsky, M., and Gardner, H.: The emergence and nurturance of multiple intelligences. In M.J.A. Howe (ed.): Encouraging the Development of Exceptional Abilities and Talents. Leicester, England, British Psychological Society, 1990.

Krechevsky, M., and Gardner, H.: Multiple intelligences, multiple chances. In D. Inbar (ed.): Second Chance in Education: An Interdisciplinary and International Perspective. Bristol, PA, Falmer Press, 1990.

Lloyd, M.: Adventures in Creative Movement Activities: A Guide for Teaching. Sdn. Bhd, Malaysia, Federal Publications, 1990.

Mitchell, R. (ed.): Measuring Up to the Challenge: What Standards and Assessment Can Do for Arts Education. New York, Americans for the Arts, 1994.

National Dance Association: Dance Education: What Is it? Why Is It Important? Reston, VA, American Alliance of Health, Physical Education, Recreation, and Dance, 1991.

Purcell, T.M.: Teaching Children Dance: Becoming a Master Teacher. Champaign, IL, Human Kinetics, 1994.

Ross, M. (ed.): Assessment in Arts Education: A Necessary Discipline or a Loss of Happiness? Elkins Park, PA, Franklin, 1986.

Stinson, S.: Dance Curricula Guidelines, K-12. Reston, VA, American Alliance of Health, Physical Education, Recreation, and Dance, 1988.

White, E., Bucek, L., and Mirus, J.: Dance Education Initiative: Curriculum Guide for Teachers. Golden Valley, MN, Minnesota Center for Arts in Education, 1992.

Winner, E.: Arts Propel: An Introductory Handbook. Cambridge, MA. Harvard Project Zero, June 1991.

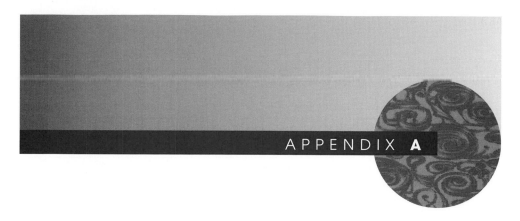

Selected Physical Fitness Test Batteries for Children and Adults

FITNESSGRAM

The FITNESSGRAM, developed by the Cooper Institute for Aerobics Research (CIAR), is a comprehensive health-related physical fitness assessment for kindergarten through college. FITNESSGRAM was endorsed by the American Alliance of Health, Physical Education, Recreation, and Dance (AAHPERD) in December 1993 as a replacement for the Physical Best fitness battery. The FITNESSGRAM is now promoted by the American Fitness Alliance as a collaborative project of CIAR, AAHPERD, and Human Kinetics Publishers.

The FITNESSGRAM system includes a test administration manual, software, computerized report forms, computer reference manual, and testing equipment. A complete technical reference manual and noncomputerized report forms are also available. The test administration manual includes suggested modifications for special populations. The American Fitness Alliance recommends that the FITNESSGRAM be used in partnership with the Physical Best fitness education system and the You Stay Active! behavior-oriented recognition system. To request the current American Fitness Alliance catalog or to order FITNESSGRAM, Physical Best, or You Stay Active! materials, please write or call:

The American Fitness Alliance
P.O. Box 5076
Champaign, IL 61825-5076
800-747-4457, ext. 2407

The FITNESSGRAM test battery is designed to assess three principal aspects of health-related physical fitness: aerobic capacity; body composition; and muscle strength, endurance, and flexibility. There are a total of six items, with alternative tests recommended for most items. Upper and lower criterion-based values are reported for the healthy fitness zone (HFZ). Examinees whose scores fall outside the HFZ are classified as needing improvement. Standards are given for both genders, ages 5 to 17 and adults.

Item 1: The Pacer

Purpose

The purpose of the Pacer is to assess aerobic capacity.

Psychometric Data

When compared with maximum oxygen uptake measures from maximal stress testing on a treadmill, concurrent validity coefficients ranged from .52 to .93. Test-retest reliability coefficients ranged from .89 to .98.

Facility Needs

The Pacer requires an outdoor or indoor running area with two lines marked by cones at a distance of 20 m (65 feet 8 inches).

Equipment

This test requires Pacer test audiotape with timed beeps or musical version (available for purchase from the American Fitness Alliance), cassette tape player, lap counter, cones, score sheets, and pencils.

Description

Examinees begin behind the starting line. A partner for each examinee is positioned to see and count laps. The examiner begins the tape. On the command to begin, examinees run to the opposite line. The examinees should pace their runs so they reach the opposite line in 9 seconds, at the first beep. Examinees touch the line, turn around, and run back toward the first line, again pacing their runs to reach the line in sync with the next beep. At the end of each minute the lap speed is increased; the increased pace is signaled to the examinees by a beep-beep-beep at the end of a lap. Examinees continue running back and forth between the lines until they can no longer maintain the pace. The test is terminated for an examinee when he or she fails to reach the opposite line in sync with the beep for three consecutive laps.

Scoring

For examinees aged 10 through 17 and adults, each completed lap is counted by the examinee's partner. Completed laps are converted to VO$_2$max values by the FIT-NESSGRAM software. Participation in the Pacer is recommended for children 5 to 9 years of age, but laps are not counted.

Evaluation

Tables A-1 and A-2 show HFZ standards for male and female participants.

Comments

Examinees must practice the timing for this test. The Pacer is especially useful for assessing the aerobic capacity of young children. Alternative tests of the mile run or the mile walk (as fast as possible while maintaining a constant walking pace) may be substituted for older children and adolescents. The FITNESSGRAM computer program converts the mile walk times to VO$_2$max values.

Item 2: Body Fat Skinfolds

Purpose

The purpose of this test is to assess body composition by measurement of skinfolds.

Psychometric Data

When compared with measures of body composition via underwater weighing, concurrent validity ranged from .70 to .90. Interrater consistency was more than .95.

Equipment

This measurement requires skinfold calipers.

Description

Skinfolds are measured at the triceps and the calf on the right side of the body (see Chapter 8). For students aged 17 and adults, the FITNESSGRAM offers an optional abdominal site measurement.

Scoring

Each skinfold is measured three times; the median value (middle score) is recorded. The skinfold values for the two or three sites are summed, then converted to percent body fat via the FITNESSGRAM computer program.

Evaluation

Tables A-1 and A-2 have HFZ standards for male and female participants.

Comments

The body mass index (BMI) may be used as an alternative test (see Chapter 8).

Item 3: Curl-up

Purpose

The purpose of this test is to assess strength and endurance of the abdominal muscles.

Psychometric Data

For several reasons the curl-up is believed to be a more valid measure of abdominal strength and endurance than the traditional sit-up. It eliminates use of the hip flexors, does not encourage use of poor form as the timed sit-up test does, and differences in body proportions affect the curl-up minimally.

Equipment

Mat; FITNESSGRAM curl-up strip (30 × 3 inches for 5- to 9-year-olds and 30 × 4.5 inches for children aged 10 to 17 and adults); audiotape of cadence and cassette player (drum or hand clap is okay).

Description

For mass testing, examinees are divided into groups of threes. The first examinee lies on the mat with knees bent and feet flat, arms and hands straight at the sides, with palms down and fingertips touching the near edge of the curl-up strip. One partner stands with both feet on the ends of the measuring strip; the other partner places both hands under the head of the examinee and counts the repetitions. Sliding the fingertips along the curl-up strip, the examinee curls up until the finger-

(text continues on page 696)

TABLE A-1   **FITNESSGRAM Standards for the HFZ for Males**

| AGE (yr) | ITEM 1 | | ITEM 2 | | ITEM 3 |
	PACER (LAPS)	MILE RUN (min:sec)	WALK TEST AND VO$_2$max (mL/kg/min)	SKINFOLDS (% BODY FAT)	BODY MASS INDEX (kg/m^2)	CURL-UPS (COMPLETE)
5	Participation	Complete run		25–10	20–14.7	2–10
6	Participation	Complete run		25–10	20–14.7	2–10
7	Participation	Complete run		25–10	20–14.9	4–14
8	Participation	Complete run		25–10	20–15.1	6–20
9	Participation	Complete run		25–10	20–15.2	9–24
10	23–61	11:30–9:00	42–52	25–10	21–15.3	12–24
11	23–72	11:00–8:30	42–52	25–10	21–15.8	15–28
12	32–72	10:30–8:00	42–52	25–10	22–16.0	18–36
13	41–72	10:00–7:30	42–52	25–10	23–16.6	21–40
14	41–83	9:30–7:00	42–52	25–10	24.5–17.5	24–45
15	51–94	9:00–7:00	42–52	25–10	25–18.1	24–47
16	61–94	8:30–7:00	42–52	25–10	26.5–18.5	24–47
17	61–94	8:30–7:00	42–52	25–10	27–18.8	24–47
17+	61–94	8:30–7:00	42–52	25–10	27.8–19.0	24–47

TABLE A-1   *(Continued)*

	ITEM 4		ITEM 5			ITEM 6	
AGE (yr)	TRUNK LIFT (in)	90° PUSH-UP (COMPLETE)	PULL-UP (COMPLETE)	FLEXED ARM HANG (sec)	MODIFIED PULL-UP (COMPLETE)	BACK SAVER SIT AND REACH (in)	SHOULDER STRETCH (PASS IF FINGERTIPS TOUCH; FAIL IF NOT)
5	6–12	3–8	1–2	2–8	2–7	±8	Fingertips touch
6	6–12	3–8	1–2	2–8	2–7	±8	Fingertips touch
7	6–12	4–10	1–2	3–8	3–9	±8	Fingertips touch
8	6–12	5–13	1–2	3–10	4–11	±8	Fingertips touch
9	6–12	6–15	1–2	4–10	5–11	±8	Fingertips touch
10	9–12	7–20	1–2	4–10	5–15	±8	Fingertips touch
11	9–12	8–20	1–3	6–13	6–17	±8	Fingertips touch
12	9–12	10–20	1–3	10–15	7–20	±8	Fingertips touch
13	9–12	12–25	1–4	12–17	8–22	±8	Fingertips touch
14	9–12	14–30	2–5	15–20	9–25	±8	Fingertips touch
15	9–12	16–35	3–7	15–20	10–27	±8	Fingertips touch
16	9–12	18–35	5–8	15–20	12–30	±8	Fingertips touch
17	9–12	18–35	5–8	15–20	14–30	±8	Fingertips touch
17+	9–12	18–35	5–8	15–20	14–30	±8	Fingertips touch

Number on left is lower limit of HFZ; *number on right* is upper limit of HFZ.

Reprinted with permission from The Cooper Institute for Aerobics Research: The Fitnessgram Test Administration Manual. Champaign, IL, Human Kinetics for the American Fitness Alliance, 1999, p. 26.

TABLE A-2 FitnessGRAM Standards for the HFZ for Females

AGE (yr)	ITEM 1				ITEM 2		ITEM 3
	PACER (LAPS)	MILE RUN (min:sec)	WALK TEST AND VO₂MAX (mL/kg/min)	SKINFOLDS (% BODY FAT)	BODY MASS INDEX (kg/m²)		CURL-UPS (COMPLETE)
5	Participation	Complete run		32–17	21–16.2		2–10
6	Participation	Complete run		32–17	21–16.2		2–10
7	Participation	Complete run		32–17	22–16.2		4–14
8	Participation	Complete run		32–17	22–16.2		6–20
9	Participation	Complete run		32–17	23–16.2		9–22
10	15–41	12:30–9:30	40–48	32–17	23.5–16.6		12–26
11	15–41	12:00–9:00	39–47	32–17	24–16.9		15–29
12	23–41	12:00–9:00	38–46	32–17	24.5–16.9		18–32
13	23–51	11:30–9:00	37–45	32–17	24.5–17.5		18–32
14	23–51	11:00–8:30	36–44	32–17	25–17.5		18–32
15	23–51	10:30–8:00	35–43	32–17	25–17.5		18–35
16	32–61	10:00–8:00	35–43	32–17	25–17.5		18–35
17	41–61	10:00–8:00	35–43	32–17	26–17.5		18–35
17+	41–61	10:00–8:00	35–43	32–17	27.3–18.0		18–35

TABLE A-2   *(Continued)*

AGE (yr)	ITEM 4 TRUNK LIFT (in)	ITEM 5 90° PUSH-UP (COMPLETE)	PULL-UP (COMPLETE)	FLEXED ARM HANG (sec)	MODIFIED PULL-UP (COMPLETE)	BACK SAVER SIT AND REACH (in)	ITEM 6 SHOULDER STRETCH (PASS IF FINGERTIPS TOUCH; FAIL IF NOT)
5	6–12	3–8	1–2	2–8	2–7	±9	Fingertips touch
6	6–12	3–8	1–2	2–8	2–7	±9	Fingertips touch
7	6–12	4–10	1–2	3–8	3–9	±9	Fingertips touch
8	6–12	5–13	1–2	3–10	4–11	±9	Fingertips touch
9	6–12	6–15	1–2	4–10	4–11	±9	Fingertips touch
10	9–12	7–15	1–2	4–10	4–13	±9	Fingertips touch
11	9–12	7–15	1–2	6–12	4–13	±10	Fingertips touch
12	9–12	7–15	1–2	7–12	4–13	±10	Fingertips touch
13	9–12	7–15	1–2	8–12	4–13	±10	Fingertips touch
14	9–12	7–15	1–2	8–12	4–13	±10	Fingertips touch
15	9–12	7–15	1–2	8–12	4–13	±12	Fingertips touch
16	9–12	7–15	1–2	8–12	4–13	±12	Fingertips touch
17	9–12	7–15	1–2	8–12	4–13	±12	Fingertips touch
17+	9–12	7–15	1–2	8–12	4–13	±12	Fingertips touch

Number on left is lower limit of HFZ; number on right is upper limit of HFZ.
Reprinted with permission from The Cooper Institute for Aerobics Research: The FitnessGram Test Administration Manual. Champaign, IL, Human Kinetics for the American Fitness Alliance, 1999, p. 26.

tips touch the far edge of the curl-up strip. He or she then lowers the upper body until the head touches the partner's hands on the mat. Repetitions are performed to a cadence of one curl-up each 3 seconds. The examinee continues to a maximum of 75 curl-ups or until too tired to do more.

Scoring
A curl-up is counted when the examinee's head returns to the partner's hands on the mat. The test score is the total number of curl-ups completed in sync with the cadence.

Evaluation
Tables A-1 and A-2 have HFZ standards for male and female participants.

Comments
When mass testing, partners must not obstruct the performance of the examinee. Partners must also keep an accurate count. Stop the test if the examinee has pain or discomfort.

Item 4: Trunk Lift

Purpose
The purpose of this test is to assess trunk extensor strength and flexibility.

Psychometric Data
Logical validity is claimed.

Equipment
This test requires a mat, ruler with colored tape at the 12-inch and 6-inch marks (9-inch mark for children aged 10 to 17 and adults).

Description
The examinee begins face down on the mat with hands under the thighs and toes pointed. The examinee lifts the head and upper body and holds the position until it can be measured. (The examinee should not be encouraged to lift higher than the 12-inch mark on the ruler.) The examiner measures to the nearest inch the distance from the floor to the examinee's chin. The examinee returns to the starting position. A second trial is administered. The higher of the two trial scores is recorded.

Scoring
The score is the greater height lifted for the two trials, recorded to the nearest inch. A score of 12 inches is recorded if the lift exceeds 12 inches.

Evaluation
Tables A-1 and A-2 have HFZ standards for male and female participants.

Comments
Despite requiring one-on-one testing, this test is very quick and easy to administer. The examiner should discourage overarching of the back.

Item 5: 90° Push-up

Purpose

The purpose of this test is to assess upper-body (shoulder girdle) strength and endurance.

Psychometric Data

Since most children can perform at least one 90° push-up, this test is believed to be more valid than the traditional pull-up test. Because many examinees cannot perform even a single pull-up, the validity of the traditional pull-up test is limited by this floor effect.

Equipment

This test requires a mat, audiotape with 20-beat-per-minute cadence, and cassette player.

Description

The examinee begins face down in a standard push-up position on the mat: hands under the shoulders, fingers straight, legs straight and parallel and slightly apart, and toes supporting the feet. The examinee straightens the arms while keeping the back and knees straight; he or she then lowers the body until there is a 90° angle at the elbows and upper arms are parallel to the mat. From this position the examinee performs as many push-ups as possible to the cadence of 20 per minute. The test ends when the examinee can no longer maintain the cadence with the correct positioning (three corrections are permitted), the examinee stops, or the examinee has pain.

Scoring

The test score is the number of correct repetitions.

Evaluation

Tables A-1 and A-2 have HFZ standards for male and female participants.

Comments

Some examinees have trouble maintaining the proper position. Examinees may be paired so one can monitor the form of the other during testing. The partner should kneel in front of the examinee for clear observation of the 90° elbow position. Partners can count for the examinee. Use of partners makes mass testing possible.

The FITNESSGRAM allows for three alternative tests: pull-ups (overhand grip), the flexed arm hang (overhand grip), or the Vermont modified pull-up (overhand grip). See the test administration manual for directions for these tests.

Item 6: Back Saver Sit and Reach

Purpose

The purpose of this test is to assess flexibility of the hamstring muscles.

Psychometric Data

Physical therapists recommend this version of the sit-and-reach test because the Back-Saver Sit-and-Reach Test is not likely to cause back or hamstring strain. Unlike the traditional sit-and-reach, however, the Back-Saver Sit-and-Reach Test assesses only hamstring flexibility, not lower back flexibility.

Equipment

Homemade or purchased sit-and-reach box 12 inches high with a ruler on top and the 9-inch mark even with the front surface of the box. (The zero point is toward the examinee.)

Description

The examinee removes shoes, then sits with one leg straight and foot flat against the front of the box. The other leg is bent with the foot flat on the floor about 2 to 3 inches from the inside of the straight leg. Hips are to be parallel to the box. The examinee places one hand on top of the other with palms down, then slowly slides the hands across the top of the box, reaching as far as possible. He or she relaxes briefly, then repeats three more times. On the fourth try the position is held for at least 1 second while the maximal distance reached is noted. The procedure is repeated for the opposite leg.

Scoring

A separate score to the nearest whole inch is recorded for each leg. Results are classified as either pass or fail.

Evaluation

Tables A-1 and A-2 have HFZ standards for male and female participants.

Comments

To prevent injuries and to maximize performances, examinees should warm up prior to taking this test. An alternative test is the shoulder stretch, in which examinees attempt to touch their fingertips together while reaching down over the shoulder with one hand and up along the back with the other hand. This is also performed on both sides and scored as pass-fail.

The Brockport Physical Fitness Test

The Brockport Physical Fitness Test is a criterion-referenced health-related physical fitness assessment battery for persons aged 10 through 17 who have physical and/or mental disabilities. This battery was developed through Project Target, a federally funded research study. Instructors can select from among 27 tests to create an individualized assessment appropriate for the student. Each test is described in detail in the test manual, along with criterion-referenced test selection guidelines and standards for assessing physical fitness. Supplementary materials include the Fitness Challenge software, technical manual, training guide, and test administration video. The Brockport Physical Fitness Test can be ordered from the American Fitness Alliance (Appendix B).

The President's Challenge

The President's Challenge, for students aged 6 through 17, is sponsored by the President's Council on Physical Fitness and Sports (PCPFS) and administered by the Amateur Athletic Union (AAU) and Indiana University. The President's Challenge battery consists of the following five tests: curl-ups or partial curl-ups; shuttle run; mile run or mile walk; pull-ups or right angle push-ups or flexed arm hang; V-sit reach or sit and reach.

Three levels of norm-based awards are given to individuals as part of the President's Challenge. The Presidential Physical Fitness Award is given to examinees who score at or above the 85th percentile on all five tests. An emblem for this award may be ordered with a number to signify consecutive years winning this award. The National Physical Fitness Award is given to boys and girls who score at or above the 50th percentile on all five tests. The Participant Physical Fitness Award is given to recognize examinees who attempt all five tests but whose scores fall below the 50th percentile on one or more of the tests. Based on enrollment categories, top performing schools may also receive the State Champion Award.

There is now an option for a criterion-referenced Health Fitness Award. This award is given for performance at or above the health criteria for the following five tests: partial curl-ups; mile run or mile walk; V-sit reach or sit and reach; right angle push-ups or pull-ups; and BMI. A convenient nomogram is provided to aid in determination of the BMI.

The manual for the President's Challenge includes guidelines for test accommodations for students with disabilities. The instructor is charged with substituting appropriate alternative test items and judging whether or not the student has performed at a level equivalent to a Presidential, National, Participant Physical Fitness, or the Health Fitness award level.

The President's Challenge Physical Fitness Packet and other support materials are free. Awards range in cost from $0.20 to $0.50 for certificates to $1.00 to $1.25 for emblems (Appendix B). All test directions and qualifying standards are available online from the PCPFS Web site at http://www.surgeongeneral.gov/ophs/pcpfs.htm. The packet and program awards may also be ordered online.

AAHPERD Health-Related Physical Fitness Test (College)

The AAHPERD Health-Related Physical Fitness Test was designed to assess the health-related fitness of college students who take classes in physical education. The battery includes four tests: a distance run of either 1 mile or 9 minutes; skinfolds at the triceps and subscapular sites; modified sit-ups; and the sit and reach. Standards are based on normative data from a large national sample of subjects. The data were collected prior to the publication date of the test manual in 1985; nonetheless, it is a useful test for many college-age populations. The test manual, *Health Related Physical Fitness Test: Norms for College Students,* with Pate as lead author (1985), is available from AAHPERD (Appendix B).

YMCA Physical Fitness Test Battery

The YMCA Physical Fitness Test Battery was designed to assess the health-related physical fitness of adults of both genders. Items include a bicycle ergometer test or step test of cardiorespiratory endurance; 3-site or 4-site skinfold assessment of body composition; a trunk flexion test of flexibility; a repeated bench press using a standard weight to assess muscular endurance; and a 1-minute sit-up test of abdominal endurance. Normative standards are provided in three categories: 35 and younger,

36 to 45 years old, and 46 and older. The test battery and norms are found in *The Y's Way to Physical Fitness*, by Golding, Myers, and Sinning (1982) from Human Kinetics (Appendix B).

AAHPERD Functional Fitness Assessment for Adults Over 60 Years

This is a field-based test of functional fitness, defined as the ability of the older person to perform ordinary and unexpected daily life activities safely and effectively. Test items include assessments of body composition, trunk and hamstring flexibility, agility and dynamic balance, eye-hand coordination, upper body muscular strength and endurance, and cardiorespiratory endurance during walking. Scores may be compared with norms based on gender and age. The tests may be repeated over time to indicate functional changes.

The test manual, *Functional Fitness Assessment for Adults Over 60 Years,* by Osness et al. (1996), and an accompanying video with demonstrations by men and women in their 80s can be ordered from AAHPERD (Appendix B).

The Canadian Standardized Test of Fitness (CSTF)

The Canadian Standardized Test of Fitness was developed as a simple, safe, and practical field test to evaluate the major components of fitness in apparently healthy adults aged 15 to 69 years of age. Before the test the Physical Activity Readiness Questionnaire (PAR-Q) (see Chapter 9) is to be given. The battery consists of the following: standardized measurements of anthropometry including height, weight, girths (chest, waist, hip, right thigh), and skinfolds (triceps, biceps, iliac crest, subscapular, and medial calf); aerobic fitness by administration of a two-step step test, the Canadian Aerobic Fitness Test (CAFT); and muscular strength, flexibility, and endurance by administration of a grip dynamometer strength test, a push-up test, a trunk forward flexion test, and a sit-up test. Gender- and age-appropriate norms are provided for ages 15 to 69.

The operations manual, interpretations manual, and copies of the PAR-Q may be ordered from the Canadian Society for Exercise Physiology (Appendix B).

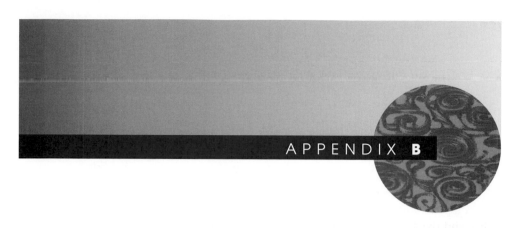

Selected Sources for Measurement and Assessment Resources: Equipment, Supplies, Books, Videos

AAHPERD
1900 Association Dr.
Reston, VA 20919
800-321-0789
http://www.aahperd.org

Testing books, videos, equipment, including manual and video for administering the *Functional Fitness Assessment for Adults Over 60 Years*, video on how to measure skinfolds, sport skill test manuals, *Dine Healthy* nutrition assessment software, *Softshare* catalog, and more. Standards for program evaluation. Source for periodicals, such as *Journal of Physical Education, Recreation and Dance, Research Quarterly for Exercise and Sport, Journal of Health Education*.

American Fitness Alliance
P.O. Box 5076
Champaign, IL 61825-5076
800-747-4457, ext. 2407

Source for FITNESSGRAM, *Physical Best*, and *You Stay Active!* materials. Also source for *The Brockport Physical Fitness Test* materials.

Best Priced Products, Inc.
P.O. Box 1174
White Plains, NY 10602
800-824-2939

Wide variety of fitness testing equipment.

Cambridge Scientific Industries
P.O. Box 265
Cambridge, MD 21613
800-638-9566

Source of Lange calipers and other equipment.

Canadian Society for Exercise
   Physiology
1600 James Naismith, Suite 311
Gloucester, Ontario, CANADA
K1B 5N4
613-748-5768

Source for the *Physical Activity Readiness Questionnaire (PAR-Q)* and materials for the *Canadian Standardized Test of Fitness*.

Computech Software
P.O. Box 107
Waconia, MN 55387
800-343-2406

Computer software for fitness testing and health monitoring, including software for *The President's Challenge*.

Consentius Technologies
8152 South 1715 East
Sandy, UT 84093
800-942-7255
yeh@xmission.com

Aerobic and metabolic testing equipment.

Country Technology, Inc.
P.O. Box 87
Gays Mills, WI 54631
608-735-4718
www.fitnessmart.com

Wide variety of fitness testing equipment.

Creative Health Products
5148 Saddle Ridge Road
Plymouth, MI 48170
800-742-4478

Wide variety of fitness testing equipment and books.

Cybex
2100 Smithtown
Ronkonkoma, NY 11779-0903
516-585-9000

Electronic and computerized testing, especially muscle strength testing.

Futrex, Inc.
P.O. Box 2398
Gaithersburg, MO 20886
800-255-4206

Body composition testing equipment.

Human Kinetics U.S.
P.O. Box 5076
Champaign, IL 61825-5076
800-747-4457
www.humankinetics.com

Books and videos for fitness and sport skill assessment for children and adults of all ages; also practice examination booklet and video for the *Certified Strength and Conditioning Specialist* certification from NCSA,

Human Kinetics Canada
475 Devonshire Rd.
Unit 100
Windsor, Ontario N8Y 2L5
800-465-7301

all YMCA fitness and sport materials such as *Y's Way to Fitness* (adult fitness testing and programming) and the *YMCA Youth Fitness Test Manual*, books from the American College of Sports Medicine, and more. Many periodicals, such as *Journal of Teaching in Physical Education* and *Journal of Sport Management*.

Calls outside the United States
    and Canada
217-351-5076

Lawrence Erlbaum Associates, Inc.
Journal Subscription Dept.
10 Industrial Ave.
Mahwah, NJ 07430-2262

Source of research periodical *Measurement in Physical Education and Exercise Science*.

Life Measurement Instruments
1980 Olivera Rd., Suite C
Concord, CA 94520
800-4 BOD POD (800-426-3763)

Source of the Bod Pod body composition system.

Monark
5612 North Western Ave.
Chicago, IL 60659
312 271 2555

Electronic testing equipment, especially bike ergometers and rowers.

Novel Products, Inc.
P.O. Box 408
Rockton, IL 61072
800-323-5143
NovelProd@aol.com

Wide variety of fitness testing equipment, including calipers, blood pressure cuffs, stethoscopes, heart rate monitors, goniometers, dynamometers, measuring tapes, scales, stopwatches, reaction time sticks, curl-up tester, flexibility tester, and more.

OARSP
Ball State University
2000 University Ave.
Muncie, IN 47306
888-278-4615

Set of 12 videotapes to help students develop observational and assessment skills in fundamental locomotor and manipulative skills. Also a set of 9 videotapes on assessment of common sports skills.

Paramount Fitness Equipment
6450 E. Bandini Blvd.
Los Angeles, CA 90040
800-421-6242

Weight training equipment, exercise cycles, treadmills, rowers.

Physio-Dyne Instrument Corp.
P.O. Box 5025
Quogue, NY 11959
physiodyne@pb.net
http://www.pb.net/~physio-dyne

Aerobic and metabolic testing equipment.

Polar CIC, Inc.
99 Seaview Blvd.
Port Washington, NY 11050
800-227-1314

Heart rate monitors.

The President's Challenge
Poplars Research Center
400 East 7th Street
Bloomington, IN 47405
800-258-8146
preschal@indiana.edu
http://www.indiana.edu/~preschal

Source for *The President's Challenge* test materials. Also distributes the *President's Council on Physical Fitness and Sports Digest*.

Quinton Instrument Co.
2121 Terry Ave.
Seattle, WA 98121-2791
800-426-0337

Electronic testing equipment, especially treadmills and bike ergometers.

Universal Gym Equipment, Inc.
P.O. Box 1270
Cedar Rapids, IA 52406
800-843-390

Weight training equipment, exercise cycles, treadmills, rowers.

Valhalla Scientific, Inc.
7576 Trade St.
San Diego, CA 92121
800-395-4565

Electronic body composition testing equipment.

Wellsource, Inc.
P.O. Box 569
Clackamas, OR 97015
800-533-9355

Computer software for fitness testing and health monitoring, including software for the *Canadian Standardized Test of Fitness*.

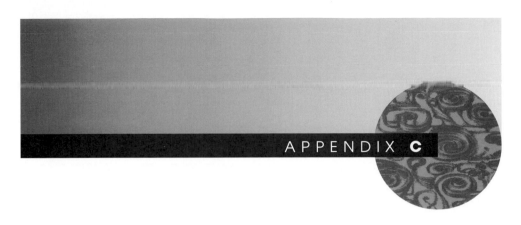

Web Sites and ListServes
for Exercise and Sport

Web Sites

Name of Organization	URL
A	
Abilities Expo	http://www.abilitiesexpo.com
Aerobics and Fitness Association of America	http://www.afaa.com
ALLSPORTS	http://204.96.64.161/allsports/ welcome.htm
Amateur Athletic Union	http://www.aausports.org
American Alliance for Health, Physical Education, Recreation and Dance	http://www.aahperd.org
American Association for Active Lifestyles and Fitness	http://www.aahperd.org/aaalf.html
American Association for Health Education	http://www.aahperd.org/aahe.html
American Association for Leisure and Recreation	http://www.aahperd.org/aalr.html
American College of Sports Medicine	http://www.acsm.org
American Diabetes Association	http://www.diabetes.org
American Heart Association	http://www.americanheart.org
American Medical Association	http://www.ama-assn.org
American Orthopaedic Society for Sports Medicine	http://www.sportsmed.org
American Physical Therapy Association	http://www.apta.org
American Running and Fitness Association	http://www.arfa.com
American Stroke Association	http://www.amhrt.org/Stroke/ index.htm
Aquatic Exercise Association	http://aeawave.com
Association for Worksite Health Promotion	http://www.awhp.org

C

Canadian Athletic Therapists Association	http://www.mtroyal.ab.ca/CATA
Canadian Association for Health, Physical Education, Recreation and Dance	http://www.activeliving.ca/cahperd
Canadian Sport and Fitness Administration Centre	http://www.cdnsport.ca/centre
Centers for Disease Control and Prevention	http://www.cdc.gov
Cooper Institute for Aerobics Research	http://www.cooperinst.org
Council for Exceptional Children	http://www.cec.sped.org
Cyber Active	http://www.tc.umn.edu

E

Educational Resources Information Center Clearinghouse on Assessment and Education	http://ericae.net

F

Fitness World	http://www.fitnessworld.com

G

Gatorade Sports Science Institute	http://www.gssiweb.com

H

Healthy People 2010	http://web.health.gov/healthy people

I

International Association of Physical Activity, Aging and Sports	http://www.members.aol.com/iapaas
International Health, Racquet and Sportsclub Association	http://www.ihrsa.org

L

Ladies Professional Golf Association	http://www.lpga.com

N

National Association for Girls and Women in Sport	http://www.aahperd.org/nagws.html
National Association for Sport and Physical Education	http://www.aahperd.org/naspe.html
National Association of Activity Professionals	http://www.naap.org
National Association of Governor's Councils on Physical Fitness and Sports	http://www.fitnesslink.com/Govcouncil
National Athletic Trainers Association	http://www.nata.org
National Coalition for Promoting Physical Activity	http://www.ncppa.org

National Council for International Health	http://www.ncih.org
National Dance Association	http://www.aahperd.org/nda.html
National Heart, Lung and Blood Institute	http://www.nhlbi.nih.gov
National Hockey League	http://www.nhl.org
National Institutes of Health	http://www.nih.gov
National Operating Committee on Standards for Athletic Equipment	http://www.nocsae.org
National Recreation and Park Association	http://www.nrpa.org
National Strength and Conditioning Association	http://www.nsca-lift.org
National Youth Sports Safety Foundation	http://www.nyssf.org

O

Office of Public Health and Science	http://www.surgeongeneral.gov/ophs

P

PE Central	http://pe.central.vt.edu
Physician and Sportsmedicine Online	http://www.physsportsmed.com
President's Council on Physical Fitness and Sports	http://www.surgeongeneral.gov/ophs/pcpfs.htm
President's Council on Physical Fitness and Sports Research Digest	http://www.indiana.edu/~preschal
Professional Golfers' Association of America	http://www.pga.org

S

Sport Information Resource Centre	http://www.SPORTQuest.com
Sporting Goods Manufacturers Association	http://www.sgma.org

U

United States Olympic Committee	http:www.usoc.org
United States Golf Association	http://www.usga.org
United States Professional Tennis Association	http://www.uspta.org
U.S. Sports Academy	http://www.sport.ussa.edu

W

Wellness Councils of America	http://www.welcoa.org
Women's National Basketball Association	http://www.wnba.com
Women's Sports Foundation	http://www.lifetimetv.com/WoSport
World Wide Web of Sports	http://www.tns.lcs.mit.edu/cgi-bin/sports

Y

Young Men's Christian Association	http://www.ymca.net
Young Women's Christian Association	http://www.ywca.org

ListServes

ListServe	How to Subscribe
ADAPT-TALK—adapted physical education and physical activity	Go to http://www.sportime.com; click on APENS
CUAC—college and university administrative issues	Send e-mail message to Hilsend@ASTRO.Temple.edu and ask to be added to the ListServe list
HEAT—technology use in health education	Send e-mail message to listproc@unc.edu with subject box blank and "subscribe heat firstname lastname" in the first line of message
HEDIR—international health education	Go to http://www.siu.edu/~kittle/HEDIR/Menu.html
HLTHPROM—health promotion	Send e-mail message to listserver@relay.doit.wisc.edu with "subscribe hlthprom" in the subject box
PE-TALK DIGEST—physical education issues	Go to Sport Time web site at http://www.sportime.com

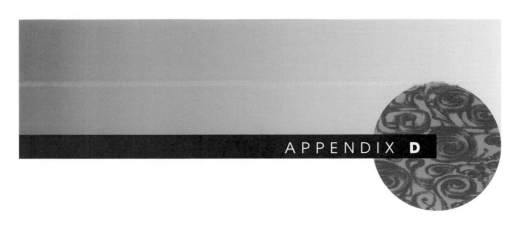

Compendium of Physical Activities

Part 1: Standardized MET Intensity Levels

CODE	MET	CATEGORY	ACTIVITY
01009	8,5	Bicycling,	Bicycling, BMX or mountain
01010	4.0	Bicycling,	Bicycling, <10 mph, general, leisure, to work or for pleasure (T 115)
01020	6.0	Bicycling,	Bicycling, 10–11.9 mph, leisure, slow, light effort
01030	8.0	Bicycling,	Bicycling, 12–13.9 mph, leisure, moderate effort
01040	10.0	Bicycling,	Bicycling, 14–15.9 mph, racing or leisure, fast, vigorous effort
01050	12.0	Bicycling,	Bicycling, 16–19 mph, racing/not drafting or >19 mph drafting, very fast, racing general
01060	16.0	Bicycling,	Bicycling, >20 mph, racing, not drafting
01070	5.0	Bicycling,	Unicycling
02010	5.0	Conditioning exercise,	Bicycling, stationary, general
02011	3.0	Conditioning exercise,	Bicycling, stationary, 50 W, very light effort
02012	5.5	Conditioning exercise,	Bicycling, stationary, 100 W, light effort
02013	7.0	Conditioning exercise,	Bicycling, stationary, 150 W, moderate effort
02014	10.5	Conditioning exercise,	Bicycling, stationary, 200 W, vigorous effort
02015	12.5	Conditioning exercise,	Bicycling, stationary, 250 W, very vigorous effort
02020	8.0	Conditioning exercise,	Calisthenics (e.g., pushups, pullups, situps), heavy, vigorous effort
02030	4.5	Conditioning exercise,	Calisthenics home exercise, light or moderate effort, general (T 150) (example: back exercises), going up & down from floor
02040	8.0	Conditioning exercise,	Circuit training, general
02050	6.0	Conditioning exercise,	Weight lifting (free weight, nautilus or universal-type), power lifting or body building, vigorous effort (T 210)
02060	5.5	Conditioning exercise,	Health club exercise, general (T 160)
02065	6.0	Conditioning exercise,	Stair-treadmill ergometer, general
02070	9.5	Conditioning exercise,	Rowing, stationary ergometer, general
02071	3.5	Conditioning exercise,	Rowing, stationary, 50 W, light effort
02072	7.0	Conditioning exercise,	Rowing, stationary, 100 W, moderate effort
02073	8.5	Conditioning exercise,	Rowing, stationary, 150 W, vigorous effort
02074	12.0	Conditioning exercise,	Rowing, stationary, 200 W, very vigorous effort
02080	9.5	Conditioning exercise,	Ski machine, general
02090	6.0	Conditioning exercise,	Slimnastics
02100	4.0	Conditioning exercise,	Stretching, hatha yoga
02110	6.0	Conditioning exercise,	Teaching aerobic exercise class
02120	4.0	Conditioning exercise,	Water aerobics, water calisthenics
02130	3.0	Conditioning exercise,	Weight lifting (free, nautilus or universal-type), light or moderate effort, light workout, general
02135	1.0	Conditioning exercise,	Whirlpool, sitting

03010	6.0	Dancing,	Aerobic, ballet or modern, twist
03015	6.0	Dancing,	Aerobic, general
03020	5.0	Dancing,	Aerobic, low impact
03021	7.0	Dancing,	Aerobic, high impact
03025	4.5	Dancing,	General
03030	5.5	Dancing,	Ballroom, fast (disco, folk, square) (T 125)
03040	3.0	Dancing,	Ballroom, slow (e.g., waltz, foxtrot, slow dancing)
04001	4.0	Fishing and hunting,	Fishing, general
04010	4.0	Fishing and hunting,	Digging worms, with shovel
04020	5.0	Fishing and hunting,	Fishing from river bank and walking
04030	2.5	Fishing and hunting,	Fishing from boat, sitting
04040	3.5	Fishing and hunting,	Fishing from river bank, standing (T 660)
04050	6.0	Fishing and hunting,	Fishing in stream, in waders (T 670)
04060	2.0	Fishing and hunting,	Fishing, ice, sitting
04070	2.5	Fishing and hunting,	Hunting, bow and arrow or crossbow
04080	6.0	Fishing and hunting,	Hunting, deer, elk, large game (T 710)
04090	2.5	Fishing and hunting,	Hunting, duck, wading
04100	5.0	Fishing and hunting,	Hunting, general
04110	6.0	Fishing and hunting,	Hunting, pheasants or grouse (T 680)
04120	5.0	Fishing and hunting,	Hunting, rabbit, squirrel, prairie chick, raccoon, small game (T 690)
04130	2.5	Fishing and hunting,	Pistol shooting or trap shooting, standing
05010	2.5	Home activities,	Carpet sweeping, sweeping floors
05020	4.5	Home activities,	Cleaning, heavy or major (e.g., wash car, wash windows, mop, clean garage), vigorous effort
05030	3.5	Home activities,	Cleaning, house or cabin, general
05040	2.5	Home activities,	Cleaning, light (dusting, straightening up, vacuuming, changing linen, carrying out trash), moderate effort
05041	2.3	Home activities,	Wash dishes-standing or in general (not broken into stand/walk components)
	2.3	Home activities,	Wash dishes, clearing dishes from table-walking
05050	2.5	Home activities,	Cooking or food preparation-standing or sitting or in general (not broken into stand/walk components)
05051	2.5	Home activities,	Serving food, setting table-implied walking or standing
05052	2.5	Home activities,	Cooking or food preparation-walking
05055	2.5	Home activities,	Putting away groceries (e.g., carrying groceries, shopping without a grocery cart)
05056	8.0	Home activities,	Carrying groceries upstairs
05060	3.5	Home activities,	Food shopping, with grocery cart
05065	2.0	Home activities,	Standing-shopping (non-grocery shopping)
05066	2.3	Home activities,	Walking-shopping (non-grocery shopping)
05070	2.3	Home activities,	Ironing
05080	1.5	Home activities,	Sitting, knitting, sewing, light wrapping (presents)
05090	2.0	Home activities,	Implied standing-laundry, fold or hang clothes, put clothes in washer or dryer, packing suitcase
05095	2.3	Home activities,	Implied walking-putting away clothes, gathering clothes to pack, putting away laundry
05100	2.0	Home activities,	Making bed
05110	5.0	Home activities,	Maple syruping/sugar bushing (including carrying buckets, carrying wood)
05120	6.0	Home activities,	Moving furniture, household
05130	5.5	Home activities,	Scrubbing floors, on hands and knees
05140	4.0	Home activities,	Sweeping garage, sidewalk or outside of house
05145	7.0	Home activities,	Moving household items, carrying boxes
05146	3.5	Home activities,	Standing-packing/unpacking boxes, occasional lifting of household items light-moderate effort
05147	3.0	Home activities,	Implied walking-putting away household items-moderate effort
05150	9.0	Home activities,	Move household items upstairs, carrying boxes or furniture
05160	2.5	Home activities,	Standing-light (pump gas, change light bulb, etc.)
05165	3.0	Home activities,	Walking-light noncleaning (ready to leave, shut/ lock doors, close windows, etc.)
05170	2.5	Home activities,	Sitting-playing with child(ren)-light
05171	2.8	Home activities,	Standing-playing with child(ren)-light
05175	4.0	Home activities,	Walk/run-playing with child(ren)-moderate
05180	5.0	Home activities,	Walk/run-playing with child(ren)-vigorous
05185	3.0	Home activities,	Child care: sitting/kneeling-dressing, bathing, grooming, feeding, occasional lifting of child-light effort

05186	3.5	Home activities,	Child care: standing-dressing, bathing, grooming, feeding, occasional lifting of child-light effort
06010	3.0	Home repair,	Airplane repair
06020	4.5	Home repair,	Automobile body work
06030	3.0	Home repair,	Automobile repair
06040	3.0	Home repair,	Carpentry, general, workshop (T 620)
06050	6.0	Home repair,	Carpentry, outside house (T 640), installing rain gutters
06060	4.5	Home repair,	Carpentry, finishing or refinishing cabinets or furniture
06070	7.5	Home repair,	Carpentry, sawing hardwood
06080	5.0	Home repair,	Caulking, chinking log cabin
06090	4.5	Home repair,	Caulking, except log cabin
06100	5.0	Home repair,	Cleaning gutters
06110	5.0	Home repair,	Excavating garage
06120	5.0	Home repair,	Hanging storm windows
06130	4.5	Home repair,	Laying or removing carpet
06140	4.5	Home repair,	Laying tile or linoleum
06150	5.0	Home repair,	Painting, outside house (T 650)
06160	4.5	Home repair,	Painting, papering, plastering, scraping, inside house, hanging sheet rock, remodeling (T 630)
06170	3.0	Home repair,	Put on and removal of tarp-sailboat
06180	6.0	Home repair,	Roofing
06190	4.5	Home repair,	Sanding floors with a power sander
06200	4.5	Home repair,	Scrape and paint sailboat or powerboat
06210	5.0	Home repair,	Spreading dirt with a shovel
06220	4.5	Home repair,	Wash and wax hull of sailboat, car, powerboat, airplane
06230	4.5	Home repair,	Washing fence
06240	3.0	Home repair,	Wiring, plumbing
07010	0.9	Inactivity, quiet	Lying quietly, reclining (watch television), lying quietly in bed-awake
07020	1.0	Inactivity, quiet	Sitting quietly (riding in a car, listening to a lecture or music, watch television or a movie)
07030	0.9	Inactivity, quiet	Sleeping
07040	1.2	Inactivity, quiet	Standing quietly (standing in a line)
07050	1.0	Inactivity, light	Recline-writing
07060	1.0	Inactivity, light	Reclining-talking or talking on phone
07070	1.0	Inactivity, light	Recline-reading
08010	5.0	Lawn and garden,	Carrying, loading or stacking wood, loading/ unloading or carrying lumber
08020	6.0	Lawn and garden,	Chopping wood, splitting logs
08030	5.0	Lawn and garden,	Clearing land, hauling branches
08040	5.0	Lawn and garden,	Digging sandbox
08050	5.0	Lawn and garden,	Digging, spading, filling garden (T 590)
08060	6.0	Lawn and garden,	Gardening with heavy power tools, tilling a garden (see occupation, shoveling)
08080	5.0	Lawn and garden,	Laying crushed rock
08090	5.0	Lawn and garden,	Laying sod
08095	5.5	Lawn and garden,	Mowing lawn, general
08100	2.5	Lawn and garden,	Mowing lawn, riding mower (T 550)
08110	6.0	Lawn and garden,	Mowing lawn, walk, hand mower (T 570)
08120	4.5	Lawn and garden,	Mowing lawn, walk, power mower (T 590)
08130	4.5	Lawn and garden,	Operating snow blower, walking
08140	4.0	Lawn and garden,	Planting seedlings, shrubs
08150	4.5	Lawn and garden,	Planting trees
08160	4.0	Lawn and garden,	Raking lawn (T 600)
08170	4.0	Lawn and garden,	Raking room with snow rake
08180	3.0	Lawn and garden,	Riding snow blower
08190	4.0	Lawn and garden,	Sacking grass, leaves
08200	6.0	Lawn and garden,	Shoveling, snow, by hand (T 610)
08210	4.5	Lawn and garden,	Trimming shrubs or trees, manual cutter
08215	3.5	Lawn and garden,	Trimming shrubs or trees, power cutter
08220	2.5	Lawn and garden,	Walking, applying fertilizer or seeding a lawn
08230	1.5	Lawn and garden,	Watering lawn or garden, standing or walking
08240	4.5	Lawn and garden,	Weeding, cultivating gardem (T 580)
08245	5.0	Lawn and garden,	Gardening, general
08250	3.0	Lawn and garden,	Implied walking/standing-picking up yard, light
09010	1.5	Miscellaneous,	Sitting, card playing, playing board games
09020	2.0	Miscellaneous,	Standing-drawing (writing), casino gambling
09030	1.3	Miscellaneous,	Sitting-reading, book, newspaper, etc.
09040	1.8	Miscellaneous,	Sitting-writing, desk work

09050	1.8	Miscellaneous,	Standing-talking or talking on phone
09055	1.5	Miscellaneous,	Sitting-talking or talking on phone
09060	1.8	Miscellaneous,	Sitting-studying, general, including reading and/or writing
09065	1.8	Miscellaneous,	Sitting-in class, general, including notetaking or class discussion
09070	1.8	Miscellaneous,	Standing-reading
10010	1.8	Music playing,	Accordion
10020	2.0	Music playing,	Cello
10030	2.5	Music playing,	Conducting
10040	4.0	Music playing,	Drums
10050	2.0	Music playing,	Flute (sitting)
10060	2.0	Music playing,	Horn
10070	2.5	Music playing,	Piano or organ
10080	3.5	Music playing,	Trombone
10090	2.5	Music playing,	Trumpet
10100	2.5	Music playing,	Violin
10110	2.0	Music playing,	Woodwind
10120	2.0	Music playing,	Guitar, classical, folk (sitting)
10125	3.0	Music playing,	Guitar, rock and roll band (standing)
10130	4.0	Music playing,	Marching band, playing an instrument, baton twirling (walking)
10135	3.5	Music playing,	Marching band, drum major (walking)
11010	4.0	Occupation,	Bakery, general
11020	2.3	Occupation,	Bookbinding
11030	6.0	Occupation,	Building road (including hauling debris, driving heavy machinery)
11035	2.0	Occupation,	Building road, directing traffic (standing)
11040	3.5	Occupation,	Carpentry, general
11050	8.0	Occupation,	Carrying heavy loads, such as bricks
11060	8.0	Occupation,	Carrying moderate loads up stairs, moving boxes (16–40 pounds)
11070	2.5	Occupation,	Chambermaid
11080	6.5	Occupation,	Coal mining, drilling coal, rock
11090	6.5	Occupation,	Coal mining, erecting supports
11100	6.0	Occupation,	Coal mining, general
11110	7.0	Occupation,	Coal mining, shoveling coal
11120	5.5	Occupation,	Construction, outside, remodeling
11130	3.5	Occupation,	Electrical work, plumbing
11140	8.0	Occupation,	Farming, baling hay, cleaning barn, poultry work
11150	3.5	Occupation,	Farming, chasing cattle, nonstrenuous
11160	2.5	Occupation,	Farming, driving harvester
11170	2.5	Occupation,	Farming, driving tractor
11180	4.0	Occupation,	Farming, feeding small animals
11190	4.5	Occupation,	Farming, feeding cattle
11200	8.0	Occupation,	Farming, forking straw bales
11210	3.0	Occupation,	Farming, milking by hand
11220	1.5	Occupation,	Farming, milking by machine
11230	5.5	Occupation,	Farming, shoveling grain
11240	12.0	Occupation,	Fire fighter, general
11245	11.0	Occupation,	Fire fighter, climbing ladder with full gear
11246	8.0	Occupation,	Fire fighter, hauling hoses on ground
11250	17.0	Occupation,	Forestry, ax chopping, fast
11260	5.0	Occupation,	Forestry, ax chopping, slow
11270	7.0	Occupation,	Forestry, barking trees
11280	11.0	Occupation,	Forestry, carrying logs
11290	8.0	Occupation,	Forestry, felling trees
11300	8.0	Occupation,	Forestry, general
11310	5.0	Occupation,	Forestry, hoeing
11320	6.0	Occupation,	Forestry, planting by hand
11330	7.0	Occupation,	Forestry, sawing by hand
11340	4.5	Occupation,	Forestry, sawing, power
11350	9.0	Occupation,	Forestry, trimming trees
11360	4.0	Occupation,	Forestry, weeding
11370	4.5	Occupation,	Furriery
11380	6.0	Occupation,	Horse grooming
11390	8.0	Occupation,	Horse racing, galloping
11400	6.5	Occupation,	Horse racing, trotting
11410	2.6	Occupation,	Horse racing, walking
11420	3.5	Occupation,	Locksmith
11430	2.5	Occupation,	Machine tooling, machining, working sheet metal
11440	3.0	Occupation,	Machine tooling, operating lathe
11450	5.0	Occupation,	Machine tooling, operating punch press

11460	4.0	Occupation,	Machine tooling, tapping and drilling
11470	3.0	Occupation,	Machine tooling, welding
11480	7.0	Occupation,	Masonry, concrete
11486	4.0	Occupation,	Masseur, masseuse (standing)
11490	7.0	Occupation,	Moving, pushing heavy objects, 75 lbs or more (desks, moving van work)
11500	2.5	Occupation,	Operating heavy equipment/automated, not driving
11510	4.5	Occupation,	Orange grove worker
11520	2.3	Occupation,	Printing (standing)
11525	2.5	Occupation,	Police, directing traffic (standing)
11526	2.0	Occupation,	Police, driving a squad car (sitting)
11527	1.3	Occupation,	Police, riding in a squad car (sitting)
11528	8.0	Occupation,	Police, making an arrest (standing)
11530	2.5	Occupation,	Shoe repair, general
11540	8.5	Occupation,	Shoveling, digging ditches
11550	9.0	Occupation,	Shoveling, heavy (more than 16 lbs·min^{-1})
11560	6.0	Occupation,	Shoveling, light (less than 10 lbs·min^{-1})
11570	7.0	Occupation,	Shoveling, moderate (10–15 lbs·min^{-1})
11580	1.5	Occupation,	Sitting-light office work, in general (chemistry lab work, light use of handtools, watch repair or micro-assembly, light assembly/repair)
11585	1.5	Occupation,	Sitting-meetings, general, and/or with talking involved
11590	2.5	Occupation,	Sitting; moderate (heavy levers, riding mower/ forklift, crane operation)
11600	2.5	Occupation,	Standing; light (bartending, store clerk, assembling, filing, xeroxing, put up Christmas tree)
11610	3.0	Occupation,	Standing; light/moderate (assemble/repair heavy parts, welding, stocking, auto repair, pack boxes for moving, etc.), patient care (as in nursing)
11620	3.5	Occupation,	Standing; moderate (assembling at fast rate, lifting 50 lbs, hitch/twisting ropes)
11630	4.0	Occupation,	Standing; moderate/heavy (lifting more than 50 lb, masonry, painting, paper hanging)
11640	5.0	Occupation,	Steel mill, fettling
11650	5.5	Occupation,	Steel mill, forging
11660	8.0	Occupation,	Steel mill, hand rolling
11670	8.0	Occupation,	Steel mill, merchant mill rolling
11680	11.0	Occupation,	Steel mill, removing slag
11690	7.5	Occupation,	Steel mill, tending furnace
11700	5.5	Occupation,	Steel mill, tipping molds
11710	8.0	Occupation,	Steel mill, working in general
11720	2.5	Occupation,	Tailoring, cutting
11730	2.5	Occupation,	Tailoring, general
11740	2.0	Occupation,	Tailoring, hand sewing
11750	2.5	Occupation,	Tailoring, machine sewing
11760	4.0	Occupation,	Tailoring, pressing
11766	6.5	Occupation,	Truck driving, loading and unloading truck (standing)
11770	1.5	Occupation,	Typing, electric, manual or computer
11780	6.0	Occupation,	Using heaving power tools such as pneumatic tools (jackhammers, drills, etc.)
11790	8.0	Occupation,	Using heavy tools (not power) such as shovel, pick, tunnel bar, spade
11791	2.0	Occupation,	Walking on job, less than 2.0 mph (in office or lab area), very slow
11792	3.5	Occupation,	Walking on job, 3.0 mph, in office, moderate speed, not carrying anything
11793	4.0	Occupation,	Walking on job, 3.5 mph, in office, brisk speed, not carrying anything
11795	3.0	Occupation,	Walking, 2.5 mph, slowly and carrying light objects less than 25 lbs
11800	4.0	Occupation,	Walking, 3.0 mph, moderately and carrying light objects less than 25 lbs
11810	4.5	Occupation,	Walking, 3.5 mph, briskly and carrying light objects less than 25 lbs
11820	5.0	Occupation,	Walking or walk downstairs or standing, carrying objects about 25–49 lbs
11830	6.5	Occupation,	Walking or walk downstairs or standing, carrying objects about 50–74 lbs
11840	7.5	Occupation,	Walking or walk downstairs or standing, carrying objects about 75–99 lbs

11850	8.5	Occupation,	Walking or walk downstairs or standing, carrying objects about 100 lbs and over
11870	3.0	Occupation,	Working in scene shop, theater actor, backstage, employee
12010	6.0	Running,	Jog/walk combination (jogging component of less than 10 min) (T 180)
12020	7.0	Running,	Jogging, general
12030	8.0	Running,	Running, 5 mph (12 min·mile^{-1})
12040	9.0	Running,	Running, 5.2 mph (11.5 min·mile^{-1})
12050	10.0	Running,	Running, 6 mph (10 min·mile^{-1})
12060	11.0	Running,	Running, 6.7 mph (9 min·mile^{-1})
12070	11.5	Running,	Running, 7 mph (8.5 min·mile^{-1})
12080	12.5	Running,	Running, 7.5 mph (8 min·mile^{-1})
12090	13.5	Running,	Running, 8 mph (7.5 min·mile^{-1})
12100	14.0	Running,	Running, 8.6 mph (7 min·mile^{-1})
12110	15.0	Running,	Running, 9 mph (6.5 min·mile^{-1})
12120	16.0	Running,	Running, 10 mph (6 min·mile^{-1})
12130	18.0	Running,	Running, 10.9 mph (5.5 min·mile^{-1})
12140	9.0	Running,	Running, cross-country
12150	8.0	Running,	Running, general (T 200)
12160	8.0	Running,	Running, in place
12170	15.0	Running,	Running, stairs, up
12180	10.0	Running,	Running, on a track, team practice
12190	8.0	Running,	Running, training, pushing wheelchair, marathon wheeling
12195	3.0	Running,	Running, wheeling, general
13000	2.5	Self-care,	Standing-getting ready for bed, in general
13009	1.0	Self-care,	Sitting on toilet
13010	2.0	Self-care,	Bathing (sitting)
13020	2.5	Self-care,	Dressing, undressing (standing or sitting)
13030	1.5	Self-care,	Eating (sitting)
13035	2.0	Self-care,	Talking and eating or eating only (standing)
13040	2.5	Self-care,	Sitting or standing-grooming (washing, shaving, brushing teeth, urinating, washing hands, put on make-up)
13050	4.0	Self-care,	Showering, toweling off (standing)
14010	1.5	Sexual activity,	Active, vigorous effort
14020	1.3	Sexual activity,	General, moderate effort
14030	1.0	Sexual activity,	Passive, light effort, kissing, hugging
15010	3.5	Sports,	Archery (nonhunting)
15020	7.0	Sports,	Badminton, competitive (T 450)
15030	4.5	Sports,	Badminton, social singles and doubles, general
15040	8.0	Sports,	Basketball, game (T 490)
15050	6.0	Sports,	Basketball, nongame, general (T 480)
15060	7.0	Sports,	Basketball, officiating (T 500)
15070	4.5	Sports,	Basketball, shooting baskets
15075	6.5	Sports,	Basketball, wheelchair
15080	2.5	Sports,	Billiards
15090	3.0	Sports,	Bowling (T 390)
15100	12.0	Sports,	Boxing, in ring, general
15110	6.0	Sports,	Boxing, punching bag
15120	9.0	Sports,	Boxing, sparring
15130	7.0	Sports,	Broomball
15135	5.0	Sports,	Children's games (hopscotch, 4-square, dodge-ball, playground apparatus, t-ball, tetherball, marbles, jacks, arcade games)
15140	4.0	Sports,	Coaching: football, soccer, basketball, baseball, swimming, etc.
15150	5.0	Sports,	Cricket (batting, bowling)
15160	2.5	Sports,	Croquet
15170	4.0	Sports,	Curling
15180	2.5	Sports,	Darts, wall or lawn
15190	6.0	Sports,	Drag racing, pushing or driving a car
15200	6.0	Sports,	Fencing
15210	9.0	Sports,	Football, competitive
15230	8.0	Sports,	Football, touch, flag, general (T 510)
15235	2.5	Sports,	Football or baseball, playing catch
15240	3.0	Sports,	Frisbee playing, general
15250	3.5	Sports,	Frisbee, ultimate
15255	4.5	Sports,	Golf, general
15260	5.5	Sports,	Golf, carrying clubs (T 090)
15270	3.0	Sports,	Golf, miniature, driving range
15280	5.0	Sports,	Golf, pulling clubs (T 080)

15290	3.5	Sports,	Golf, using power cart (T 070)
15300	4.0	Sports,	Gymnastics, general
15310	4.0	Sports,	Hacky sack
15320	12.0	Sports,	Handball, general (T 620)
15330	8.0	Sports,	Handball, team
15340	3.5	Sports,	Hang gliding
15350	8.0	Sports,	Hockey, field
15360	8.0	Sports,	Hockey, ice
15370	4.0	Sports,	Horseback riding, general
15380	3.5	Sports,	Horseback riding, saddling horse
15390	6.5	Sports,	Horseback riding, trotting
15400	2.5	Sports,	Horseback riding, walking
15410	3.0	Sports,	Horseshoe pitching, quoits
15420	12.0	Sports,	Jai alai
15430	10.0	Sports,	Judo, jujitsu, karate, kick boxing, tae kwan do
15440	4.0	Sports,	Juggling
15450	7.0	Sports,	Kickball
15460	8.0	Sports,	Lacrosse
15470	4.0	Sports,	Moto-cross
15480	9.0	Sports,	Orienteering
15490	10.0	Sports,	Paddleball, competitive
15500	6.0	Sports,	Paddleball, casual, general (T 460)
15510	8.0	Sports,	Polo
15520	10.0	Sports,	Racquetball, competitive
15530	7.0	Sports,	Racquetball, casual, general (T 470)
15535	11.0	Sports,	Rock climbing, ascending rock
15540	8.0	Sports,	Rock climbing, rapelling
15550	12.0	Sports,	Rope jumping, fast
15551	10.0	Sports,	Rope jumping, moderate, general
15552	8.0	Sports,	Rope jumping, slow
15560	10.0	Sports,	Rugby
15570	3.0	Sports,	Shuffleboard, lawn bowling
15580	5.0	Sports,	Skateboarding
15590	7.0	Sports,	Skating, roller (T 360)
15600	3.5	Sports,	Sky diving
15605	10.0	Sports,	Soccer, competitive
15610	7.0	Sports,	Soccer, casual, general (T 540)
15620	5.0	Sports,	Softball or baseball, fast or slow pitch, general (T 440)
15630	4.0	Sports,	Softball, officiating
15640	6.0	Sports,	Softball, pitching
15650	12.0	Sports,	Squash (T 530)
15660	4.0	Sports,	Table tennis, ping pong (T 410)
15670	4.0	Sports,	Tai chi
15675	7.0	Sports,	Tennis, general
15680	6.0	Sports,	Tennis, doubles (T430)
15690	8.0	Sports,	Tennis, singles (T 420)
15700	3.5	Sports,	Trampoline
15710	4.0	Sports,	Volleyball, competitive, in gymnasium (T 400)
15720	3.0	Sports,	Volleyball, noncompetitive, 6–9 member team, general
15725	8.0	Sports,	Volleyball, beach
15730	6.0	Sports,	Wrestling (one match = 5 min)
15731	7.0	Sports,	Wallyball, general
16010	2.0	Transportation	Automobile or light truck (not a semi) driving
16020	2.0	Transportation	Flying airplane
16030	2.5	Transportation	Motor scooter, motor cycle
16040	6.0	Transportation	Pushing plane in and out of hanger
16050	3.0	Transportation	Driving heavy truck, tractor, bus
17010	7.0	Walking,	Backpacking, general (T 050)
17020	3.5	Walking,	Carrying infant or 15-lb load (e.g, suitcase) level ground or downstairs
17025	9.0	Walking,	Carrying load upstairs, general
17026	5.0	Walking,	Carrying 1- to 15-lb load, upstairs
17027	6.0	Walking,	Carrying 16- to 24-lb load, upstairs
17028	8.0	Walking,	Carrying 25- to 49-lb load, upstairs
17029	10.0	Walking,	Carrying 50- to 74-lb load, upstairs
17030	12.0	Walking,	Carrying 74+-lb load, upstairs
17035	7.0	Walking,	Climbing hills with 0- to 9-lb load
17040	7.5	Walking,	Climbing hills with 10- to 20-lb load
17050	8.0	Walking,	Climbing hills with 21- to 42-lb load
17060	9.0	Walking,	Climbing hills with 42+-lb load
17070	3.0	Walking,	Downstairs

17080	6.0	Walking,	Hiking, cross country (T 040)
17090	6.5	Walking,	Marching, rapidly, military
17100	2.5	Walking,	Pushing or pulling stroller with child
17110	6.5	Walking,	Race walking
17120	8.0	Walking,	Rock or mountain climbing (T 060)
17130	8.0	Walking,	Up stairs, using or climbing up ladder (T 030)
17140	4.0	Walking,	Using crutches
17150	2.0	Walking,	Walking, less than 2.0 mph, level ground, strolling, household walking, very slow
17160	2.5	Walking,	Walking, 2.0 mph, level, slow pace, firm surface
17170	3.0	Walking,	Walking, 2.5 mph, firm surface
17180	3.0	Walking,	Walking, 2.5 mph, downhill
17190	3.5	Walking,	Walking, 3.0 mph, level, moderate pace, firm surface
17200	4.0	Walking,	Walking, 3.5 mph, level, brisk, firm surface
17210	6.0	Walking,	Walking, 3.5 mph, uphill
17220	4.0	Walking,	Walking, 4.0 mph, level, firm surface, very brisk pace
17230	4.5	Walking,	Walking, 4.5 mph, level, firm surface. very, very brisk
17250	3.5	Walking,	Walking, for pleasure, work break, walking the dog
17260	5.0	Walking,	Walking, grass track
17270	4.0	Walking,	Walking, to work or class (T 015)
18010	2.5	Water activities,	Boating, power
18020	4.0	Water activities,	Canoeing, on camping trip (T 270)
18030	7.0	Water activities,	Canoeing, portaging
18040	3.0	Water activities,	Canoeing, rowing, 2.0–3.9 mph, light effort
18050	7.0	Water activities,	Canoeing, rowing, 4.0–5.9 mph, moderate effort
18060	12.0	Water activities,	Canoeing, rowing, >6 mph, vigorous effort
18070	3.5	Water activities,	Canoeing, rowing, for pleasure, general (T 250)
18080	12.0	Water activities,	Canoeing, rowing, in competition, or crew or sculling (T 260)
18090	3.0	Water activities,	Diving, springboard or platform
18100	5.0	Water activities,	Kayaking
18110	4.0	Water activities,	Paddleboat
18120	3.0	Water activities,	Sailing, boat and board sailing, windsurfing, ice sailing, general (T 235)
18130	5.0	Water activities,	Sailing, in competition
18140	3.0	Water activities,	Sailing, Sunfish/Laser/Hobie Cat, keel boats, ocean sailing, yachting
18150	6.0	Water activities,	Skiing, water (T 220)
18160	7.0	Water activities,	Skimobiling
18170	12.0	Water activities,	Skindiving or SCUBA diving as frogman
18180	16.0	Water activities,	Skindiving, fast
18190	12.5	Water activities,	Skindiving, moderate
18200	7.0	Water activities,	Skindiving, SCUBA diving, general (T 310)
18210	5.0	Water activities,	Snorkeling (T 320)
18220	3.0	Water activities,	Surfing, body or board
18230	10.0	Water activities,	Swimming laps, freestyle, fast, vigorous effort
18240	8.0	Water activities,	Swimming laps, freestyle, slow, moderate or light effort
18250	8.0	Water activities,	Swimming, backstroke, general
18260	10.0	Water activities,	Swimming, breaststroke, general
18270	11.0	Water activities,	Swimming, butterfly, general
18280	11.0	Water activities,	Swimming, crawl, fast (75 yards·min^{-1}), vigorous effort
18290	8.0	Water activities,	Swimming, crawl, slow (50 yards·min^{-1}), moderate or light effort
18300	6.0	Water activities,	Swimming, lake, ocean, river (T 280, T 295)
18310	6.0	Water activities,	Swimming, leisurely, not lap swimming, general
18320	8.0	Water activities,	Swimming, side stroke, general
18330	8.0	Water activities,	Swimming, synchronized
18340	10.0	Water activities,	Swimming, treading water, fast vigorous effort
18350	4.0	Water activities,	Swimming, treading water, moderate effort, general
18360	10.0	Water activities,	Water polo
18365	3.0	Water activities,	Water volleyball
18370	5.0	Water activities,	Whitewater rafting, kayaking, or canoeing
19010	6.0	Winter activities	Moving ice house (set up/drill holes, etc.)
19020	5.5	Winter activities	Skating, ice, 9 mph or less
19030	7.0	Winter activities	Skating, ice, general (T 360)
19040	9.0	Winter activities	Skating, ice, rapidly, more than 9 mph
19050	15.0	Winter activities	Skating, speed, competitive
19060	7.0	Winter activities	Ski jumping (climbing up carrying skis)

19075	7.0	Winter activities	Skiing, general
19080	7.0	Winter activities	Skiing, cross-country, 2.5 mph, slow or light effort, ski walking
19090	8.0	Winter activities	Skiing, cross-country, 4.0–4.9 mph, moderate speed and effort, general
19100	9.0	Winter activities	Skiing, cross-country, 5.0–7.9 mph, brisk speed, vigorous effort
19110	14.0	Winter activities	Skiing, cross-country, >8 mph, racing
19130	16.5	Winter activities	Skiing, cross-country, hard snow, uphill, maximum
19150	5.0	Winter activities	Skiing, downhill, light effort
19160	6.0	Winter activities	Skiing, downhill, moderate effort, general
19170	8.0	Winter activities	Skiing, downhill, vigorous effort, racing
19180	7.0	Winter activities	Sledding, tobogganing, bobsledding, luge (T 370)
19190	8.0	Winter activities	Snow shoeing
19200	3.5	Winter activities	Snowmobiling

Part 2: Guidelines for Assigning Activities by Major Purpose or Intent

1. Conditioning exercises include activities with the intent of improving physical condition. This includes stationary ergometers (bicycling, rowing machines, treadmills, etc.), health club exercise, calisthenics, and aerobics.
2. Home repair includes all activity associated with the repair of a house and does not include housework. This is not an occupational task.
3. Sleeping, lying, sitting, and standing are classified as inactivity.
4. Home activities include all activities associated with maintaining the inside of a house and includes house cleaning, laundry, grocery shopping, and cooking.
5. Lawn and garden includes all activity associated with maintaining the yard and includes yard work, gardening, and snow removal.
6. Occupation includes all job-related physical activity where one is paid (gainful employment). Specific activities may be cross-referenced in other categories (such as reading, writing, driving a car, walking) and should be coded in this major heading if related to employment. Housework is occupational only if the person is earning money for the task.
7. Self-care includes all activity related to grooming, eating, bathing, etc.
8. Transportation includes energy expended for the primary purpose of going somewhere in a motorized vehicle.

Part 3: Guidelines for Coding Specific Activities

A. General guidelines: All activities should be coded as "general" if no other information about the activity is given. This applies primarily to intensity ratings. If any additional information is given, activities should be coded accordingly.
B. Specific guidelines
  1. Bicycling
    a. Stationary cycling using cycle ergometers (all types), wind trainers, or other conditioning devices should be classified under the major heading of Conditioning Exercise, stationary cycling specific activities (codes 02010 to 02015).
    b. The list does not account for differences in wind conditions.
    c. If bicycling is performed in a race, classify it as general racing if no descriptions are given about drafting (code 01050). If information is given about the speed or drafting code as 01050 (bicycling, 6–19 mph, racing/not drafting or >19 mph drafting, very fast) or 01060 (bicycling, ≥ 20 mph, racing, not drafting).
    d. Using a mountain bike in the city should be classified as bicycling, general (code 01010). Cycling on mountain trails or on a BMX course is coded 01009.
  2. Conditioning Exercises
    a. If a calisthenics program is described as a light or moderate type of activity (e.g., performing back exercises) but indicates a vigorous effort on the part of the participant, code the activity as calisthenics, general (code 02030).
    b. Exercise performed at a health club that is not described should be classified as health club, general (code 02060). Other activities performed at a health club (e.g., weight lifting, aerobic dance, circuit training, treadmill running, etc. at a health club) should be classified under separate major headings.
    c. Regardless of whether aerobic dance, conditioning, circuit training, or water calisthenics programs are described by their component parts (i.e., 10 min jogging in place, 10 min sit-ups, 10 min stretching, etc.) code the activity as one activity (e.g., water aerobics, code 02120).
    d. Effort, speed, or intensity breakdowns for the specific activities of stair-treadmill ergometer (code 02065), ski machine (code 02060), water aerobics or water calisthenics (code 02120), circuit training (code 02040), and slimnastics (code 02090) are not given. Code these as general, even though effort or intensities may vary in the descriptions of the activity.

3. Dancing
   a. If the type of dancing performed is not described, code it as dancing, general (code 03025).
4. Home Activities
   a. House cleaning should be coded as light (code 05040) or heavy (code 05020). Examples for each are given in the description of the specific activities.
   b. Making the bed on a daily basis is coded 05100. Changing the bed sheets is coded as cleaning, light (code 05040).
5. Home Repair
   a. Any painting outside of the house (i.e., fence, the house, barn) is coded, painting, outside house (code 60150).
6. Inactivity
   a. Sitting and reading a book or newspaper is listed under the major heading of Miscellaneous, reading, book, newspaper, etc. (code 09030).
   b. Sitting and writing is listed under the major heading of Miscellaneous, writing (code 09040).
7. Lawn and Garden
   a. Working in the garden with a specific type of tool (i.e., hoe, spade) is coded as digging, spading, filling garden (code 08050).
   b. Removing snow may be done by one of three methods: shoveling snow by hand (code 08200), walking and operating a snow blower (code 08130), or riding a snow blower (code 08180).
8. Music Playing
   a. Most variation in music playing will be according to the setting (i.e., rock and roll band, orchestra, marching band, concert band, standing on the stage, performance, in a church, etc.) The compendium does not consider differences in the setting (except for marching band and guitar playing).
9. Occupation
   a. Types of occupational activities not listed separately under specific activities (e.g., chemistry laboratory experiments), should be placed into the types of energy expenditure classifications best describing the activity. See sitting: light (code 11580), sitting: moderate (code 11590), standing: light (code 11600), standing: light to moderate (code 11610), standing: moderate (code 11620), standing: moderate to heavy (code 11630).
   b. Driving an automobile or a light truck for employment (taxi cab, salesman, contractor, ambulance driver, bus driver), should be listed under the major heading of Transportation, automobile or light truck (not a semi) driving (code 06010).
   c. Performing skin or SCUBA diving as an occupation is listed under the major heading of Water Activities, and the specific activity of skindiving or SCUBA diving as a frogman (code 18170).
10. Running
    a. Running is not classified as treadmill or outdoor running. Running on a treadmill or outdoors should be coded by the speed of the run (codes 12030 to 12130). If speed is not given, code it as running, general (code 12150).
11. Self-care
    a. The compendium does not account for effort ratings. All items are considered to be general.
12. Transportation
    a. Being a passenger in an automobile is coded under the major heading of inactivity, sitting quietly (07020).
13. Walking
    a. Household walking is coded 17150, regardless if the subject identified a walking speed.
    b. If the walking speed is unidentified, use 3.0 mph, level, moderate, firm surface as the standard speed (code 17190). This should not be used for household walking.
    c. Walking during a household move, shopping, or for household work is coded under the major heading of Home Activities. Walking for job-related activities is coded under Occupational Activities.
    d. If a subject is backpacking, regardless of descriptors attached, the code is backpacking, general (code 17010).
    e. The compendium does not account for variations in speed or effort while carrying luggage or a child.
    f. Mountain climbing should be classified as general (rock or mountain climbing, code 17120) if no descriptors are given. If the weight of the load is described, code the activity as climbing hills with the appropriate load (codes 17030 to 17060).
    g. Walking on a grassy area (golf course, in a park, etc.) should be coded as walking, grass track (code 17260). The compendium does not account for variations in walking speed on a grassy area, so ignore recordings of walking speed or effort. If the walking is not on a grassy area, code the activity according to the walking speed (codes 17150 to 17230).
    h. Walking to work or to class should be coded as 17270. The compendium does not account for walking speed or effort in this activity. Even though a speed or effort is given for the walking, do not code walking to work or to class in any other walking category.
    i. Hiking and cross-country walking (code 17080) should be used only if the walking activity lasts 3 h or more. Do not use this category for backpacking, but for day hikes.
14. Water Activities
    a. Swimming should be coded as leisurely, not lap swimming, general (code 18310) if descriptors about stroke, speed, or swimming location are not given.
    b. Lap swimming should be coded as swimming laps, freestyle, slow (code 18240) if the activity is described as lap swimming, light or moderate effort, but stroke or speed are not indicated.

Swimming laps should be coded as swimming, laps, freestyle, fast (code 18230) if the activity is described as lap swimming, vigorous effort, but stroke or speed are not indicated.

c. Swimming crawl should be coded as swimming, crawl, slow (50 yards·min⁻¹) if speed is not given and the effort is rated light or moderate (code 18290). Swimming crawl should be coded as swimming, crawl, fast (75 yards·min⁻¹) if speed is not given, but the effort is rated as vigorous (code 18280).

d. The swimming strokes of backstroke (code 18250), breaststroke (code 18260), butterfly (code 18270), and sidestroke (code 18320) are coded as general for speed and intensity.

e. If a swimming activity is not identified as lake, ocean, or river swimming (code 18300), assume that the swimming was performed in a swimming pool.

f. If canoeing is related to a canoe trip, code as canoeing, on a camping trip (code 18020). Otherwise, code it according to the speed and effort listed.

Glossary

aesthetic response—movement that meets universal standards of beauty.

analysis—ability to identify the elements or parts of the whole, to see their relationships, and to structure them into some systematic arrangement or organization.

analysis of variance (ANOVA)—statistical test used to determine whether two or more means are significantly different at a preselected probability level.

anthropometry—science of measuring the human body.

application—ability to use knowledge and understanding in a particular concrete situation.

assessment—process of subjectively quantifying or qualitatively describing an attribute of interest; it can also refer collectively to both the processes of measurement and assessment.

athletic ability—one's acquired level of learning in skills common to athletic performance.

authentic assessment—assessment characterized by lack of artificiality; assessment that (*a*) measures skills that are essential for successful performance and (*b*) is scored according to real rather than arbitrary standards.

battery—collection of related tests administered within a specified time frame to obtain information about a multidimensional attribute.

between-group variance—variability among the sample means.

bioelectrical analysis—method for determining body composition calculated from the measure of resistance to electrical current plus the square value of the client's height.

blood pressure—measure of the force or pressure exerted by the blood against the interior walls of the arteries.

Bod Pod—body composition procedure for estimating body density from a measure of air displacement.

body composition—relative contributions of fat and lean body tissues to the overall weight of the body. Together with bone density, body composition constitutes morphological fitness.

body image—psychological construct that develops from thoughts, feelings, and perceptions about one's own general appearance, body parts, and physiological structures and functions.

body mass index—ratio of total body weight in kilograms to the square of height expressed in meters.

bone density—consistency of the skeleton. Together with body composition, it constitutes morphological fitness.

bradycardia—resting heart rate lower than 60 bpm.

caliper—tool used to measure the thickness of a skinfold to estimate body fat.

cardiorespiratory fitness—submaximal exercise endurance, maximal aerobic power, heart and lung functions, and blood pressure.

CD-ROM—laser disk that stores large volumes of information accessed by computer. CD-ROM is short for compact disk read-only memory.

change score (improvement score)—numerical value that represents the gain or loss between measures taken at different times.

checklist—dichotomous rating scale used to aid observation.

chi square—statistical test that determines the significance of the pattern of the number of persons, objects, or responses that fall into two or more categories.

choice—possible response to a multiple-choice question.

closed skills—skills performed in a stable, unchanging environment; the practice goal of closed skills is consistency.

Compendium of Physical Activities—comprehensive alphabetized listing of physical activities and their standardized MET levels.

comprehension—ability to interpret knowledge and to determine its implications, consequences, and effects.

concentric muscular contraction—contraction that occurs when muscle shortens as bony levers draw together.

concurrent validity—measure of accuracy of a test and a form of criterion validity; a correlation coefficient of .70 or higher (between the test and an older standard of measure) adequately demonstrates concurrent validity.

confidence interval—range of scores that provides the estimated bounds for a true population parameter.

construct validity—measure of accuracy of a test; the degree to which a norm-referenced instrument accurately assesses an attribute that cannot be measured directly.

content analysis—research technique for making replicable and valid inferences from qualitative data.

content validity—measure of accuracy of a test; the degree to which the items or tasks sampled from a norm-referenced instrument are representative of a defined universe or domain of content.

continuous data—data that can take on any value within a range.

contract grading—practice of agreement between teacher and students at the beginning of an instructional unit regarding goals and standards for grades.

creeping obesity—tendency for aging adults to accumulate gradually greater amounts of body fat.

crepitation—palpable or audible sound, such as crunching, grating, creaking, rattling, or crackling.

criterion validity—measure of accuracy of a test; the degree to which a norm-referenced instrument assesses the true or criterion behavior of examinees; concurrent and predictive validity are two forms of criterion validity.

criterion-referenced evaluation—interpretation of an examinee's score by comparing it with a predetermined standard defined by a behavior.

criterion-referenced grading—practice of assigning grades to students' performance in accordance with a specific standard of achievement.

critical value—value of test statistic at and beyond which the null hypothesis is rejected.

database—filing system that organizes information into records and fields.

decision validity—measure of accuracy of a test; the degree to which a criterion-referenced instrument accurately classifies examinees as masters or nonmasters. The C (contingency) value of .80 or higher adequately demonstrates evidence of decision validity.

degree of freedom—number of observations minus the number of restrictions placed on them.

descriptive statistics—statistics used to describe or summarize characteristics of a set of data.

diagnosis—comprehensive process that identifies strengths and weaknesses of a person to determine appropriate placement and intervention.

diagnostic assessments—assessments designed to identify weaknesses.

diastolic blood pressure—measure of force of blood at diastole (when the heart muscle is relaxed and chambers are filling with blood), traditionally written as the second number in a blood pressure measurement, e.g., 80 is the diastolic blood pressure in 120/80.

difficulty rating—numerical value of a test item based on the proportion of students who answered that item correctly.

discrepancy score—difference between the perceived body size and shape and the ideal body size and shape.

discrete data—data that take on only distinct values, usually representing whole events.

discrimination—ability of a grade or score to differentiate among students who are truly different in levels of attainment.

distorting image techniques—techniques that allow a person to alter an image of himself or herself so that it reflects that person's body image.

distractor (foil)—incorrect response to a multiple-choice question.

documentation—written records. (If it isn't written down, it didn't happen!)

domain-referenced validity—measure of accuracy of a test; the degree to which items or tasks sampled by a criterion-referenced instrument adequately represent the domain of items or tasks.

due process (procedural safeguards)—requirement that parents, guardians, and clients be informed of their rights and allowed to challenge decisions that they consider unfair.

dynamometer—spring-loaded device for measuring muscular force; force in pounds or kilograms is read off an index or recording scale.

eccentric muscular contraction—contraction that occurs when the muscle lengthens during exertion of force against resistance.

edema—excessive accumulation of serous fluid in the tissues, that is, swelling.

electronic reference database—extremely large file of reference information that is accessible via a networked computer.

elements of dance—variations in space, time, and force created by the movements of the body.

energy expenditure—transfer of chemical energy to work and heat energy. Daily energy expenditure depends on the resting metabolic rate, the thermogenic effect of food consumed, and one's level of physical activity.

essential body fat—minimal level of fat necessary for maintenance of normal functions of the body.

evaluation—process of making judgments based on quantitative and/or qualitative measurement or assessment data; ability to form judgments with respect to the value of information.

field assessment—assessment that requires no prohibitively expensive equipment or extremely specialized training of the administrator or evaluator.

flat-slope syndrome—tendency of subjects to overestimate actual underconsumption and to underestimate actual overconsumption of food and beverages.

flexibility—ability of a joint to move through an optimal range of movement.

foil—see *distractor*.

foreseeable hazard—condition that is obvious enough that a reasonably prudent facility manager would recognize and correct it before someone is injured.

formative assessment—assessment that occurs while skills, knowledge, and/or attitudes are still being formed, not at the end of a program; it is the process of gathering evidence of learning during the instructional process.

freedom from assessment bias—impartiality of an assessment instrument. An instrument that is free of assessment bias is appropriate for examinees from all groups for whom the instrument is intended.

frequency distribution—tabulation of scores from high to low or low to high, showing the number of occurrences of each score value.

frequency polygon—line graph of a frequency distribution in which score values or score intervals are charted on the horizontal axis and associated frequencies are given on the vertical axis.

frequency table—tabulation of nominal scale data, showing the number of occurrences within each category.

function (of a response choice)—proportion of test takers who selected that choice as the correct answer.

functional testing—performance-based assessment procedures.

gender-fair grading—practice of assigning grades in such a way that grade distributions for both genders are approximately the same.

goniometer—protractorlike instrument that measures joint range of motion in degrees.

grade—symbol used to denote an estimate of students' status, progress, and/or achievement.

grade inflation—systematic increase in grades given for work of a constant quality or quantity.

grade point (grade point average)—numerical evaluation of scholastic achievement based upon a formula of equivalents that assigns varying credit with the grade attained, for example, 4 points for an A, 3 for a B, and zero or negative points for failure.

graded exercise test (GXT)—laboratory test of cardiovascular functioning; cardiovascular and respiratory responses of the GXT examinee are monitored during progressive increases in workload.

grouped frequency distribution—tabulation of score intervals from high to low or low to high, showing the number of occurrences within each score interval.

histogram—bar graph of a frequency distribution that charts scores or score intervals on one axis and frequencies on the other axis.

hypertension—disease characterized by chronically elevated blood pressure, i.e., systolic blood pressure above 140 mm Hg and/or diastolic blood pressure above 90 mm Hg.

inadequate intake—consumption of a nutrient at or below a level that is less than approximately two-thirds of the RDA for that nutrient.

independent samples t-test—statistical test used to compare the means of two samples that were randomly formed.

index of discrimination—correlation coefficient of a test item that reveals the relationship between students' overall performances on a test and their performance on the particular item.

inferential statistics—statistics used to make inferences about populations based on characteristics of the sample data.

injury assessment—evaluation of a possible injury by nonmedical personnel, such as athletic trainers.

internal consistency reliability—measure of consistency of a test; the degree to which examinee scores are consistent across parts or trials of a norm-referenced instrument.

Internet—vast network of computers linking individual and organizational computers in most parts of the world. The World Wide Web, one Internet application, allows the user access to information from computers anywhere in the world.

inventory—assessment instrument used to obtain information about an affective attribute of an examinee; examinee responses typically are *not* judged as correct or incorrect.

item analysis—process of examining students' responses to a test item to discern the level of difficulty and the discriminatory quality of the item.

knowledge—awareness of specific facts, universals, and information; it requires remembering and the ability to recall.

laboratory test—test that requires specialized equipment and training of examiners and/or evaluators; laboratory tests may be time consuming because only one examinee is tested at a time.

ListServe—electronic mailing list that allows subscribers (i.e., those who sign up through an e-mail account) to communicate with each other about a common topic of interest.

mainframe computer—multiuser system composed of large pieces of hardware that have huge memory capacities; the system is accessed through a terminal consisting of a keyboard and a monitor.

mass testing—the practice of simultaneously administering an assessment instrument to a group of examinees.

maximal aerobic power—upper limit or maximal rate at which oxygen can be taken in, distributed, and used during exercise; measured by maximal oxygen consumption (VO_2max).

measurement—process of systematically assigning numerical values to an attribute of interest.

median—value that divides an ordered data set into two equal halves so that half of the scores are greater than the median and the other half of the scores are less than the median.

medical diagnosis—identification of the nature and severity of an injury or illness by a physician.

metabolic equivalent (MET)—measure of energy expenditure; one MET is the basal metabolic rate of a subject at rest; also, the ratio of the metabolic rate for an activity divided by the resting metabolic rate; 1 MET is equivalent to 1 kcal per kg body weight per hour, or about 3.5 $mL \cdot kg^{-1} \cdot min^{-1}$.

microcomputer—stand-alone computer to serve a single user; it consists of hardware including a central processing unit, a keyboard, a monitor, and sometimes a printer and other peripheral devices.

mode—most frequently occurring value in a data set.

moderate intensity—performance of a physical activity at 40 to 60% of VO_2max or at 50 to 75% of maximum heart rate reserve.

morphological fitness—bone density and body composition taken together.

motor ability—level to which a person has developed his or her innate capacity.

motor capacity—person's innate potential for motor performance.

motor educability—ease with which one learns new motor skills.

motor fitness—result of optimal development of agility, balance, coordination, muscular power, and speed.

multiple grades—practice in which two or more grades are reported to represent a student's status in different areas of concern within a teaching unit. For example, one grade is reported for motor skill, another for participation, effort, and discipline, and a third grade for improvement.

multiple-repetition tests—sport skill tests that require the examinee to perform a particular skill repeatedly: to manipulate a ball or other object that rebounds from a wall target. Also sometimes called repeated wall volley tests.

musculoskeletal fitness—result of the optimal development of muscular strength, muscular endurance, and flexibility.

NewsGroup—Internet application that allows users to exchange news and views about a common topic of interest.

norm-referenced evaluation—interpretation of an examinee's score by comparing it with the scores of similar examinees.

normal distribution—distribution that produces a bell-shaped frequency polygon with known characteristics.

null hypothesis *(H_o)*—initial statement about the value of the population parameter; it states that there is no difference (or relationship) between variables. Any observed difference (or relationship) is a chance difference (or relationship) caused by sampling errors.

nutrient dense—characteristic of food with high levels of nutrients relative to its number of calories.

obesity—level of excess fat at which fat-related health risks begin to increase.

objectivity—accuracy of the scoring system of an assessment instrument. An objective assessment instrument can be used consistently by different scorers to obtain similar results. Correlation coefficients of .80 or higher adequately demonstrate evidence of objectivity.

one repetition maximum (1RM, one rep max)—maximum weight that can be lifted only one time (i.e., one repetition).

open skills—skills performed in an unstable, changing environment; the practice goal of open skills is successful adaptation to the environmental conditions.

orthopaedic—pertaining to bones, joints, muscles, tendons, ligaments, and related soft tissues of the body.

paired samples t-test—statistical test used to compare the means of two samples formed by some type of matching.

palpation—examination or exploration of an area of the body by touching.

parallel forms reliability—measure of consistency of a test; degree of consistency in scores on two forms of a norm-referenced assessment instrument.

parameter—characteristic of an entire population.

PAR-Q (Physical Activity Readiness Questionnaire)—brief, self-administered questionnaire used to identify adults for whom physical activity might be inappropriate.

physical activity—any bodily movement produced by skeletal muscles that results in energy expenditure, including all active pursuits and many sedentary pursuits.

physical self-worth—general feeling of pride, self-respect, satisfaction, and confidence in one's physical self.

population—complete group of persons or objects that have in common at least one defining characteristic.

portfolio—compilation of dance work intended to demonstrate the developing skills and knowledge of a student.

post hoc multiple comparison—procedure used after a significant analysis of variance to determine which pair or pairs of means are significantly different.

power (of a computer)—memory capacity and processing speed.

prediction—process of estimating a score on one variable from knowledge of a score on another variable.

predictive validity—measure of accuracy of a test and a form of criterion validity; a correlation coefficient of .60 or higher (between the test and a future measure) adequately demonstrates predictive validity.

procedural safeguards—see *due process*.

proficiency assessment—assessment designed to determine placement in or exemption from a required program.

prognostic assessment—assessment designed to predict potential for development of a human attribute.

psychomotor taxonomy—classification scheme for motor abilities and skills.

psychometry—academic specialization in testing and assessment; validity, reliability, objectivity, and freedom from assessment bias are psychometric qualities.

qualitative data—words or illustrations used to describe an attribute according to kind or quality.

quantitative data—numerical information. They describe an attribute according to amount or number.

random sampling—process of selecting a sample in such a way that each element of the population has an equal chance of being selected.

range—value of the spread of scores in a distribution; it is the numerical difference between the highest and lowest scores.

rating scale—test that provides a subjective estimate of an attribute based on observation and/or self-appraisal; it provides for degrees of the attribute being examined.

RDA—see *recommended dietary allowance*.

real limits—upper and lower values of score intervals in a frequency distribution, defined so that no numerical area is unaccounted for between the score intervals.

recommended dietary allowance (RDA)—level of an essential nutrient deemed to be adequate to meet the nutrient needs of most healthy persons.

reflection—use of serious and persistent thought so as to act intentionally rather than routinely or impulsively.

reliability—dependability of an assessment instrument. A reliable instrument assesses an attribute consistently so that scores consistently reflect differences between examinees. A correlation coefficient of .80 or higher adequately demonstrates evidence of reliability.

repeated mastery reliability—measure of consistency of a test; degree to which a criterion-referenced assessment instrument consistently classifies examinees as masters and nonmasters.

risk management—formal process of assessing exposure to risk and taking whatever actions are necessary to minimize its effect.

risk treatment—determining the best method *(a)* to eliminate a hazard or *(b)* to make the situation as safe as possible.

rubric—set of criteria for judging quality of performance; it usually contains specific statements that define the performance at various levels of proficiency.

sample—portion of a population.

sampling error—expected variation in statistical values that occurs when a sample is selected from a population.

scattergram—graph that visually depicts the relationship between two quantifiable variables whose values are paired. Individual data points are plotted at the intersection of the appropriate values for the variables charted on the horizontal and vertical axes.

screening—use of quick and simple tests or procedures to identify those who may have special learning and/or performance needs; screening tests are usually followed by more precise forms of assessment.

search engine—device that scans Web sites to find matches with the keyword or keywords entered for a search. The Web site rated as the best match is listed first on the results list.

self-referenced evaluation—interpretation of an examinee's score by comparing it with his or her score from another administration of the same assessment instrument.

semi-interquartile range—measure of the variability of the middle 50% of the scores in a distribution.

sign—single specific condition that indicates a single specific injury or illness, e.g., Battle's sign.

skewness—tendency of a distribution to depart from symmetry of balance around the mean. If more than half of the scores fall below the mean, distribution is positively skewed. If more than half of the scores fall above the mean, distribution is negatively skewed.

skinfold—double fold of skin and the immediate layer of subcutaneous fat.

social physique anxiety—psychological construct resulting from uncomfortable feelings associated with the perception that one's body is being scrutinized by others.

special-needs populations—individuals whose physical, mental, and/or emotional characteristics interfere with their optimal development and/or performance.

split half reliability—measure of consistency of a test; consistency of examinees' scores on two halves of a norm-referenced assessment instrument.

sport skill test—instrument or procedure that elicits an observable response that provides information about a motor skill used in a sport.

stamina—see *submaximal exercise endurance.*

standard deviation—theoretical measure of the spread of the middle 68% of the scores taken from the mean.

standard error—standard deviation of the distribution of sample estimates of a population parameter.

statistic—characteristic of a sample that may be used to estimate the value of a population parameter.

statistical significance—conclusion that results are unlikely to be due to chance; the observed difference or relationship is probably real.

stem—preliminary statement or question in a multiple-choice item.

studio activity—structured task that requires students to use their dance knowledge and skills in defining a problem, generating a solution, evaluating choices based on criteria, or demonstrating a final dance.

submaximal exercise endurance (stamina)—level of tolerance to low-intensity exercise demands for prolonged periods.

submaximal exertion—level of physical exertion that is less than one's maximal possible exertion level.

summative assessment—assessment conducted at the end (summation) of an identified program.

symptom—condition or behavior associated with a number of injuries or illnesses, e.g., swelling.

synthesis—ability to structure a whole from understanding of the relationships among specific elements or parts.

systolic blood pressure—measure of force of blood at systole (when the heart muscle is contracting and pumping blood into the aorta and pulmonary artery), traditionally written as the first number in a blood pressure measurement, e.g., 120 is the systolic blood pressure in 120/80.

t-test—statistical test used to determine whether two sample means are significantly different at a preselected probability level.

table of specifications—two-way table used to depict the content emphasis and the cognitive taxonomic placement of items on a test of knowledge.

tachycardia—resting heart rate higher than 100 bpm.

test—instrument or procedure that elicits an observable response to provide information about a specified attribute of a person or persons.

test consumer—someone who uses test results to make informed decisions.

test of significance—statistical test used to determine whether or not a sample statistic is likely to represent a particular population parameter.

test specificity—term used to explain measurement differences caused by differences in the nature or demands of various tests.

test-retest reliability—measure of consistency of a test; the degree to which a norm-referenced assessment instrument yields consistent scores over time.

type I error—error that occurs if a true null hypothesis is rejected on the basis of the sample evidence.

type II error—error that occurs if a false null hypothesis is accepted on the basis of the sample evidence.

universal resource locator (URL)—address for a particular computer file that can be accessed via the World Wide Web.

validity—veracity of an assessment instrument. A valid instrument accurately assesses the attribute it claims to assess and allows meaningful inferences to be made from the assessment results.

Valsalva maneuver—holding one's breath during physical exertion, causing an increase in intrathoracic pressure that slows the pulse, decreases return of blood to the heart, and increases venous pressure.

vigorous intensity—performance of a physical activity at more than 60% of VO_2max or at 75 to 85% of maximum heart rate reserve. In absolute terms, it is more than 6 METs.

waist-to-hip ratio—waist circumference divided by the hip circumference.

weighting—comparative valuing of various components of a grade.

within-group variance—variability among individual scores within the sample.

World Wide Web—one of the newest and most exciting Internet applications that allows the user to access information from computers anywhere in the world.

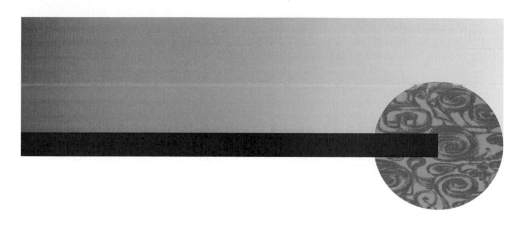

Index

Page numbers in *italics* followed by *f* denote figures; those followed by *t* denote tables.

Robertson Modified Curl-up Test, 294–297, *297t*
Rockport Fitness Walking Test, 33, 264–265
Rogers, Frederick Rand, 30
Roger's strength test, 30
Romberg's sign, 506
Rosentsweig Revision of the Fox Swimming Power Test, 387–388
Rosser, Phyllis, 70
Rubric, 606, *608f*
Rummel, Rose M., 236
Running/walking tests, 33, 264–265, 270
Ryan, C., 606

S
Sacroiliac compression test, 516, *518f*
Samples
 ANOVA, 149–156, *152t-154t*, 167–168, *167f, 168f*
 computers for, 164–169, *165f, 166f, 167f, 168f, 169f, 170f*
 confidence interval, 137, *137t*
 critical values, 141, *147t, 152t-154t*
 null hypothesis, 139, *140t*
 one-way analysis of variance (ANOVA), 149–156, *152t-154t*
 one-way chi square, 160–162, *161f, 163t*, 169, *170f*
 Pearson correlation, 157, *158t*, 159–160, 168–169, *169f*
 population sample, 106
 random sampling, 134–135, 145
 representative, 133–135, *134f*
 sample size, 134, *135t*
 sample size and degrees of freedom, 141
 sampling errors, 135–136
 standard error, 136–139, *137t, 138f*
 statistical significance, 141, 142–143
 t-test, 144–149, *147t*, 164–166, *165f, 166f*
 tests of significance, 139, 140–141, *142f*, 143–163
 two-tailed test, 141, *142f*
 type I and type II errors, 140
Sargent, Dudley Allen, 28, 29
SAS (Statistical Analysis System), 101, 102, 128
Scales of measurement, 89, 91, *91t*
Scattergrams, *124f*, 128
Schneider, E. C., 32
Scholastic Achievement Test (SAT), 38
 as formal test, 12

gender bias and 1987 version of, 70
predictive validity assessment of, 60
Scholastic Aptitude test, 38, 662
School program evaluation instruments, 37–38
Schultz, Ellen E., 23
Screening, 620
Screening tests
 Denver II: Revision of the Denver Developmental Screening Test, 620–621, *622f-623f, 624f*
 Purdue Perceptual-Motor Survey, 624, 626, *627f, 628f*
 Sherrill Perceptual-Motor Screening Checklist, 621, 624, *625f, 626f*
Search engines, computer, 55
Sebren, A., 592
Second International Consensus Symposium, 243
Seidel, S., 668
Self-evaluations, for grading, 188
Self-referenced evaluations, 10–11, *11f*
Self-report scales and inventories, 20
Semi-interquartile range, 114, *115t*
Semiquantitative serving sizes, 447
Senate Select Committee on Nutrition and Human Needs, U.S., 455
70% of Maximum Strength Testing Protocol, 292
Shannon, B. J., 325
Shareware programs, 102
Sherrill Perceptual-Motor Screening Checklist, 621, 624, *625f, 626f*
Shick-Berg Indoor Golf Skill Test, 353–355, *355f*
Shifflett and Shuman Criterion-Referenced Archery Test, 327–328
Short-answer questions on essay tests, 575–576
Shoulder injuries, 517, *519f*, 520–521, *521f, 522f, 523f*
Shoulder rotation test, 305–306, *306t*
Siedentop, D., 604
Signs and symptoms in injury assessment, 501
 evaluation of, *500f*, 505–507, *506f*
Silhouette rating scales, 413–415, *414f, 415f*
Simple frequency distributions, 94–95, *95t*
Simple linear prediction, 159–160
Skeletal nuclear imaging, 524
Skewness, 111, *112f*
Skinfold, 207–208